Catherine Price has spent much of her workin[g life] humble beginnings and few expectations in [life to] work with women and their families througho[ut] hood in hospitals birth centres and at homebirths 'catching over 1000 babies. She still works casually in a Sydney birth centre but now devotes much of her time running the www.birth.com.au website, with her business partner and close friend, Sandra Robinson. She is married to a wonderful man, Peter, and has two sons, Hugh and Callum.

Since 1991 Sandra Robinson has worked as a childbirth educator in Sydney. She continues to support pregnant women and their partners with their options and choices for pregnancy care and their preferred environment for labour and giving birth. In 1999 she created the concept for Internet childbirth classes. With the tireless help of her close friend of 25 years, Catherine Price, a business partnership and website were born. This website provided the inspiration for the idea, writing and ultimate publishing of this book. Sandra is married to her loving friend and partner, Stephen, and has one daughter, Alice, and two sons, Liam and Declan.

For further information please visit www.birth.com.au

BIRTH

CONCEIVING, NURTURING
AND GIVING BIRTH TO YOUR BABY

CATHERINE PRICE & SANDRA ROBINSON

Foreword by Robin Barker

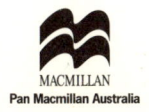

Metric conversion table

The birth weight of babies can be measured in both imperial and metric measurements.

1 inch	2.54 millimetres	1 centimetre	0.394 inches
1 ounce	28.3 grams	1 gram	0.0353 ounces
1 pound	454 grams	1 kilogram	2.20 pounds

First published 2004 in Macmillan by Pan Macmillan Australia Pty Ltd
1 Market Street, Sydney

Reprinted 2005, 2006

Copyright © 2004 Catherine Price and Sandra Robinson

All rights reserved. No part of this book may be reproduced or transmitted in any form or by any means, electronic or mechanical, including photocopying, recording or by any information storage and retrieval system, without prior permission in writing from the publisher.

National Library of Australia cataloguing-in-publication data:

Price, Catherine A. (Catherine Anne).
Birth: conceiving, nurturing and giving birth to your baby.

ISBN 1 4050 3612 5.

1. Pregnancy – Popular works. 2. Childbirth. I. Robinson, Sandra. II. Title.

618.2

Text design by Liz Seymour, Seymour Designs
Internal illustrations copyright © Travis Tischler 2004
Typeset in 11/14pt Fairfield Light by Post Pre-press Group
Printed in Australia by McPherson's Printing Group

Papers used by Pan Macmillan Australia Pty Ltd are natural, recyclable products made from wood grown in sustainable forests. The manufacturing processes conform to the environmental regulations of the country of origin.

Foreword

I have been involved in the care of families and the under-threes all my working life, as a paediatric nurse, midwife and child and family health nurse. During this time I have been acutely aware how much the unique perspective and detailed knowledge hands-on health professionals bring to families is needed in the marketplace, ideally in easily accessible books. The wide-ranging experience of these particular practitioners is essential in order to help parents keep sanity and balance in the face of the avalanche of information available on pregnancy, birth and the first three years.

Historically, there has been a paucity of Australian information for Australian families, although to a large extent that has been addressed in the last ten years. Thankfully we no longer need to rely on books from overseas to tell us how to give birth, breastfeed and handle toddler tantrums.

My books were written with this in mind and for some time I have been hoping a pregnancy and birth book might appear driven by the same philosophy. A book written by a committed, experienced hands-on professional based not only on his or her academic background but on the hours spent one-on-one with parents over many years. A book written by a caregiver who listens to parents and understands their hopes, their fears and their concerns right down to the tiniest details. A book that reflects the many different dimensions of pregnancy and birth, acknowledging that no two pregnancies, births or babies are the same. A book with no agenda and no bias that provides safe, balanced options but is not afraid to confront the difficult issues. A respectful book, a positive and joyful book, clearly laid out with a good index.

Birth, written by midwife, Catherine Price and birth educator/doula, Sandra Robinson is all of the above and I am delighted and excited that Australian parents will have access to Catherine and Sandra's years of knowledge and experience, painstakingly assembled in this authoritative book.

Birth is a mighty tome that covers every aspect and offers every choice available to prospective parents. The information is meticulously researched. The language is warm and, if it is possible to imagine in a book, *Birth* discusses, listens and gives answers.

Birth has many strengths but in particular I love the way it addresses the emotional issues throughout for women and their partners. It will also be invaluable for prospective parents who haven't a clue how the Australian healthcare system works and need to know how to find their way around it to get what they want.

Catherine and Sandra, I salute you. Being dedicated hands-on health professionals, wives and mothers leaves little time for much else in life let alone writing a book so wide-ranging and detailed it is surely destined to become an Australian classic.

I highly recommend *Birth* to all women and men on the road to parenthood and to anyone whose work is related to pregnancy, birth and the wellbeing of the families who come to them for help.

Robin Barker, August 2004
Registered nurse, midwife, child and family health nurse
Author of *Baby Love, Baby and Toddler Meals, The Mighty Toddler*

CONTENTS

Introduction.........xiii

Chapter 1 ~ Preparing to conceive your baby.........1
Emotional readiness and your relationship • Financial and work considerations

Preparing your body for pregnancy – 4
*A nutritious diet • Vitamins and minerals • Lifestyle changes - what to avoid
Physical activity before pregnancy • Physical activity when conception occurs • Healthy weight range • Managing stress • Preconceptual health check*

Conceiving your baby – 29
*The female and male reproductive systems • A woman's menstrual cycle
Charting your Fertility • Detecting the fertile days • Timing sex for conception
When conception is not straightforward • Choosing the sex of your baby*

Difficulty conceiving – 44
*Causes of infertility • Investigating infertility • Treatment options
Emotional considerations*

Chapter 2 ~ A new pregnancy: Conception to 12 weeks.........48

Your unborn baby's growth and development – 48

Confirming your pregnancy – 52
*Urine pregnancy tests • Blood pregnancy tests • Calculating your baby's due date
Implantation bleeds • Ultrasound dating • Twins, triplets or more*

Early pregnancy – 58
'Morning' sickness

Your diet during pregnancy – 62
*Listeria • Mercury in fish • Cravings • Vegetarian and vegan diets • Weight gain
Exercise*

Emotions in early pregnancy – 66
Emotions for the woman • Emotions for the partner • Your relationship

Taking care – 68
Lifestyle changes • Prescribed medications • Over-the-counter treatments • Natural therapies • Environmental and occupational hazards

In the beginning – 88
*Announcing your pregnancy • Choosing a caregiver and birthplace
Transfer for the woman or baby • What to expect at your first pregnancy visit
Tests you may be offered • Genetic testing*

Early pregnancy variations – 109
*Bleeding during early pregnancy • Miscarriage • Ectopic pregnancy • Excessive vomiting
Retroverted uterus*

Chapter 3 ~ The middle of pregnancy: 13 to 28 weeks.........119

Your unborn baby's growth and development – 119

Middle pregnancy – 122
Physical changes • Aches and pains • Growing belly • Maternity clothes • Baby's movements

Adapting to change – 137
Emotions in the middle months • Body image, sexuality and libido

As the pregnancy progresses – 141
What to expect at your caregiver pregnancy visits • Tests you may be offered • Ultrasounds

Middle pregnancy variations – 150
High blood pressure • Asthma • Diabetes • Epilepsy • Heart disease • Thyroid conditions Blood disorders • Urine infection • Antenatal depression • Twin variations • Baby dying during pregnancy

FAQs – 158
What about travel during pregnancy? • Can I lie on my back? What will I do with my belly piercing?

Chapter 4 ~ The final months: 29 weeks till birth.........162

Your unborn baby's growth and development – 162

Physical changes in preparation for birth – 164
The uterus • The cervix • Membranes and amniotic fluid • The placenta • The umbilical cord • The pelvis • The pelvic floor muscles • The perineum

The final weeks – 170
Physical changes • Aches and pains • Your baby's movements

Emotions and sex during late pregnancy – 182
Emotions for the woman • Emotions for the partner • Sex during late pregnancy

Monitoring more closely – 185
What to expect during the remaining pregnancy visits

Getting ready for baby – 188
Feeding your new baby • Sleeping arrangements • Buying for baby Cloth or disposable nappies • Planning childcare arrangements

Late pregnancy variations – 200
Premature baby • Breech baby • Small baby • Too much or too little fluid around the baby Pre-eclampsia • Gestational diabetes • Bleeding during late pregnancy • Isoimmunisation Cholestasis

FAQs – 214
When should I stop work? • Do I need raspberry leaf? • What about clicking or popping noises? • Should I be concerned about my belly feeling cold?

Chapter 5 ~ Preparing for birth 217

*Childbirth classes • Do I need a support person? • Preparing your other children
When considering a water birth • What to pack for the birth • Writing a birth plan*

Prelabour – 231
*Physical signs of prelabour • Support strategies • Emotions
What to expect from your caregiver during prelabour
Admission to the delivery suite or birth centre • Should I stay or should I go?*

Variations for prelabour – 241
Waters breaking, no contractions • Dehydration and ketosis

Chapter 6 ~ First stage of labour.........244

Early first phase • Active first phase • End of first stage or transition • Physical signs

Support strategies – 250
Support strategies for the woman • Support strategies for the partner/support person

Expectations for care – 254
What to expect from your caregiver • Continuous monitoring

Variations for the first stage – 257
*Continual vomiting • Fever • Difficulty urinating • Posterior labour • Slow progress
Baby distressed • Anterior lip • Shoulder presentation • Heavy bleeding • Cord prolapse*

Chapter 7 ~ Second stage and birthing your baby.........268

Resting phase • Active pushing phase • Crowning phase • Birthing phase

Support strategies – 275
*Support strategies for the woman • Support strategies for the partner/support person
Positioning for birth*

Expectations for care – 279
Vaginal examinations • Time limits

Variations for the second stage – 280
*Tearing • Episiotomy • Fast birth • Baby distressed • Baby's presentation
Forceps and ventouse • Shoulder dystocia • Giving birth to twins
Baby born before arrival at the birthplace • Stillborn baby*

Chapter 8 ~ Third and fourth stages of labour.........296

The third stage – 296
*Natural vs. active management • Clamping and cutting the cord • Checking the placenta
Emotions • Issues and controversies*

The fourth stage – 304
Physical recovery • Emotions • Support strategies • Expectations for care

Variations for third and fourth stages – 309
*Difficulty urinating • Feeling faint • Haematomas • Primary postpartum haemorrhage
Retained placenta • Third and fourth degree tears • Anal fissures • Uterine inversion*

Chapter 9 ~ The pain of labour.........318

The physiology of pain – 318
The pain of labour and birth

The woman's perception of her labour pain – 320
*Fears and concerns • Psychological approach and pain threshold • Expectations
Feeling in control • Social, cultural and spiritual beliefs • Other factors
Exploring beliefs and perceptions • Helpful tools*

Medical forms of pain relief – 331
Gas • Pethidine • Epidural and spinal anaesthesia

Natural therapies and other methods of pain relief – 347
*Acupuncture • Acupressure, shiatsu and reflexology • Aromatherapy
Bach flower and Australian bush flower essences • Breathing and birthing noises • Herbs
Homeopathy • Hypnosis • Massage • Movement • Music
Transcutaneous Electrical Nerve Stimulation (TENS) • Visual focus • Visualisation
Water • Water Injections*

Chapter 10 ~ Inducing or augmenting the labour.........354

Induction – 354
Going 'overdue' • Readiness for labour

Induction methods – 357
*Pharmacological methods • Mechanical methods
Risks and problems with medical inductions • Natural methods • Coping strategies
Emotional considerations*

Augmentation – 371
Medical methods • Natural therapies • Support strategies

Chapter 11 ~ Caesarean birth 377

What a caesarean operation involves – 378
Before the operation • Anaesthetic used • The operation • The recovery room

Early care and physical recovery – 386
*First 24 to 48 hours • Next one to two weeks • Two to eight weeks
Two months and beyond*

Risks and problems associated with caesareans – 390
Possible variations for the woman • Possible variations for the baby

Emotional reactions – 393
Emotions for the woman • Emotions for the partner/support person

Vaginal birth after caesarean – 396
*Health factors relating to VBAC • Arguments for and against VBAC
Achieving the optimal outcomes • Emotions when planning a VBAC*

Chapter 12 ~ Your baby soon after birth.........405

The role of the birthing environment – 406

Routine procedures and possible interventions – 407
*The Apgar score • Routine interventions at birth • Identification and observations
Weighing, measuring and bathing • Vitamin K • Hepatitis B vaccination
Well babies needing further observations*

Early parenting – 416
*Bonding with your baby • The first feed • Early parenting skills
Introducing the baby to their siblings*

Your newborn baby's physical appearance and behaviours – 422
*A newborn's appearance • Early physical variations • Normal newborn behaviour
A newborn's physical reflexes*

What to expect from your caregiver – 430
Newborn examinations • Routine screening blood test

Variations for the baby – 434
Unwell baby • Jaundice

FAQs – 437
Should my son be circumcised? • At what age can a newborn travel by plane?

Chapter 13 ~ The woman's recovery after birth.........440

Physical recovery – 440
Nutrition and good health • Exercise

Feeding your baby – 445
Breastfeeding • Bottle feeding • Sterilising feeding/expressing equipment

Emotional changes and support strategies – 457
Support during the early weeks

Expectations for care – 461
Your six to eight week postnatal check • Unexpected outcomes/unmet expectations

Variations for the woman – 464
*Breastfeeding variations • Infections • Thrush and Gardnerella • Heavy bleeding
Thrombosis • Postnatal depression • Post-traumatic stress disorder • Postnatal psychosis*

Chapter 14 ~ Transition to parenting.........477

The birth of a parent – 477
*Realistic parenting expectations • Relationship survival tips • When caring for your baby
'Advice', take it or leave it? • Sibling rivalry*

Sex, sexuality and contraception – 486
Resuming your sexual relationship • Sexuality and intimacy • Contraception

Settling in with your new baby – 500
*Sleeping and feeding patterns • Getting your baby to sleep • Settling your crying baby
Caring for twins, triplets or more*

Lifestyle and breastfeeding – 508
*Expressing and storing breast milk • Breastfeeding while out and about
Breastfeeding with work or study • Weaning your baby from the breast*

Returning to work or study – 514
Partner returns • Mother returns • Stay-at-home dads

Variations – 518
Breast milk supply

Conclusion – 522

Appendices – 523
*Visualisation techniques – 523 • Acupressure points – 526 • Natural therapies – 530
Birth plan – 542 • Labour support guide – 550*

**Support resources – 554
Further reading – 565
Glossary – 568
Endnotes – 575
Acknowledgments – 584
Index – 585**

Introduction

Birth: Conceiving, Nurturing and Giving Birth to Your Baby was conceived in 1999 as a website for online childbirth education classes. After four years of nurturing, it developed into a comprehensive reference library spanning preconception, pregnancy, birth and early parenting, until finally giving birth to this book.

When we set out on our adventure, we had many hopes and aspirations for our 'baby'. We wanted it to be practical and up-to-date, accurate and research-based. We wanted it to be reader-friendly and as much for partners and support people as for women themselves. We wanted it to be as relevant for those choosing an obstetrician and private hospital as for those choosing midwifery care, public hospitals, birth centres or homebirth. We wanted to explain all the physical changes, yet explore the range of emotions that reflect the journey to parenthood. We wanted to include possible medical treatments, as well as helpful natural therapies. We wanted to present a wide range of options, without being biased or condescending, and include sensible, achievable support strategies. We wanted to empower parents to make informed decisions about their care and respect their choices, yet provide realistic expectations of what this can mean. We wanted to address every major concern, as well as all those endless worries, and try to put them in perspective in a reassuring way. We wanted to deal with issues that have only been glossed over by others, like managing labour pain.

Actually, what we really wanted was the best pregnancy and birth book we had ever read. And here it is!

DISCLAIMER: All care has been taken to provide accurate and safe information, however, this book is for educational purposes only and is not a substitute for medical, counselling or other professional advice or services for you, your partner or your baby. You should consult your professional caregiver or practitioner before relying on any information provided by this book.

CHAPTER 1

Preparing to conceive your baby

Deciding to have a baby can kindle an array of emotions such as excitement, joy, apprehension or simply relief that the decision has been made. Having a baby now is very different from when our parents conceived us, often being a lifestyle choice that considers career, education, travel, and financial issues, as well as the spacing of siblings (if having more than one child). However, despite this cultural shift, 50% of pregnancies still remain unplanned.

In many cases feeling it is 'the right time' is the biggest emotional step, although 'the right time' may never come! Women are increasingly delaying their parenting, with some financially independent women choosing to have babies on their own. This decision may also involve a sense of urgency, if it is felt that the 'biological clock' is ticking.

Even though people say, 'Nothing can ever prepare you for having a baby', there are many things you can do to help with your planning. Identifying any foreseeable issues before starting (or extending) your family can be a very worthwhile exercise. If your intention is to be a sole parent, sourcing people for reliable, practical and emotional support during the pregnancy, birth and early parenting is particularly important.

EMOTIONAL READINESS AND YOUR RELATIONSHIP

Being emotionally prepared means different things to different people. For some, it is simply feeling ready. For others, it is a natural step after financial, travel and career needs are fulfilled. You may have yearned for a child for years, or perhaps find yourself suddenly wanting a baby. A few people don't ever feel emotionally ready, but take a leap of faith with the hope that it will fall into place once the baby comes.

If you say to other parents, 'My life will not change when I have a baby', you'll probably receive looks of disbelief, smirks, or even an outright laugh (famous last words). Part of your emotional preparation is learning to deal with change. Change as the pregnancy progresses; change as the labour and birth unfold; and change as you take on your parenting role. Change can be confronting and scary, but it can also be exciting and rewarding. Being open to change, and flexible in your approach, will help you to cope with these adjustments as they unfold. It is true that babies place a whole new perspective on your life, but this is often for the better, and the journey to parenthood can be an amazingly wonderful experience.

Realistic relationship expectations

You may be excited to have a baby, perhaps seeing this as reinforcing your commitment to your relationship, or you may not be sure it is what you really want. A baby entering the dynamics of a one-on-one relationship means meeting the needs of this new person, as well as your own and each other's needs. Newborns are very demanding and the first few months can be particularly tiring. Being clear with each other about how you expect your roles to change is important. If you have mismatched expectations, this can place incredible demands on even the most stable of relationships. Deciding to have a baby in the hope of solving problems within a relationship usually only magnifies them and introduces new ones. Before conceiving, try to be honest about how you both feel. Some aspects to consider are:

- Am I ready to be a parent? Am I prepared to be less selfish and more giving? Can I put another person first? Do we want another child (if this is not your first child) and how long do we wish to wait?
- Am I happy with my partner? Is our relationship strong and flexible enough to support this baby? Are we prepared to have less time for each other as a couple?
- How will the household tasks be divided?
- Who will take time off paid work and for how long? Who will care for the baby if we both return to work? If going from two wages to one, how do I feel about being financially dependent on my partner, or vice versa?
- Do we agree on the child's surname, discipline, religious teachings, education?
- Are there concerns about a previous labour or birth experience, a pregnancy loss or the death of a baby? Sometimes professional counselling is needed to help with these issues, before moving on to plan another child.

NOTE: Communication skills don't come naturally to everyone and may involve considerable effort and self-awareness. Sharing your feelings can be an art in itself, sometimes requiring you to change long-term communication patterns. It is important to talk openly and respectfully from the start and appreciate each other's history, feelings and ideals. From this understanding you can learn to grow as a family.

FINANCIAL AND WORK CONSIDERATIONS

New babies invariably affect all areas of your life. In many cases, the question of affordability is the deciding factor. Clothing, nappies, baby equipment, food, childcare, healthcare and education are ongoing financial commitments for 18 years or more. Parents generally spend at least 20% of their earnings (or pension) on child-related expenses, regardless of their income. So you may want to think about what you want for your child(ren) and how you intend to support them. If working, you need to estimate how much time you can afford to take off. Make sure you factor in unexpected pregnancy complications which may require leaving work earlier (such as a premature baby).

When planning finances you might consider:
- Saving more money.
- Paying extra off the mortgage, or reducing payments while on maternity/paternity leave.
- Realistically budgeting when buying for baby.
- Assessing whether you need to move house, renovate or buy a new car.
- Finding out health costs for the pregnancy and birth.
- Checking life insurance entitlements.
- Investigating government benefits and housing allowances.
- Researching the cost of childcare.

Health insurance

You may want to review, or take out, private health insurance. As a guide:
- Find out the minimum waiting period before claiming maternity services. Most funds require 12 months membership before the baby is born (3 months before conceiving).
- Shop around. Some funds pay gap fees, charge an excess for each claim or require you to use certain caregivers or hospital services. Check what is covered by Medicare.
- Find out what the fund covers and what out-of-pocket expenses you'll face. Take into account hospital accommodation, obstetrician's and possibly anaesthetist's fees (for epidural or caesarean), paediatrician, ambulance, intensive care, blood tests and ultrasounds.

Work considerations

Employers usually require you to work continuously for 12 months or more before considering you eligible for paid maternity or paternity leave (if available). You should find out:
- Your entitlements and length of leave (paid or unpaid leave, or a mixture of both). Unpaid leave is usually 12 months from the birth date of your baby (not from the time you leave work).
- Whether you have other leave owing, such as long service leave.
- Your job options when you return to work, such as part-time or working from home. Also, clarify your job – you may only be guaranteed an equivalent position in a different department.

Discrimination

The Australian Sex Discrimination Act 1984 means you should not be discriminated against because you intend to become pregnant, are pregnant or need to take leave. It is important to understand your rights. As a guide, pregnancy discrimination can occur if someone:
- Refuses to employ or promote you.
- Dismisses or retrenches you.
- Excludes you from training.
- Transfers or demotes you.
- Refuses you accommodation, or goods or services.

In-depth information can be found in *Pregnancy Guidelines*, a booklet put out by the Human Rights and Equal Opportunity Commission.[1]

Preparing your body for pregnancy

To assist conception, and give your baby the best possible start, both parents need to take steps towards preparing themselves, both physically and emotionally. Ideally, you should begin preparing about three months before trying to conceive, and bear in mind it takes a healthy, fertile couple an average of six months to achieve a pregnancy.

A NUTRITIOUS DIET

Both men and women need to have a well-balanced, nutritious diet to support their ability to conceive, and help ensure the woman has adequate stores of essential vitamins, minerals and nutrients to support her unborn baby.[2]

Planning your diet

It can be difficult to change poor eating habits, such as skipping meals, eating fast foods, grabbing quick snacks and alleviating cravings for things like coffee and chocolate. However, if you can eat healthier food for four to six weeks, you can usually break these bad habits. To help make the transition easier:
- Only have nutritious foods in the house. Take fresh fruits, yoghurts, muesli snacks, nuts or dried fruits to work.
- Eat healthy takeaway foods (sandwiches, salads, pasta, rice or noodle dishes).
- Have a bottle of water handy.
- Keep a daily diary of what you eat and read it at the end of the week.

Have food that is:
- Recently prepared and as fresh as possible.
- High in fibre (wholegrain instead of processed).
- Organic or free range, if possible.
- Varied, to gain all essential vitamins and minerals.
- Low in fat, sugar and salt.
- Complemented with six to eight glasses of water per day. Keep tea, coffee and fizzy drinks to a minimum, replacing them with fruit juices, milk or herbal teas.
- Not high in preservatives and chemical additives.
- Not genetically modified? The jury is out on that one!

The five food groups

For healthy eating, nutritionists recommend proportional amounts from the five food groups. Grains (or complex carbohydrates) are what we need most of, followed by fruits and vegetables, then dairy, meat, eggs, fish, chicken and vegetable alternatives, with fats, sugars and salt kept to a minimum.

Five food groups

Food group	Suggested servings
Group 1 – breads, cereals and grains (complex carbohydrates). Preferred source for long-lasting energy (better than sugars or simple carbohydrates). Provides fibre, protein, essential B group vitamins (especially folic acid) and some iron.	**1 serve** = 1 slice of bread or $1/2$ a bread roll or bagel or $1/2$ cup of cereal/porridge or 2 Weet-Bix or $1/2$ cup of cooked pasta, rice, noodles, Polenta or couscous or 2 large cracker biscuits. *NOTE: Cakes, biscuits, pies and pastries are also carbohydrates, but contain sugars and fats with excess calories and little nutritional value.* **Non-pregnant women** need 6 servings a day. **Men and physically active women** need 8 servings a day. **Active men and athletic women** need 11 servings per day (or more).

6 BIRTH: CONCEIVING, NURTURING AND GIVING BIRTH TO YOUR BABY

Group 1 (cont.)	**Pregnant women** need 8 servings each day to cater for increased metabolism and the unborn baby's needs. **Breastfeeding women** need 8 to 9 servings per day for the first 6 months. **Pregnant with twins** – 10 servings per day. **Triplets** – 12 servings per day. **Breastfeeding twins** – 11 servings per day. **Breastfeeding triplets** – 13 servings a day (for the first 6 months).
Group 2 – fruits and vegetables. Provides many vitamins and minerals. Increases absorption of iron present in other foods. High in fibre. Optimises health for fertility, pregnancy and the baby's growth and development.	**1 serve of fruit** = 1 apple or banana or orange or a bunch of grapes or 4 pieces of dried fruit or a handful of sultanas or $1/2$ cup of canned or frozen fruit or $1/2$ cup of 100% fruit juice (unsweetened). **1 serve of vegetables** = $1/2$ cup of cooked or raw vegetables or $1/2$ cup of legumes (beans, lentils, split peas) or 1 cup green leafy vegetables or $1/2$ cup of tabouli or 1 small carrot or 1 tomato or 1 cup 100% vegetable juice. **Both men and women** need 2 to 4 servings of fruit and 3 to 5 servings of vegetables each day. **Pregnancy** – 4 servings of fruit and 4 servings of vegetables each day. **Breastfeeding** – 4 servings of fruit and 4 to 5 servings of vegetables. **Pregnant with twins** – 6 to 7 servings of fruit and 4 to 5 servings of vegetables. **Triplets** – 8 servings of fruit and 5 servings of vegetables. **Breastfeeding twins** – 5 servings of fruit and 4 to 5 servings of vegetables. **Breastfeeding triplets** – 5 servings of fruit and 5 servings of vegetables.
Group 3 – meat, chicken, fish, eggs and vegetable alternatives. Provides protein to build healthy new body cells and a range of essential vitamins and minerals (iron, B12, B6, zinc, niacin, thiamine). Helps produce haemoglobin, to prevent anaemia. Helps produce healthy eggs and sperm for conception and growth and development of the unborn baby.	**1 serve of meat, chicken, fish or eggs** = 70 to 100 g of cooked meat, chicken, fish or shellfish or 1 egg (raw or cooked) or 1 chop. **1 serve of vegetable alternatives** = $1/2$ of a cup of cooked lentils or 1 handful of peanuts or 4 tablespoons of peanut butter or $1/2$ cup of sesame, pumpkin, sunflower seeds or linseed or 120 g of tofu. **Recommended daily protein intake** is 0.75 g/kg of body weight per day. (Eg. if you weigh 60 kg, 60 x 0.75 g = 45 g per day). One serving provides 7 to 8 g of protein. However, protein is also in breads, cereals, grains (1 serving = 3 g), dairy foods (1 serving = 8 g) and some vegetables (1 serving = 2 g). A typical meal has 20 g or more of protein. **Pre-conception** – 2 to 3 servings per day. **Pregnancy and breastfeeding** – 2 to 3 servings per day. **Pregnant with twins** – 3 to 4 servings per day, reduced back to 2 to 3 servings a day when breastfeeding. **Triplets** – 4 to 5 servings per day, reduced to 3 serving a day when breastfeeding.

Group 4 – dairy foods (foods containing cow's milk). Main source of calcium for growth and strength of bones and teeth, protects against high blood pressure, important for muscle functioning. Provides protein and vitamins A, D and riboflavin.

1 serve = 1 glass of milk or 1 tub of yoghurt or 1 slice of cheese or 5 heaped tablespoons of powdered milk. (1 serve of dairy food = 300 mg of calcium.) **Men and non-pregnant women** – 2 to 3 servings (choose low-fat dairy products). If you do not eat dairy products (or very little), eat alternative foods high in calcium (see vitamins and minerals table, page 14).
Pregnancy and breastfeeding – 3 to 4 servings of dairy a day to have adequate calcium. Continue this while breastfeeding. Pregnant and breastfeeding women under 20 years need at least 4 servings per day, because their body is still building bone density for later life.
Pregnant with twins – 4 to 5 servings a day, continue this while breastfeeding. **Triplets** – 5 to 6 servings a day, with similar amounts while breastfeeding. Your caregiver may prescribe calcium supplements to help you keep up with your body's needs.

Group 5 – fats. Supply fat-soluble vitamins (A, D and E) for body tissue repair, hormone manufacture and some body energy. Unsaturated vegetable fats are healthier than saturated animal fats (except for palm or coconut oil). **Sugars** – for short bursts of body energy. **Salt** – our bodies contain 9% salt.

Fats – naturally present in many foods, so there is no need to add to your diet. **Sugars** – found naturally in fruits, fruit juices, honey and milk. Provides extra calories without additional vitamins and minerals. Not recommended in large quantities. **Salt** – naturally present in many foods. You should have salt to taste. Don't restrict but don't add extra salt to foods or when cooking.
Pregnancy and breastfeeding – Fats and sugars only needed in small amounts, even if having twins or more. Excess salt has been linked with higher blood pressure and fluid retention (or swelling). Salt restriction has been linked with leg cramps. Aspartame (artificial sweetener) in diet soft drinks is considered safe in pregnancy (no more than 2800 mg a day). Saccharin (another artificial sweetener) is also considered safe for pregnant women.

Daily diet examples

You may choose to meticulously follow the five food group portions, or just use them as a guide. However, to some people it seems all too hard. So, to give you an idea, we have suggested some daily diets. (Men and very active women need two extra servings of carbohydrates, eg. two slices of bread).

Breakfast	A bowl of cereal, cup of milk and glass of orange juice **or** Fruit salad, yoghurt, bagel with peanut butter, and cup of tea **or** Baked beans on toast and glass of milk **or** Bacon, eggs, tomato, mushrooms on Turkish bread, pineapple juice and coffee **or** Porridge, milk and orange juice

Morning tea	Cheese, cracker biscuits, cup of tea **or** Apple, handful of nuts, glass of water **or** Yoghurt and mandarin **or** Carrot sticks, crackers, Vegemite
Lunch	Chicken and tabouli sandwich, bunch of grapes, and diet drink **or** Tuna and salad on pita bread, dried fruits, cheese, glass of blackcurrant juice **or** Egg and lettuce bread roll, and orange juice **or** Beef kebab with lettuce, tomato and cheese, and mineral water **or** Japanese rice cakes with tuna, slice of melon, cup of tea
Afternoon tea	Banana and yoghurt **or** Banana smoothie **or** Nuts, dried fruits, coffee and water **or** Muesli bar, milk shake **or** Fresh popped corn and apple juice
Dinner	Beef and vegetable stir-fry, rice, fruit and custard or ice cream **or** Spaghetti bolognaise, grated cheese, side salad **or** Chicken burritos with tomato, lettuce, cheese, guacamole **or** Grilled fish, rosemary potatoes, carrots, beans **or** Tandoori lamb cutlets, dhal, naan, tomato and mint side salad

VITAMINS AND MINERALS

Vitamins and minerals are essential for health, especially during preconception, pregnancy and breastfeeding. Most vitamins and minerals can be obtained through eating a variety of nutritious foods, but sometimes caregivers suggest supplements.

NOTE: *Never self-prescribe vitamin and mineral supplements. Always check with your health practitioner about appropriate dosages.*

Folic acid

During early pregnancy women need twice as much folic acid or folate to support the rapid growth of thousands of new body cells. It is now recommended that women take folic acid supplements for 1 to 2 months before conceiving, until 12 weeks of the pregnancy, to help prevent neural tube defects in their developing baby.[3]

Neural tube defects

Neural tube defects (NTD) occur when there are problems with the development of the baby's brain, skull and spinal cord, mainly during the first six weeks of pregnancy (or four weeks after conception). Adequate daily intakes of folate during early pregnancy reduce the chances of having a baby with an NTD by about 70%. In Australia, the rate of NTD is 1.6 per 1000 (or 0.0016%), about 400 babies each year. Adequate folate may also reduce the chances of other abnormalities, such as cleft lip and/or palate.

Women at increased risk of having a baby with an NTD are those who:
- Have had a previous baby with an NTD.
- Have close relatives who have had a baby with an NTD.
- Are insulin-dependent diabetics.
- Take certain medications that interfere with folic acid metabolism (for example, anti-epileptics and anti-malarials).

Women in these higher risk categories are prescribed 5 mg (5000 ug) by a doctor, to be taken under medical supervision.

Folic acid in foods
It is possible to have adequate folic acid through diet alone, if you eat foods rich in folic acid on a daily basis. Be aware that:
- You only absorb 50 to 60% of folic acid from natural food sources (but 100% from folate supplements).
- Heating and processing foods can destroy folic acid by up to 50%.
- Drinking alcohol interferes with folic acid absorption.

Some commercially prepared foods have folate added. These include certain brands of flour, bread, cracker biscuits, breakfast cereals, pasta, rice, yeast extracts, fruit and vegetable juices, soy drinks and tofu. The folic acid added to these foods is thought to be 100% absorbed by the body.

Folic acid supplements
The recommended daily folic acid supplement for preconception and early pregnancy is 0.4 mg (400 ug). Some caregivers recommend 0.5 mg (500 ug). Supplements can be purchased from pharmacies without a prescription.

If you are taking a multivitamin, READ THE LABEL. Many brands don't have enough folic acid, or too much. Don't take two tablets to have the 'correct' amount of folic acid, as you can overdose on other vitamins that can be harmful to your baby. Also, specialised brands 'for women' or 'for pregnancy' aren't necessarily better, and they're usually more expensive. Not every woman has the luxury of planning her pregnancy, or finding out she is pregnant early. As a guide, starting folate supplements:
- At least one month before conception provides the maximum benefits, but two months prior is ideal.
- Any time between conception and six weeks of pregnancy can still be of benefit.
- After six weeks of pregnancy may be helpful, but probably not as effective.
- After 12 weeks of pregnancy is of no benefit.

Vitamins and minerals

Vitamins	Recommended daily intake (RDI)
Vitamin A (retinol or beta-carotene) **Needed for:** healthy vision, resisting infection, growth and development of cells in lining of the mouth, throat, stomach, intestines, lungs, uterus, vagina and bladder. Supports reproductive organs and development of healthy sperm in men. Acts like a hormone during pregnancy, regulating cell growth and development of the unborn baby.	750 ug or 2500 IU of retinol. Adequately gained through a normal or vegetarian diet.
Vitamin B1 (thiamine) **Needed for:** metabolising carbohydrates for energy for body tissues. Facilitating normal nerve functioning. Helping growth and functioning of the unborn baby's body organs and nervous system.	1 mg. Adequately gained through a normal or vegetarian diet.
Vitamin B2 (riboflavin) **Needed for:** metabolism and releasing nutrients into body cells. Growth of the developing baby, especially in the first few weeks.	1 to 1.5 mg. Adequately gained through a normal or vegetarian diet.
Vitamin B3 (niacin) **Needed for:** effective metabolism and energy transfer of glucose and fat in the body, for general health and emotional stability. Helps the unborn baby's brain development.	15 to 20 mg. 50% of niacin comes from the breakdown of proteins eaten, and 50% comes from foods with niacin.
Vitamin B5 (pantothenic acid) **Needed for:** metabolism of fats, nerve transmitters, steroid hormones and the production of haemoglobin, to prevent anaemia. Helps the unborn baby's growth and development.	5 to 10 mg. Adequately gained through a normal or vegetarian diet.

Preconception, pregnancy, breastfeeding	Found in
Pregnancy – Vitamin A supplements containing retinol (from animal products), and should not be taken. High levels during the first 12 weeks of pregnancy may cause birth defects in some babies. Accutane taken for acne (or isotretinoin) contains high amounts of vitamin A and should be ceased for at least 1 month prior to conceiving. Skin products with Retin-A are not as toxic but should be avoided if possible. Take care with fish liver oil and multivitamins with vitamin A. Check the labels. **Breastfeeding** – Breast milk is high in fat, and excess vitamin A can pass to the baby, who is more susceptible to vitamin A toxicity. **Overdosing** – You can't overdose on beta-carotene (from vegetables and fruit). However, eating large amounts of carrots can make your skin look orange. This is not harmful.	Carrots, tomatoes, rockmelon, watermelon, mangoes, apricots, peaches, sweet potato, pumpkin, prunes, broccoli, spinach, prawns, liver (pâté), kidneys, fish liver oils, eggs, dairy products (cow's milk, cheeses, ice cream). Added to most margarines and some breakfast cereals. *NOTE: Not generally lost with normal cooking.*
Pregnancy – 1.5 mg, because the woman's metabolism and energy needs are increased. However, supplementing is not required because adequate amounts are available through diet alone. **Overdosing** – There is no evidence that you can overdose on thiamine.	Wholegrain bread, cereals, oatmeal, wheatgerm, rice, spaghetti, flour, yeast, nuts, kidney beans, pulses, peas, spinach, tomato juice, watermelon, soymilk, ham, pork and steak. *NOTE: Thiamine is almost completely removed in refined and processed foods. It can be destroyed at very high temperatures and dissolves into cooking water.*
Pregnancy – About 1.5 mg. Supplementing is not required. **Overdosing** – There is no evidence that you can overdose on riboflavin.	Milk, yoghurt, cheese, eggs, whole grains, cereals, wheatgerm, dark green vegetables (spinach, asparagus, broccoli). Vegans must rely on ample intakes to obtain adequate riboflavin. *NOTE: Cooking does not destroy riboflavin, but it is affected by exposure to sunlight.*
Pregnancy – Too much niacin during the first 12 weeks may lead to birth defects. Supplementing is not recommended. **Breastfeeding** – Supplementing is not recommended. **Overdosing** – More than 35 mg per day can cause serious illness.	Whole grains, cereals, wheatgerm, rice, spaghetti, flour, yeast, potatoes, avocados, legumes, peanuts, mushrooms, spinach, eggs, milk, cheese, tofu, tuna, codfish, bluefish, prawns, chicken, ham and steak. *NOTE: Niacin can be destroyed if food is overcooked.*
Pregnancy and breastfeeding – Helps prevent anaemia. Supplementing is not required. **Overdosing** – There is no evidence that you can overdose on vitamin B5.	Beef, chicken, whole grains, cereals, wheat bran, yeast, peanuts, potatoes, tomatoes, broccoli, mushrooms, avocados, cheese. *NOTE: Vitamin B5 can be readily destroyed by freezing, canning and refining foods.*

Vitamin B6 (pyridoxine)
Needed for: metabolising proteins and fats for cell building, producing haemoglobin (to prevent anaemia), producing white blood cells, to fight infection. Helps mental and cognitive performance and steroid hormone activity. Helps growth and development of new cells in the unborn baby.

1 to 1.5 mg. The oral contraceptive pill may slightly decrease the amount of vitamin B6 available to the body from foods.

Folic acid (folate, folacin, pteroylglutamic acid or PGA)
Needed for: growth of healthy, new body cells, especially lining of the intestines. Vital for forming haemoglobin (along with iron and vitamin B12). Thought to play a role in preventing cancer.

0.2 to 0.4 mg or 200 to 400 ug. Alcohol and smoking can inhibit the body's use of folate as well as some medications, including antacids, aspirin and the contraceptive pill.

Vitamin B12 (cobalamin)
Needed for: metabolism of protein, carbohydrates and fats. Contributes to producing haemoglobin, to prevent anaemia. Maintains the protective cover around nerves and promotes their growth. Helps the healthy development of the baby's brain and nervous system. Vitamin B12 and folic acid rely on each other to enable the body to use them.

4 to 6 ug. Gained easily from a diet with meats and/or dairy products. Vegans may need a daily B12 supplement (generally 4 ug).

Vitamin C (ascorbic acid)
Needed for: wound healing and scar formation. Increases absorption of iron from foods. Assists resistance to infection and helps with stress. High dose supplements may combat colds and other illnesses (although the possible benefits are unclear). Helps form a healthy placenta.

70 to 90 mg a day. Easily obtained through a normal diet with fruit and vegetables. Smoking and the contraceptive pill can deplete vitamin C. Smokers need 30 to 40 mg extra per day.

Pregnancy and breastfeeding – Too much vitamin B6 (more than 100 mg per day), during the first 12 weeks of pregnancy may be linked with birth defects involving the baby's arms, legs and nerve development. Unborn babies can also develop a dependency and withdrawal after birth, if their mother supplements daily for the weeks just before birth. Low dose supplements may be prescribed for morning sickness. There is conflicting evidence as to whether it helps with carpal tunnel syndrome or sleep disorders.
Overdosing – Taking more than 2 g per day, for 2 months or more, can lead to irreversible nerve damage.

Whole grains, cereals, wheat bran, yeast, potatoes, kidney beans, tomatoes, bananas, broccoli, watermelon, avocados, prune juice, milk, yoghurt, chicken, turkey, eggs, ham, steak and tuna. *NOTE: Foods can lose some vitamin B6 when heated.*

Preconception and pregnancy – Supplementing with 0.4 to 0.5 mg (400 to 500 ug) of folic acid per day is recommended for 1 month before conceiving and the first 6 to 12 weeks of pregnancy to reduce the chances of the baby developing neural tube defects (NTD).
Overdosing – Taking more than 1000 mg per day can be dangerous because it masks a deficiency in vitamin B12 (which is not common). If a person takes high doses of folic acid and is B12 deficient, they can develop irreversible nerve damage. Vegetarians or vegans can sometimes be vitamin B12 deficient. Ideally, a blood test should be done to screen for vitamin B12 deficiency before being prescribed higher doses.

Oranges, bananas, strawberries, tomatoes, asparagus, avocados, beetroot, broccoli, brussels sprouts, spinach, green leafy vegetables, leeks, parsley, parsnip, potato, cauliflower, green beans, peas, spring onions, milk, red kidney beans, lentils, chickpeas, soy beans, almonds, hazelnuts, walnuts, cashew nuts, peanut butter, wholemeal bread, rice, pasta, bran, wheatgerm and wheat cereals, salmon, tuna, Vegemite, Marmite, Bonox and Bovril. *NOTE: Cooking and processing can destroy some folic acid available in foods; depending on the food and the way it is cooked, it can be as high as 50%.*

Pregnancy – Women with a vegan diet need B12 supplements. Babies born to mothers who are B12 deficient are at risk of spinal cord damage and possibly a severe inability to move well.
Breastfeeding – If the mother is B12 deficient while breastfeeding, her baby may start to exhibit limited movement. A paediatrician may prescribe vitamin B12 supplements to help reverse the majority of these signs, but there can be permanent learning and language delays.
Overdosing – There is no evidence that you can overdose on vitamin B12.

Meat, fish, chicken, shellfish, eggs, milk, cheese, yoghurt. Foods fortified with B12 include some brands of soymilk, yeast extracts, veggie burgers and cereals. Contrary to popular belief, yeast, miso (soybean paste), mushrooms and sea algae (spirulina) do not contain active vitamin B12. They are present in these foods but not able to be absorbed by the body. *NOTE: B12 is destroyed by microwave cooking but may be preserved by cooking on a stove top or in an oven.*

Pregnancy – Doses above 200 mg are not recommended. At this stage there is no evidence that higher doses during early pregnancy causes birth defects. Small supplements may be prescribed with iron supplements (or drinking orange or blackcurrant juice). Vitamin C readily crosses the placenta to the baby. Taking more than 200 mg per day during late pregnancy, till the birth, can create a dependency for the baby, making them experience a withdrawal (vitamin C deficiency) soon after birth, similar to scurvy. Supplements have been prescribed by some doctors to help prevent high blood pressure and premature birth. However, this has not been definitely proven effective.
Overdosing – More than 2000 mg per day can lead to kidney stones and a dependence on vitamin C, with physical signs of deficiency if suddenly stopped. Cutting down slowly is recommended.

Oranges, limes, grapefruits, watermelon, pawpaw, rockmelon, strawberries, blackcurrants, kiwi fruit, mangoes, pineapple, bananas, avocados, apples, capsicum, tomatoes, bean sprouts, brussels sprouts, spinach, peas, green beans, corn, potatoes, sweet potatoes, broccoli. *NOTE: Vitamin C is fragile and easily lost through heat and cooking. Raw fruits and vegetables tend to provide higher amounts.*

Vitamin D (calciferol)
Needed for: the absorption of calcium and phosphorus into the bones, making them stronger and denser. Assists the growth and development of a baby's bones.

10 ug. Gained from diary products or 1 to 2 hours of sunlight exposure each week.

Vitamin E (alpha-tocopherol or alpha-TE)
Needed for: the health of cell membranes. May play a role in protecting against heart disease and possibly cancer. *NOTE: Claims that vitamin E increases physical performance, slows aging, improves male sexual function or inhibits Parkinson's disease are not proven.*

10 to 15 mg per day. A normal and vegetarian diet contributes about 30 mg per day (more if wheatgerm oil is included).

Vitamin K (menadione)
Needed for: blood clotting and preventing excessive bleeding. Thought to play a role in building strong bones.

None recommended. The body manufactures its own vitamin K through synthesising bacteria in the bowel, then storing in the liver. Supplements should only be prescribed by a doctor.

Minerals

Calcium (Ca)
Needed for: healthy bones and teeth; muscle contraction, blood clotting, nerve impulse conduction and the regulation of hormones. Adequate calcium may help prevent high blood pressure, high cholesterol, heart disease, diabetes and bowel cancer. Assists the development of the baby's bones.

600 to 900 mg per day for men and non-pregnant women.

Pregnancy and breastfeeding – Vitamin D deficiency can occur in women who have little sun exposure, especially if they don't eat dairy products. This can lead to the development of osteomalacia (a bone disorder) and the baby being at risk for low calcium (hypocalcaemia) at birth, possibly experiencing seizures and a slowing of their heart rate. If you think you may be vitamin D deficient, ask your doctor about the possible need for a supplement. A blood test can show what your levels are.
Overdosing – Excess vitamin D (with supplementing) can quickly produce toxic effects. Foods naturally containing vitamin D and/or extended sun exposure do not create excess vitamin D in the body. Never take vitamin D supplements unless prescribed by a doctor. Keep supplements out of the reach of children.

Milk, cheese, butter (some margarines have vitamin D added), egg yolks, fish liver oils, swordfish, salmon, tuna and sardines. Small exposures to sunlight (the hands, arms and face for 10 to 15 minutes a few times a week). People with dark skin need 4 times longer sun exposure than people with fair skin, to produce the same amount of vitamin D. *NOTE: Sunscreens (SPF 8+ or more) prevent vitamin D synthesis. However, take care not to become sunburnt. People with a vegan diet may not obtain vitamin D through their diet, and should rely on sun exposure.*

Pregnancy – Contributes to the health of new cells in the developing baby. Mothers pass vitamin E to their babies during the last 12 weeks of pregnancy (about 20 mg in total). Some very premature babies (less than 28 weeks) show signs of vitamin E deficiency soon after birth, possibly leading to haemolytic anaemia. Vitamin E has sometimes been prescribed (combined with vitamin C) to help prevent high blood pressure during pregnancy and premature birth.
Overdosing – There appears to be no ill effects from taking doses up to 200 mg per day.

Wheatgerm oil, vegetable oils (peanut, olive, safflower, sunflower and canola), margarine, salad dressings, nuts, sunflower seeds, pumpkin seeds and sesame seeds. *NOTE: Vitamin E can be destroyed at deep-frying temperatures.*

Pregnancy – Supplements are not necessary. Pregnant women taking medications that can interfere with vitamin K in the body (antibiotics, anti-epileptics, barbiturates, tuberculosis drugs and Warfrin) may be prescribed supplements for the last 4 weeks of their pregnancy (about 10 mg per day). This aims to decrease the chances of their baby experiencing vitamin K deficiency. Newborns have a natural degree of vitamin K deficiency at birth, which is normal, but are usually given an injection (or 3 oral doses) of vitamin K soon after birth.

Vitamin K produced in the bowel is called K2 (menaquinone), this is more than adequate to protect us from bleeding, even if our diet is inadequate. A small amount of vitamin K comes from foods (K1 or phylloquinone) – fresh green leafy vegetables, cabbage, spinach, green vegetables, brussels sprouts, cauliflower, soy beans, eggs, milk, meats, liver, cereals and fruits. *NOTE: Vitamin K can be destroyed by prolonged exposure to light but is not lost by cooking.*

Pregnant and breastfeeding – The unborn baby draws on their mother's calcium in her bones for growth and development. To keep these stores adequate, to help prevent osteoporosis (weakened bones) later in life, you need 900 to 1200 mg of calcium a day, and continue this while breastfeeding. Pregnant and breastfeeding women under 20 years need 1200 mg, because their body is still building bone density for later life. **Pregnancy with twins** – 1200 to 1500 mg, and continued while breastfeeding. **Triplets** – 1500 to 1800 mg, continue while breastfeeding. Your caregiver may prescribe calcium supplements to help keep up with your body's needs. Calcium may help prevent high blood pressure during pregnancy and possibly premature birth.

Dairy foods tend to contain the highest amounts of calcium (milk, yoghurt, cheeses). Women who dislike or are allergic to dairy foods need to have alternative foods with calcium such as raw spinach, sardines, raw cabbage, prawns, sesame seeds, molasses, tinned salmon (with the bones), tofu fortified with calcium, soy beans, almonds, seafood scallops, nuts, broccoli, blackberries, pineapple juice, oranges, fish, baked beans, carrots, pumpkin, seaweed. Some commercially prepared

Calcium (cont.)

Iodine (iodide)
Needed for: thyroid hormones to regulate metabolism, body temperature, reproduction, growth, blood cell production, nerve and muscle function. Essential for the baby's growth and development. Lack of iodine can lead to hypothyroidism, affecting a person's general health, fertility and the ability to carry a pregnancy.

120 to 150 ug. Readily available through a normal or vegetarian diet.

Iron (Fe, ferrous iron or ferric iron)
Needed for: the production of haemoglobin, to prevent anaemia (working in partnership with folic acid and vitamin B12).

7 to 10 mg for men; 15 to 18 mg for non-pregnant women aged 19 to 50 years; 10 to 13 mg for teenagers; 22 to 27 mg during pregnancy.

Magnesium (Mg)
Needed for: muscle contraction and blood clotting (in partnership with calcium); regulating blood pressure and functioning of the lungs. Necessary for energy metabolism (body's use of glucose, protein and fat) and normal functioning of the immune system. Keeps calcium in tooth enamel to prevent decay. May be protective against heart disease and high blood pressure when taken with calcium.

250 to 300 mg, which can easily be provided with a normal or vegetarian diet.

Phosphorus (Ph or phos)
Needed for: cell growth and healthy muscle function. Combines with calcium in the bones and teeth and is part of DNA (or genes).

1000 mg. Readily available through a normal and vegetarian diet.

Overdosing – Supplements should not exceed 1000 to 1500 mg a day and should be taken under medical supervision. When combined with calcium-rich foods, the total intake should not exceed 2500 mg per day.

foods have added calcium, such as some brands of orange juices, cereals and tofu.

Pregnancy – Prolonged lack of iodine during pregnancy can affect the baby's growth and development, possibly leading to intellectual and physical disabilities (known as cretinism). Too much iodine (through supplements) can cause the unborn baby to develop a goitre in their throat. Pregnant women should take care with kelp tablets and iodised vitamins. The normal amount of iodine required is obtained through diet.
Overdosing – Excessive iodine can cause hyperthyroidism.

Seafood, kelp, seaweed, some breads and cow's milk products. Vegetables grown in iodine-rich soils (coastal regions). Added to salt in most western countries. Foods high in salt (particularly fast foods) have a high iodine content, although generally not at toxic levels.

Preconception and pregnancy – Anaemia may inhibit conception for the woman and sperm production for the man. Iron is needed to prevent anaemia to support the pregnancy and growth of the baby. This reduces the chances of the baby becoming distressed during labour, helps the woman tolerate a normal blood loss at birth (or more) and assists in recovery after the birth and helps breast milk production. During the last 3 months of pregnancy, the unborn baby stores iron in their liver to use during the first 6 months of their life, before starting solid foods. Iron supplements are not routine during pregnancy, but blood tests are performed twice (or more) to see if they are required.
Overdosing – The body automatically absorbs less iron when its iron stores are full. However, excess iron supplements (especially when taken with vitamin C) can overwhelm the intestines, leading to 'iron overload', causing similar signs to anaemia (tiredness, apathy, lethargy), but tissue damage can also occur, especially the liver. Supplements should not exceed 45 mg of elemental iron per day. *NOTE: If a small child takes adult iron supplements, they can have iron poisoning, with nausea, vomiting, diarrhoea, a rapid heart rate, weak pulse, dizziness, shock and confusion. As little as 5 x 200 mg tablets can cause heart failure and death in a young child. Keep iron tablets out of the reach of children.*

Red meat (beef, veal, lamb), with lesser amounts in chicken, fish, pork, ham, eggs and shellfish (all known as haem sources, which are readily absorbed by the body, up to 25%). Breads, grains, cereals, dark green leafy vegetables, spinach, broccoli, parsley, potatoes, dried fruits, beans (baked, green, kidney, black), peanuts, sunflower seeds and tofu. These are nonhaem sources, which are not as readily absorbed (up to 10%). Absorption can be increased up to 4 times if they are eaten with vitamin C–rich foods or drinks. When haem and nonhaem foods are eaten together, they interact with each other to maximise the body's ability to absorb the iron they contain. *NOTE: Excess calcium foods (or calcium supplements) and tannic acid in tea and coffee can inhibit iron absorption.*

Pregnancy and breastfeeding – Needed for tissue growth for mother and baby, and is passed to the baby through breast milk. Low magnesium may be linked to leg cramps, fluid retention and restless legs during pregnancy. Magnesium sulphate can be prescribed by a doctor for very high blood pressure during late pregnancy (given in hospital through an intravenous drip), to help prevent seizures that may eventuate from extremely high blood pressure.
Overdosing – Magnesium toxicity is rare but can lead to low blood pressure, drowsiness, diarrhoea and dehydration. Intake should not exceed 350 mg per day.

Wholegrain breads, cereals, rice, pasta, oatmeal, wheatgerm, nuts, peanut butter, soybeans, kidney beans, baked beans, bran, bananas, corn, artichokes, potatoes, sweet potatoes, watermelon, dried fruits, oranges, grapefruit, limes, avocados, broccoli, seaweed, dark green leafy vegetables, spinach, milk, yoghurt, cheeses, meats, chicken, fish, eggs and chocolate!

Pregnancy and breastfeeding – Essential for the overall development of the baby and to support the pregnancy and breastfeeding.
Overdosing – Phosphorus is only toxic when calcium levels are extremely low (which is rare). Intake should not exceed 4000 mg per day.

Phosphorus is part of all cells and abundant in all natural foods. Main sources include hard cheeses, milk, yoghurt, meat, fish, chicken, eggs, legumes, breads, rice, pasta, tofu, seeds, beans, fruits and vegetables. Phosphorus is also a common food additive.

Potassium (K)
Needed for: regulating the levels of potassium, sodium and water in the body (has a balancing relationship with salt). Regulates fluids, nutrients and waste products in and out of cells. Allows muscles and nerves to conduct 'electric charges' for movement and functioning. Controls and regulates the heartbeat. Seems to protect against high blood pressure and stroke.

50 to 140 mmol/L. Most diets provide adequate potassium. Dehydration or prolonged vomiting and diarrhoea can create a potassium deficiency, as well as certain medications (diuretics, steroids and strong laxatives).

Sodium (Na, salt, sodium chloride)
Needed for: regulating fluids, nutrients and waste product movement in and out of cells (has a balancing relationship with potassium). Helps muscles and nerves to conduct 'electric charges' for movement and functioning. Helps balance body fluid. When you eat foods high in salt, your thirst sensation is triggered, so your body keeps the sodium–water balance at its desired level.

40 to 100 mmol/L. Most people eat more salt than required. Limit foods with a high salt content.

Zinc (Zn)
Needed for: protein synthesis, growth, insulin regulation, blood clotting, vitamin A usage by the body and learning performance. Assists taste sensations, vision, conception, reproduction and wound healing. Contributes to a strong immune system. Strengthens the cells' resistance to free radicals.

10 to 12 mg a day, generally obtained through a well-balanced diet.

• Recommended daily intakes based on the Australian Natural Health and Medical Research (NHMRC) guidelines.

Pregnancy – Some remedies used to relieve fluid retention during pregnancy may cause a loss of extra potassium. Cell salts may help with this imbalance (available at health food stores).
Overdosing – Toxicity can occur if a person takes too many potassium salts or supplements with potassium (including some 'energy fitness shakes').

Most fresh fruits and vegetables, meats, chicken, fish, dairy foods, breads and cereals, tomatoes, oranges, carrots, potatoes, artichokes, bananas, legumes, liquorice, chocolate, molasses, milk and yoghurt. Processed foods tend to contain less potassium (and more salt).

Pregnancy – Sodium contributes to the natural fluid in the blood (or plasma) increasing during pregnancy (up to 50%) and the woman's normal water balance. Research no longer supports restricting salt to help with high blood pressure, leg cramps or fluid retention during pregnancy. Salt intake should not be excessive, but also not restricted (generally determined by personal taste).
Overdosing – Excess sodium can contribute to fluid retention and a temporary high blood pressure. Poor kidney function can also cause sodium toxicity, especially if the body's water needs are not met. You should drink more water when you have fluid retention, rather than restricting fluids to help with this imbalance. High salt intakes in the long term can contribute to high blood pressure later in life.

Processed foods, bacon, ham, corned beef, salami, kidneys, sausages, anchovies, caviar, dried cod, sardines, smoked salmon, olives, pickles, processed cheeses, sundried tomatoes, soy sauce, salted nuts, chips, crackers, pretzels, popcorn, milk, seafoods, some vegetables, pastes and drinks such as Vegemite, Marmite, Promite, Bovril and Bonox.

Preconception – Vital for conception and reproduction, the healthy development of sexual organs during puberty and adequate sperm production in adult men.
Pregnancy and breastfeeding – You need 4 to 6 mg of extra zinc a day. Unborn babies needs zinc for cell division and tissue growth and use it to utilise protein for growth and development. Early research indicated that zinc may be protective against a prolonged labour, premature labour, going past the due date (reducing the need for induction) and high blood pressure. However, evidence is conflicting and has not been proven. Some caregivers recommend zinc supplements to boost the immune system for illnesses such as the common cold or for herpes outbreaks (along with garlic and vitamin C). There appears to be no adverse effects from sensible supplementing, up to 20 mg per day.
Overdosing – High doses of zinc (50 to 450 mg) can cause vomiting, diarrhoea, dizziness, drowsiness, headaches, exhaustion, loss of appetite, muscle pain, fever and a lowered immune system. Supplements should not exceed 40 mg per day.

Meat, fish, oysters, shellfish, prawns, crab, turkey, chicken, ham, milk, yoghurt, cheeses (especially ricotta), beans (green, kidney, baked), peanut butter, nuts, tofu, lentils, eggs, breads, cereals, pasta, rice, wheatgerm, bran, onions, ginger and sunflower seeds.
NOTE: Some zinc may also be obtained if you cook with galvanised pots.

Taking folic acid supplements:
- May slightly increase your chances of conceiving twins. For every 176 pregnancies, one extra woman supplementing with folic acid will conceive twins.[4]
- May decrease your chances of feeling dizzy or experiencing morning sickness.
- Does not enhance your fertility or help you conceive a baby sooner.
- Does not cause miscarriage or ectopic pregnancy.
- Does not prevent stillbirth.

NOTE: *Folic acid can reduce the effectiveness of anti-epileptic medications, possibly causing seizures. Consult with your doctor, a neurologist or genetic counsellor.*

Lifestyle changes — what to avoid

When planning to have a child, it is not unusual to have renewed motivation to look after your body by stopping (or cutting back) any unhealthy lifestyle habits. Making positive changes can improve your chances of conceiving sooner, and hopefully enable you to continue them during the pregnancy, and when the new baby arrives.

People can take a range of legal and illegal substances for recreational use, or because they have an addiction. While we know about the possible effects on conception and pregnancy of common substances (caffeine, alcohol and cigarettes), less is known about harder drugs such as marijuana, amphetamines, tranquillisers, benzodiazepines, LSD, hallucinogens, cocaine, ecstasy, and heroin, to name but a few. However, it probably comes as no surprise that these should not be taken by men or women who are trying to conceive a baby.

NOTE: *The resource section at the back of the book lists organisations to help overcome addictions. Maternity hospitals also have health professionals who work with pregnant women who are addicted to various substances. Ask your caregiver.*

Caffeine

Caffeine is a mild stimulant contained in coffee, chocolate, cocoa, cola, energy drinks, many teas, some herbal remedies and medicines for headaches, colds, allergies, weight loss and staying awake. Having it in moderation is not harmful to your health, although it does interfere with the body's ability to absorb iron from foods.

About 24 hours after stopping caffeine (or greatly cutting back), you may experience withdrawal symptoms for up to a week or so. Many people reduce their intake gradually, perhaps replacing it with decaffeinated products. If you smoke, you need twice the amount of caffeine to feel the same effects as people who don't smoke. Therefore if you stop smoking, the effects of caffeine on your body double.

Preconception – Both men and women should limit their caffeine intake to 200 mg a day or less when trying to conceive.

Pregnancy – More than 300 mg of caffeine a day is possibly linked with miscarriage, but there is no evidence it causes birth defects. Caffeine passes from the mother to the unborn baby within 20 to 30 minutes, possibly stimulating them to be more active in the uterus. It mildly constricts blood vessels and may decrease blood flow to the baby for short periods. Heavy intakes during the weeks leading up to the birth can cause the newborn baby to experience withdrawal symptoms for 24 to 48 hours afterwards, being more unsettled, crying and irritable.

Breastfeeding – Caffeine passes to the baby through breast milk, with high intakes making the baby irritable, cry more and sleep less.

Content of caffeine	
1 cup of espresso	150 mg
1 cup of instant coffee	80 mg
1 cup of decaffeinated coffee	3 mg
1 cup of tea	50 mg
1 can of iced tea	70 mg
1 can of cola drink	40 mg
1 cup of hot chocolate	10 mg
1 cup of chocolate milk	5 mg
30 g of milk chocolate	5 mg
30 g of dark chocolate	20 mg
30 g of chocolate syrup	5 mg

Alcohol

Alcohol is medically classified as a sedative. It interferes with the body's absorption of B group vitamins (especially folic acid) and makes you pass more urine, losing many essential vitamins and minerals. Alcohol takes 24 hours to be fully excreted by the body. So people who drink daily are never alcohol-free.

Preconception – Alcohol decreases the chances of conception by 50% for both men and women. Most caregivers say NO alcohol when trying to conceive. Some say one drink a week is acceptable. Others allow up to four drinks a week (with no more than one drink in a single session).

Pregnancy – The World Health Organisation (WHO) suggests there is NO safe level of alcohol consumption during pregnancy. Some caregivers say half to one drink on the odd occasion may be okay. More than one to two drinks on a regular basis (several times a week), may contribute to miscarriage, the baby growing slowly or being premature. Fetal alcohol syndrome

(FAS) may occur with two to four drinks a day. This is an irreversible and untreatable condition causing the baby to develop unusual facial features, mental and development delays, poor coordination and hyperactivity as a child. Fetal alcohol effects (FAE) is less severe than FAS, but may be caused by regularly having one drink a day (or seven drinks a week).

Breastfeeding – Alcohol inhibits the let-down reflex and passes into breast milk within an hour of the mother drinking. The baby's immature liver and their small body size means it takes longer for them to get rid of it from their system. More than one drink (or regular daily intakes) can be harmful for your baby. Some caregivers suggest limits of half to one drink on the odd occasion AFTER the baby has breastfed, and then delaying the baby's next feed for about two hours.

Cigarettes

Tobacco smoke contains over 4000 toxic chemicals which can cause cancer, heart and lung disease. Smoking depletes vitamin stores in the body and can harm the health of others who inhale the fumes (known as passive smoking). There is NO safe level of smoking, and 'light' or 'mild' cigarettes don't prevent health effects. Also, people tend to breathe in the smoke of light cigarettes more deeply, smoke them more often and smoke right down to the butt, absorbing the same amounts of chemicals as regular brands.

Smoking is very addictive and many people return to it after periods of abstinence, often requiring assistance and guidance to quit for good. When stopping (or greatly cutting back), you may experience headaches, coughing, muscle spasms, stomach and bowel problems, irritability, tension and/or nervousness, difficulties sleeping and concentrating, an increased appetite, a slight weight gain (about 4 to 5 kg) and frequent cravings for cigarettes.

Preconception – Smoking decreases fertility by 20 to 30%. The chemicals interfere with hormonal balance, decreasing sperm counts and their ability to 'swim' for men, and affecting healthy egg production for women. It takes three months after stopping for your fertility to return to normal.

Pregnancy – Smoking may cause miscarriage. After 16 weeks of pregnancy, smoking can lead to complications such as bleeding, placental abruption and premature birth. The baby is more likely to be distressed during labour (needing forceps, ventouse or a caesarean). Smoking reduces oxygen and nutrients available to the unborn baby, making them smaller and accounting for up to 25% of stillbirths and 20% of newborn baby deaths.

After the birth – If a woman smokes up until the birth, her baby is more likely to have low temperatures, breathing problems, low blood sugar levels and may require intensive care. The baby often experiences withdrawal symptoms for up to a week, crying more, sleeping less and being more difficult to comfort. Parents who smoke increase the risk of their baby dying from SIDS (sudden infant death syndrome). Always smoke outside, away from your baby.

Breastfeeding – Smoking is not a reason to stop breastfeeding. However, some women find their milk supply slowly declines after the first couple of months, possibly due to less blood supply to the breasts. Small amounts of nicotine do pass to the baby through breast milk. Try to limit your smoking to soon after a breastfeed and avoid it for one hour before the next breastfeed.

Marijuana

Marijuana, cannabis or hashish contains tetrahydrocannabinol (THC), which gives a 'high' within minutes of inhaling (or half an hour to an hour after eating), lasting for up to five hours (12 hours after eating). THC is stored in the body's fat cells and takes one month to fully leave the body. Women store more THC than men. Daily or weekly use means THC is always present in the body. THC has been linked with triggering (or worsening) depression and other psychiatric illnesses (such as schizophrenia) in people who are predisposed to these. If cannabis is combined with tobacco, the health effects of cigarettes also occur.

Cannabis is addictive and a 'safe level' is difficult to estimate because plants contain various levels of THC. If suddenly stopped after regular use, it can cause mild, flu-like symptoms such as headaches, nausea, upset stomach, feeling irritable, depressed, anxious and generally have difficulty sleeping. Sometimes professional assistance and counselling is needed to quit.

Preconception – The effects on fertility are not fully known. THC does decrease sex drive and may reduce sperm counts in men and make the menstrual cycle irregular in women.

Pregnancy – THC does not cause birth defects but can affect the baby's growth and the development of their brain and nervous system, possibly causing behavioural changes in older children (impulsive, hyperactive, attention and learning difficulties). If the mother smokes during the month before the birth, the baby may take longer to adjust to light in the room, startle more easily, have tremors (the shakes) in the early days and initially not sleep well.

Breastfeeding – Smoking cannabis is not a reason to stop breastfeeding, but THC can pass to the baby through breast milk for several hours after the mother smokes. This may increase the risk of delayed physical development (holding objects, coordination, crawling and walking) because the baby's brain and nervous system is still maturing (until 18 months of age). Babies should be kept away from cannabis smoke to help prevent SIDS. Always smoke outside, away from your baby.

Physical activity before pregnancy

Regular physical activity is healthy and may help with conception. Other benefits include:
- Balancing hormones in (men and women).
- Supporting emotional wellbeing to help deal with stress.
- Better sleep and more energy.
- Preparing a woman's body for the physical demands of pregnancy and labour.
- Preparing both partners for the physical demands of early parenting.
- Helping maintain a healthy weight range.

Physical activity doesn't have to be hard work, just regular. Often, once you get into a pattern, activities become easier and more enjoyable. Convincing your partner (or a friend) to exercise with you commits you to exercising more regularly, but finding time can be a barrier. Try to be creative; perhaps plan social gatherings around bushwalking or bicycling. If you have another child, schedule exercise when your partner is home, organise a babysitter, or attend a facility with childminding services.

Daily physical activity is ideal but not always achievable. Several times a week is excellent, but whenever you get the chance is better than not at all. Ideally, exercise for at least 20 minutes each session, 30 to 45 minutes if you can.

Swimming, yoga, Pilates, belly dancing, bike riding or walking can be good activities to get started. When exercising for the first time (or resuming after three to four weeks break), begin with short, gentle sessions, gradually building up over a few weeks. Remember to do some warm-up exercises for at least 10 minutes beforehand, to help prevent injuries. Stretch and warm down for 5 to 10 minutes at the end of each session to enhance flexibility and lessen muscle soreness.

Too much exercise can affect your fertility. Elite female athletes may experience irregular menstrual periods or stop menstruating altogether, and male athletes may have reduced sperm counts. If you are training at a strenuous level, you could experience difficulties conceiving, until you wind down. Discuss your plans for having a baby with your caregiver and/or coach. You may also need to modify your training once you are pregnant.

Physical activity when conception occurs

Your pregnancy won't be confirmed for at least two to three weeks after conceiving. Therefore, it may be wise to modify your exercise for the last two weeks of your menstrual cycle, after ovulation. Use your own judgment, but consider avoiding:

- Prolonged, strenuous exercise which increases your body temperature above 37.5°C for more than 20 minutes.
- Deep-sea scuba diving, as pressure changes can stress your body and the bends can induce a miscarriage.
- Flying at altitude in small, nonpressurised aeroplanes or being at more than 3000 metres above sea level. These conditions reduce oxygen to your body.
- Activities that may induce serious injury; for example, skydiving, abseiling, horse riding, water or snow skiing, bungy jumping.

HEALTHY WEIGHT RANGE

Both men and women tend to be less fertile if they are underweight or overweight. Being outside your healthy weight range does not mean you are unable to conceive, but being within it may help you conceive sooner.

Before conception, aim to stabilise your weight into the desired healthy weight range. This is calculated as a body mass index (BMI), estimating your ideal weight in relation to your height.

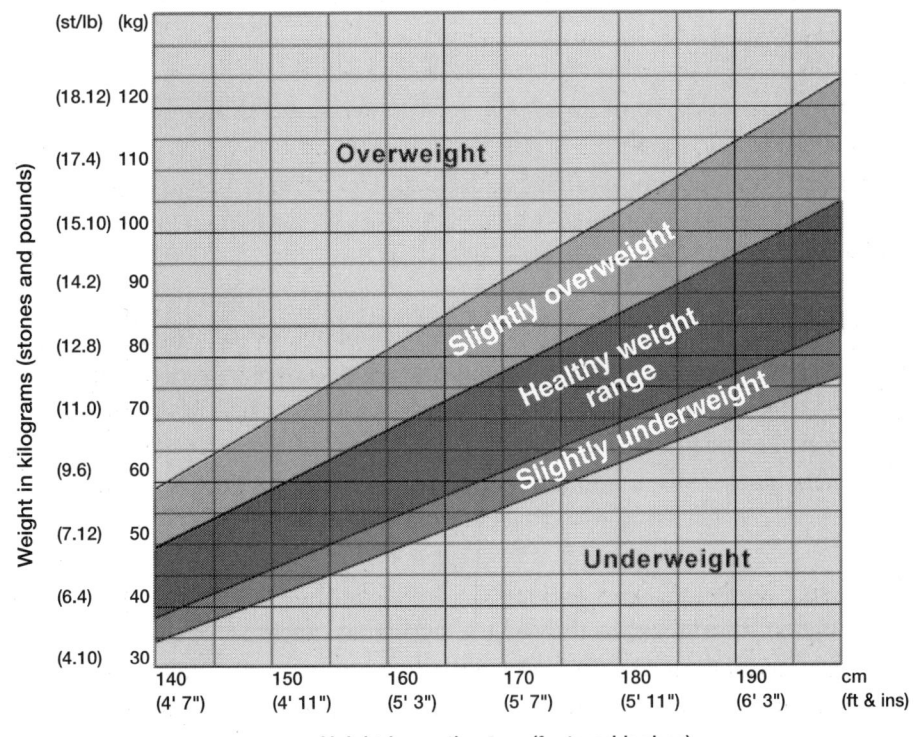

Your caregiver may calculate your BMI by dividing your weight by your height squared. For example, if you are 70 kg and 168 cm tall, this is calculated as:

$$BMI = \frac{70}{(1.68)^2}$$
$$= \frac{70}{2.82}$$
$$= 24.8$$

As a guide, a BMI of:
- Less than 20, means you are underweight for your height.
- 20 to 25, means you are within a healthy weight range.
- More than 25, means you are overweight for your height.

For women, a BMI of between 20 and 27 is thought to be ideal for supporting normal fertility and pregnancy.

Managing stress

It is impossible to rid our lives of stress altogether; however, severe and ongoing stress can negatively affect your health and wellbeing, including your fertility. People who are chronically stressed tend to:
- Eat less well and have less of an appetite.
- Be tired and less enthusiastic about doing enjoyable things in their life.
- Spend less quality time with people close to them and feel less like having sex.
- Suffer from ailments such as headaches, migraines and heartburn.
- Have a lowered immune system and be less able to fight off infections.
- Feel depressed and be unhappy with their lives.

As the spiral continues, the stress increases. Managing stress with caffeine, cigarettes, alcohol and/or recreational drugs is common. You may even feel that stopping these could make you even more stressed; however, learning to manage stress with healthy but enjoyable alternatives can support you during the immense adjustments of pregnancy, labour, birth and early parenting.

Aim to put in place some easy, reliable techniques that allow you to unwind on a daily basis. The first step is making time to relax each day, which may initially take some effort, but even 10 minutes can make a real difference. Some strategies include:
- Going out for dinner, to the movies, away for a day or a weekend. Spending quality time with your partner to nurture your relationship.
- Having a regular massage. Swap one with your partner or a friend if you can't afford to pay for one.

- Having a warm bath.
- Walking or other regular physical activity.
- Stimulating your mind with hobbies or activities outside work.
- Using natural therapies (hypnosis, meditation, homoeopathic or herbal remedies).
- Trying herbal teas such as chamomile, passion flower, valerian, rosehip or dandelion. Add honey or milk to taste.
- Using a quick muscle relaxation exercise. Intentionally tense your neck and shoulder muscles, while taking a breath in; hold for five seconds; release and breathe out, letting your muscles flop or relax. Repeat this three times.
- Using visualisation (see visualisation appendix).

Systematic muscle release techniques can also be very effective. An easy example follows:
- Sit comfortably or lie down.
- Close your eyes (if possible).
- Bring all your attention to your natural breath, breathing in and out rhythmically.
- Starting with your toes and feet, consciously relax them, visualising them being heavy and floppy. Move up to the calves of your legs, then your thighs and so on, until you reach your neck, facial muscles and head.
- Let the heaviness be felt in your relaxed muscles each time you breathe out. Once your whole body is completely relaxed, remain still and feel heavy for a few minutes. Maintain an even, slow, breathing pattern, in and out.
- If you don't fall asleep, slowly give your hands and feet a shake. Wait a moment before getting up.

PRECONCEPTUAL HEALTH CHECK

You may consider seeing a health professional for a physical check-up – as well as advice, information and support – before conceiving your baby, as a couple or separately. This can be performed by your local doctor, family planning centre, women's health nurse, public maternity hospital, fertility clinic or private obstetrician/gynaecologist.

Most preconceptual consultations aim to discuss your general health, assess your fertility and identify any potential problems. They also provide an opportunity for you to ask questions and discuss any concerns, so write down a list of questions to take with you.

Caregivers vary in how much they do at a preconceptual health check, but there are some common components, such as checking your blood pressure and weight; asking about your health history and family's health; noting your age, if you take regular medications, the details of previous operations, injuries or sexually transmitted infections; and discussing your diet, lifestyle habits, stress levels, exercise regimes and occupational hazard exposures.

Women are asked about the details of past pregnancies, their menstrual cycles, past use of contraception and past pap test results, and will probably be recommended to start taking daily folic acid supplements.

Men may be asked their health and medical history and past injuries to the groin area, with the caregiver possibly opting to perform a genital examination if an injury has occurred.

In most cases tests are not required, but some caregivers offer women:
- A blood test for rubella (German measles) immunity. If you are not immune, vaccination may be recommended but you will need to delay conception for one to two months after having this.
- A pap test, if you are due for one.
- A full blood count for haemoglobin levels, which indicate iron deficiencies and anaemia.
- A midstream urine test for infection.
- Blood tests for sexually transmitted viruses (Hepatitis B, C or HIV/AIDS) and/or swabs of the vagina or penis for other sexual infections if it is thought these might be present.

Health conditions

Women with health conditions such as diabetes, high blood pressure, epilepsy, heart or kidney disease, thyroid, blood or mood disorders should see a specialist physician before conceiving a baby. This is in order to plan the management of the condition during pregnancy, as well as to discuss the use of medications, which may need to be slowly reduced, changed or adjusted.

NOTE: *It is important you do not discontinue prescribed medications without first seeking advice from your doctor.*

Genetic counselling

Some couples see a genetic counsellor if they hold concerns about conceiving a child with a genetic disorder. This may be because:
- They are aware, or suspect, they suffer from, or carry, a genetic disorder.
- Their previous baby had a genetic disorder, or a close family member has.

- They have experienced recurrent miscarriages or their previous baby died.
- Their partner is a close family relative (for example, a first cousin).
- They are older (women over 40 and men over 55).
- They feel strongly about seeking the advice of a genetic counsellor before conception.

Genetic counsellors are employed by most large public maternity hospitals or may work in private practice. They generally discuss risk factors and estimate the likely statistical chances of conceiving a baby with a specific health condition, as well as provide information about various conditions and available screening tests. Counsellors offer assistance in the decision-making process and provide resources and local contacts for further information and support.

Conceiving your baby

A healthy, fertile couple have a one in five chance (20%) of becoming pregnant each menstrual cycle. Therefore it is normal to take up to 6 to 12 months to conceive, even with well-timed, unprotected sex. It is generally recommended that couples seek medical advice after trying to conceive for 12 months without success. However, some women in their late thirties (or older) prefer to seek advice sooner (after six to eight months), in order to allow more time to investigate any possible fertility problems.

> **Did you know?**
> A woman's fertility peaks at age 20, then gradually declines, decreasing dramatically after 40 years.

THE FEMALE AND MALE REPRODUCTIVE SYSTEMS

Our reproductive systems are amazing gifts of nature. A man and woman each contribute half the genetic material for conception, which then mixes and shuffles to create a unique baby.

The female reproductive system

A woman's reproductive system produces an egg each month, ready to be fertilised. Once conception occurs, her body provides a nurturing environment to protect, nourish and grow her new baby.

The vagina is a muscular canal, extending upwards and slightly backwards from the vaginal opening to reach the womb. It sits between the bladder (at the front) and rectum (at the back) and is lined with folds of mucous skin that allows it to stretch.

The uterus (or womb) is a hollow, pear-shaped organ, with thick, muscular walls, about the size of a clenched fist. It sits within the pelvic bones and usually leans forward, to rest almost on top of the bladder. However, 20% of women have a retroverted or tipped uterus that leans backwards. This is a normal, individual difference and does not affect conception, pregnancy or birth.

The cervix is the entrance to the uterus (or the neck of the womb), which extends down into the top of the vagina. It is approximately 2.5 cm long, 2 to 3 cm thick, and is firm and closed.

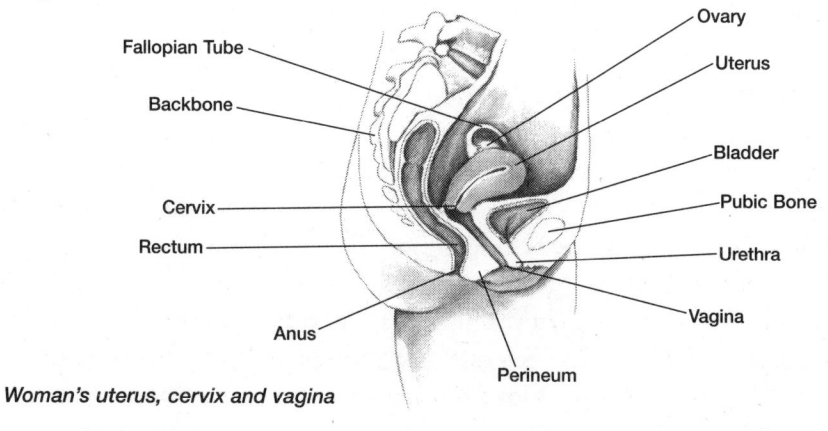

Woman's uterus, cervix and vagina

The endometrium is the inner lining of the uterus, which is shed through menstruation each month, before regenerating and thickening in readiness for a fertilised egg to implant.

The fallopian tubes are two narrow, hollow tubes leading from the top of the uterus each side, spreading outward and downward towards the ovaries, ending in long, finger-like tentacles (or fimbria). These gently sweep the ovary to draw a mature egg inside the fallopian tube each month. The egg is transported to the uterus by small, hair-like structures lining the tubes (called cilia). It is in the fallopian tube that a man's sperm meets the egg and fertilisation occurs.

The ovaries are two white almond-shaped organs positioned each side of the uterus, under the end of each fallopian tube. They store thousands of eggs, of which 300 to 500 mature during a woman's lifetime. Each month around 20 eggs ripen, but only one dominates to maturity, before being released into the fallopian tube. This process is called ovulation. The left ovary releases one month, then the right ovary releases the next month, and so on. If both ovaries release an egg in the same month, the woman may conceive twins.

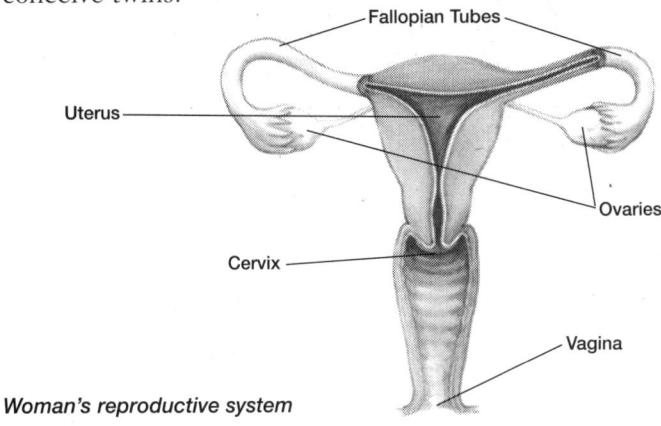

Woman's reproductive system

The male reproductive system

A man produces millions of sperm, but only one successfully fertilises an egg at conception. Each sperm determines the sex of a child, with half carrying the female gene (X chromosome) and half carrying the male gene (Y chromosome).

The penis is formed from three cylindrical columns of spongy erectile tissue filled with thousands of small spaces. When the man is sexually aroused, blood fills the spaces in the penis making it erect for sexual intercourse, enabling semen to be deposited into the woman's vagina when the man ejaculates.

The testes are a pair of oval organs within the scrotal sac. Immature sperm are manufactured here, before moving to the epididymis, a small organ on top of each teste, for storage and nourishment to create mature spermatozoa. This process takes about 70 days. If sperm are not ejaculated, they break down and are reabsorbed by the man's body. The scrotum (or sac) holds the testes away from the man's groin, at 2 to 3°C below body temperature. It naturally relaxes in hot weather and contracts in cold weather, to regulate the ideal temperature for sperm production.

> **Did you know?**
> Approximately 300 million sperm are produced in the testes each day, from the time a boy starts puberty and for the rest of his life, although the quality and quantity of healthy sperm decrease as the man passes 40 years.

The vas deferens tubes run upwards from the epididymis into the man's pelvic area. During ejaculation, rapid waves of contractions push sperm up into the seminal vesicles, two pouches behind the man's prostate gland. These secrete a sticky fluid containing glucose, prostaglandins and anti-infective agents, which mix with the spermatozoa to make 60% of semen. Two pea-sized structures behind the prostate (called Cowper's glands) secrete a clear mucus that drains into the man's urethra before ejaculation, acting as a lubricant for sexual intercourse.

The prostate gland is about 3 cm wide and sits at the base of the man's bladder, surrounding the urethra. During sexual arousal it produces a thin, milky fluid containing calcium and enzymes, which mix with the spermatozoa and other fluids to form the semen that is eiaculated during intercourse.

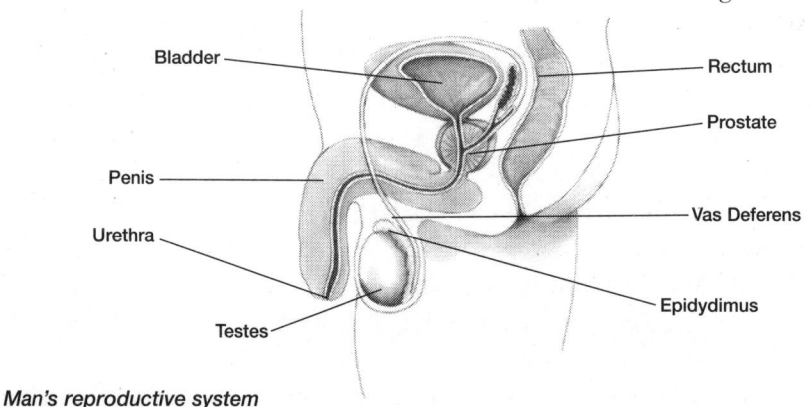

Man's reproductive system

Did you know?
One ejaculation is about 3 to 6 ml and contains 60 to 200 million sperm. About 60 to 80% of these sperm are capable of fertilising an egg, but 50% lose their motility (movement) after 1 hour at the woman's body temperature. Only one sperm is needed to conceive a baby!

A WOMAN'S MENSTRUAL CYCLE

Girls become fertile when their period commences (called menarche). From menarche till menopause, women have the potential to bear children. The average menstrual cycle is 28 days (ranging from 20 to 40 days) and patterns can change over a lifetime. Changes may also be noticed when you stop hormonal contraception, or after having a baby.

NOTE: *To work out your menstrual cycle length, start counting from the first day of your period (or bleeding) until the first day of your next period.*

Menstrual cycles can be temporarily disrupted, delayed or missed altogether (called amenorrhoea) through factors such as:
- Being unwell.
- Not eating properly, and losing or gaining excessive weight.

- Excessive exercise.
- Travelling and experiencing time differences and climate changes.
- Extreme emotional stress.
- Being pregnant (of course) and breastfeeding.
- Hormonal contraception, such as the minipill or Implanon.

If you do miss a period, it is important to see your doctor to rule out other possible health problems and/or have a pregnancy test.

Charting your fertility

A baby is conceived during the fertile days of a woman's menstrual cycle. It is possible to observe various physical and emotional changes in your body to estimate when ovulation is likely to occur. Keeping a daily record, or charting your cycle, can create a greater awareness of your fertility so intercourse can be timed effectively.

Charting can also be handy if conception proves difficult. Having three to six months of menstrual cycle patterns can greatly assist caregivers to determine possible reasons for infertility.

NOTE: If you want to chart your cycle before trying to conceive, you need to use non-medicated forms of contraceptives (condoms, diaphragm, intrauterine device), as hormonal contraception (the pill, minipill, progesterone injections or implants) overrides your body's natural menstrual cycle with 'pretend' periods (or no periods) and no fertile days.

The following is a guide to the physical signs and how to chart your fertility.

Temperature

Soon after ovulation your temperature rises slightly and stays elevated for at least 10 days. This cannot predict ovulation but confirms it has happened, giving you an idea of when it occurs in relation to the rest of your cycle. You take your Basal Body Temperature, or temperature on waking, first thing in the morning. To record this accurately:

- Use a thermometer that measures small temperature changes (10 levels between each degree; eg. 37.1 to 37.9°C). Mercury thermometers need to be left in place for at least three minutes. Follow the manufacturer's instructions for electronic thermometers. Don't change thermometers in the middle of a cycle, wait until the next cycle starts.
- Take your temperature as soon as you wake and before getting out of bed, after at least three hours sleep and before eating, drinking or smoking.

You can take your temperature orally (under the tongue) or vaginally. But if you

Fertility chart

DATE:

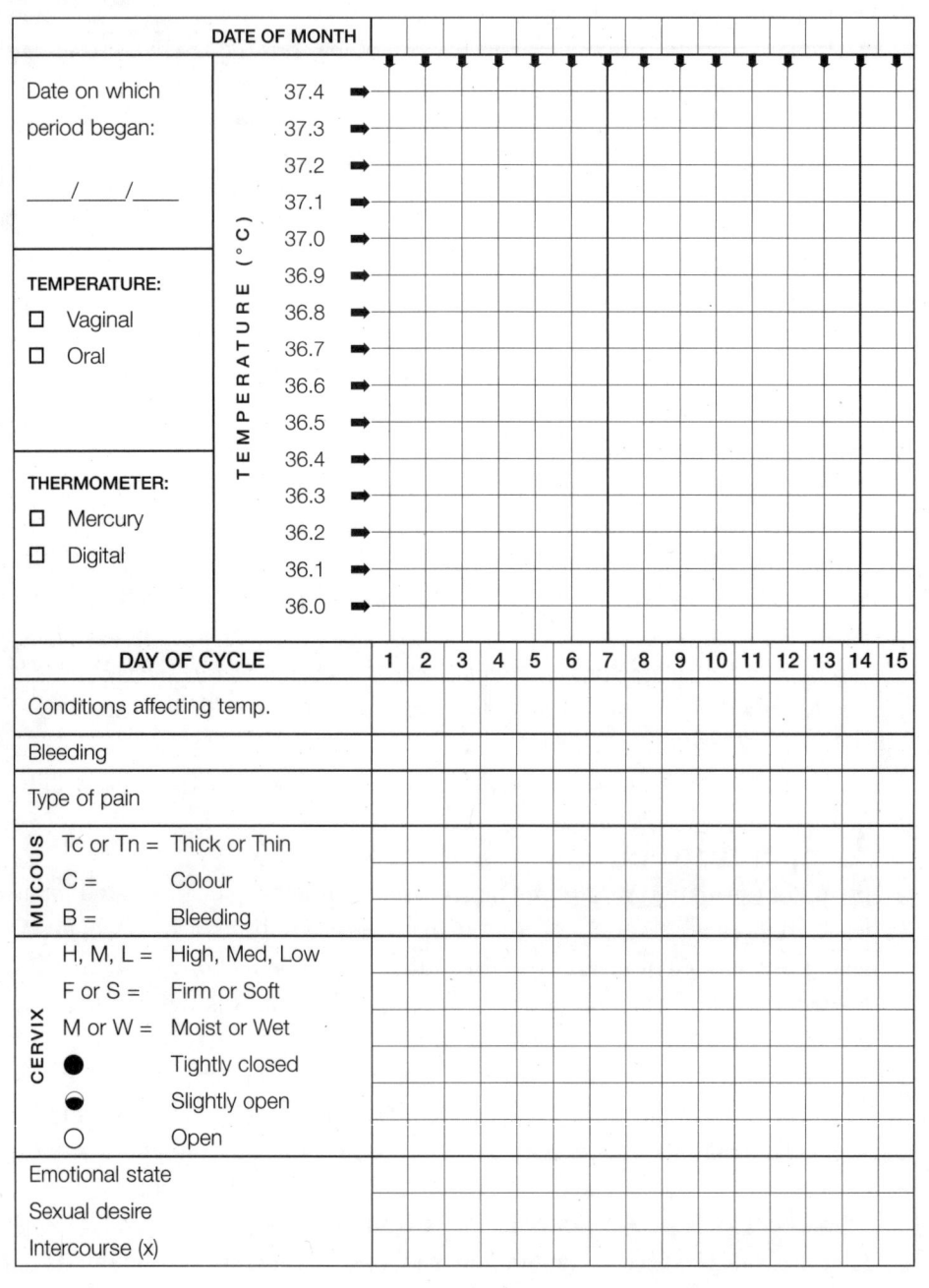

	DATE OF MONTH															
Date on which period began: ___/___/___	37.4															
	37.3															
	37.2															
	37.1															
	37.0															
TEMPERATURE: ☐ Vaginal ☐ Oral	36.9															
	36.8															
	36.7															
	36.6															
	36.5															
	36.4															
THERMOMETER: ☐ Mercury ☐ Digital	36.3															
	36.2															
	36.1															
	36.0															

TEMPERATURE (°C)

DAY OF CYCLE	1	2	3	4	5	6	7	8	9	10	11	12	13	14	15
Conditions affecting temp.															
Bleeding															
Type of pain															
MUCOUS Tc or Tn = Thick or Thin															
C = Colour															
B = Bleeding															
CERVIX H, M, L = High, Med, Low															
F or S = Firm or Soft															
M or W = Moist or Wet															
● Tightly closed															
◐ Slightly open															
○ Open															
Emotional state															
Sexual desire															
Intercourse (x)															

PREPARING TO CONCEIVE YOUR BABY 35

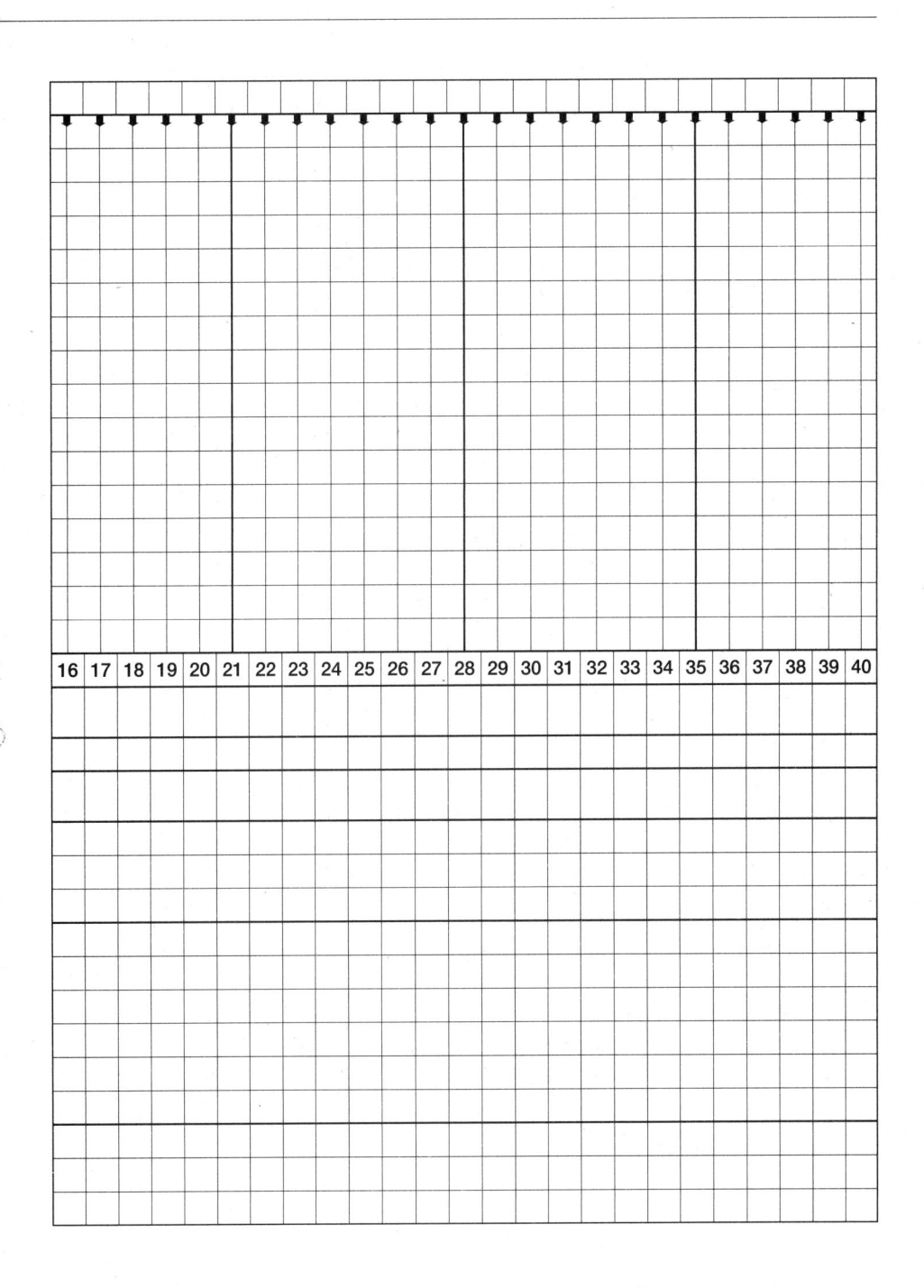

| 16 | 17 | 18 | 19 | 20 | 21 | 22 | 23 | 24 | 25 | 26 | 27 | 28 | 29 | 30 | 31 | 32 | 33 | 34 | 35 | 36 | 37 | 38 | 39 | 40 |

start using one method, continue taking it this way for the rest of the cycle (vaginal temperatures are always a little higher). Record your temperature on your fertility chart by drawing a small dot at the temperature level on the relevant day. Then connect the dots from day to day to show the month's pattern. Be aware that your temperature can be unusually high or low if you are:
- Unwell and have a fever.
- Travelling, with climate and time changes.
- Feeling unusually stressed.
- Doing shift work.
- Having interrupted sleep.

The odd high or low reading is okay. Just make a note in the 'conditions affecting temp.' column. Usually, an average of four consecutive temperatures is indicative of what is happening. Be patient. It may take a few menstrual cycles before a typical pattern is visible and ovulation can be estimated fairly accurately.

Vaginal mucus

The cervix normally produces different types of mucus throughout a menstrual cycle. Monitoring these changes can be helpful in predicting ovulation, especially if you have irregular periods. You need to observe:
- Colour (whitish, yellowish, cloudy, clear, bloodstained).
- How it feels (pasty, thick, tacky, sticky or flaky and crumbly or thin, wet and slippery, like raw egg white).
- The amount.

Check your mucus each day, when not menstruating, by placing your fingers at the opening of your vagina, or looking for it on your underwear or toilet paper. Try checking at around the same time each day (ideally afternoons or early evenings, prior to sex), as it can change over the course of a day. If you don't produce much mucus, try doing a series of pelvic floor exercises before checking, or perhaps placing a finger inside your vagina to touch your cervix. Record your findings on the fertility chart.

NOTE: Semen can remain in the vagina for 24 hours after sex, making vaginal mucus hard to identify. It may be useful to use condoms for one or more menstrual cycles to help read your vaginal mucus more accurately. Also, vaginal infections (such as thrush) can make your vaginal discharge more difficult to interpret. Make a note of these on your chart as appropriate.

Feeling your cervix

Feeling your cervix each day, when not bleeding, is an additional observation to help detect ovulation, particularly for women who don't experience obvious mucus changes, or only have small amounts. However, if you feel uncomfortable about checking your cervix, it is not absolutely necessary.

If you have never felt your cervix before, it may take a little practice. As a guide:
- First wash and dry your hands.
- Get into a comfortable position to help you to relax (sitting on the toilet, standing with one leg up on the bath, kneeling or squatting, lying down).
- Gently insert one or two fingers into your vagina. Slowly move them upwards and slightly backwards (towards your tailbone), until you reach a smooth bump. This is your cervix. It usually feels similar to the tip of your nose. The actual opening to the womb can feel like a small dimple, or be large enough to surround your fingertip.

The cervix gradually changes during the menstrual cycle, but it may take a while to notice this. Compare daily features, noting whether the cervix feels:
- Lower or higher.
- Firmer or softer.
- More open or closed.
- Slightly moist or wetter.

Write these down on your chart.

Detecting the fertile days

Day 1 of your cycle is the first day of your period. Once bleeding finishes, you can observe your temperature, vaginal mucus and perhaps cervix changes, to work out when you are most fertile.

The fertility cycle

Cycle phase

Bleeding phase – The start of the period is Day 1 of your menstrual cycle. Bleeding lasts from 2 to 8 days (usually 4 to 6 days). Oestrogen and progesterone are at their lowest levels now. If you conceive a baby later this cycle, Day 1 of your period is used to calculate your baby's due date, even though conception does not occur until about 2 weeks later.

Physical changes

Temperature – There is no need to take your temperature during the bleeding phase.

Vaginal mucus – Just record your bleeding on your fertility chart by putting a 'B' in the mucus column.

Cervix – There is no need to feel your cervix during this time.

Emotions/sexual desire – Some women feel anxious, irritable and/or short-tempered. You

Bleeding phase (cont.)

may be feeling upset, disappointed or depressed if you wanted to conceive but this has not happened.

Pre-fertile phase – After the bleeding stops, there is usually a few days (to a week or more) before the fertile phase begins. The lining of the uterus starts to thicken and a group of eggs in one ovary starts to ripen. Both oestrogen and progesterone remain low. *NOTE: If you have a shorter menstrual cycle (21 to 26 days), you may not have a pre-fertile phase, being fertile as soon as your period finishes.*

Temperature – Your daily temperature should be fairly stable, somewhere around 36.5 to 36.7°C.

Vaginal mucus – Most women feel dry, with no noticeable vaginal mucus. There may be small amounts of thick, whitish, flaky or crumbly mucus, or possibly thick, sticky, tacky, cloudy white or yellowish mucus, which feels very pasty.

Cervix – Your cervix should feel relatively low, firm and only slightly moist (or even dryish) and tightly closed (compared to other times in the menstrual cycle).

Emotions/sexual desire – This phase may bring feelings of relief and wellbeing, because the period has now finished.

Fertile phase – This is the time you can conceive (or become pregnant). One egg outperforms the others and matures as it prepares to be released from the ovary. Oestrogen levels start to rise, peaking to its highest level just before ovulation (progesterone remains low). The uterus and cervix produce a special fertile mucus, capable of protecting the man's sperm and helping transport it into the woman's fallopian tubes to fertilise the egg. The woman releases a surge of lutenising hormone about 30 hours prior to ovulation.

Temperature – Your temperature should remain fairly stable, somewhere around 36.5 to 36.7°C. Some women notice a small drop in their temperature of about 0.2 to 0.3°C, 12 to 24 hours before they ovulate. However, this is not essential.

Vaginal mucus – Vaginal mucus usually increases, making you feel damp or wet. It may look cloudy or clear and colourless. It is usually thinner and more runny in consistency (when compared to the previous days). *NOTE: Not all women produce large amounts of mucus during their fertile phase. You may need to feel your cervix to detect it. If you don't notice fertile mucus, this does not mean you are less fertile or unable to conceive, it is just that your mucus stays well contained within your cervix and uterus.*

Cervix – The cervix should feel higher, softer, wetter and slightly more open.

Emotions/sexual desire – Many women notice an increase in their libido and naturally feel more like having sex when they are fertile. Some women experience a pain on one side of their lower abdomen or back, called Mittelschmerz (meaning 'middle pain') about 24 to 48 hours before they ovulate.

Ovulation – A mature egg is released from one ovary into the adjacent fallopian tube, surviving for around 12 to 24 hours.

Temperature – Your temperature starts to rise just before, during or after the egg is released, usually by about 0.2 to 0.4°C. It should stay elevated until just before your next period begins (10 to 14 days after ovulation). If your temperature does not stay elevated for at least 10 days, you may not have ovulated.

Vaginal mucus – Vaginal mucus remains clear (or slightly cloudy), slippery and wet just prior to (and during) ovulation. There is usually more of it, closely resembling egg white, being stretchy and see-through or perhaps pinkish or a bloodstained tinge (from releasing the egg). If you put this mucus between your fingers and then move your fingers slowly apart, it often stretches up to 5 to 10 centimetres. Again, not all women produce large amounts of mucus like this.

Cervix – The cervix is at its highest point and may even be difficult to reach. It should feel very wet, soft and open.

Emotions/sexual desire – A woman's sex drive is at its highest level during ovulation, although some women experience slight nausea.

Post-fertile phase – From ovulation until the next period starts, lasting 14 days (ranging from 12 to 16 days). Also called the luteal phase, as a capsule is left in the ovary where the egg was released (*corpus luteum*), which produces progesterone to thicken the lining of the uterus. A small cyst forms on the ovary (usually disappearing by 16 weeks of pregnancy, if pregnant). This is also called the secretory phase, as the lining of the uterus secretes glucose to nourish the developing baby before full implantation. Progesterone rises to its highest level, dropping to trigger a period to start. But if you have conceived, progesterone continues to rise. Oestrogen drops dramatically after ovulation, but slowly rises until the period starts (or continues to rise if you are pregnant). The last day of the post-fertile phase is the last day of the menstrual cycle.

Temperature – Your temperature should stay elevated for at least 10 days after ovulation, or stay elevated until the period begins. If your temperature continues to be elevated past the time your period was due (14 to 16 days), you are probably pregnant.

Vaginal mucus – Vaginal mucus decreases, feeling dry again, and changes to small amounts of thick, white, flaky, crumbly or sticky, tacky, cloudy, yellowish mucus until the bleeding begins (or you may not notice any mucus at all).

Cervix – The cervix should feel lower, firmer, only slightly moist or even dry, and tightly closed again. Similar to the pre-fertile phase.

Emotions/sexual desire – The few days after ovulation may see a decrease in sexual desire. As the period draws closer, premenstrual symptoms may be noticed (nausea, breast tenderness, bloating, skin changes, headaches and emotional mood swings), which may be confused with early pregnancy symptoms. The 'two week wait' after ovulating can be an agonising one when trying to conceive.

Did you know?
A recent Canadian study observed the ovaries of 63 healthy women not on fertility treatments. In six cases, an egg was released twice in one cycle, which was previously thought to be impossible. 'Waves' of maturing and regressing eggs happened two to three times before ovulation. Occasionally a pre-ovulation wave ended with a mature egg being released, as well as another at normal ovulation.[5]

Ovulation prediction kits

Ovulation prediction kits (OPK) work by testing saliva or urine to alert you to the fact you may be fertile. Care needs to be taken to use them effectively, and they are not meant to completely replace the other methods discussed above.

Saliva tests detect an oestrogen rise, two to four days before ovulation, which makes saliva more salty. Saliva is placed on a glass slide each day to dry. When you are fertile, it should crystallise in a fern-like pattern (when viewed under a microscope). However, sometimes 'ferning' happens at other times in the cycle. Saliva OPKs are an expensive outlay, but reusable over several months.

Urine tests detect the lutenising hormone (LH) surge, about 20 to 44 hours (average 30 hours) before ovulation. It takes 8 to 12 hours for LH to filter from the bloodstream to the urine (to test positive), and testing between 11 am and 3 pm tends to be most accurate, with ovulation occurring about 24 hours later.

Urine OPKs are expensive and may be used only once; a kit usually contains five to nine tests, depending on the brand. If your cycle is longer or shorter than 28 days, you may need two kits. They are about 90% effective, if the manufacturer's directions are followed. However, factors that make them inaccurate include:
- The urine not being concentrated enough. Don't drink fluids for two hours before the test.
- Testing starting too late with a short menstrual cycle (less than 26 days), or testing stopped too early with a longer cycle (35 days or more).
- Exposing the kit to extreme heat or cold.
- The kit is past its use-by date.
- Ovulation not occurring during that menstrual cycle.
- Having hyperthyroidism, ovarian cysts or approaching menopause (often giving false positive results).
- Taking fertility drugs (Pergonal, Danazol and Metrodin). Clomid (Serophene) does not affect LH urine tests.

Timing sex for conception
Once you observe, and perhaps chart, your physical signs, you can estimate when ovulation occurs to plan some well-timed sex to conceive your baby. As a guide:
- A man's sperm can survive for up to six days in a woman's fertile mucus before she ovulates, but one to three days is more likely.
- The woman's egg only survives for 12 to 24 hours after ovulation.
- A woman's most fertile time is thought to be one to three days (but up to five days) before she ovulates and within 12 to 24 hours after ovulation. As ovulation commonly occurs between 4 pm and 7 pm, it's helpful to time sex the day before this, so sperm are already present in the fallopian tubes (lying in wait, so to speak).

Counting the days
If your menstrual cycle is fairly regular, then counting the days can help you estimate when you are fertile. As a general rule, ovulation occurs around 12 to 16 days *before* your next period is due.
- **28 day cycle** – Ovulate days 12 to 16; most fertile days 6 to 17, but more likely days 9 to 15.
- **26 day cycle** – Ovulate days 10 to 14; most fertile days 4 to 15, but more likely days 7 to 13.
- **35 day cycle** – Ovulate days 19 to 23; most fertile days 13 to 24, but more likely days 16 to 22.

This is only a rough estimate, so combine it with observing other physical signs; otherwise, if your menstrual cycle is longer or shorter than expected, you will not know for sure when you ovulated until your period arrives.

Helpful hints
Other things that may increase your chances of conceiving sooner include:
- The man abstaining from ejaculation for two or three days beforehand, to increase his sperm count; or have sex every second day during the fertile phase.
- Not using artificial lubricants (or having sex in water).
- The woman experiencing orgasm before, or at the same time as, the man ejaculates.
- Deep penetration of the penis into the vagina. This can be achieved by the man's penis entering the woman's vagina from behind her.
- Leaving the penis in the vagina after ejaculation (until the penis is soft).
- The woman remaining in bed for 20 to 30 minutes after intercourse.

Some women place a pillow under their buttocks to elevate their hips slightly.

Emotional considerations

The decision to have a baby can bring much excitement and enthusiasm. Ceasing contraception can feel liberating and the sexual act may take on a new and intimate meaning. However, timing conception to fit in with your plans is not always easy.

If neither of you have ever achieved a pregnancy before, you may approach the process with an open mind, perhaps expecting it to take a while, only to be shocked (or pleasantly surprised) if you are pregnant in the first month. If you have previously conceived on your first attempt or by accident, you may feel disappointed or frustrated if it takes a while.

When attempts to become pregnant continue for several months, it is common to question your and your partner's ability to conceive. The longer this takes, the more likely there will be feelings of depression, guilt, anger, anxiety, distress, blame and resentment, which can be destructive to your relationship. Sex can become a timed chore, with pressure to perform on cue, removing spontaneity from what should be a pleasurable and loving activity.

It is important to keep an open mind and accept that conception can't be controlled. Some strategies to help you deal with your feelings include:

- Communicating openly with each other, rather than leaving things unsaid. Perhaps seek professional counselling if you are finding communication difficult.
- Trying to have impromptu sex at other times of the menstrual cycle. Remember, your sexual relationship is more than just for procreation.
- Not trying to conceive for a month (or longer) to take the pressure off for a while.
- Making lifestyle changes together (diet, stopping smoking, exercising) to reinforce your commitment to working towards your pregnancy as a couple.
- Using natural therapies to enhance your health and wellbeing, such as massage, acupuncture, herbs or homeopathy. Try visualisations or hypnotherapy for relaxation.

Did you know?
Women who take the pill for more than six months and conceive the month after stopping have double the chance of having twins![6]

When conception is not straightforward

Various circumstances, such as stopping contraception and breastfeeding, can make conceiving a baby less straightforward (discussed further in Chapter 14). If you are having very irregular periods, see your local doctor for advice.

If you have experienced a miscarriage or stillbirth, it is normal to have an instinctive urge to conceive again soon. This may be an emotional response to grieving, or a personal decision that just feels right. Information on miscarriage can be found in Chapter 2, and stillbirth is dealt with in Chapter 7.

If you would like to conceive another baby soon, your fertility should return within two to six weeks after a miscarriage (less than 20 weeks gestation) and up to 4 to 10 weeks after giving birth (later than 20 weeks). Be aware that you will ovulate before your next period is due. So you may conceive before getting a period. Some caregivers recommend delaying another pregnancy for one or several months, especially if you were unwell or lost a lot of blood (and are possibly anaemic). Discuss this with your caregiver and consider how you feel about this.

Choosing the sex of your baby

The notion of being able to control the sex of a baby has fascinated the human race for centuries. It was originally thought that the woman's body determined the baby's sex, but we now know it is the man's sperm that decides the gender of a child.

> **Did you know?**
> Hippocrates thought the man's right testicle produced boys and his left produced girls, leading men to tie string around one testicle during sex to prevent the 'undesired' sperm leaving their body. During the eighteenth century some aristocrats asked doctors to remove their left testicle to ensure a male heir!

Choosing the sex of your baby is a hot, ethical debate in many societies, but in western countries it tends to be linked with wanting to create gender balance in the family. However, concerns centre on 'unsuccessful' couples experiencing anger, depression, guilt, relationship difficulties or rejecting their new child because they are the 'wrong' gender. The bottom line is, you need to want to have a baby, whether a boy or a girl, and be fully prepared if your baby is not the sex you desire.

Fertility clinics sometimes facilitate sex selection for couples carrying debilitating sex-linked genetic disorders (such as haemophilia or muscular dystrophy). However, the process is complex and expensive. The woman's eggs are harvested and fertilised using in-vitro fertilisation, then female or male embryos are selected before placing them into the woman's uterus.

There are many sex-selection methods promoted by books and commercial fertility clinics. However, no technique currently offered is supported by research, and the few available studies are conflicting. What's more, medical approaches involve artificial insemination, which reduce the chances of conceiving a baby at all, let alone one of the sex you desire. This often leads parents to be disappointed, at great financial and emotional expense.

Natural conception creates 49% girls and 51% boys in any given population. Sceptics of sex selection methods suggest that parents already have about a 50% chance of 'succeeding', making it hard to know the real chances of a method actually working.

The most common natural theory followed by couples is the Shettles method, which is based on timing sexual intercourse. The 'boy method' advocates having sex close to ovulation and abstaining from sex for several days beforehand, and the 'girl method' recommends timing sex for the two to four days before ovulation, then abstaining until a few days after ovulation. Shettles claims an 80% success rate for boys and a 75% success rate for girls.[7]

Difficulty conceiving

People take it for granted that part of their lives will be devoted to raising children, if that is their choice. However, having a child is not always straightforward, and as months of trying to conceive pass, hopes can turn into despair every time the woman's period arrives. About 60% of couples conceive within 6 months of trying, and a further 25% by 12 months, but around 10 to 15% do not conceive naturally, with a small percentage of these couples achieving a pregnancy through fertility treatments.

The medical definition of infertility is not conceiving after 12 months of unprotected intercourse during the woman's fertile phase each month. Primary infertility refers to difficulty conceiving when you have never had a child, and secondary infertility refers to difficulty conceiving after having had previous children, or conceiving but continually miscarrying.

CAUSES OF INFERTILITY

Physical causes for infertility can be identified in up to 80% of couples; about 40% are related to the man, and 40% related to the woman. The

remaining 20% are due to both, or the infertility is regarded as unexplained. A healthy woman's fertility is also governed by her age. As a guide, fertility problems are approximately:
- 3% for women aged 20 to 24 years.
- 5% for women aged 25 to 29 years.
- 8% for women aged 30 to 34 years.
- 15% for women aged 35 to 39 years.
- 32% for women aged 40 to 44 years.
- 69% for women aged 45 to 49 years.

Success rates of medical fertility treatments also declines as the woman's age increases, being about 80% for women under 35 years, 74% for women between 35 and 39 years and 60% for women aged 40 years and over[8].

Female factors

Infertility in women (or recurrent miscarriages) can relate to:
- Hormonal imbalances, irregular periods, disorders of ovulation or early menopause.
- Blocked or scarred fallopian tubes, possibly due to a past sexually transmitted infection or an ectopic pregnancy.
- Endometriosis, when parts of the lining of the uterus grow in other places around the woman's reproductive organs.
- Polycystic ovarian syndrome (PCOS), when cysts form on the ovaries, affecting the woman's hormonal balance. Eggs often mature but are not released.
- The woman's fertile mucus producing antibodies against the man's sperm.
- Environmental exposures to toxins, chemicals, pesticides, gases, radiation, some drugs and smoking.
- Health conditions, such as diabetes, hypothyroidism, auto-immune, genetic or inherited disorders.

Male factors

Infertility in men normally relates to their semen production, affecting the number, shape and motility of their sperm. Factors affecting semen production include:
- Environmental exposures to toxins, chemicals, pesticides, radiation, heavy metals (lead, mercury), some drugs, excessive heat and smoking.
- Sexually transmitted infections or mumps contracted as an adolescent or adult.
- Health disorders that cause hormonal imbalances (diabetes, hypothyroidism, antibody, auto-immune, genetic or inherited disorders).

- Undescended testes into teenage years.
- Blockage of the vas deferens due to injury or vasectomy.
- Inefficient ejaculation, possibly due to a health condition or disability.

INVESTIGATING INFERTILITY

There are many tests available to help determine medical causes of infertility. A referral to a fertility specialist or clinic can be obtained from your local doctor or family planning clinic. Both partners should attend the first consultation. Take any previously performed tests or ultrasound results and menstrual cycle charts.

The initial visit usually involves being asked many personal questions about your health and medical history (similar to a preconceptual health check), as well as the frequency and timing of sexual intercourse in relation to the woman's menstrual cycle. The specialist may physically examine one or both partners and perhaps offer tests, depending on individual circumstances. Often the woman is asked to chart her cycle for a few months, if she hasn't already done this. Sometimes no obvious problem can be detected.

Tests can include:
- Semen analysis to look at the number (normally 20 million per millilitre), how well they move (motility) and correct shape (morphology).
- Blood tests for both partners to investigate their general health and hormone levels.
- An ultrasound of each partner's reproductive organs.
- Sperm and mucus test, in which a sample of the man's sperm and the woman's fertile mucus are placed together on a slide under a microscope to observe how they react with each other.

TREATMENT OPTIONS

Treatments for infertility are complex and varied and will usually depend on the diagnosis. If considering medical treatments, it is very important you obtain as much information as possible about the various approaches being offered – how likely they are to succeed, their cost and the possible side effects. Be aware that the success rates of achieving a viable pregnancy (one that ends in the birth of a baby), and the possibility of a multiple birth, varies considerably between different clinics. Only about 10 to 20% of couples actually require assisted conception (eg. IVF), but these have relatively low success rates (usually less than 20%).

Fertility treatments can be time-consuming, inconvenient and expensive. They may cause undesirable side effects and in some cases lead to long-term health consequences. They can also place incredible strain on a couple's relationship and life. All these things need to be weighed up. Most fertility clinics have counsellors and social workers to help support couples making decisions about the treatments they will accept and how long they are willing to continue. However, this information and advice can be very biased towards what the clinic offers. So it may be worthwhile to do some independent research, and possibly contact other couples through infertility support groups.

A natural approach

Natural fertility specialists use a holistic approach to work on both an emotional and physical level, involving diet, exercise, lifestyle, stress management, vitamins and mineral supplements and perhaps herbs, acupuncture, homeopathy and so on. These specialists are often used as a first step, prior to medical treatments (or combined with them), or as an alternative if infertility is unexplained. Bear in mind, these treatments may not work if either of you have significant reproductive health problems.

Emotional considerations

Infertility is a major life crisis, which can be amplified by the inconvenience and stress of fertility treatment. It can also be emotionally isolating, with many women finding it increasingly difficult to be around pregnant women, parents or attend family gatherings. Others often judge and give advice, telling couples to relax or have a holiday. However, there is no research to support that emotional factors cause infertility, making these comments hurtful and confusing.

Coming to terms with not having children usually means acknowledging and accepting an enormous loss. However, because it is an ongoing situation, often accompanied by continuous glimmers of hope, there is no significant event (such as a miscarriage) to mark the grief, yet it is very real and traumatic. For some people there is never a feeling of acceptance or closure; for others there is a growing sense of being free to move on, to make the best of life and their relationships without a child. Occasionally, adopting a child becomes the next step. However, couples who do conceive as planned are faced with an entirely different journey over the next nine months, as they approach impending parenthood.

CHAPTER 2

A new pregnancy: conception to 12 weeks

The journey of life starts well before birth, entailing an amazing, intricate sequence of growth and development within the life-giving environment of a woman's uterus. From conception to 12 weeks, called the first trimester, a truly magnificent feat of biology takes place to create a new person. By the start of the thirteenth week, most of your baby's organs are formed, or well on the way.

Your unborn baby's growth and development

This week-by-week guide shows how your baby is developing. Bear in mind, this can vary, depending on your menstrual cycle and when sperm and egg met.

Week 3 – Two weeks before the next period is due. Your baby is two microscopic cells becoming one!

Within 24 hours after ovulation, the woman's egg is fertilised by a single sperm in her fallopian tube, making a conceptus. Within hours, the conceptus splits into two identical cells, then these two cells split into four cells, and so on. By four days after conception, 16 to 20 cells form a ball shape called a morula. By the fifth day, these cells group on one side of the morula, leaving a sac of fluid (which the baby will float in) on the other side. The group of cells start to change (or differentiate) in preparation for performing their individual functions, each destined to become a different part of the baby's body (as well as the placenta). By day six, the morula becomes a blastocyst and leaves the fallopian tube to enter the uterus, where it implants in its thick lining. It is now one week before the woman's next period would have been due.

Week 4 – The beginning of week 4, or 7 to 13 days after conception. Your baby is now called a blastocyst and is like a ball, about 4 mm in width.

The blastocyst fully implants into the lining of the uterus, taking about six days to complete (finishing 12 days after fertilisation). The baby now taps into their mother's blood supply, as their cells continue to multiply and differentiate to create a flat disc with three distinct layers: 1. **the endoderm** forms their internal organs (lungs, liver, bowel and bladder); 2. **the mesoderm** forms their skull, bones, sex organs, muscles and heart; 3. **the ectoderm** forms their skin, hair, eyes, ears, brain and spinal cord. At the same time, the outside of the blastocyst divides onto two layers, one forming the beginnings of the placenta, and the second forming the amniotic sac, which slowly fills with amniotic fluid.

Week 5 – 14 to 21 days after conception, when your next period would have been due (and is now late!). Your baby is now called an embryo, measuring about 1.5 mm.

On day 18 after conception, the neural tube begins to form along the baby's back (which will house their spinal cord). The top end of the tube balloons out and enlarges to form the beginnings of the baby's brain (although quite primitive at this point). At the same time, the endoderm (or bottom layer of cells) balloons out in front of the baby at chest level, to form a yolk sac. A body stalk protrudes from their waistline to make the beginnings of an umbilical cord. In the meantime, the yolk sac supplies nourishment, before eventually being reabsorbed into the baby's body to form their bowel, liver, lungs and bladder. It also starts the manufacture of the baby's own blood supply.

Week 6 – 21 to 28 days after conception, your period is one week late. Your baby is curled in the shape of the letter C (looking like a tadpole). This makes it difficult to measure them from head to toe, so they are measured from the top of their head to the base of the back (crown to rump length or CRL), around 2 to 4 mm. Your baby's heart develops and begins beating, around 24 days after conception. At this stage, the heart is simply a long tube, rhythmically expanding and contracting. Their bloodstream starts to develop, being completely separate from their mother's, often with a different blood type. Their neural tube closes over at the top (over their brain) and over the base of their spinal cord, and small hand and feet buds start sprouting from their upper and lower body. The body stalk from their belly elongates and starts to form two arteries and one vein inside, creating the umbilical cord. This transports oxygen and nutrients from mother to baby and takes away carbon dioxide and waste products from baby to mother. Philosophers and scientists in early times believed the moment the baby's heart began beating was the time the 'spark of life' and spirit entered their body.

Week 7 – 28 to 35 days after conception, your period is two weeks late. Your baby's crown to rump length is about 5 mm.

Their facial features gradually build up around a wide mouth, with their lower jaw forming first, shortly followed by their upper jaw. Their head and forehead are comparatively large, as their brain forms within and eyes start bulging on each side of their head. Their limbs begin to lengthen, firstly their arms, then their legs, with hands and feet resembling ridged paddles. Internal organs are taking shape – their gullet (oesophagus), stomach, kidneys and bowel are being defined, as well as two small buds which will form lungs. Their heart is forming chambers and is beating away efficiently, up to 200 beats per minute.

Week 8 – 35 to 42 days after conception. Your baby has more than doubled in size and is just over 1 cm long.

Each eye now has an optic cup, retina and lens and they move from the side of the baby's head to the front. Your baby's nasal pits are now present, which will extend to become nostrils, and their inner ears and tongue start to form. Their upper jaw and palate come together, fusing as one and their 'tadpole' tail recedes, as their body becomes slightly straighter. Their pancreas, appendix and the beginnings of their reproductive organs are now present, although not distinctly male or female yet. By the end of this week, a fine, transparent layer of skin covers their body. And although their fingers are still webbed, they have distinct fingers and thumbs.

Week 9 – 42 to 49 days after conception, the time your second period would have been due. Your baby has grown to measure 1.5 cm and their head makes up 25% of their entire body.

Your baby's face is now recognisably human. Their cheeks, mouth, lips and chin are more defined. Their nasal passages create the tip of their nose, and eyelids have developed (but remain fused and closed until 24 weeks). Their external ears and middle ear (responsible for hearing and balance) begin to form, but your baby cannot hear until about 19 to 24 weeks. Immature tastebuds are on their tongue and many tiny blood vessels can be seen networking through their body under smooth, translucent skin. Their skeleton starts to form, with arms and legs growing longer, extending forwards and across their body, appearing slightly bent. Their webbed fingers and toes start to separate.

Did you know?
Webbing between your baby's fingers and toes undergoes degeneration (the dying-off of cells) to allow their body to 'sculpture'. For an unborn baby's development to unfold, both cell growth and death are necessary. A supreme adaptation of nature!

Week 10 – 49 to 56 days after conception. Your baby now measures more than 2.5 cm from crown to rump and is now called a foetus, a Latin word meaning 'young one'.

The webbing between their fingers and toes has disappeared, creating separate digits. Nail beds start to form but actual nails are not present until 20 weeks. Their heart has four distinct chambers and valves and their aorta and pulmonary blood vessels directing blood flow one way, to and from their body and lungs. Their yolk sac has disappeared and their blood is produced by their liver (which will eventually be taken over by their bone marrow, once bones fully mature). Their lungs are growing bronchi, which branch out, spreading through their chest. Elbows, knees, wrists and ankles are now forming and muscles appear between their skin and soft, flexible bones. Their neck is more developed, allowing them to slightly lift and turn their head. Your baby may now touch their own face with their hand (the beginnings of thumb sucking!). Their anus, ovaries or testes are now well developed, but both sexes look the same at this early stage, because their external sex organs are just beginning to form.

Week 11 – 56 to 63 days after conception. Your baby now measures 3.5 cm and weighs about 5 g.

By the end of this week all your baby's major organs will be in place. Their legs are longer than their arms, with muscles forming thick bands of padding between their skin and underlying bones. Their brain and nervous system are maturing, with nerves now facilitating their first movements, although small, jerky and uncoordinated (far too small to be felt by their mother just yet). They have primitive reflexes and can respond to touch if the palm of their hands or the soles of their feet are stroked. Their jaw can now open and stretch. Their body is straighter and small ribs can be seen through their chest. Their digestive system is developing rapidly, as they prepare for a growth spurt.

Week 12 – 63 to 70 days after conception. Your baby is now 5 cm long from crown to rump and weighs about 8 g – nearly doubling in size during the last week.

Immature sucking and swallowing movements are present and their tastebuds are mature enough to taste the amniotic fluid. Their kidneys are now functioning and secrete fluid into their bladder, which they will soon pass as a type of urine. The cycle of swallowing and urinating amniotic fluid continues until birth. Amniotic fluid is also breathed into their lungs, strengthening their diaphragm and allowing your baby to regularly practise rhythmic expansion of their lungs. Their stomach now produces gastric juices and they have 20 baby teeth in their gums. Sex organs are still developing but not yet obvious to the naked eye. Increased testosterone (for boys) or lack of testosterone (for girls) makes them take shape. Their gonads move into place as either testes or ovaries and a shaft of tissue either enlarges to become a penis, or reduces in size to become a clitoris (usually by 15 weeks). Bags of tissue on each side become either the scrotum or labia. Movements are now more coordinated, purposeful and regular (daily, when they are awake). These are important for growth and development, otherwise muscles would waste, joints would seize and bones would become brittle.

Confirming your pregnancy

Around 6 to 12 days after conception, your new baby implants in the lining of the uterus and starts physically interacting with your body by releasing human gonadotrophin hormone (HCG) into your bloodstream. Pregnancy tests detect HCG. The level begins at 5 IU/L, roughly doubling every two to three days. At 50 to 80 IU/L, a urine pregnancy test will show positive, usually around the time the next period is due. HCG causes some physical signs of early pregnancy. However, increasing levels of progesterone and oestrogen contribute to sore breasts and bloating, which are often confused with pre-menstrual signs. You may not realise you are pregnant for a while, or perhaps you know even before the test shows positive.

Urine pregnancy tests

Urine pregnancy tests can be used at home or your caregiver may use one to confirm your pregnancy. Make sure you follow the manufacturer's instructions. Coloured markings show within minutes of your urine soaking the test. If only one marking is visible the test is **negative**. If two markings are visible (even if the second marking is very faint) then it is **p sitive** and you are pregnant – congratulations!

It is possible to get a negative urine result yet still be pregnant because:
- The test is done too soon. Up to 10% of women take longer to build up adequate HCG levels because the baby took longer to implant or the menstrual cycle was longer. Repeating the test in a few days time usually brings a positive result.
- The urine is not concentrated. Tests are up to 97% accurate if the urine is concentrated (first thing in the morning after waking is best). A diluted urine sample makes tests only 75% accurate.

It is rare for a pregnancy test to show positive if you are not pregnant. However a faintly positive test followed by a late period usually means a very early miscarriage which you probably would not have been aware of had you not tested. Women having HCG injections for fertility treatment can have high HCG levels for two to three weeks afterwards making a pregnancy test positive even though they are not pregnant.

Blood pregnancy tests

Your caregiver may do a blood pregnancy test. About 5% of pregnant women show positive as early as eight days after conception but it usually takes 11 to 12 days after conception, similar to urine tests. A HCG of 5 IU/L indicates a possible pregnancy or early miscarriage, 25 IU/L (or more) is definitely positive. If the test is repeated in two to three days time the level should have roughly doubled confirming the pregnancy is continuing. If the second test is lower or only slightly increased it is likely a miscarriage is inevitable.

Normal HCG blood levels vary widely so be careful when interpreting the numbers. The level itself is not as important as how much it is rising by every few days. Some healthy normal pregnancies start off with quite low HCG levels. A higher than expected level may indicate the pregnancy is more advanced or perhaps twins!

NOTE: HCG can stay in a woman's blood for four to six weeks after a miscarriage.

Guide to normal HCG levels

Weeks of pregnancy	Days after conception	HCG level for single baby (mIU/ml or IU/L)
Week 3	7	0 to 5
Week 4 – next period due	14	5 to 426
Week 5	21	18 to 7340
Week 6	28	1 080 to 56 500
Weeks 7 to 8	35 to 42	7 650 to 229 000
Weeks 9 to 12	49 to 70	25 700 to 288 000
Weeks 13 to 16	77 to 100	13 300 to 254 000
Weeks 17 to 24		4 060 to 165 400
Weeks 25 to birth		3 640 to 117 000
4 to 6 weeks after birth		Less than 5

Calculating your baby's due date

After your positive pregnancy test you'll want to know when your baby is due. This is the estimated date of delivery (EDD) or estimated date of confinement (EDC). However it is precisely that an *estimate*! Only 5% of babies are born on their due date and any time from 37 to 42 weeks is regarded as on time. Most babies are born between 39 and 41 weeks more commonly after 40 weeks.

A human pregnancy lasts about 38 weeks (266 days) from conception or 280 days from the first day of the last period (for a 28 day cycle). The chart on pages 56–57 estimates your baby's due date (and star sign) for a 28 day cycle. Find the first day of your last period on the top line (in grey) and then look at the day below.

You can adjust the due date for different menstrual cycle lengths by adding or subtracting the appropriate amount of days. For example:
- If you have a 26 day cycle subtract 2 days from the estimated due date.
- If you have a 32 day cycle add 4 days to the estimated due date.

If you are unsure when your last period was but know your baby's conception date calculate the baby's due date from conception then minus 14 days.

Implantation bleeds

Some women experience implantation bleeds which can be confused with a period making them believe they are not pregnant (for a while anyway) or assume their pregnancy is less advanced than it actually is. An implantation bleed is light bleeding as the baby implants in the lining of the uterus, about 8 to 12 days after conception. These are common, but not experienced by every woman. Sometimes it is impossible to estimate the baby's due date, unless an ultrasound is performed.

ULTRASOUND DATING

If you don't have a 'last period' or conception date, your caregiver may order a dating ultrasound. This measures the baby's physical size to roughly calculate their gestation and estimate when they may be due. Generally speaking, the earlier the ultrasound, the more precise the estimated due date.

Between 6 and 12 weeks of pregnancy they are within 3 to 5 days of accuracy. If the ultrasound estimates more than 7 days from the calculated due date the EDD is readjusted. From 12 to 22 weeks ultrasounds can be up to 10 days out. After 22 weeks they can be 2 to 3 weeks out and shouldn't be used to estimate the due date, unless this is all you have to go on. If you are given several different ultrasound dates, use the earliest estimate.

TWINS, TRIPLETS OR MORE

Ultrasound can also be used to detect the presence of more than one baby. Before the widespread use of ultrasound, up to 50% of twins were discovered at the time of birth. This is because the physical signs of a multiple pregnancy are not always obvious. Even the most experienced obstetricians and midwives can miss a twin pregnancy. However, you may have an intuitive feeling, or experience more severe morning sickness, or perhaps get an abnormally high pregnancy blood test. Ultrasounds cannot definitely confirm twins until 10 to 12 weeks, when two heartbeats and two heads are seen, although two sacs may be visible from 6 weeks.

The incidence of multiple pregnancies in Australia has nearly doubled over recent decades, despite the overall birth rate being fairly static. This is attributed to women delaying their childbearing (at 20 years the chance of twins is 0.6%, compared to 2.2% from 35 to 40 years), and the increased use of fertility treatments, which can increase the chances of twins to 25%.

Twins can be:

Non-identical twins – These include fraternal, dizygotic or binovular twins, where the woman inherits the ability to release two eggs in one menstrual cycle, and both are fertilised; 50% are boy–girl, 25% boy–boy and 25% girl–girl combinations. They always have two separate placentas and

Due date calculator chart

January	1	2	3	4	5	6	7	8	9	10	11	12	13	14	15
October	8	9	10	11	12	13	14	15	16	17	18	19	20	21	22

Libra

February	1	2	3	4	5	6	7	8	9	10	11	12	13	14	15
November	8	9	10	11	12	13	14	15	16	17	18	19	20	21	22

Scorpio

March	1	2	3	4	5	6	7	8	9	10	11	12	13	14	15
December	6	7	8	9	10	11	12	13	14	15	16	17	18	19	20

Sagittarius

April	1	2	3	4	5	6	7	8	9	10	11	12	13	14	15
January	6	7	8	9	10	11	12	13	14	15	16	17	18	19	20

Capricorn

May	1	2	3	4	5	6	7	8	9	10	11	12	13	14	15
February	5	6	7	8	9	10	11	12	13	14	15	16	17	18	19

Aquarius

June	1	2	3	4	5	6	7	8	9	10	11	12	13	14	15
March	8	9	10	11	12	13	14	15	16	17	18	19	20	21	22

Pisces

July	1	2	3	4	5	6	7	8	9	10	11	12	13	14	15
April	7	8	9	10	11	12	13	14	15	16	17	18	19	20	21

Aries

August	1	2	3	4	5	6	7	8	9	10	11	12	13	14	15
May	8	9	10	11	12	13	14	15	16	17	18	19	20	21	22

Taurus

September	1	2	3	4	5	6	7	8	9	10	11	12	13	14	15
June	8	9	10	11	12	13	14	15	16	17	18	19	20	21	22

Gemini

October	1	2	3	4	5	6	7	8	9	10	11	12	13	14	15
July	8	9	10	11	12	13	14	15	16	17	18	19	20	21	22

Cancer

November	1	2	3	4	5	6	7	8	9	10	11	12	13	14	15
August	8	9	10	11	12	13	14	15	16	17	18	19	20	21	22

Leo

December	1	2	3	4	5	6	7	8	9	10	11	12	13	14	15
September	7	8	9	10	11	12	13	14	15	16	17	18	19	20	21

Virgo

A NEW PREGNANCY: CONCEPTION TO 12 WEEKS

16	17	18	19	20	21	22	23	24	25	26	27	28	29	30	31
23	24	25	26	27	28	29	30	31	Nov 1	2	3	4	5	6	7

Scorpio

16	17	18	19	20	21	22	23	24	25	26	27	28
23	24	25	26	27	28	29	30	Dec 1	2	3	4	5

Sagittarius

16	17	18	19	20	21	22	23	24	25	26	27	28	29	30	31
21	22	23	24	25	26	27	28	29	30	31	Jan 1	2	3	4	5

Capricorn

16	17	18	19	20	21	22	23	24	25	26	27	28	29	30
21	22	23	24	25	26	27	28	29	30	31	Feb 1	2	3	4

Aquarius

16	17	18	19	20	21	22	23	24	25	26	27	28	29	30	31
20	21	22	23	24	25	26	27	28	Mar 1	2	3	4	5	6	7

Pisces

16	17	18	19	20	21	22	23	24	25	26	27	28	29	30
23	24	25	26	27	28	29	30	31	Apr 1	2	3	4	5	6

Aries

16	17	18	19	20	21	22	23	24	25	26	27	28	29	30	31
22	23	24	25	26	27	28	29	30	May 1	2	3	4	5	6	7

Taurus

16	17	18	19	20	21	22	23	24	25	26	27	28	29	30	31
23	24	25	26	27	28	29	30	31	Jun 1	2	3	4	5	6	7

Gemini

16	17	18	19	20	21	22	23	24	25	26	27	28	29	30
23	24	25	26	27	28	29	30	Jul 1	2	3	4	5	6	7

Cancer

16	17	18	19	20	21	22	23	24	25	26	27	28	29	30	31
23	24	25	26	27	28	29	30	31	Aug 1	2	3	4	5	6	7

Leo

16	17	18	19	20	21	22	23	24	25	26	27	28	29	30
23	24	25	26	27	28	29	30	Sep 1	2	3	4	5	6	7

Virgo

16	17	18	19	20	21	22	23	24	25	26	27	28	29	30	31
22	23	24	25	26	27	28	29	30	Oct 1	2	3	4	5	6	7

Libra

amniotic sacs, although at birth, the placentas can look like one large placenta because they have fused. Fraternal twins are more common than identical twins (66% vs 33%).

Identical twins – These include monozygotic or uniovular twins, where one fertilised egg spontaneously splits into two identical babies, which is not inherited. Identical twins are always the same sex. They look the same and often have similar personality traits. Some identical twins are mirror-imaged, meaning one is right-handed and the other left-handed, or their hair parts on opposite sides. Identical twin types are categorised according to how long after conception the fertilised egg separated to create two babies.

- **Dichorionic and diamniotic twins** – There are two separate placentas and two separate amniotic sacs (similar to non-identical twins). The fertilised egg has separated before three days after conception.
- **Monochorionic and diamniotic twins** – These share one placenta, but develop two separate fluid sacs (75% of identical twins). Separation occurred three to eight days after conception.
- **Monochorionic and monoamniotic twins** – These share one placenta and one amniotic sac (rare). Separation occurred 8 to 13 days after conception.
- **Conjoined or Siamese twins** – Very rare; separation is delayed until 13 to 15 days after conception. The babies are physically joined on some part of their body, as well as sharing the one placenta and amniotic sac (monochorionic, monoamniotic).
- **Acardiac twins** – Similar to conjoined twins but the babies share one heart (very rare).

Triplets or more – When a woman releases three eggs, she may conceive non-identical triplets (and so on for quads, etc). Although uncommon, if one fertilised egg splits into three, identical triplets are conceived (6% of triplets). In many cases, two babies are identical and the third is not. Identical triplets are categorised as trichorionic and triamniotic (three placentas and three amniotic sacs) and can have various combinations of sharing placentas and/or sacs.

Early pregnancy

Pregnancy brings many new physical sensations. Your early physical signs may be obvious, or quite subtle, or may only become clearer in retrospect –

'So that's why I've been so sick and tired!' It is common to feel unsure about what is normal. While missing your menstrual period is generally expected, you may experience all, none or just some of the following physical changes:

- **Breast and nipple changes** – From four to six weeks of pregnancy, the breasts' milk ducts grow and mature, making them larger. Increased blood supply makes the veins under the skin more noticeable. They can feel tender and fuller, and possibly tingle. The nipples often become more prominent and may feel quite sensitive (or even sore).
- **Passing urine more frequently** – Passing more urine is normal. Blood flow to the kidneys increases, making them produce 25% more urine. This peaks by 9 to 16 weeks, before settling down. Pressure from the growing uterus may also make you urinate more often, but to a much lesser degree (until the last three months of pregnancy).
- **Increased temperature** – Your metabolism increases by 20%, creating more body heat and slightly raising your temperature from 37°C to about 37.8°C. Blood flow also increases up to 50%, making your skin warmer; you may notice you sweat more.
- **Constipation and wind** – Constipation in early pregnancy is caused by hormones slowing the digestive processes, as well as dietary changes from morning sickness and possibly slight dehydration. (Strategies for dealing with constipation are discussed in Chapter 4.) Your bowel often produces more gas during pregnancy, causing occasional wind pains. Peppermint water or tea can help.
- **Aches and pains** – Mild cramps, bloating, tugging and pulling and perhaps slight backache is common as the uterus starts to grow. This often causes women concern, but if there is no heavy bleeding, it is probably normal.
- **Increased saliva** – Excess saliva (ptyalism) is often associated with morning sickness. This usually improves as the nausea subsides (by 12 to 14 weeks). Eating dry, plain cracker biscuits may help. Homeopaths may prescribe Mercurius solubilis or Veratrum album. Check with your practitioner.
- **Dizziness and fainting** – Pregnancy hormones make your blood vessels relax and dilate, lowering your blood pressure, which may in turn make you feel dizzy and faint. Drink plenty of fluids and eat regular meals. Get up slowly after sitting or lying down, and avoid hot, crowded environments.
- **Tiredness** – Feeling extremely fatigued and lethargic is common. Once your body adjusts to the metabolic changes necessary to grow your baby, the tiredness usually subsides (around 12 to 14 weeks), bringing renewed energy and vigour. In the meantime, rest as much as possible.

- **Headaches** – Headaches may be caused by increased blood flow through the brain, or tension and stress, especially if you are struggling to adjust emotionally to the new pregnancy. However, some women find they suffer less from headaches or migraines during pregnancy. Try to find a cause (lack of sleep, eye strain, skipping meals, dehydration, caffeine withdrawal, anxiety or concerns). Often rest and relaxation techniques help. Have a neck massage, or apply a cool cloth to the back of your neck or forehead. Some women rub tiger balm into their temples. A chiropractic or osteopathic treatment may help if your neck is out of alignment. Herbs, homeopathy or acupuncture may be the answer. See your practitioner. Avoid painkillers where possible, especially during the first 12 weeks. Contact your caregiver if the headache becomes severe. Avoid aspirin or codeine (unless prescribed) and don't take migraine medications.

'Morning' sickness

Morning sickness (or all day and all night sickness!) typically starts around 6 weeks of pregnancy and continues until 12 to 14 weeks (or beyond if you are unlucky – about 15% of women are nauseated beyond 20 weeks of pregnancy). You may experience constant nausea or waves of it, perhaps vomiting at times. Some women find they don't initially gain weight, or perhaps lose weight for several weeks. This is normal and your baby relies on your fat stores to grow. Once the sickness settles and your appetite returns, your body 'catches up'.

We don't really know why morning sickness occurs, or why some women but not others suffer from it. Hormonal changes (high HCG levels) may play a role, but an increased body metabolism, which lowers your blood sugar levels, is more likely to blame. This is probably why eating often helps and why the nausea tends to be worse in the mornings, after not eating overnight. However, emotional stress, certain smells or even accidentally pushing the toothbrush too far down your mouth can trigger nausea and vomiting.

> **Did you know?**
> Severe morning sickness does not predict whether you are having a girl or a boy.

Remedies

Morning sickness is an individual experience and the effectiveness of remedies varies. You may need to try some different approaches before finding a strategy that works for you.

- Eat small, regular meals and chew food thoroughly. Some women find not drinking anything half an hour before and after eating helps. Snack on dry cracker biscuits, nuts or fruit. Have something light before going to bed and again first thing on waking. Try eating a plain piece of toast and having a cup of sweet tea or a glass of juice, half an hour before getting up. Avoid fatty and spicy foods. Pickled Asian plums (*umeboshi*) may help.
- Liquid meals, such as banana smoothies, or fresh fruit and vegetable juices, may be more palatable. Mineral water and sports drinks help balance your mineral intake and avoid dehydration. Try lemon and honey drinks or hot water with honey (and milk). Perhaps add a teaspoon of cider vinegar.
- Stress and anxiety may contribute to the intensity of your morning sickness and perhaps make it linger beyond 16 weeks (or return later in pregnancy). Deep breathing, yoga, meditation, massage and/or relaxation exercises may be beneficial. Look at ways to take the pressure off. Perhaps talk with someone you trust about how you honestly feel about the pregnancy, or seek professional counselling.

Natural therapies

- Vitamin B6 may reduce nausea, but not necessarily vomiting. Caregivers sometimes prescribe 10-20 mg, 3 times a day.
- Ginger sweets or biscuits, flat ginger ale or powdered ginger (1g daily in water). Try cutting fresh ginger and placing it in boiling water to make a tea.
- Lollipops can help with low blood glucose.
- Acupressure applied to the wrist with your fingers, or a seasickness wristband (available from pharmacies). The point is shown in the Acupressure appendix.
- Herbalists may suggest peppermint, anise and fennel seed or chamomile teas; slippery elm before meals or remedies with wild yam root or dandelion root. Check with your practitioner. Avoid raspberry leaf tea or tablets, which may cause nausea.
- Homeopaths may prescribe Ipecacuanna, Nux vomica, Sepia or Pulsatilla.

NOTE: *Essential oils (such as sniffing peppermint oil on a handkerchief) are generally not recommended during the first 12 weeks of pregnancy.*

Medical treatments

Most anti-nausea medications are not proven to be completely safe during early pregnancy. However, they may be prescribed if the morning sickness is very severe. For medications such as Maxalon and Phenergan, the small amount of research done so far has not shown any adverse effects for the unborn baby.[1]

Your diet during pregnancy

Your body is home to your baby for the next 40 weeks. So a healthy, well-balanced diet is important. There is no need to eat for two, and women carrying twins or more don't need to double or triple their food intake. If you have a medical condition (such as diabetes), you should consult a dietician at your maternity hospital. An in-depth guide to diet during pregnancy (for single and multiple babies) is contained in Chapter 1.

LISTERIA

In recent years there has been increased awareness about pregnant women possibly contracting listeriosis from contaminated foods. Listeriosis is fairly rare (60 to 70 cases a year in Australia), but unborn babies are particularly at risk from it. The listeria monocytogenes bacteria are readily found in soil and vegetation and are usually transmitted to humans through contaminated food. Recorded outbreaks are linked to some dairy products and pre-cooked meats. Listeria can multiply at temperatures as low as 0.5°C. Therefore, refrigerating does not always help. However, cooking contaminated foods at high temperatures does kill the bacteria.

Listeria can also be transmitted through handling the miscarried foetuses of animals. Pregnant women working with animals should not touch these products, or wear gloves if they cannot be avoided. Most people don't notice physical symptoms of listeriosis and there is no test available to detect listeria infection. The best strategy is to avoid eating foods that may carry the bacteria.[2]

As a guide:
- **AVOID** soft cheeses such as brie, camembert, feta, blue-vein, Havarti and ricotta. All hard and processed cheeses including mozzarella, cheese slices, spreads, cream cheese and cottage cheese are safe. Ensure the packaging is intact when you buy it, and store in the fridge. Fresh, pasteurised and UHT milk and yoghurt is safe. Make sure they are not past their use-by date.
- **AVOID** ready-made coleslaw and salads (from salad bars or packaged), or salads stored in the fridge for more than 24 hours. Washed fresh fruit and vegetables are safe. After making a salad, store it in fridge and use within 12 hours.

- **AVOID** dips and salad dressings, that have been previously exposed to raw vegetables, even when refrigerated. Salad dressings are safe. Store opened containers in the fridge.
- **AVOID** cold meats from supermarkets or sandwich bars, and pates or meatloaf products. Cold meats (roasted or boiled) are safe, if home cooked. Use within 12 hours of cooking or freeze. Unused portions can be thawed in the fridge and used immediately. Canned meats are safe. Once opened, refrigerate and use within 12 hours.
- **AVOID** pre-sliced chicken loaf and cooked diced chicken (used in sandwich shops). Chicken cooked at home is safe. Cook thoroughly and use immediately or store in fridge and use within 12 hours. Hot take-away chicken is safe. Make sure it is steaming hot when you buy it. Use immediately or store in fridge and use within 12 hours.
- **AVOID** uncooked or smoked seafood (chilled or frozen), smoked shellfish, and raw seafood (oysters, sashimi or sushi). Canned fish (tuna, salmon, etc) is safe. Once opened, store in the fridge and use within 12 hours.

Preparation tips include:
- Taking care when reheating foods. Make sure leftovers are well heated. Microwaves heat unevenly, so mix it at intervals, or use your oven or stove top to reheat.
- Prepare and store foods safely. Keep raw meat separate and don't store it where meat juices could drip onto other foods. Keep all stored food in the fridge individually covered.
- Wash your hands, knives and cutting boards well with hot soapy water after dealing with raw foods (especially meats).
- Cook all animal products right through. Avoid rare or medium rare steaks and runny eggs.

Mercury in fish

Pregnant women should avoid eating fish high in mercury, which can affect the development of the baby's brain. The types to avoid are swordfish, ray, shark, barramundi, gemfish, ling, orange roughy and southern bluefin tuna. Canned tuna is safe.

Cravings

Pregnancy is synonymous with weird and wonderful food cravings. These are very normal and may come and go. Changes in your taste and smell sensations are thought to be due to hormonal changes, not your body needing certain foods. Take care that your cravings don't impinge on having a nutritious diet. Sugary, fatty and salty foods can be acceptable as occasional treats, but should not be eaten excessively.

Vegetarian and vegan diets

Women with vegetarian or vegan diets can have normal, healthy pregnancies. The key is having a wide variety of foods so you obtain all the nutrients you and your baby require. As a guide:

- Make sure you have sufficient energy by eating breads, rice, pasta and grains to maintain your weight and help your baby grow.
- Be conscious of obtaining adequate calcium, vitamin B12, vitamin D and zinc (see Chapter 1).
- Combine several vegetables, whole grains, soy products, pulses, legumes, nuts and seeds (and possibly dairy foods and eggs) to provide adequate protein. Soy protein alone can fall short in meeting your needs.
- If you become iron deficient, you may require supplements. However, pregnancy makes a woman's body naturally adapt to absorb more iron from foods, so supplements are not routine.

Weight gain

Being pregnant means you will inevitably gain weight. Yet weight gain often becomes the focus of concern. In recent years, routine weighing by caregivers has all but stopped, as it has no known health benefits and avoids anxiety about not enough or too much weight!

Each woman's body responds differently to pregnancy. As a guide:

- Underweight women often naturally adjust by putting on more weight in addition to their normal pregnancy weight gain, to reach their ideal weight.
- Overweight women may not put on very much, or even naturally lose weight, as their metabolism increases for the physical needs of pregnancy.
- Retaining fluid can cause extra weight gain after 20 weeks of pregnancy.

A common pregnancy weight gain pattern is to:

- Gain a few kilograms up until 12 to 16 weeks (or lose weight if experiencing morning sickness).

- Have a growth spurt during middle pregnancy, up to about 32 weeks.
- Slowly gain weight over the following four to eight weeks.
- Lose 1 to 2 kg just prior to starting labour.

However, some women gain most of their pregnancy weight during the first 20 weeks, and only small amounts after this.

Normal pregnancy weight gains can be as little as 8 kg or as much as 20 kg. However, the average is around 12 to 14 kg, which is attributed to:

Baby: 3 to 4 kg
Placenta: 0.5 kg
Amniotic fluid: 1 kg
Uterus: 1 kg
Blood volume: 1.5 kg
Breasts: 0.5 kg
Fat stores for breastfeeding: 3.5 kg
Fluid retention: 1.5 kg

Women carrying twins, triplets or more do tend to put on more weight, but not double or triple. In fact, weight gain may be similar to women having a single baby. As a guide, women having:

- Twins may gain up to 15 to 20 kg (or more).
- Triplets may gain up to 20 to 25 kg (or more).

Be aware that most triplets and quads (and 50% of twins) are born premature (less than 37 weeks). Therefore weight gain naturally increases more rapidly during early pregnancy.

Exercise

Moderate exercise during pregnancy, at least three times a week, has been shown to improve a woman's physical fitness and her perceived body image, without harming her baby.[3] Therefore, if you are well and healthy and your pregnancy is progressing normally, you can exercise.

Women with multiple pregnancies need to be more cautious about strenuous physical activity. Be guided by your caregiver. (Information on getting started with your exercise program, and what to avoid during early pregnancy, is given in Chapter 1.)

NOTE: Being fit can go some way towards assisting you to cope with the physical demands of labour. However, don't feel guilty if you don't get much exercise during your pregnancy, as most women still cope very well without having had regular exercise.

Be aware that:
- Increased progesterone softens muscles and ligaments, making them

more flexible and prone to sprains, strains and injury. Always stretch and warm up before and after exercise. Also, aggressive contact sports make you vulnerable to injuries and falls.
- If you experience dizziness or fainting, have something to eat an hour before exercising. Drink plenty of water and make sure you can sit down if you start feeling light-headed.
- Very strenuous sports can slightly increase your risk of premature labour. Seek the advice of your caregiver and use your own judgment.
- Keep your heart rate below 140 beats per minute.

Emotions in early pregnancy

Discovering a new pregnancy is a life-changing event, whether planned or a surprise. It inevitably triggers many emotions, with feeling unsure or ambivalent being most common. It is normal to feel as though you are on an emotional rollercoaster moving through excitement, shock, happiness, relief, anxiousness, pride, fear and concern as the reality sinks in.

Talking with your partner, friends, family and/or other parents may help work through these responses. However, it can be overwhelming if your news triggers horror stories of agonising labours, sleepless nights and dirty nappies. Sometimes professional counselling is more helpful.

EMOTIONS FOR THE WOMAN

Early pregnancy can bring powerful, shifting emotions (often rekindling memories of puberty) as unpredictable feelings and responses surface without rhyme or reason. Many women cry unexpectedly, catching themselves, and others, by surprise! Remember, you are in the midst of a profound, intense period of change and your emotions will reflect this. Try not to feel guilty, or that you need to justify your tears. It is a normal process that ultimately passes as the pregnancy progresses. Some concerns can include:
- Worrying about becoming a mother and feeling you won't know what to do with a baby.
- Wondering how you will manage with an extra child (if this is not your first).
- Fear of miscarriage or the impending labour and birth.
- Feeling overwhelmed by the prospect of single parenting and/or negotiating involvement from the father.

EMOTIONS FOR THE PARTNER
Becoming a father can initially feel quite surreal, because the baby is not part of your body, and your life has not dramatically changed. Common concerns centre around increased responsibility, taking on additional domestic chores, and financial issues. Others can include:
- Worrying about supporting your partner during labour, or repeating a previous negative birth experience. Maybe not wanting to go to birth classes!
- Going through it all again, if this is not your first child.
- Wondering whether the baby is yours, especially if the relationship is not an established one.

YOUR RELATIONSHIP
New pregnancies impact on relationships, whether long-term or relatively new. Assessing your own emotions and accepting your partner's may strengthen your relationship or place a strain on it. Listening to each other can help you work towards support strategies for the coming months, and eventually into the parenting years. Having an open, honest line of communication is important, even if this causes anxious moments when your partner's feelings are not what you want to hear. However, if things are left unsaid, bottled up or ignored, they will tend to come out in other (usually destructive) ways. If the difficulties seem impossible to resolve, seeing a counsellor (preferably together) may be the answer.

Sex during early pregnancy
Making love throughout pregnancy is perfectly safe, unless the woman has heavy vaginal bleeding (or her waters break during later pregnancy). Libido changes are common, some women feel more like having sex, as extra blood flow to their breasts and genitals increases their sensitivity and sexual arousal. Others find they are too tired or sick to even think about it. Concerns about miscarriage may also interfere with sexual desire, especially if the woman has miscarried before. She may feel like wrapping herself in cotton wool, or her partner may be afraid to touch her in case he causes a problem.

Penetrative sex does not cause miscarriage; even so, it is important to follow your instincts and do what feels right for you. Abstaining from sex for a while may make you feel more comfortable. Try to be patient and honest with your partner about how you are feeling. Cuddling and reassuring each other can help you both feel loved, as well as keeping you emotionally close until sexual desire returns.

Taking care

Most pregnant women try to make a conscious effort to do everything they can to have a healthy baby. However, well-meaning family, friends, caregivers and the media tend to focus on what you can or can't do. This can make you feel you are tip-toeing through a minefield of potential dangers, or that you have to give up *everything* in order to be a 'good mother' and have a perfect baby.

Pregnancy is an emotionally vulnerable time and this popular 'thou shalt not' mind-set can lead to many women experiencing stressful pregnancies, and suffering guilt and anxiety about things they may have done, perhaps even before they knew they were pregnant.

Let's put it in perspective. The human population carries a 3% baseline risk of producing babies with an abnormality or birth defect. Of these babies, 37% are due to inherited disorders, 3% are from infectious viruses (such as rubella) and less than 1% is attributed to recreational, prescribed or over-the-counter drugs. For the remaining 60% the cause is unknown.

Pregnant women exposed to known harmful substances (drugs, alcohol, radiation, chemicals or certain viruses) can increase their baseline risk to 5 or 10%, depending on the substance, how much and how often the mother was exposed and at what stage during the pregnancy, but 90 to 95% of babies will be fine.

Coming to terms with possible harmful exposures can be difficult. However, bear in mind that not all environment risk factors are avoidable (eg. pollutants, electronic communication waves, pesticides and food chemicals). Some things that have helped other women deal with their concerns are:

- Remembering that most babies are born well and healthy.
- Taking the attitude, 'What's done, is done. I cannot change the past. I will feel positive for my baby and myself.'
- Repeating reassuring statements like, 'I am a good mother. I am doing the best I can.'
- Ignoring the often misinformed suggestions from others.
- Trying not to blame yourself if something does go wrong.

NOTE: *If you are concerned about a serious exposure (radiation, medications, drugs, or a viral infection such as rubella), then obtaining accurate information and advice is imperative, particularly if your caregiver is suggesting you terminate your pregnancy. Ask to speak with a genetic counsellor if you need more information about any possible effects on your baby.*

LIFESTYLE CHANGES

Pregnant women are always advised to stop (or reduce) potentially harmful habits, because these things *are* controllable and can help improve a baby's chances of being healthy. However, there are no guarantees. The possible effects of caffeine, alcohol, cigarettes and marijuana are covered in Chapter 1.

Caffeine, alcohol and cigarettes are physically and socially addictive, especially if associated with shared activities or rituals (a coffee and cigarette at morning tea, Friday night drinks, winding down after work). Dealing with the social part of your habit is a good starting point when making lifestyle changes. Some strategies include:

- Planning outings to places other than bars or parties. Try going to the movies, out to dinner or catching up with friends over breakfast.
- Trying deep breathing, reading a magazine, keeping busy by knitting, drawing, or going for a walk.
- Discussing with your partner the possibility of them stopping their habits to support you.
- Replacing alcohol with nonalcoholic soft drinks or juices in a wine glass. Having a fruit cocktail without the alcohol.
- Replacing colas with mineral waters.
- Replacing tea and coffee with decaffeinated, herbal or green teas.

In Australia, 25% of pregnant women smoke and 25% of these give up before their first pregnancy visit (perhaps because they were not heavy smokers). Women who continue to smoke often feel guilty and become closet smokers to avoid criticism.

Giving up smoking before 16 weeks of pregnancy reduces the risks of complications. However, if you are finding it extremely difficult to stop, or have the occasional relapse, bear in mind that cutting back to five cigarettes a day or less will help greatly. Contacts for information and support on quitting in Australia and New Zealand are in the resources section.

PRESCRIBED MEDICATIONS

In an ideal world no pregnant woman would ever take medications. However, this is not always possible or desirable, creating difficult decisions for women and their caregivers.

As a general guide medications should only be prescribed during pregnancy if the expected benefits for the mother are thought to be greater than any risks to the unborn baby. Where possible, medications should be avoided during the first 12 weeks of pregnancy and when a woman is trying to conceive.

While this is a starting point it doesn't reflect the lack of information we have about the possible risks of many drugs. Doctors often prescribe medications with a degree of uncertainty, because in many cases there is insufficient evidence to prove a substance is completely safe.

Some drugs are backed by thorough research, or have such dramatic (or tragic) side effects that making the decisions to use or avoid them is easy. However:

- Up to two-thirds of prescribed drugs have little or no background data on them and it is not ethical or desirable to test them on pregnant women. Drug companies label products 'Not recommended for pregnant women', not because they are necessarily harmful but often because their safety is unknown.
- Reliable human studies are few and far between.
- Most new drugs are tested on pregnant animals, which cannot reliably indicate what is safe or harmful for human babies.
- Birth defects are obvious, but long-term effects on a child's development, behaviour and intellectual abilities are less visible and under-researched.

With only vague guidelines, doctors normally opt for drugs that have been used for several years and *seem* to have no effect on unborn babies. These are regarded as relatively safe but are not 100% fail-safe. For example, phenobarbitone was prescribed for pregnant women with epilepsy from 1912, but it was not until the 1990s that accumulated evidence linked it with higher risks for birth defects.[4]

These dilemmas make some doctors reluctant to prescribe anything at all unless a woman's health condition is urgent or life-threatening. This can be frustrating if a woman feels she needs to be treated or is not given the option of considering the risks herself.

To help caregivers prescribe medications during pregnancy, there is a category rating system (A, B, C, D and X – from safest to least safe). Medications can move up or down categories as new research comes to hand. This system is helpful but not ideal, with doctors who research teratogens (substances that may cause birth defects) criticising it because it gives the impression that category A drugs are completely safe, rather than safer than other categories. Even category A medications should be avoided unless absolutely necessary, especially during the first 12 weeks of pregnancy.

NOTE: *Up to 10% of pregnant women take antibiotics at some stage during their pregnancy, with most commonly prescribed antibiotics thought to be relatively safe.*

A few women require continued medications during their pregnancies to treat chronic health conditions (epilepsy, asthma, diabetes) or pregnancy complications (such as high blood pressure). Generally, the risks of these conditions not being treated far outweigh the risks of taking the medications. The general aim is to have a healthy mother so the baby can also be healthy. Consult your doctor or specialist.

OVER-THE-COUNTER TREATMENTS

Over-the-counter products are not always associated with being potentially unsafe for unborn babies. However, any substance that can affect your body is classified as a drug, including medical and natural self-help remedies and other day-to-day substances such as beauty products, teas, tinctures, creams, drops, sprays and inhalants. As a general rule, the less you take the better, especially during the first 12 weeks of pregnancy. However, if this is unreasonable, contact your caregiver, pharmacist or pregnancy information service in your State.

Hair dyes

Chemicals used in hair dyes are many and varied, and there is little concrete evidence to estimate the real risks. However, they are absorbed through the scalp (or the skin on your hands if you don't use gloves) and can be detected in your urine within hours of applying them to your head. There are questions as to whether hair dying may be linked to birth defects, especially during the first 12 weeks of pregnancy. However, many caregivers think that the amount of chemicals used and the frequency of their use during pregnancy is not enough to be of concern.

What you can do — While there are no clear guidelines to minimise any possible risks you can:
- Avoid dying your hair during the first 12 weeks of pregnancy. If you are trying to conceive, dye your hair during the first two weeks of your cycle and avoid it after ovulating (until the next period).
- Space the timing of hair dyes as much as possible.
- Ask your hairdresser to place a rubber cap on your head and pull as much hair through the holes as he or she can, so the dye does not come in contact with your scalp.
- Have foils, which help keep the dye off your skin.
- If dyeing at home, follow the manufacturer's instructions and always wear gloves.

Hair removal

Chemical depilatories work by breaking the disulfide bonds in hair, breaking off each hair shaft at the level of the skin. Chemicals used include barium sulphide or calcium thioglycolate preparations. Both are classed as category C drugs, meaning their safety during pregnancy has not been established.

What you can do – Use mechanical methods to remove hair such as shaving, laser, electrolysis or epilady machines, especially during the first 12 weeks of pregnancy.

Intestinal worms

Pregnant women can have worms, particularly if they have other children. In developing countries, having them for several months can contribute to malnutrition, anaemia and a lowered immune system during pregnancy. In industrialised countries, they tend to be just annoying and easily passed on to others. Medications include:

- Pyrantel embonate (Combantrin, Early bird), which has been researched in animals, but not humans. It is not really known whether it is capable of causing birth defects if used during the first 12 weeks of pregnancy.
- Mebendazole (Vermox) has recently been researched, showing a very slight increase in birth defects when used during the first 12 weeks of pregnancy, but better health outcomes for mother and baby if used after 12 weeks.
- Albendazole (Zental, Albenza or Eskazole) is ***not*** to be taken when trying to conceive or during pregnancy.

What you can do – If possible, wait to treat worms until after 12 weeks. In the meantime, eat nutritious foods and wash your hands thoroughly after going to the toilet and before handling foods, to decrease the chance of passing them on to others. A natural approach is chewing a handful of raw rice for breakfast (eating nothing else); eat other meals during the day normally; between meals, eat one clove of garlic and one small handful of pumpkin seeds (crush garlic and mix with other foods or miso, to help you swallow); about two hours or more after the last meal of the day, drink one cup of nettle tea. Continue this for 10 days, stopping for 7 days, then resuming for a final 10 days to remove parasites that have hatched from eggs after the initial treatment.

Lice, nits and scabies

Up to 10% of chemicals contained in head lice and scabies treatments can be absorbed into the body. As a guide, avoid preparations containing lindane during pregnancy, as it has been linked with birth defects. Lindane should also be avoided when breastfeeding. If you do use it, express your milk and discard it for four days afterwards feeding your baby with previously expressed breast milk or formula.

What you can do – Some natural products on the market contain lavender and tea tree oils. A simple (but messy) method for treating nits is to cover your hair and scalp with a generous amount of olive oil and leave for 10 minutes. Using a special fine nit comb run through your hair section by section. After each comb wipe the excess oil and any nits onto a piece of tissue or absorbent paper. Continue this until you have combed through all your hair and then wash your hair with regular shampoo. You may need to repeat this in 10 days time. Wash pillow cases and towels in hot water adding a few drops of tee tree oil to the water to help prevent them spreading.

Pain killers

Using analgesics during pregnancy essentially comes down to your own personal decision about whether the pain is severe enough to warrant a painkiller, and/or worth any possible risks. Caregivers often recommend paracetamol. Prescribed painkillers for severe pain depends on the individual situation. Avoid aspirin, unless prescribed by your doctor, as it can interfere with normal blood clotting. Do not use non-steroidal anti-inflammatory drugs (NSAIDs – such as naproxen or ibuprofen). These are associated with possible birth defects during early pregnancy and can affect the baby's heart and lungs if taken during the last three months of pregnancy. Migraine medications should be avoided, unless prescribed by your doctor, knowing you are pregnant.

What you can do – Depending on how you are feeling, you may want to try to put up with as much pain as you can without taking anything, or you may feel you are suffering so much that any small risks associated with the painkiller are acceptable. It is all about balance and what you feel emotionally and physically comfortable with. If you do take painkillers, try to leave taking them until you really need it and minimise your intake as much as possible. Be guided by your caregiver and never exceed the recommended dose on the packet.

Skin disorders and aching muscles

Many creams lotions and ointments contain chemicals and medications that can be absorbed through the skin and into your bloodstream (reaching your baby). Most plain moisturising creams and oils are fine; however you need to take care with skin products containing medicated additives. Treatments for acne and skin conditions should be checked with your caregiver, especially when trying to conceive or are pregnant. Avoid creams containing vitamin A and don't use creams containing antibiotics unless prescribed by your doctor. Use steroid creams sparingly and only when prescribed. Try to avoid antifungal creams during the first three months of pregnancy.

What you can do — Sorbelene cream is best to keep dry skin moisturised. Try alternatives like pawpaw ointment for minor skin irritations. Deep heat type creams or ointments for muscular pains can be replaced with heat packs and massage (particularly during the first 12 weeks of pregnancy).

Tanning

There is little concrete evidence to estimate the real risks involved with tanning beds and self-tanning products during pregnancy. Most caregivers err on the side of caution and recommend avoiding them. Tanning creams and lotions contain dihydroxyacetone (DHA), which is absorbed through the skin, passing into your bloodstream and to the baby. The amount transmitted varies, depending on how much is applied, the frequency used and if there are any abrasions or sores on the skin. Increased oestrogen and melanocyte stimulating hormone (MSH) causes many pregnant women to experience darkened areas on their skin, especially their face (called chloasma). UV radiation and tanning beds should be avoided.

What you can do — As always, use sunscreen and wear a hat when out in the sun, to avoid permanent skin damage and reduce the risks of skin cancer developing in later life.

Vaginal deodorants

Vaginal deodorants should not be used during pregnancy because they can contain chemicals (such as hexachlorophane) that have been linked with birth defects, particularly if used during the first 12 weeks. If you are concerned about the odour of your vaginal discharge, you should see your caregiver to rule out an infection.

NATURAL THERAPIES

Natural therapies are increasingly accepted as mainstream and are often used instead of, or in combination with, traditional medical treatments. However, many people don't associate them with being harmful, even though some remedies and treatments are capable of creating unwanted (or even dangerous) side effects for you or your baby. Take care: don't assume that because it is 'natural' it is safe.

Ideally you should:
- Take time to find a qualified practitioner to advise you, preferably one who has specialist knowledge and experience with preconception, pregnancy and breastfeeding. Contact the relevant professional association for a list of local practitioners.
- Avoid self-prescribing.
- Always let your caregivers (medically trained or natural practitioners) know about other prescribed or over-the-counter medications and/or natural remedies you are currently using. These can interact with each other, making them less effective (or ineffective) or produce potentially harmful side effects. (See the Natural therapies appendix.)

Environmental and occupational hazards

Many women express concerns about environmental or occupational hazards during pregnancy (eg. toxins, air pollution, radiation, chemicals, heavy metals, infectious diseases, pesticides and electronic equipment). Caregivers find it difficult to answer questions about these because there is little scientific information to accurately determine the risks. At this stage, most caregivers, employers, government bodies and manufacturers take the blanket approach of avoiding or minimising exposure to anything that may potentially cause problems wherever possible during pregnancy.

Exposure during the first 12 weeks is generally of more concern than during later pregnancy. Risk levels also depend on how much toxin has reached the woman's body (and her unborn baby) and for how long she is exposed.[5] Some things are known to be relatively safe, others are definitely harmful, but in most cases we don't know enough to make a firm judgment. As a guide:

- **Televisions, visual display units or terminals** emit low levels of radiation and weak electromagnetic fields, but much less than natural sources (such as the sun), and below levels considered harmful by the International Radiation Protection Association. Research so far indicates there is no reliable or convincing evidence to support any links between miscarriage or birth defects and using VDUs.[6] There is also no evidence that **photocopiers** are unsafe, if used in a well-ventilated room.
- There is no evidence that **microwaves** (or other household appliances) affect a woman's pregnancy or her unborn baby.
- We don't yet know whether electromagnetic fields from **mobile phones** affect unborn babies. Keep your phone away from your belly as much as possible and turn it off whenever you can.[7]

- **Magnetic resonance imaging (MRI)** creates pictures of muscles, ligaments, nerves and body organs using a strong magnet. They slightly heat the body, but the effects on the unborn baby are not fully known. In general, avoid them during pregnancy unless absolutely necessary, especially during the first 12 weeks. Ultrasounds are preferable, but MRIs are better than X-rays. Discuss the benefits and risks with your doctor.
- **X-rays and CT scans** emit ionising radiation that potentially affects a person's fertility and is capable of causing birth defects or miscarriage (if used before 12 weeks of pregnancy). It also increases the chances of childhood cancer for the unborn baby later. The maximum dose for an entire pregnancy should not exceed 1 millisievert, especially between 2 and 6 weeks of pregnancy. Female and male radiographers (or those who work with irradiation to prepare foods) need to be mindful of their work environment and exposures, which do accumulate.[8]

Chemicals

Over 200 chemicals and solvents are known to have health effects, including reducing fertility, increasing the incidence of birth defects or inhibiting the growth and development of unborn babies. Thousands more agents have unknown effects. Harmful chemicals at work or home may include pesticides; cleaning agents; paint products; chemicals used in industrial production, machinery maintenance and agriculture; solvents and plastics; dyes used in hairdressing, clothing and printing; anaesthetic medical gases and ethylene oxide used to sterilise; laboratory chemicals and embalming fluids. If dealing with chemicals, check the labels, wear protective clothing and have adequate ventilation. Follow occupational health and safety policies and procedures at work to minimise risks.

Lead

Lead poisoning can cause serious long-term health problems, especially for babies and young children. It accumulates in the body, is stored in the bones and can be released during pregnancy, passing to the unborn baby (or while breastfeeding). Lead levels can increase if the woman is further exposed during pregnancy, especially if her diet lacks calcium, iron and zinc, because lead is more easily absorbed when these essential minerals are lacking. Very high lead levels can cause miscarriage, premature birth or the baby being stillborn.[9]

If you think you are at risk, ask your caregiver for a blood test. Signs of moderate lead poisoning include muscle pains, prickly or itchy feelings, tiredness, aggressiveness, irritability and abdominal discomfort. Severe lead poisoning can cause joint pain, fatigue, poor concentration, tremor, headache, abdominal pain, constipation and weight loss.

The Environment Protection Authority (EPA) provides extensive information about reducing and/or removing lead exposure. See our resource section.

Overheating

Unborn babies cannot sweat and have no way of cooling themselves down. They essentially rely on their mother's body to regulate their temperature. If the woman's body temperature rises above 38.5°C for several hours, the risk of miscarriage or abnormal development of the baby is increased. Later in pregnancy, it can make the baby distressed. As a guide:

- If you have a fever, contact your caregiver. Generally they will advise paracetamol and other interventions to bring your temperature down.
- Avoid very hot spas, baths and saunas.
- Don't have prolonged, strenuous exercise sessions.

Physical hazards

Pregnant women need to be aware of the way they sit, bend, move and lift objects. Hormones make your muscles and ligaments more flexible and prone to injury. Depending on your occupation, you may need change from a standing job to one with more sitting (or be provided with a stool). However, even sitting for long periods can be uncomfortable.

Try:
- Taking regular breaks, moving around frequently and varying tasks.
- Placing your feet on a foot stool while sitting.
- Having a small pillow supporting your lower back.
- Using lifting aids or getting others to lift for you.
- Reducing very strenuous, physical work as the pregnancy progresses.
- Avoiding excessive physical vibrations and exposure to very loud noise.

As your belly enlarges, your posture and centre of gravity change, often causing momentary loss of balance. Take care when negotiating stairs, stepping over obstacles or walking on slippery floors.

Infections

Infectious hazards (usually viruses) can affect a woman's pregnancy, or pass to her unborn baby, depending on her immunity and the stage of pregnancy.

Common infections

Infection	Physical signs
Chicken pox (Varicella-zoster virus) – An infection spread by coughing and sneezing or contact with an infected person's contaminated items (tissues, drinking glasses or soiled hands) early in the illness, and then by direct contact with skin sores. Infectious for 1 to 2 days before the rash appears, until 5 days after the rash stops and all the blisters have all scabbed over. People rarely get chicken pox twice. **Shingles** is a reactivation of the chicken pox virus many years after the initial illness (usually when the immune system is lowered). **Incubation** – 2 to 3 weeks.	Up to 90% of adults have had chicken pox. Physical signs are slight fever, runny nose, feeling generally unwell for 1 to 2 days, then a skin rash appearing as raised, pink spots on various parts of the body over 3 to 4 days. The spots form blisters, which break and form crusts and scab. **Shingles** causes painful skin eruptions on an area on one side of the body, which persist for 2 weeks (occasionally 3 to 5 weeks) and is spread through direct contact with skin eruptions.
Chlamydia – A sexually transmitted infection. Using condoms when having sex with new or different partners helps prevent infection. **Incubation** – 7 to 21 days.	**Women** – May have no, or mild, physical signs. Chlamydia may cause an unusual vaginal discharge and possibly painful intercourse. It can spread to the uterus and fallopian tubes causing pelvic inflammatory disease (PID), leading to lower abdominal pain, fever and feeling generally unwell. Chlamydia can live in the cervix undetected for months, flaring up at any time in the future, possibly leading to chronic pain, infertility and/or ectopic pregnancies. **Men** – Infects the urethra leading to pain when passing urine, and possibly a discharge. However, many men do not notice symptoms. It can spread to the prostate and testes, sometimes causing chronic pain and/or fertility problems.
Cytomegalovirus (CMV) – A viral infection that is not highly contagious. Acquired through close, personal contact with saliva or urine from young children or sexual intercourse and kissing with an infected adult. **Incubation** – 28 to 60 days, averaging 40 days.	Most adults do not show physical signs. If they do occur, it can be similar to glandular fever, with headache, sore throat, weakness and fatigue.
Gonorrhoea (the clap) – A sexually transmitted bacterial infection that can only be transmitted through sexual intercourse (or oral sex). Using condoms when having sex with new or different partners helps prevent infection. **Incubation** – 2 to 7 days.	**Women** – Physical signs can be very mild, or even absent for some time, may cause burning or discomfort when passing urine and/or an abnormal vaginal discharge (often yellow-green in colour). If the gonorrhoea remains untreated, it can spread to the uterus and fallopian tubes causing pelvic inflammatory disease (PID), possibly leading to fertility problems.

Effects on the pregnancy or baby	Tests and treatments
Pregnant women should avoid exposure when possible. Chicken pox experienced early in the pregnancy has a very low chance of infecting the unborn baby (0.4% from conception to 13 weeks, 2.2 % from 13 to 20 weeks). However, if the baby is infected, this increases the chance of miscarriage, slow growth of the baby and sometimes abnormalities of their bones, muscles, fingers, toes, eyes or brain. Infections after 20 weeks may cause the unborn baby to develop chicken pox in the uterus (including a rash with skin scarring). Newborn babies are most at risk of developing severe chicken pox if their mother has a rash 4 days before, or 2 days after, the birth (30% chance). If an older baby develops chicken pox, the infection is usually mild.	Pregnant women who think they are not immune and have been exposed to chicken pox need to have a blood test for IgG and IgM** antibodies. This may need to be repeated in 7-10 days. A rising titre shows the infection has been recent. A zoster immunoglobulin (ZIG) injection can be given within 96 hours of exposure to help make the infection milder. Sometimes antiviral medication is prescribed. Newborn babies may be given ZIG to decrease the severity of the infection (or help prevent it). Vaccination (2 doses 1 to 2 months apart) is available for children over 12 months of age. A blood test is usually done to check immunity in adolescents and adults before vaccination. You may decide to have this when planning a pregnancy, but you will need to delay conception for 2 months. Vaccination is not advised during pregnancy.
Pregnant women may experience their waters breaking prematurely (before 37 weeks) and/or premature labour. If Chlamydia is present during the birth, there is a 5 to 25% chance the baby will become infected, possibly leading to eye, ear and lung infections (pneumonia) during the first few weeks after birth. Blindness may occur if eye infections are not treated. Chlamydia may cause a uterine infection after the birth.	A swab test needs to be taken of the woman's cervix or the man's penis. Sometimes it can be detected in a urine sample. Chlamydia tests need to be delayed at least 7 days from the recent sexual contact. Antibiotics are prescribed. Sexual partners also need to be treated and sex needs to be avoided while taking antibiotics, to avoid infecting others or becoming reinfected yourself.
CMV is rare during pregnancy, but if it does occur, 40 to 50% of babies become infected. If the pregnancy is less than 20 weeks, 5 to 15% of babies develop birth defects and up to 30% of babies die soon after birth. Of the babies who survive, 85–90% have long-term health effects (hearing loss, blindness and/or mental delays). If the baby is infected at birth or while breastfeeding, they rarely become unwell. Women previously infected with CMV do not necessarily have immunity. However, the unborn baby is less likely to be affected.	Testing is difficult as a single high IgG** titre cannot show if an infection is new (primary), or a reinfection (secondary). Usually 2 tests are done 4 weeks apart to try to detect rising titres. A current infection may be detected through testing urine or saliva samples. There are no treatments or vaccinations available for CMV.
Pregnant women may experience their waters breaking prematurely (before 37 weeks) and/or premature labour. If gonorrhoea is present during a vaginal birth, 30 to 47% of babies are infected (more likely if the waters have been broken for more than 24 hours). Gonorrhoea can cause a severe infection of the uterus after birth. The	A swab test is taken from the woman's cervix or the man's penis. Tests need to be delayed at least 7 days from the recent sexual contact. Gonorrhoea is effectively treated with antibiotics. Sexual partners also need to be treated and sex avoided while taking the antibiotics, to avoid infecting others or becoming reinfected yourself. Depending on where

Gonorrhoea (cont.)

Men – May lead to burning or discomfort when passing urine and possibly a discharge. If the infection remains untreated, it can spread to the prostrate and testes, possibly leading to fertility problems. Gonorrhoea can also cause a sore throat, if a person becomes infected after oral sex.

Genital herpes – A sexually transmitted virus (herpes simplex virus 2 or HSV2), which is different from oral herpes or cold sores (herpes simplex virus 1 or HSV1). Transmitted through skin-to-skin contact with a herpes sore during sexual intercourse, oral sex or touching the genitals of a person with an outbreak. It is most infectious during the prodromal symptoms (tingling, pain, feeling unwell or irritable, before the actual sore appears), but the person remains infectious until the sore completely heals (about 6 to 7 days).
Incubation – The virus enters the body, travels down the nerves to the genital area and lies dormant. It is 'reactivated', causing an outbreak, 2 to 20 days after first being infected, or months or years later. Some people carry the virus and never have an outbreak.

Produces periodic outbreaks of sores on the genitals, buttocks or around the anus. It does not affect a person's fertility and is not transmitted by sperm. Outbreaks may be sporadic, usually when tired, run down, premenstrual, stressed or not eating well. Signs of a baby having neonatal herpes include blisters anywhere on their body, a fever, and the baby being extremely irritable and not wanting to feed. Seek medical attention if you think your baby has contracted neonatal herpes.

Hepatitis A – A viral infection that inflames the liver. It is transmitted by contact with contaminated bowel motions in water supplies, foods washed in contaminated water, eating oysters and shellfish contaminated with sewerage, eating utensils handled by the unwashed hands of an infected person, changing the nappy of an infected baby, or anal or oral sex with an infected person. Bowel motions are infectious for 2 weeks before physical signs are apparent, until 1 to 2 weeks after jaundice is first visible (3 to 4 weeks in total).
Incubation – Between 2 and 7 weeks, with an average of 4 weeks.

Physical signs are nausea, vomiting, loss of appetite, weight loss, abdominal pain, diarrhoea, mild fever, aching joints, headaches, jaundice, dark coloured urine, pale bowel motions, an enlarged liver. Jaundice can last from 1 to 6 weeks, before making a full recovery. Hepatitis A does *not* cause long-term liver problems and once a person has experienced an infection they have lifelong immunity.

Hepatitis B – A viral infection that inflames the liver. It is transmitted by coming into contact with the infected blood of another person (sharing injecting equipment, razors, contact with open wounds, tattooing or body piercing with non-sterile equipment, occupational

Physical signs include tiredness, fatigue, abdominal pain, fever, aching joints and muscles, skin rashes, nausea, vomiting, jaundice, dark coloured urine, pale bowel motions and an enlarged liver. About 50% of infected adults show physical signs. The remaining 50% are not visibly ill but are capable of newborn baby can experience conjunctivitis within a week of birth, possibly causing partial or complete blindness if not treated. *NOTE: It is normal for many newborn babies to have sticky eyes, which may require regular cleansing with sterile saltwater, or squirting breastmilk into their eyes.*

you have your baby, treatments for them can include silver nitrate eye drops, antibiotic eye drops, iodine-based medications or giving the baby antibiotics.

Up to 25% of pregnant women (and/or their partners) have genital herpes. Many women experience more frequent outbreaks, or notice a first outbreak during pregnancy. Transfer of the virus from mother to baby is low risk if the woman already had genital herpes before conceiving. Antibodies pass to the baby providing a degree of natural immunity, but having cold sores does not protect the baby. About 0.25% of babies born to women carrying herpes develop neonatal herpes (5% if the waters are broken for more than 4 hours during an active outbreak). If there are no signs of an outbreak during labour, it is very rare. Women infected for the first time before 28 weeks of pregnancy can develop antibodies to protect their baby at birth. However, premature babies less than 28 weeks have no protection, with at least 50% of these babies being infected. Babies who develop neonatal herpes after birth may experience eye infections, fits or seizures and possibly mental delays, which can sometimes be life-threatening. Antiviral medications help 50% of babies recover well.

Women who have herpes for the first time during pregnancy need a viral swab of any visible sores. A blood test can let you know if it is HVS1 or HSV2. However, it may not be able to determine a new or old infection. A routine caesarean is often advised for women experiencing an outbreak when labour starts, or once the waters break. About 16% to 30% of babies born by caesarean are infected (usually if the waters break first). Some women cover their sores with a plastic-backed bandaid or dressing during a vaginal birth, to increase protection for their baby. Antiviral medications may be prescribed to lessen the chances of the baby being infected and may be routinely prescribed during the last few weeks of pregnancy to reduce the chance of an outbreak during labour. The safety and effectiveness of this is not known. Natural therapies† can be used from 37 weeks to boost the immune system and discourage an outbreak. You may try using betadine (from chemists) or diluted tea tree oil in a carrier oil or Aloe vera gel or calendula tincture or ointment on sores. *NOTE: Babies can develop neonatal herpes from being kissed by someone with a cold sore. People with cold sores can hold your baby. If you have genital herpes, wash your hands before touching your baby.*

Pregnant women with hepatitis A do not generally infect their unborn babies. However, vaccination is advised 2 weeks before if travelling to countries with high rates of hepatitis A. Immunity lasts for 12 months after 1 vaccination and 20 years if revaccinated. If exposed to hepatitis A an injection of immunoglobulin (NIGH) and hepatitis A vaccine may be prescribed within 2 weeks of contact to try and reduce physical symptoms. Most children up to 6 years remain well, or only have very mild physical signs, but are still infectious. Breastfeeding women infected with hepatitis A are encouraged to breastfeed, but should wash their hands thoroughly with warm water and soap after changing the baby's nappy or going to the toilet before touching their breasts and nipples.

A blood test for anti-HAV IgM** antibodies can detect an infection, but only during the 2 weeks before physical signs appear, or while the person is ill (2 to 5 weeks after being exposed). Positive anti-HAV IgG antibodies means you have had hepatitis A in the past and are immune. Treatments include rest, fluids and a nutritious diet. Some women use natural therapies† to help boost their immune system. You should not share eating and drinking utensils, linen or towels (which need to be washed separately in warm, soapy water in a washing machine). If possible, don't prepare food for others, including baby bottles. If this is not possible, wash your hands thoroughly with warm water and soap before handling food, or wear clean (preferably disposable) gloves.

Pregnant women exposed to hepatitis B may be prescribed an injection of hep B immunoglobulin (HBIG) within 72 hours, as well as the hepatitis B vaccine (within 7 days of exposure). A second vaccination is given 1 month later and a third around 6 months after

A blood test for hepatitis B is routinely done at your first pregnancy visit. If you carry hepatitis B, the blood test is positive for HBsAg. A positive anti-HBs or HBsAb means you are immune to hepatitis B (after vaccination or a past infection). There is a 3 month window period between the time of first

Hepatitis B (cont.)
needle stick injuries) and through sexual intercourse, and to a lesser extent saliva.
Incubation – 6 to 25 weeks.

infecting others. About 5% continue to carry the virus in their bodies for years (called carriers); 25% experience long-term liver disease, and 15 to 25% develop liver cancer later in life.

Hepatitis C – A viral infection that inflames the liver. It is transmitted by contact with the blood of an infected person (sharing injecting equipment, tattooing or body piercing with non-sterile equipment, sharing toothbrushes or razors, occupational needle stick injuries or blood transfusions before February 1990 in Australia). It is *not* transmitted through saliva and very rarely through sex. 50% of people who find out they have hepatitis C do not know how they became infected.
Incubation – 3 to 20 weeks, averaging 6 to 10 weeks.

Physical signs include a mild fever, feeling tired, loss of appetite, nausea, vomiting, diarrhoea, muscular aches and possibly a mild body rash and occasionally jaundice. Only 25% of people become unwell with hepatitis C. The remaining 75% are capable of infecting others (called carriers). 15 to 20% of adults clear the virus within 2 to 6 months and stop being infectious. 80 to 85% continue to carry the virus in their bodies for years. Of these, 60 to 65% develop long-term liver damage (after 15 years) and 20 to 25% develop liver cirrhosis (after 20 to 40 years), while a minority of people develop liver cancer.

HIV/AIDS – A person can be infected by coming in contact with blood, semen or vaginal fluid of an infected person, needle stick injuries, blood splashes, a blood transfusion before May 1985 in Australia. It is *not* spread by kissing or contact with sweat, tears, vomit or bowel motions and cannot be transmitted by mosquitoes.
Incubation – 1 to 6 weeks.

Physical signs are initially a flu-like illness, tiredness, headache, sore throat, fever, mild rash, enlarged lymph nodes, vomiting and diarrhoea. This is a temporary primary HIV infection. After recovering, the person carries HIV and can infect others and may progress onto AIDS within 8 to 10 years. AIDS weakens the immune system, making normal infections, like the common cold or diarrhoea, life-threatening. Some people who are HIV positive, are not ill and never progress to AIDS.

HPV (Human Papilloma Virus) – A common wart virus. There are over 100 different types. Some cause genital warts, others may lead to cell changes in a cervix. Up to 80% of the population carry some type of wart virus, which is thought to be spread through close body contact (not necessarily sexual).
Incubation – Unknown, possibly a month to several years.

Most people carry HPV for many years but don't have physical signs. Genital warts (condyloma) can develop as tiny, flat, flesh-coloured bumps or small, soft, cauliflower-like clumps at the entrance of the vagina and around the anus in women, and the penis, scrotum and anus in men. Individual warts only measure 1 to 2 mm, but clusters can cover a large area. They are usually not uncomfortable, but sometimes itch, burn, feel tender or bleed. Most people's immune system eventually make the warts disappear without treatments (within weeks, months or sometimes years). For a few people, the warts continue to appear and spread for several years, despite treatments. Being immune to one type of HPV does not mean immunity to other types of HPV. HPV may be detected with a Pap test, if it is causing minor cell changes in the cervix which usually heal on their own, but can occasionally progress to cancer of the cervix if not monitored, about 5 to 15% of the time.

this. Pregnant women who carry hepatitis B do not infect their unborn baby. However, the baby may be exposed and infected at birth (up to 40%, vaginal or caesarean), or through breastfeeding. The baby is given an injection of hepatitis B immunoglobulin (HBIG) soon after birth, before their first breastfeed and their first (of 3) hepatitis B vaccinations within 7 days of birth. Mothers who carry the hepatitis B virus are encouraged to breastfeed their baby.

being exposed to when blood tests show positive. There are no treatments for hepatitis B, except rest, fluids and a nutritious diet. Some people use natural therapies[†] to help boost their immune system. Carriers of hepatitis B virus need to practise safe sex (using condoms) and should not share toothbrushes, razors or other personal items that may transmit blood or saliva to another person.

Pregnant women with hepatitis C have a 5 to 10% chance of infecting their baby. However, this is increased if the woman is first infected during pregnancy. Hepatitis C is not passed through breast milk and breastfeeding is encouraged, unless the nipples are cracked or bleeding. The baby may have a blood test at 6 to 8 weeks of age, to measure hepatitis C virus in their blood. If the baby is infected, the outlook for their health is similar to infected adults.

Testing for hepatitis C during pregnancy is increasingly routine. However, it is not compulsory. If you carry the virus, the blood test is antibody positive. There is a 3 month window between being first exposed and a blood test showing positive. There is no cure or vaccination for hepatitis C. Treatments to fight the virus (Interferon and Ribavirin) have a high risk of causing birth defects. Women are advised not to conceive for at least 6 months after stopping Ribavirin and not take it while breastfeeding. Some women also use natural therapies[†] to help boost their immune system.

About 50% of all HIV positive women in Australia are mothers. Babies born to HIV positive mothers have about a 15 to 30% risk of becoming infected, but with treatments available, this can be as low as 2%. Caesarean birth may lower infection for the baby by up to 50% when compared to vaginal birth. Breastfeeding can double the risk of the baby becoming infected and is usually advised against.

A blood test for HIV during pregnancy is increasingly routine but is not compulsory. Women who carry HIV show as antibody positive. There is a 3 month window between first being exposed and the blood test showing positive. There is no cure for HIV and no vaccine. A variety of medications can slow the progress of HIV and reduce the chances of the baby being infected. These include antiretroviral medications such as Zidovine (AZT), which appear to be safe for the baby, and Protease inhibitors, the effects of which are unknown.

Genital warts is fairly common during pregnancy. Hormones lower the immune system and encourage them to grow and flourish. In most cases they disappear after the birth. Treatments are not required, but may be done as a personal choice. Newborn babies usually do not show physical signs. In very rare cases, the baby or small child can develop laryngeal papillomatosis, where small warts grow on their vocal chords (0.04%). This can be treated. The baby may be infected by the mother or through contact with others after birth. A caesarean is not recommended, as it does not prevent the transmission of the virus from mother to baby. Treating visible warts during pregnancy does not decrease the chances of a baby being infected (if delivered vaginally or by caesarean), as the underlying viral infection is still present. Genital warts do not affect whether a woman has a vaginal tear at birth and is not a reason to routinely perform an episiotomy.

Most people carry HPV and it is only routinely tested for indirectly through routine Pap tests. The success of genital wart treatments varies and is unpredictable, making it hard to know if they have helped, or if the person's immune system made them go away. The only chemical thought to be safe during pregnancy and while breastfeeding is Trichloroacetic acid (TCA), which needs to be applied by a health professional. *NOTE: Do not treat genital warts yourself with non-prescription drugs meant for wart removal on other parts of the body. Freezing, burning, laser or surgical removal may be used if they are large and may be considered after the birth if they don't disappear. Many women use natural therapies[†] to boost their immune system or treat genital warts.*

Measles (ordinary measles or rubeola) – A highly contagious virus spread by the infected person coughing and sneezing or by coming in contact with their contaminated items (eg. tissues, drinking glasses or soiled hands). The person is infectious from the first symptoms, until about 5 days after the rash appears. Then they have lifelong immunity.
Incubation – 7 to 14 days averaging 10 days for early symptoms, a rash appearing 4 days later.

Most adults are immune to ordinary measles. Non-immune adults and children may experience sneezing, tiredness, runny nose, slight fever, dry cough, headache, and sore, red watery eyes, followed by a blotchy, red rash that starts on the face before spreading down towards the feet until the whole body is covered (taking about 36 hours). The rash turns brownish, then fades after 5 days. About 3% of people develop pneumonia or ear infections and about 0.1% develop an infection of the brain (encephalitis), which may be life-threatening.

Mumps (myxovirus) – Infects the parotid glands, which produce saliva, and is spread by a person coughing and sneezing or contact with their contaminated items (eg. tissues, drinking glasses or soiled hands). The person is infectious for 1 to 2 days before symptoms start, until 9 days after the swelling appears. Usually infects children between 5 and 15 years, but occasionally non-immune adults.
Incubation – 12 to 28 days, averaging 18 days.

Most adults are immune, 15% to 20% of people do not have physical signs. Those who do become ill can experience fever, headache, loss of appetite, swollen, tender glands, pain and soreness around the jaw and neck, possibly abdominal pain and back pain. Up to 30% of adult men develop swollen, painful testicles (orchitis) up to a week or so later. Very rarely this can lead to fertility problems. Women may have inflamed ovaries (oophoritis). This does not affect their fertility. In very rare cases, mumps can infect the brain, although most people recover well without treatments. Another very rare complication is hearing loss.

Parvovirus B19 (5th disease or slapped cheek syndrome) – A viral illness spread by the infected person coughing and sneezing, or by coming in contact with their contaminated items (eg. tissues, drinking glasses or soiled hands). It is most infectious before the rash appears. Once the rash is evident the person is no longer infectious. After the illness the person is usually immune for life.
Incubation – 4 to 20 days, averaging 14 days.

Up to 40 to 60% of adults are immune, especially those working with children (childcare, teachers etc.). Many people are not aware of having had the illness as a child, because their physical signs are mild. These are often flu-like including fever, tiredness, possibly a cough, red cheeks (giving a 'slapped cheek' appearance), an itchy lace-like rash on the body, arms and legs, joint pain and swelling. The rash disappears in 7 to 10 days.

Rubella or German measles – A milder form of ordinary measles, but not as infectious. It tends to be seasonal (late winter, spring and early summer) and is spread by the person coughing and sneezing, or by coming in contact with their contaminated items (eg. tissues, drinking glasses or soiled hands). The person is infectious for 4 to 5 days after the rash appears. Vaccinated immunity (if successful) is believed to last for 16 years. A natural rubella infection provides longer immunity, but may not be lifelong.
Incubation – 14 to 21 days, averaging 18 days.

About 95% of women are immune (due to vaccination programs). Physical signs are very mild and many people are not aware they have rubella, but can include a headache, sore throat, runny nose, mild fever, followed by a mild rash (small pink spots) starting on the face and scalp, then spreading to the arms and body, occasionally spreading to the legs, fading after 2 or 3 days. May have swollen glands behind the ears and the neck or stiff, painful joints. Can rarely cause temporary thrombocytopenia (low platelet blood cells).

Ordinary measles does not cause abnormalities in unborn babies (like rubella). However, it may increase the chances of miscarriage, low birth weight or premature birth. If the mother has measles close to the time of the baby's birth, the baby is at risk of being infected.

The type of measles you have can only be determined by a blood test. Some caregivers prescribe an immunoglobulin injection, usually within 3 days of exposure, aiming to make the infection milder. There is a measles vaccine, usually given in combination with mumps and rubella (MMR) vaccines, as part of the immunisation schedule for children (given at 1 and 5 years of age). Measles vaccinations are not recommended during pregnancy, and conception should be delayed for at least 2 months after vaccination. Treatments include rest and drinking plenty of fluids. Some people use natural therapies† to help them recover.

Natural mumps infection during pregnancy does not cause birth defects or premature birth, but if the woman is infected during the first 12 weeks, the risk of miscarriage is increased. Mumps is rare in babies less than 12 months of age, because they usually gain temporary immunity from their mother.

There is a mumps vaccine, usually given in combination with measles and rubella (MMR) vaccines, as part of the immunisation schedule for children (given at 1 and 5 years of age). Mumps vaccination is not recommended during pregnancy, and conception should be delayed at least 2 months after vaccination. Treatments include rest, eating soft foods, soups and drinking plenty of fluids. Some people use natural therapies† to help them recover.

Pregnant women who become infected with parvovirus usually only experience a mild illness. It does not cause birth defects. However, if a woman is infected during the first 20 weeks of pregnancy, this can increase her chances of miscarrying. Up to 5% of babies develop anaemia, which may be severe enough to lead to a condition called fetal hydrops. This can sometimes be life-threatening, although most unborn babies become well on their own without treatments. A few require a blood transfusion while still in the uterus.

Pregnant women can be tested for IgG and IgM antibodies**, to see if they are immune, or have recently been infected. Some caregivers recommend more ultrasounds and more frequent pregnancy visits. There are no vaccinations or treatments. If an older sibling has parvovirus, careful hand washing and avoiding sharing drinks can help prevent infection. Isolating the child is not necessary, as they are not infectious once the rash appears. Staying away from work during pregnancy if there is an outbreak is not generally recommended, as the woman has most likely already been exposed. However, this is a personal decision after discussions with your family, employer and caregiver.

Women infected before 20 weeks of pregnancy may have a baby with abnormalities. During the first 8 to 10 weeks of pregnancy, there is a 90% chance of having multiple abnormalities (deafness, blindness, mental delays and heart abnormalities). Infections between 10 and 16 weeks have a 10 to 20% chance of abnormalities, but usually not as severe. From 16 to 20 weeks, effects on the baby are rare. Infections after 20 weeks should not affect the baby. Women with past immunity to rubella (even if this has diminished over time) have only a very small chance of their baby being affected, no matter what stage of the pregnancy. It is

A blood test for rubella immunity is routine during pregnancy. Women who are not immune are offered a vaccination after their baby is born to boost their immunity for future pregnancies. This can produce mild rubella symptoms about 1 to 3 weeks afterwards, but this is **not** infectious and does not affect the baby if breastfeeding. The vaccine is usually given in combination with measles and mumps (MMR) vaccines, as part of the immunisation schedule for children (given at 1 and 5 years of age). Rubella vaccination is not recommended during pregnancy, and conception should be delayed at least 2 months after vaccination. Non-immune women exposed to the

Rubella or German measles (cont.)

Toxoplasmosis – An infection caused by a small parasite called toxoplasmosis gondii. Cats acquire it from eating infected animals such as mice and birds. Humans can be infected by coming in contact with cat faeces (or faeces of other infected animals) and then not washing their hands thoroughly before eating. Faeces can remain infective in water or moist soil for up to 1 year. You can also become infected by eating raw or undercooked meat infected by toxoplasmosis. Once the meat is cooked the toxoplasmosis dies. A person can only be infected once, they then have immunity for life. An infected person cannot pass toxoplasmosis on to another person.
Incubation – Not really known. Toxoplasmosis parasites can grow and multiply within 5 to 23 days after entering the body, but it can take many weeks or months before signs of infection appear (if they appear at all).

Most healthy adults, children and babies are not bothered by a toxoplasmosis infection and do not become unwell. Pregnant women and people with lowered immune systems are more susceptible and may experience swollen glands, muscle pains, and a fever that may come and go and generally feeling unwell.

Trichomonas – A common sexually transmitted infection caused by a protozoan parasite called Trichomonas vaginalis. Can only be transmitted through sexual intercourse. Using condoms when having sex with new or different partners helps prevent infection.
Incubation – 4 to 20 days.

Women – A vaginal infection, with a frothy yellow-green discharge, and an unusual vaginal odour. Possibly feeling itchy or sore and experiencing pain when urinating or having sex. Although these physical signs can be quite severe, there is no long-term health problems.
Men – Usually showing no physical signs. May have mild discomfort when urinating or a minor discharge.

**IgG and IgM antibodies both show positive shortly after being infected. IgM often disappears several months later but IgG stays positive forever. If you test positive for IgG, but not IgM, the infection happened more than several months ago. If you test positive for IgG and IgM, then the infection was more recent, but it is difficult to pinpoint the exact time.
†Natural therapies to boost the immune system include: cloves of raw garlic or garlic capsules; eating lysine-rich foods (potatoes, brewer's yeast, fish, beans, eggs, foods with vitamin B, C or zinc); rest and relaxation (massage, acupressure, meditation, visualisation, yoga); herbal echinacea or teas with chamomile, St John's wort, scullcap, burdock root, dandelion, nettle or passionflower; homeopathic remedies such as Natrum muriaticum, Rhus toxicodendron, Sepia, Dulcamera or Hepar sulphuris; avoiding fatigue, eating too many sugars or arginine-rich foods (eg. peanuts, chocolate, cola).

important to speak with a genetic counsellor. Ultrasounds after 18 to 19 weeks may detect some abnormalities, but the extent of effects (such as deafness or blindness) are not fully known until the child is older.

Newborn babies usually have no symptoms or only experience a very mild illness after birth. If a woman is infected for the first time during pregnancy, this can increase her chances of miscarrying or infecting her unborn baby and causing congenital toxoplasmosis, which is rare. The more developed the baby is, the less likely they will become unwell. Before 13 weeks of pregnancy, about 17% of babies become infected, of which 14% are severely ill (anaemia, jaundice, small head size, fluid on the brain, vision impairment, blindness, deafness, recurrent seizures or fits, mental delay). After 28 weeks, 65 to 72% of babies are infected, but hardly any of them become unwell. It is very important to speak with a genetic counsellor.

It is unclear whether Trichomonas affects a woman's pregnancy or her unborn baby. It used to be thought that it may cause premature labour, but this has now been disproved. At this stage, Trichomonas is not thought to cause any health concerns for mother or baby.

rubella virus during pregnancy are usually prescribed an immunoglobulin injection. This does not stop the infection from occurring, but may slightly delay the incubation period.

Up to 90% of people have immunity to toxoplasmosis. A new infection may be detected by a blood test. However, it may show positive, when in fact it is actually negative, because you are immune. Two or more tests need to be done days apart, to look for rising IgM** antibody levels. There is no toxoplasmosis vaccination. Treatments for non-immune women infected with toxoplasmosis include antibiotics, but it is not clear whether these are capable of successfully treating unborn babies, or if they do more harm than good, because they can themselves cause birth defects. The baby is usually given a blood test soon after birth. Ways to avoid toxoplasmosis during pregnancy include: not cleaning cat litter trays without wearing gloves; disposing of litter daily, trays should be washed with boiling water; feeding the cat dry, canned or boiled foods and not letting it out for hunting and scavenging; cooking meat thoroughly. Wash your hands and kitchen utensils thoroughly with hot, soapy water. Children's sandpits should be covered when not in use.

A swab test of a woman's vaginal discharge is placed on a glass slide for the caregiver to view under a microscope. This can be done at the time of the consultation. Treatments include a single dose of metronidazole (Flagyl) antibiotic, often repeating the dose 2 weeks later. The woman's partner also needs to be treated and sex needs to be avoided for 24 hours after treatment. Although Flagyl is thought to be relatively safe during pregnancy, caregivers usually recommend delaying treatment until after 12 weeks. Some caregivers prescribe antifungal vaginal medications (similar to those used to treat thrush), which can be effective and safe.

In the beginning

ANNOUNCING YOUR PREGNANCY

Finding out you are pregnant can bring excitement mixed with tentative feelings about how the pregnancy will unfold. Some women tell everyone as soon as they know. Others prefer to wait a while. If you only want some people to know, make sure they will keep your secret for you!

Telling family and friends

A pregnancy often means your family becomes more involved in your life, which may be positive or negative. Depending on your circumstances, it can be difficult to know exactly the right time to tell those close to you. It helps if couples agree about when and how the pregnancy will be made known. You may want a joint announcement, or perhaps a one-on-one conversation with particular people, rather than telling everyone over Christmas lunch!

An unintended pregnancy can trigger a range of feelings for yourself and your partner, and may mean you have to deal with other people's reactions as well. Many women withdraw into themselves for a while, to integrate the reality of having a baby, before telling others. Take your time. Try not to feel rushed or pressured before you are ready.

Apprehension about the permanence of the pregnancy makes some parents, especially those who have experienced a pregnancy loss, reluctant to share their news until the magic 12 weeks, when the likelihood of miscarriage is considerably less. However, keeping a pregnancy quiet may not necessarily be the best thing, particularly if a miscarriage does occur. Many couples find they lack the support and understanding they need when grieving, because nobody knew. As one couple shared: 'Losing our baby was a very lonely experience. Everyone carried on as usual, not knowing what we were going through. We were left to mourn on our own.'

Not telling others can be a way of protecting yourself. However, it may increase feelings of stress, as you go about your day-to-day life under a cloud of concern. Consider sharing your feelings – it may not take your fears away but it might provide love and support at this vulnerable time.

Parents who choose genetic tests may not tell others about their pregnancy until the results are known. If the outcome is unfavourable, then agonising decisions about whether to end the pregnancy can make dealing with others' opinions difficult (especially if they conflict with your own). Take into consideration your emotional needs and bear in mind that grieving for your baby may be lonely and isolating if others aren't able to give you the support you need.

Telling your other children

When to tell your children is a very personal choice. You may share the news straightaway, or when the pregnancy starts showing, or once other family members know (in case it is blurted out to Grandma!). Research suggests that children should be made aware of a pregnancy as soon as possible, to help them clear any confusion they may feel about things being different.[10] They know and understand more than we give them credit for and are often aware of a pregnancy before being told. Giving simple explanations lets them share in your joy (or even loss, if the pregnancy miscarries) and helps them understand your emotions, providing life skills for dealing with positive and negative experiences.

Children are usually quite accepting, and generally go through periods of talking a lot about the baby, or not mentioning it at all. Many parents worry about their young child being impatient, or not understanding how long they must wait to see the baby. Sometimes giving them an event (like 'after Christmas' or 'after your birthday') helps, or telling them, 'I had to wait a long time to see you before you were born.' If they ask questions like 'How did the baby get in there?' or 'How will it get out?', answer them in a straightforward way, preferably using the correct terminology.

Older children and teenagers may feel put out, or express real joy and excitement. If the baby is part of a new relationship, it may be more difficult for them to accept. Give them space and just play it by ear. A new pregnancy is something everyone has to adjust to.

Telling employers and work colleagues

Telling your employer and others at work is entirely at your discretion. Even though pregnant women should not be discriminated against, it still happens in subtle ways. You may want to consider your career prospects or attend a job interview first. Some women prepare a contingency plan outlining when and how they will return to work and present this along with their good news.

CHOOSING A CAREGIVER AND BIRTHPLACE

Now you are pregnant, there are many decisions to make about where to have your baby and who will care for you. Your choices may be wide-ranging or limited by:
- Where you live and the services available.
- Your preferred caregiver(s), their availability and how early they book up.
- Whether your chosen caregiver attends your preferred birthplace.

- What you can afford and private health insurance (if you have it and choose to use it).

Your overall health, and whether your pregnancy is expected to progress normally, also play a role, especially if considering midwifery care, birth centres or homebirth.

If you've never had a baby before, it can be difficult to know what choice to make straight off. Often once you do some research and talk to others, it becomes clearer. Try to keep in mind that the choices your relatives or friends made may not be suitable for you. Perhaps ask them what they liked (or did not like) about their care and take it from there.

Shop around. Take on the role of a consumer, rather than patient. You should feel you are working in partnership with your caregiver. Before making a final decision, compile a list of questions. If you are not comfortable with the answers you are given, then look elsewhere.

Some questions to ask may include:

- Who will do my pregnancy checks? Is it the same person or a group of different caregivers? Is there flexibility to choose a caregiver?
- Who will attend the birth and what happens if my chosen caregiver cannot be there (if sick or on holidays)?
- What approach do you have to pregnancy and birth care? Are there routine procedures (continuous monitoring of the baby's heart rate, or an episiotomy)?
- Can I give birth in any position I choose (or in the shower or bath)?
- What are my pain relief options (natural and medical)?
- Are there limits to how many support people I can have? Can they be with me if I need a caesarean? Can I bring my other child(ren) to the labour?
- If complications arise, will I (or my baby) need to transfer to another ward or hospital?
- What about postnatal care? Can my partner stay overnight? Can I go home early and have home visits? Are mothers and babies separated for any reason after birth? What are the hospital's attitudes towards breastfeeding and bottle feeding?
- Are there any costs (whether insured or not)?

These can be starting points to work from. Perhaps write down your ideal situation and try to find a birthplace that most fits your expectations.

After a decision is made, remember, it is a woman's prerogative to change her mind! If you become dissatisfied, or find something better, you *can* change (if other options are available). While most women are loath to do this, it may be better than continuing with your original arrangements.

Partners should also feel comfortable about the choices being made. Make time to discuss your preferences, but ultimately it is the woman who labours and gives birth. Therefore, her needs are paramount.

Hospital antenatal clinic

Antenatal clinics are staffed by obstetric consultants, registrars, residents and midwives. The hospital also provides dieticians, physicians, social workers, genetic counsellors, ultrasonographers, physiotherapists, pathologists and childbirth educators. These services can also be accessed with a referral from other maternity caregivers (such as a GP or obstetrician), or you may use private services in your local community. Antenatal clinics care for normal and complicated pregnancies, as well as multiple pregnancies. Smaller and rural hospitals may only care for relatively normal pregnancies.

Pregnancy visits – You may see a mixture of caregivers, with a different person each time. Some hospitals offer the option of sharing care with your local doctor. Wait times for appointments can be long, depending on the hospital, as appointments may not be strictly scheduled.

Labour and birth – In the hospital's delivery suite, midwives monitor and facilitate most of the labour and birth care. Obstetric registrars and residents oversee the process, providing medical services as required. Senior obstetric registrars and consultants become involved if complications arise or if forceps, ventouse or a caesarean is required. Paediatric registrars or residents are present at the birth if the baby is premature or expected to be unwell. If you require stitches after the birth, this may be done by the midwife, or an obstetric resident or registrar attending the birth.

Pain relief options – These are natural forms such as heat packs, showers and possibly a bath. Not many delivery suites facilitate water births (ask them). Medical forms include gas, narcotic injections and epidurals. The rostered anaesthetic registrar inserts the epidural. Some smaller hospitals don't provide epidurals, or only make them available for caesareans or complications (such as very high blood pressure).

Postnatal care – This takes place on the postnatal ward of the hospital. Your stay will normally be three to five days after a normal birth, or five to seven days after a caesarean (longer if there are health complications or breastfeeding problems). This may be in a single or shared room. Your partner may be permitted to stay overnight if you are not sharing your room. Most public hospitals offer early discharge, which involves going home within 24 to 48 hours after the birth and being visited daily by a midwife, for an hour or so, for several days. If complications develop at home, you and/or your baby are re-admitted to the hospital.

Six to eight week postnatal check – This may be done at the hospital clinic or you may prefer to see your local doctor, women's health nurse or family planning clinic.

Fees – All services are bulk-billed to Medicare.

Midwives' clinic

Many public hospitals have a midwives' clinic, caring for relatively normal pregnancies. If you have a pre-existing health condition such as diabetes or a multiple pregnancy, you need to attend the antenatal clinic. If complications arise as the pregnancy progresses, the midwife refers you to the obstetric registrar or consultant. Depending on the condition, your care may be transferred to the doctors in the antenatal clinic for the remainder of the pregnancy.

Pregnancy visits – You usually see the same midwife for every visit, or two to three midwives at various times. They take blood tests and order ultrasounds as required. Waiting times for appointments are generally reasonable with scheduled times. Some midwives' clinics are conducted at convenient venues in the local community.

Labour and birth – In the hospital's delivery suite, although different midwives are rostered on to provide care. The hospital doctors only become involved if complications arise (similar to the hospital antenatal clinic).

Pain relief options – Pain relief options are the same as those explained previously.

Postnatal care – Postnatal care options are the same as explained previously. If you choose early discharge, the visiting midwife is usually different again from the midwife who provided your pregnancy visits and those who attended your labour and birth.

Six to eight week postnatal check – This may be with the midwives' clinic, or you may prefer to see a hospital doctor, local doctor, women's health nurse or family planning clinic.

Fees – All services are bulk-billed to Medicare.

Birth centres

Birth centres are staffed by 8 to 10 midwives, who provide total pregnancy, labour and birth care for normal pregnancies. Birth centres are usually part of a major public maternity hospital, but a few are privately run. Shared care with your GP, obstetrician or private midwife is usually offered.

Pregnancy visits – These are performed at the birth centre. You meet different midwives at various visits, with the aim of meeting them all, so you have someone you know caring for you during the labour and birth. They take blood tests and order ultrasounds as required. Waiting times for appointments are usually reasonable, as visits are scheduled. If complications arise, or the baby is breech, you are referred to the antenatal clinic doctors.

Labour and birth – The midwife rostered on provides all your labour and birth care (midwives change shifts every 8 to 10 hours). If complications arise (such as the baby being premature, the labour not progressing or the baby becomes distressed), transfer to the hospital's delivery suite is required. This is also necessary if the birth centre is full. If you require stitches after the birth, the birth centre midwife does this. A paediatric registrar comes to the birth centre if the baby unexpectedly needs medical attention.

Pain relief options – Birth centres support labour and birth as a normal, physical process requiring minimal intervention. Therefore pain relief is focussed on heat packs, showers, baths, acupressure, massage, TENS machines and other natural therapies. Most birth centres facilitate water birth if you want this. Medical forms of pain relief, such as gas and narcotics, are available if necessary. If you want, or need, an epidural, transfer to the hospital's delivery suite is required.

Postnatal care – You may be able to stay with your partner in the birth centre for several hours, or possibly overnight. Otherwise you move to the hospital's postnatal ward. If you choose early discharge, visits are done by different midwives. A few women choose to transfer to a private hospital.

Six to eight week postnatal check – Some birth centres provide this, usually with the midwife who was present at the birth. Otherwise you can see your local doctor, women's health nurse or family planning clinic.

Fees – Public birth centres are bulk-billed to Medicare. Private birth centres charges fees like private hospitals.

Midwifery teams and caseloads

Team midwifery involves 8 to 10 midwives working rostered shifts and being on-call to provide total pregnancy, labour, birth and postnatal care for normal pregnancies. Midwifery caseloads involve two or three midwives sharing total care of a few women.

Pregnancy visits – You meet all the midwives at various pregnancy visits. They take blood tests and order ultrasounds as required. Waiting times for appointments are reasonable, with scheduled times. Sometimes visits are conducted at convenient venues in the local community, or perhaps at your home.

Labour and birth – Usually at the hospital's delivery suite, but a birth centre may be used (if available) and occasionally homebirth is offered.

When labour starts, the midwife on call comes to provide labour and birth care (midwives change shifts every 8 to 12 hours). Hospital doctors only become involved if there are complications. If you are in a birth centre, transfer to the delivery suite is necessary if medical attention is required. If you need stitches, the midwife who attends the birth does this.

Pain relief options – These are the same as for a delivery suite or birth centre, depending on where you are labouring. Homebirths use natural forms of pain relief. Gas or narcotic injections can sometimes be arranged. Water births are usually facilitated (if a bath is available).

Postnatal care – Again, the same as provided by the public hospital delivery suite or birth centre. The team or caseload midwives provide home visits if you choose early discharge or have a homebirth.

Six to eight week postnatal check – This is often provided by the midwife who attended the birth. Alternatively, you can see your local doctor, women's health nurse or family planning clinic.

Fees – All services are bulk-billed to Medicare.

Local doctor

Some GPs provide pregnancy care. If they are accredited to the hospital or birth centre you are attending, they may offer shared care with the antenatal or midwives' clinic or birth centre. In rare cases, they may attend homebirths. GPs usually care for normal pregnancies (similar to midwifery services) and refer to doctors at the hospital if complications arise. Depending on the condition, your care may be transferred to the antenatal clinic for the rest of the pregnancy.

Pregnancy visits – These are provided at the doctor's rooms. Some visits are performed at the hospital or birth centre with shared care. Waiting times for appointments depend on how busy the doctor is. You will need to visit the hospital or birth centre by 12 to 14 weeks for a booking visit.

Labour and birth – Care is provided by the hospital delivery suite or birth centre, depending on where you plan to go. Usually the GP is not involved in labour and birth care, except in some rural areas, or if attending a homebirth.

Pain relief options – The same as the delivery suite or birth centre.

Postnatal care – Again, the same as for the public hospital or birth centre. Local doctors do not usually provide home visits with early discharge. This is provided by the hospital's midwives.

Six to eight week postnatal check – This can be done by your local doctor, or you may prefer to go to the hospital or birth centre, women's health nurse or family planning clinic.

Fees – Your local doctor may bulk-bill to Medicare, or charge a gap fee for each visit.

Private obstetrician

Private obstetricians provide pregnancy and birth care for normal, complicated and multiple pregnancies and attend public or private hospital delivery suites. A few attend birth centres if the pregnancy is progressing normally. Rarely do they attend homebirths. If your obstetrician is away on holidays, or at another birth, they organise another obstetrician to care for you. You may ask to meet this obstetrician during the pregnancy.

Pregnancy visits – These are provided at the obstetrician's rooms. They may take blood tests or ask you to attend a private pathologist. Waiting times for appointments are usually reasonable with scheduled times, but may be delayed or re-scheduled, if they are called away to deliver a baby.

Labour and birth – The midwives in the public or private delivery suites, or the birth centre, provide most of the labour care. They communicate with the obstetrician over the phone, who comes in for the birth, or before this, if complications arise. Obstetricians perform a forceps delivery, ventouse or a caesarean if required. A paediatric specialist is present at the birth if the baby is premature or needs medical attention. If you require stitches, the obstetrician does this.

Pain relief options – These are the same as the hospital delivery suite or birth centre. Private hospitals provide similar forms of pain relief to public hospitals. A specialist anaesthetist is on-call to insert an epidural if required. Most obstetricians do not facilitate water births.

Postnatal care – This is provided in the hospital's postnatal ward, with a single room in private hospitals and priority for a single room in public hospitals (but not guaranteed). Most private hospitals do not provide early discharge, but may give you contact numbers for private midwives who can. You should arrange this before you have your baby.

Six to eight week postnatal check – This is provided by the obstetrician or you may prefer to see your local doctor, women's health nurse or family planning clinic.

Fees – These vary widely and are partly covered by Medicare and private health insurance, often with large gap fees. Ask for a quote when booking. Health services do not attract GST in Australia and costs exceeding $1500 are presently tax deductible.

Private midwife

Private midwives provide all pregnancy, labour, birth and postnatal care for homebirth and sometimes attend birth centres or delivery suites, if accredited to them. They may work alone, or in partnership with another midwife, who covers for them if they are sick, on holiday or at another birth. You can ask to meet this midwife during the pregnancy. Independent midwives generally care for normal pregnancies, but in Australia they are not regulated and have their own criteria. For example, some will care for twins or breech babies.

NOTE: *One midwife should not care for more than five women a month.*

Pregnancy visits – These are provided at your home and/or at the midwife's home or their rooms. If complications arise, they refer you to a supportive obstetrician, or the hospital's doctors. Your local doctor usually orders blood tests and ultrasounds, unless the midwife is authorised to do this. If your appointment coincides with the midwife delivering another baby, the visit is rescheduled.

Labour and birth – Your midwife is on-call and provides all labour and birth care at your home (or birth centre or delivery suite), staying for two to three hours after the birth. A back-up midwife may be called if the labour is prolonged (18 to 24 hours or more), to give them a break for a few hours.

Pain relief options – Homebirths use natural forms of pain relief. Gas or narcotic injections can sometimes be arranged through your local doctor. Water births are usually facilitated.

Postnatal care – If you have your baby at the hospital or birth centre, you may stay in the postnatal ward. Otherwise your midwife visits you at home daily for one to two weeks, depending on your needs.

Six to eight week postnatal check – Your midwife usually provides this at your home, or you may prefer to see your local doctor, women's health nurse or family planning clinic.

Fees – Fees vary and are not covered by Medicare, although plans are underway to change this. Some private health funds partially rebate midwifery services. Check with your insurer. Health services do not attract GST in Australia and costs exceeding $1500 are presently tax deductible.

Booking in

Women usually see their local GP (or family planning clinic) first, to confirm their pregnancy and obtain a referral to a local maternity service or preferred obstetrician. Many GPs also provide pregnancy care (or shared care with other maternity caregivers). Be aware that your GP may not know all the services or obstetricians available (especially in metropolitan areas), or may only recommend services they prefer (for example, not offer homebirth or a birth centre). Talk to other pregnant women and parents and/or ring your local maternity hospital to find out more.

When booking in, your first antenatal visit is usually scheduled between 10 to 14 weeks of pregnancy. Ring for an appointment around six to eight weeks (or as soon as possible) and find out what you need to bring (eg. copies of test results, Medicare card or a written referral). If you want genetic tests, or require an early dating ultrasound, ask about this as well (or your GP may organise it). Some private hospitals book up early but will take tentative bookings by phone before your appointment with the obstetrician.

Transfer for the woman or baby

Birth is a normal process for up to 85% of women, and most babies are born on time and healthy. However, transferring from your planned birthplace may be required, which can be unsettling and unexpected. In Australia, 2.5% of pregnant women and 4% of babies (after birth) transfer to a specialist public maternity hospital for various reasons, including:
- The woman being seriously ill, during pregnancy or after the birth.
- The baby(s) being very premature (less than 34 weeks) or seriously ill.

Transfer to a hospital delivery suite is also possible when planning to have your baby in a birth centre or at home, mainly when the mother or baby requires closer monitoring and medical attention.

Intensive care nurseries for babies

Maternity hospitals have intensive care nurseries for unwell and premature babies. However, the 'level' of nursery provided is often the deciding factor as to whether transfer is necessary.

Level 1 is for relatively well babies requiring closer observation or minor treatments. Just about every maternity hospital has a level 1 nursery.

Level 2 is for babies who are unwell, requiring involved medical treatments such as an intravenous drip, humidicrib, oxygen, feeding with a tube and monitoring of the heart rate and breathing. Some private and smaller public hospitals and all major public maternity hospitals have a level 2 nursery.

Level 3 is for very sick and premature babies who require a ventilator (a machine that breathes for the baby) and advanced medical treatments. They have specialised staff and are only available at selected large public maternity and children's hospitals.

NOTE: *If transfer is required after the birth, caregivers will try to keep mother and baby(s) together. However, this is not always possible and you may need to be separated. Your partner (or support person) will then need to make the difficult decision to be with the baby(s), or with you, until you can be reunited.*

When having twins, triplets or more

If you find you are having twins, or more, your planned pregnancy care and birthplace may need to be reconsidered. Birth centres and midwifery services do not deliver twins, but sometimes shared care can be organised between these services and an obstetrician (or an obstetrician and GP). Occasionally a woman will plan a homebirth with a supportive midwife, if this is her strong preference and the pregnancy is otherwise progressing normally.

Depending on where you live, most caregivers recommend care by an obstetrician or a public antenatal clinic when having twins (and insist on it for triplets or quads). In some cases they also recommend the babies be born in a large public maternity hospital with a level 3 intensive care nursery capable of caring for very premature babies. Smaller public and rural hospitals, or private hospitals, may accept twins if there are no complications and the babies are born after about 34 weeks.

WHAT TO EXPECT AT YOUR FIRST PREGNANCY VISIT

You may look forward to your first pregnancy visit with excitement, or anticipate it with a degree of nervousness and apprehension. If you have never been pregnant before, it is hard to know what is involved. For many women this is their first real contact with hospitals, which can seem mysterious, intimidating and/or scary.

At the first visit your caregiver will ask you many questions and hopefully provide a lot of information. This can feel overwhelming and it may be difficult to absorb everything you are told. Consider writing down a list of questions beforehand and perhaps taking a few notes during the visit. You may take your partner if you have one, or a close relative or friend. This can be a good way to get them involved too and they can help you form first impressions.

NOTE: *You will be asked very personal questions about your health, past pregnancies and lifestyle habits. Therefore you may want to ask your caregiver to conduct some of the visit alone and then invite your partner, relative or friend in for the remainder of the consultation. If English is not your first language, ask for an interpreter. Don't rely on family and friends to interpret.*

The caregiver obtaining information – This includes your age, weight, height, general health, family medical history; allergies, past operations, mood disorders (eg. depression), past sexually transmitted infections, abnormal Pap tests and treatments; lifestyle habits (diet, exercise, smoking, alcohol, caffeine), past intravenous drug use; tattooing, body piercing (to assess risks for Hepatitis B, C or HIV/AIDS), exposures to environmental hazards, whether you are taking any prescribed medications, vitamin supplements or natural remedies.

You will be asked the details of past pregnancies (miscarriages, abortions, adopted babies); past contraceptive use, fertility treatments; the date of your last menstrual period, whether you have had any vaginal bleeding since then; when you first noticed pregnancy symptoms; what you are experiencing at the moment and perhaps ways to manage any unpleasant symptoms. Other topics include: whether the pregnancy was planned; whether you have good emotional and practical support; social and financial issues; as well as any relevant concerns, such as domestic violence.

NOTE: *You can request that very personal information is **not** recorded on your pregnancy record card. But your caregiver will make a note of them on their records.*

Physical examination – This usually entails:
- Taking your blood pressure.
- Feeling your belly. However, before 12 weeks of pregnancy the uterus is still contained within the bones of the pelvis and cannot be felt.
- Listening to your baby's heartbeat (only possible after 12 weeks and if your caregiver has a Doppler machine).
- Some caregivers do an overall physical health check by listening to your heart and lungs, and checking for breast lumps, etc.

NOTE: *You do not need to undress for a first pregnancy visit, but it may be helpful to wear clothes that allow your caregiver easy access to your belly. Unless you need a Pap test, there is really no reason to have a vaginal examination.*

Information and resources – Caregivers usually provide information and contact numbers for other services, depending on your needs:
- Further options for care during pregnancy, labour, birth and afterwards.
- Childbirth, early parenting and/or breastfeeding education classes.
- Physiotherapy services, pregnancy exercise or yoga classes.
- A dietician.
- Social worker for advice on financial issues, government support, housing or for counselling.
- Staff specialising in stopping, or cutting back, addictions.

At the end of the visit your caregiver should answer any questions you have and tell you the timing of subsequent visits for the remainder of the pregnancy, as well as book your next appointment. They should provide a 24-hour contact number in case you have urgent health concerns (usually a direct line to the hospital's delivery suite or birth centre). Private caregivers may provide a personal pager or mobile number, or ask you to ring their secretary.

Tests you may be offered

The first visit entails many routine tests, and possibly some optional ones, depending on your preferences and your caregiver's. Routine tests aim to identify potential or existing health conditions before any obvious physical signs emerge, so treatments can be started to prevent or minimise their effects. Some previously routine tests are now obsolete and new tests have been introduced. If you have a medical condition (such as diabetes), additional tests may be required.

Blood tests

Group and antibodies consists of three tests:
- Identifying your blood group (A, B, AB or O), in case you require a blood transfusion.
- Identifying your blood group's Rhesus factor, written as 'positive' (+) or 'negative' (–); for example 'A positive'.
- Screening for antibodies (or agglutinins). Ideally the result should be 'negative' or 'nil antibodies detected'.

Full blood count (FBC) looks at many cells in the blood, mainly:
- Haemoglobin (Hb), which indicates iron levels, with normal levels being 10.5 to 15.0 gm% (105 to 150 g/L).
- Platelets (thrombocytes), which relate to blood clotting and control of bleeding. Normal levels are 140,000 to 450,000.
- A serum ferritin may also be done (but not routinely), to measure iron stores. Normal serum ferritin is 20 to 150 ng/ml.

Rubella titre, to check immunity to the rubella virus. A rubella vaccination may be offered after the baby is born if you are not immune (less than 10 to 20 IU/ml).

Syphilis, 'VDAL/RPR and TPHA' routinely tests for this sexually transmitted infection, which often has no physical signs and can be carried for years. The result should be 'nonreactive' for no infection, but if it is present the result is 'reactive'. Antibiotics are prescribed (usually penicillin) to prevent the unborn baby being infected. The partner also needs to be tested and treated.

Hepatitis B and C, and HIV/AIDS screening is becoming increasingly accepted as routine. However, they are not compulsory and you may decline them if you wish. Your caregiver should provide pre-test counselling and an opportunity to discuss the social, physical and emotional implications of receiving a positive result.

Urine tests

You may be asked to provide a sterile urine specimen to test for mild bladder infections, which may occur without any physical signs during pregnancy. If an infection is detected, a course of antibiotics may be prescribed in case the infection worsens and causes premature labour later in the pregnancy.

Ultrasounds

An ultrasound may be performed in early pregnancy if you are bleeding (to check the baby's wellbeing) or to date the pregnancy if you're not sure how many weeks pregnant you are. A nuchal translucency scan may be done to screen for genetic abnormalities in the unborn baby. Some caregivers have ultrasound machines in their rooms to perform informal ultrasounds. These generally provide a limited amount of information, and you would still need additional ultrasounds performed by a qualified ultrasonographer to confirm your caregiver's findings. Informal ultrasounds are not essential and you can decline them if you prefer.

GENETIC TESTING

Genetic tests screen for, or detect, inherited disorders in unborn babies. They are increasingly being accepted as routine, especially for women in their late thirties and early forties. However, they *are* optional, no matter what your age. In fact, up to 40% of women over 37 years choose not to have genetic tests.

Screening tests

Screening tests aim to identify babies that **may** be at increased risk of having a genetic disorder. They are only an estimate and not 100% accurate. Many screening tests show high risk, yet the woman's baby is born healthy and normal, while a few tests show low risk, but the baby has a genetic disorder. Low risk does not mean no risk!

Diagnostic tests

Diagnostic tests are medically invasive procedures that hold small risks of:
- Miscarriage.
- Injury to the baby.
- Vaginal bleeding.
- Rupturing the waters.
- Infection of the uterus.

They obtain cells from inside the woman's uterus (the placenta, amniotic fluid or the baby's umbilical cord) to grow cells in a laboratory. The baby's genes are mapped and examined to confirm or rule out a genetic disorder. Diagnostic tests are up to 99% accurate, but cannot detect every problem a baby may have as there are over 5000 genetic markers for various disorders; realistically, not all of these can be looked for. However, if you know your family carries a rare disorder, your caregiver can request this specific marker be looked for.

Diagnostic tests can confirm whether your baby is a boy or a girl with 100% accuracy. Therefore, if you do not wish to know the gender of your baby, tell your caregiver. Normal results are stated as 46 XX (a girl) or 46 XY (a boy) and 'normal karyotype'.

Considerations

Genetic tests have far-reaching implications and many caregivers don't clearly spell out what they involve or, more importantly, what they can lead to. The bottom line is, if an abnormality is detected, there are no cures or treatments, the only options for parents are to:

1. Continue the pregnancy with the knowledge that their baby has a genetic disorder, but have the opportunity to prepare mentally and emotionally for this.
2. Terminate the pregnancy.

This may not be clear when having a screening test, but it can become more significant if the result of this test is 'high risk'; often creating enormous pressure to have a further diagnostic test. Parents then have to weigh up their need to find out whether their baby has a genetic disorder, with the possible risks of losing a potentially healthy baby. In fact, some parents do this statistically, depending on the results. For example, the chances of miscarrying from an amniocentesis is 1:200 (0.5%), more than twice as risky as the 1:500 (0.2%) chance of a genetic disorder.

It is important to consider all the issues carefully. Seeing a genetic counsellor can help with the decision-making process, but you should feel free to refuse tests if you don't want them. Some parents find genetic counselling biased towards having the tests, so you may need to take this into consideration.

Understanding the numbers

Screening tests don't provide absolute yes or no answers and these uncertainties can be frustrating for many parents. High or low risk results are statistically expressed as odds (eg. 1 in 100), with the aim of helping you understand the likelihood of having a child with a genetic disorder. However, odds can be difficult to grasp fully and most people understand percentages much better (1 in 100 = 1%). Therefore, when looking at odds, bear in mind that:

- They refer to the probability of an outcome for a single event. Therefore, a person with a one in four chance of having a baby with a genetic disorder has this chance with each separate pregnancy. It does **not** mean that if a person has four children, three will be normal and one will not.
- They refer to the likelihood of the abnormality occurring, not to the likelihood of having a normal baby. For example, if a woman has a 1 in 300 chance of having a baby with an abnormality, she has a 299 in 300 chance of having a normal baby.

Also, if you look at the percentage of an event **not** happening, this may be more reassuring. For example, a 1 in 100 (or 1%) chance means you have a 99% chance that it will not occur.

NOTE: *To convert an odd to a percentage, divide 1 by the odd and then multiply by 100. For example, if the odds are 1:650 the calculation is:*

$$\frac{1}{650} = 0.0015 \text{ then } 0.0015 \times 100 = 0.15\%$$

Age-related risk

A woman's age-related risk is a comparison with the expected risk for other women the same age. This calculates whether you are at a higher or lower risk. As an example, the normal age-related risk for having a baby with Down syndrome is:

- 1 in 1500 (0.06%) for women under 21 years.
- 1 in 1000 (0.1%) for women at 29 years of age.
- 1 in 300 (0.3%) for women at 36 years of age.
- 1 in 100 (1%) for women at 40 years of age.
- 1 in 30 (3.3%) for woman at 45 years of age.

The age-related risk is combined with the results of the screening test to calculate an overall risk for the baby having a specific genetic disorder.

NOTE: *Be aware that measurements on the higher level of 'normal' are still normal; statements like this often create unnecessary concern.*

Genetic tests

Screening tests

Nuchal translucency (NT) – Uses ultrasound to visualise and measure a fluid-filled sac at the back of the unborn baby's neck, usually between 11 weeks and 14 weeks. A blood test is often done as well. This increases the accuracy of the NT scan from 75% to 85%. (Blood tests are not done for multiple pregnancies, because they are not accurate.)

AFP blood test (alpha-fetoprotein) – Assesses the likelihood that an unborn baby will have a neural tube defect, but cannot definitely tell if a defect exists.

Triple test – A blood test that measures alpha-fetoprotein (AFP) for neural tube defects and 2 hormones to estimate the risk of the baby having Down syndrome. Other names are maternal serum test or Bart's test.

Quadruple test (or triple test plus) – A triple test with an extra blood test looking for an enzyme (alkaline phosphatase) in the white cells of the blood. This is quite expensive and not widely used, but increases the accuracy of the triple test from 80% to 90%.

How is it done?

A specially trained ultrasonographer places the transducer on your lower abdomen to measure the baby's nuchal fluid. It can take up to 30 minutes to obtain an adequate measurement, especially if the baby is in an awkward position. Occasionally, the NT scan is performed vaginally, to look more closely at the baby. However, you are not obliged to consent to this if you feel uncomfortable about having a transvaginal ultrasound.

A blood test is done between 16 and 18 weeks of pregnancy. After 18 weeks it cannot be relied upon. The accuracy depends on the unborn baby's age being calculated correctly.

A blood test is taken at about 16 weeks of pregnancy (can be done between 14 and 21 weeks). The accuracy depends on the unborn baby's age being calculated correctly.

What will it tell me?

Generally, the larger the measurement (or depth of fluid), the greater the chance the baby may have a genetic disorder, such as Down syndrome, Edward's syndrome or Patau syndrome. There is no normal measurement because it varies widely between babies. The NT measurement, blood test results, woman's age and estimated age of the baby are combined to calculate a risk estimation. As a guide, low risk is considered more than 1 in 300, high risk is considered less than 1 in 300. The results may be given to you after the test or sent to your caregiver, taking several working days. If your risk is 'high', you will be offered further genetic counselling to discuss the options of having a diagnostic test (CVS or amniocentesis).

Results take 3 to 4 working days and are adjusted to take into account the woman's age, ethnic race, weight (thinner women have higher AFPs) and the gestational age of the baby. The result is expressed as risk or MOM (multiple of median), which is essentially an individual woman's risk in relation to the general population. AFP is about 90% accurate. It has a high false positive rate, meaning the result is high, but the baby is actually healthy and normal (50% of 'high' results). This can be caused by:
- The pregnancy being more advanced than calculated.
- Carrying twins or more (higher if the twins are identical).
- The woman has experienced bleeding during the pregnancy.
- The baby has another physical abnormality involving the kidneys or bowel (very rare).

Baby boys tend to have higher AFP levels than baby girls (but still within the normal range). If the AFP level is high, you may be offered a repeat AFP and/or a detailed ultrasound of the baby, specifically looking for a neural tube defect. Ultrasounds usually detect 100% of anencephaly, but only 70 to 85% of spina bifida.

Results take 3 to 4 working days. The 3 tests are combined with the woman's age and expressed as low (or screen negative), meaning the baby is probably not affected, or high (screen positive), meaning the baby is thought to be at risk of having a disorder. You may also be given a statistical number similar to the nuchal translucency. An abnormally high AFP may indicate the baby has a neural tube defect, and you will be offered a more detailed ultrasound of the baby at 18 weeks to specifically look for this. An abnormally low AFP may indicate the baby has Down syndrome, and you would be offered further genetic counselling to

Risks and problems

The more experienced the ultrasonographer, the more likely the test will be accurate. Health risks are only those that may possibly be related to having an ultrasound. It can be stressful having a high risk result and you may feel pressured to go on and have further diagnostic tests.

No health risks for the pregnancy or unborn baby.

No health risks for the pregnancy or unborn baby.

Triple test (cont.)

Diagnostic tests

CVS (chorionic villus sampling) – Takes a small sample of cells from the unborn baby's placenta, usually between 10 and 12 weeks of pregnancy.

CVS can be done vaginally through the cervix, or with a needle inserted through the abdomen into the uterus (transabdominal), depending on the caregiver's preferences, the method they have most experience in, as well as the position of the uterus and where the baby's placenta is implanted.
Vaginal CVS. An abdominal ultrasound locates the placenta, and the caregiver uses a speculum to view the cervix. A thin instrument is passed through the cervix and into the uterus and a small biopsy is taken to obtain a sample of the placenta. No anaesthetic is required. It may be slightly uncomfortable, possibly with cramping during the procedure and for a few hours afterwards. Sometimes more than one attempt is required. The whole process takes about 30 minutes, taking the sample itself lasts about 5 minutes. It is not unusual to experience a small amount of vaginal bleeding afterwards. Make sure you rest for a day or so. If your blood group is Rhesus negative, you need an injection of anti-D immunoglobulin. Vaginal CVS has a small risk of introducing infection from the vagina. The caregiver may take a swab test a few days before the procedure, to make sure no infection is present.
Abdominal CVS. The caregiver passes a needle through the lower abdomen into the uterus. Under ultrasound guidance, a small biopsy of the placenta is obtained. No anaesthetic is required, but it may be slightly uncomfortable, possibly with cramping during the procedure and for a few hours, or a couple of days afterwards. Make sure you rest for a day or so. The whole process takes 30 minutes, with the sample itself taking 5 minutes. Sometimes more than one attempt is required. There may be some bruising around the area and a small amount of vaginal bleeding may occur. If your blood group is Rhesus negative, you need an injection of anti-D immunoglobulin.

Amniocentesis – Takes a sample of amniotic fluid that the baby floats in from inside the woman's uterus. The fluid has cells naturally shed from the baby. It is usually performed around 15 weeks, but can be performed up to 18 weeks or later.

Ultrasound images guide the insertion of the needle through the abdomen into the uterus, to where a pool of fluid surrounding the baby is, avoiding the baby and placenta. The needle often has to be manoeuvred several times to obtain the fluid required. Sometimes more than one needle insertion is required to collect enough fluid. At least 10 to 20 ml (4 teaspoons full) is needed, which is less than 10% of the baby's total fluid volume. Laboratory failure happens in up to 6% of amniocentesis done at 15 weeks or over, and up to 18% if done before 15 weeks. Some caregivers filter the amniotic fluid to obtain the cells before reinjecting the fluid back into the uterus. The fluid sample may be clear or straw-coloured, but about 10%

discuss the options of having a CVS or amniocentesis. A triple test is about 70% accurate. It is also possible (5%) to have a false positive result, where the risk is high, yet the baby is actually healthy and normal.

The results take 10 to 14 days. If a genetic disorder is detected, you will meet with the genetic counsellor and/or your caregiver to discuss your options. It is possible to get inconclusive results (2%). Occasionally, the cells develop subtle changes from the original cells, giving them a slightly different appearance making them impossible to interpret. This means repeating the CVS, or having an amniocentesis.

CVS holds small risks for the unborn baby. Complications are less likely if the doctor is experienced (doing at least 50 or more a year). However, even the most experienced doctor can have problems. Overall, abdominal CVS has less complications than vaginal CVS. However, it is preferable that the doctor uses the method they are accustomed to. If the position of your uterus, or the location of the placenta, favours one method over the other, then this is the most preferred method.

The main risk is miscarriage within days, or a week or so afterwards, 2 to 3% for vaginal CVS and 1.5 to 2% for abdominal CVS. (This increases to 5% if the CVS is done before 10 weeks). The cause may be excessive bleeding or infection (or unknown). Sometimes the miscarried baby is found to have a genetic disorder and it is felt the miscarriage may have happened anyway. If the CVS is done before 9 weeks there is a 2% chance of injuring the baby, compared to 0.05% if done after 10 weeks.

Results take up to 14 to 21 days. If they detect a genetic disorder, you will meet with the genetic counsellor and/or your caregiver to discuss your options. Inconclusive results can happen if the cells do not grow (0.2%). Occasionally the cells develop subtle changes from the original cells, giving them a slightly different appearance making them impossible to interpret. This means repeating the amniocentesis, or a cordocentesis may be considered.

Amniocentesis holds small risks for the unborn baby. This is less likely if the doctor is experienced (at least 50 or more per year). Yet even the most experienced doctor can have problems. The main risk is miscarriage within days, or a week or so afterwards, or not for several weeks, 0.5 to 1% if done at 15 weeks or more, or 2 to 5% if done before 15 weeks. The cause may be infection, the waters breaking, the uterus contracting, or excessive bleeding (or unknown). Direct injury to the baby with the needle is very rare. If the baby is inadvertently pricked, this does not usually cause any

Amniocentesis (cont.)

are bloodstained. This is not a problem, just indicating that a small blood vessel in the woman had been punctured. No anaesthetic is required. The procedure may be slightly uncomfortable for some women, with cramping or contractions during the procedure, and for up to two days afterwards. A small amount of vaginal bleeding may occur afterwards or the waters may leak (not common). It is recommended you take complete rest for 24 hours.

Cordocentesis – Takes a blood sample from the unborn baby's umbilical cord and can only be done later in the pregnancy (18 to 24 weeks), when the umbilical cord has adequately developed. Usually done if an amniocentesis was unsuccessful, or the tests results were inconclusive.

Ultrasound images guide the insertion of a long, thin needle through the woman's belly and uterus and into the baby's umbilical cord, at the end closest to the placenta. A small blood sample is taken and the needle is removed. The baby's heartbeat is continuously monitored during the procedure, which can take up to 1 hour. No anaesthetic is required. The procedure may be slightly uncomfortable, with cramping or contractions during the procedure and for a few hours to a day or two afterwards. Some women experience a small amount of vaginal bleeding (although uncommon) and a few women experience the waters leaking. It is recommended you take complete rest for about 24 hours after the procedure.

Things to consider

People make decisions based on their personal beliefs, values, culture, concerns and individual circumstances. Some parents are quite accepting of, or very keen to have, genetic tests. Others have no desire for them, or perhaps see them as unethical.

Couples can have different points of view on genetic testing, which may place immense strain on the relationship when making complex and serious decisions. It is important you both share your thoughts and feelings and attend genetic counselling together, to help come to a decision you can both live with. Be aware that some women allow the weeks to pass without making a decision. However, this ends up being a decision in itself.

Parents expecting twins (or more) can be faced with the even greater dilemmas if one baby shows 'high risk'. This is something you need to discuss in depth with your caregiver and genetic counsellor.

Emotional reactions

The process of genetic testing can be a very emotional one and has been shown to delay a woman's emotional and psychological connections with her unborn baby. This may be by not announcing the pregnancy or not wearing maternity clothes, or even not tuning in to her baby's movements, because the pregnancy is put on hold.[11] Besides an emotional withdrawal, there can also be feelings of anxiety, distress, guilt, sadness or depression. However, some women feel that not knowing is worse and are anxious until they have their test results.

noticeable or long-term injury. Talipes (club foot) is increased when an amniocentesis is done before 14 weeks (1.8%). Breathing problems at birth are also increased by 1%, as amniotic fluid plays an important role in the development of a baby's lungs.

Test results are available within 48 hours. Cordocentesis can also be used to detect blood disorders such as haemophilia, or to check the baby for suspected viral infections (rubella, toxoplasmosis, cytomegalovirus), or to see if the baby is anaemic (with isoimmunisation).

Cordocentesis has a miscarriage (or premature birth) rate of about 1 to 2%, as well as a small risk of infection. Sometimes the baby's heartbeat temporarily slows during the procedure. If the pregnancy is quite advanced (more than 26 weeks) and the baby becomes distressed during the procedure, an emergency caesarean would be required. However, this is a very rare complication.

If complications from a diagnostic test lead to losing a normal, healthy baby, anger, grief, guilt, rage and depression can follow as parents try to come to terms with their decision. Genetic counsellors are also trained to provide support for parents experiencing these devastating outcomes.

Did you know?
Scientists at the University of Queensland have developed a Pap-smear-type test to obtain cells from the woman's cervix that trickle down from the placenta. These cells can be used to diagnose genetic abnormalities in the unborn baby without the health risks of diagnostic tests. It is thought the test will be widely available by 2005–2006.

Early pregnancy variations

BLEEDING DURING EARLY PREGNANCY

Vaginal bleeding during early pregnancy is referred to as a threatened miscarriage and is experienced by up to 30% of women before 14 weeks. Bleeding is always of concern, but does not necessarily mean there is a problem. About 50% of women continue to have a healthy pregnancy and baby after bleeding, but 50% go on to miscarry.[12] Bleeding can range from a light pink discolouration when wiping yourself, to bright red spotting, to quite heavy period-like bleeding, sometimes associated with mild cramping pains and/or backache. The bleeding can be a one-off incident, or may come and go over a period of weeks. A common pattern is to have a day of fresh red blood, followed by a several days of old brown blood as the remnants of the original bleed come away.

NOTE: *Any vaginal bleeding during pregnancy should be communicated to your caregiver.*

Around 30% of women find no reason for their bleeding. However, possible causes can include:
- An imminent miscarriage.
- An ectopic pregnancy.
- A polyp (skin tag) growing inside the vagina, which may bleed spontaneously or after rubbing (with sexual intercourse). They are not a problem and usually disappear after the birth.
- An infection or irritation of the vagina (thrush or Gardnerella), or a sexually transmitted infection.
- Hormonal bleeds, around the time your period would have been due (at 4, 8, 12 and 16 weeks of pregnancy).
- Bleeding after sex, as the woman's cervix softens with an increased blood supply. On *very rare* occasions this may be a sign of cell changes in the cervix. You may need a Pap test if you haven't had one for a year or two.
- Loss of a twin or triplet baby. Up to 50% of multiple pregnancies involve the death of one baby in early pregnancy. This may go unnoticed (as the baby is reabsorbed – called a vanishing twin), or involve bleeding as the baby miscarries.
- A molar pregnancy.

Care and treatments

Bleeding during early pregnancy triggers immense uncertainty and anxiety for parents. Unfortunately, often all you can do is wait and hope that the bleeding stops and your baby will be all right. If the bleeding continues or increases, your caregiver may want to see you for a check-up (or ask you to go to the hospital for this), which may involve:
- Using a speculum to check the vagina and cervix.
- Two HCG blood tests a few days apart, to see whether the levels are rising. Perhaps a progesterone blood test to see whether this is normal (9 to 47 ng/ml up to 12 weeks).
- An ultrasound (if more than six to seven weeks) to try to detect the baby's heartbeat. If the heartbeat is seen, the chances of the baby surviving are up to 85% (but 15% still miscarry).[13]

In the past, women were advised to rest in bed (at home or in hospital). However, current research suggests this does not prevent a miscarriage occurring (if this is the final outcome). The general advice is to avoid strenuous activity, and possibly sexual intercourse, until the bleeding stops. Be guided by your caregiver.

MISCARRIAGE

A miscarriage is when a baby dies before 20 weeks gestation and/or is less than 400 g in birth weight. About 80% are early miscarriages (before 13 weeks) and 20% are late miscarriages (between 13 and 20 weeks). Miscarriages affect up to 15 to 20% of women and their families and tend to be more common around the times that subsequent periods would have been due (4, 8 and 12 and 16 weeks of pregnancy).[14]

Around 97% of women who miscarry go on to have a healthy baby with the subsequent pregnancy, and up to 75% of women who have 3 or more miscarriages have a subsequent, normal pregnancy and baby.

NOTE: *The medical term for miscarriage is 'abortion' (eg. 'threatened abortion'), which can be distressing to hear. Other terms that can sound harsh and uncaring are the baby being referred to as an 'embryo' or a 'foetus', or 'products of conception' for the baby and placenta passed with a miscarriage.*

Reasons for miscarriage

It is estimated that 50% of miscarriages are due to genetic or physical abnormalities in the baby, usually occurring at the time of fertilisation. This prevents the baby from developing properly, or causes the baby to die after several weeks, before being naturally expelled from the uterus.

For the other 50%, finding reasons for a miscarriage can be frustrating. In most cases no cause is found. This can make dealing with the loss very difficult, often bringing up feelings of helplessness, guilt and doubt about your body's ability to carry a baby, as well as a lot of fear and anxiety about future pregnancies. While these are normal reactions to grief, it is important to remember that it is very rare for a woman to miscarry because of something she may or may not have done. Sometimes a reason is found, such as:

- A viral or bacterial infection (rubella or listeria).
- An infection of the uterus.
- A complication of a CVS or amniocentesis.
- A weakened cervix which opens spontaneously, usually between 14 and 28 weeks (known medically as cervical incompetence).

- The baby implanting on a very large fibroid in the uterus or on a septum (with a heart-shaped or bicornuate uterus).
- A serious car accident or blow to the lower stomach, or abdominal surgery.
- Exposure to certain drugs, medications, smoking, excessive alcohol, radiation, chemicals or pesticides.
- Health conditions for the woman (eg. auto-immune diseases, blood-clotting disorders, diabetes, kidney disease, low thyroid function).
- Increased age. About 10% of women in their twenties miscarry compared to about 50% of women over 40 (or the man being over 55 years).

Inevitable miscarriage

An inevitable or spontaneous miscarriage means losing the baby is imminent, or in the process of happening. This may follow vaginal bleeding, or happen suddenly with little warning.

Up to 6 weeks – Miscarriage can be similar to experiencing a very heavy period, possibly with small blood clots and mild cramping. The baby can miscarry naturally and the process rarely requires medical intervention. At six weeks the baby is about 0.5 to 1 cm long, or the size of your little fingernail.

Emotions: Women bond very early with their baby. Early miscarriages can be very distressing, isolating and lonely, often because others don't give the loss much significance. A few women take comfort in the fact that they know they can conceive, although this reassurance is often mixed with anger and sadness, because the pregnancy did not continue.

6 to 13 weeks – This is the most common time to miscarry.
- **A complete miscarriage** – The woman's body expels all the pregnancy naturally, without medical interventions (80% of inevitable miscarriages). This causes bleeding, often accompanied by blood clots and mild to moderate cramping, with waves of pain, until everything has passed. The process may take a few hours, or be on and off for a few days, before the bleeding eases, continuing lightly for one to three weeks. The physical signs of pregnancy (tender breasts, nausea, etc) disappear after one to two weeks, but a pregnancy test can remain positive for four to six weeks. If an ultrasound is done, the uterus is empty, with no sign of the baby or placenta.
- **An incomplete miscarriage** – Some of the baby and/or the placenta remain inside the uterus, requiring an operation or D&C (20% of inevitable miscarriages). The bleeding and blood clotting may become heavier or sometimes it subsides, but if a D&C is not done, an infection

may develop in the uterus within days (or weeks), causing lower abdominal pain, fever, and/or an offensive-smelling vaginal discharge. An ultrasound can detect whether any of the pregnancy remains.

NOTE: *If you are soaking pads every half an hour for more than an hour or two, and/or continuously passing large blood clots, and/or feeling faint, nauseated or dizzy, you need to seek medical attention as soon as possible.*

The baby. What will I see?: At this stage, the baby and placenta may, or may not, be identifiable within blood clots (which resemble liver). If you require an operation to remove the baby, this process makes the baby non-identifiable. Babies at 7 weeks are about 1.8 cm in length; by 12 to 13 weeks, they are about 8 to 10 cm, but their sex is not obvious yet.

Emotions: Losing your baby can come as quite a shock, or turn fears and anxiety into a horrible reality. You may feel empty, sad, angry, confused or bewildered, or very lonely, if others were not yet aware of your pregnancy. Many parents feel overwhelmed by a profound sense of loss, often made worse by other people's attitudes of 'It was for the best' or advice to 'Just try again.' Talk openly and honestly about your feelings and respect your partner's expression of their grief. You may end up seeking professional counselling, or a support group, to help you cope.

14 to 20 weeks – These miscarriages are more likely to be incomplete, requiring medical intervention, because the baby and placenta are more developed. While the baby may be passed easily, often the placenta is fully or partially retained within the uterus, requiring a D&C to remove it. Physical signs can be similar to an early miscarriage, but more severe, with the pain being labour-like. A late miscarriage due to a weakened cervix is relatively painless, with little warning. If you start miscarrying after 14 weeks, contact your caregiver or seek medical attention as soon as possible.

The baby. What will I see?: Depending on how developed your baby is, you may be able to identify them and possibly make out their sex. You may even be able to hold them. However, if the baby has died weeks beforehand, or if you require an operation, this may not be possible.

Emotions: Late miscarriages are very unexpected. The grief and sadness that follows can be overwhelming and confusing, often mixed with feelings of disbelief, anger, sadness, guilt and heartache, similar to women experiencing a stillbirth. If the pregnancy miscarries quickly, this can be very frightening and extremely upsetting, particularly as you are witnessing your loss in front of your own eyes. Things to consider when dealing with a late miscarriage are included in Chapter 7.

Missed (or 'silent') miscarriage

Sometimes the baby dies but the woman's cervix stays closed and there is no bleeding. The baby remains inside the uterus and the death not discovered until days or weeks later. A few women notice their pregnancy signs disappear, but others still feel pregnant, as the placenta continues to release hormones. At some stage, brown or red vaginal bleeding may be noticed and the miscarriage becomes inevitable, or an ultrasound may detect a baby that is smaller then expected, with no heartbeat visible.

NOTE: *Once the baby dies, they shrink at the same rate they would have grown by had the pregnancy progressed normally. For example, if the baby died at 12 weeks and the miscarriage was found at 14 weeks, the baby shrinks to about a 10 week size.*

Once a missed miscarriage is discovered, you may choose to wait and see whether the pregnancy miscarries naturally (this can take several days or weeks). An operation is advisable if you start to bleed heavily or don't want to wait. You may choose to have a few days to come to terms with the miscarriage before having an operation. If the pregnancy is more than 15 weeks, medications are used to induce labour and expel the baby naturally. However, because the placenta is comparatively small, it may remain within the uterus after the baby is born, requiring an operation to remove it.

Emotions: Some women instinctively know their pregnancy is not quite right. Others have no inkling that anything is wrong. Grappling with the idea that your baby has died days or weeks earlier can be hard to believe, often making you wonder how you were not aware of it and creating nervousness for future pregnancies. Emotional reactions can include shock, emptiness, confusion and bewilderment, as you come to terms with what has happened.

Blighted ovum

A blighted ovum (or anembryonic pregnancy) occurs when the fertilised egg implants but the cells don't divide and differentiate as they should. The pregnancy test is positive and pregnancy symptoms are felt, but the baby miscarries, usually between 7 and 12 weeks (or becomes a missed miscarriage). If an ultrasound is done, a small, empty sac is seen, with no baby inside. Treatments are similar to an inevitable or missed miscarriage.

Emotions: The beginnings of a pregnancy connect you with your unborn baby. However, being told there is no baby can feel confusing and disconcerting. The term 'blighted ovum' itself is very impersonal, because it is a medical way of saying your baby was not a real person. However, there was a baby (the very beginnings of one) to create your pregnancy and you will need time to grieve for your loss.

Considerations when having a D&C

A few women don't feel ready (or feel pressured) to have an operation soon after their miscarriage has been discovered. Sometimes they find the miscarriage difficult to comprehend, believing their baby may still be alive. If you are well, and the bleeding is not excessive, the operation can be delayed, or you may choose to miscarry naturally, if this is what you want. It is important that you feel comfortable with what is happening. However, heavy bleeding will make an operation necessary. Some options to consider are having:

- Two blood HCG tests, two to three days apart, or
- Two ultrasounds a week or more apart.

This can confirm (or disprove) the miscarriage and may reassure you in accepting the loss.

Women with a Rhesus negative blood group (eg. O negative) need to have an injection of anti-D immunoglobulin within 72 hours of heavy bleeding, or after an operation to remove a miscarried pregnancy. This prevents antibodies developing in the blood and lasts for three months. Anti-D is not necessary if the pregnancy was less than six to seven weeks.

Recurrent miscarriage

About 1 to 2% of women experience recurrent miscarriages, which is three or more consecutive miscarriages. As a general rule, tests are only done to try to find a physical cause after a third miscarriage, mainly because in the majority of cases no cause is found after one or two miscarriages.

Over the last 60 years, medicine has tried several therapies to prevent recurrent miscarriage, such as hormones (Diethylstilbestrol or 'DES' and progesterone), human chorionic gonadotrophin (HCG) or immunotherapy. So far none of these have shown any benefits, and in some cases they are harmful.[15]

If late miscarriages are thought to be caused by a weakened cervix, caregivers may suggest placing a stitch in the cervix (called a cerclage) at around 12 weeks of pregnancy. This is controversial, with research finding no reduction in pregnancy loss, or pre-term delivery rates, when stitches are used electively (just in case), or as an emergency (when the woman's cervix is seen to be shortening or 'funnelling' on ultrasound). However, if you have lost one or more babies, this approach may feel right for you, despite the risks involved; these can include:

- Uterine contractions.
- The waters breaking prematurely (1 to 9% of cases).[16]
- Vaginal bleeding.
- Infection of the amniotic fluid sac.
- Trauma to the cervix, sometimes leading to it not dilating during labour.

Physical recovery from miscarriage

If you lost a lot of blood, it may take a while to recover. Rest as much as possible, eat regular, nourishing meals, take time off work or have help with your other children. Your doctor may recommend a check-up three to six weeks after the miscarriage, to make sure you have recovered physically. If you are anaemic, feeling tired, lethargic or irritable, iron supplements may help. Natural therapies can include:
- Homeopathic remedies – Arnica, Ferrum metallicum or Calcarea phosphoricum.
- Herbal remedies for the immune system (nettle tea, vitamin C, Echinacea, garlic).
- Acupuncture, to support recovery and balance hormones.

Sex and future pregnancies

You can resume sexual intercourse once the bleeding stops (one to three weeks), or later, when you feel physically and emotionally ready. There are no clear guidelines as to when you can conceive again, but if you feel well, then it really depends on what you would like to do (Chapter 1 deals with conceiving after miscarriage). If you don't want another baby soon speak with your caregiver about appropriate contraception.

ECTOPIC PREGNANCY

An ectopic (or 'out of place') pregnancy occurs when a fertilised egg implants before it reaches the uterus, usually in the fallopian tube (98%), but occasionally outside the uterus on the ovary, or in the lower abdomen. About 1% of pregnancies are ectopic, but 50% of these spontaneously miscarry, or are naturally absorbed by the woman's body, leaving her unaware of the pregnancy.

The causes of an ectopic pregnancy are often unknown, but usually relate to a damaged or scarred fallopian tube after a pelvic infection (possibly sexually transmitted) or a past abdominal operation (appendectomy or caesarean). Other causes are:
- Some contraceptives (eg. the minipill or an intra-uterine contraceptive device).
- Taking fertility medications that stimulate ovulation.
- Smoking.[17]

The normal signs of pregnancy are usually experienced, but some women are not aware they are pregnant. Between 5 and 12 weeks (more commonly 6 to 8 weeks), pain starts on one side of the lower abdomen, which may be persistently mild to moderate, or become increasingly intense over hours or

days. Sometimes it is sudden and severe. Other physical signs can include:
- An unusually light or heavy period, or dark, watery blood (similar to prune juice).
- Shoulder tip pain and/or pain when passing urine or opening the bowels.
- Feeling light-headed, dizzy and/or nauseated.
- Looking pale, a fast pulse and possibly collapsing (in late stages).

If an ectopic pregnancy goes untreated, it can be life-threatening for the woman.

If you suspect an ectopic pregnancy, seek medical attention as soon as possible. An ultrasound is usually performed, as well as a blood pregnancy test. The caregiver may take a wait-and-see approach, particularly if you are feeling well and don't have much pain, but if the pain worsens, you may need a laparoscopy operation to remove the fallopian tube and pregnancy. Sometimes the doctor can preserve the fallopian tube, but this is not always possible. Removing a fallopian tube reduces a woman's fertility by 50%. A more recent experimental approach is to inject a small amount of methotrexate into the pregnancy (chemotherapy used to treat cancer). This breaks down the pregnancy so it can be reabsorbed (taking a couple of days), but may avoid an operation. However, its success is not guaranteed.[18]

For women who conceive again, the risk of experiencing a second ectopic pregnancy rises from 0.5% to 7–10%. If you think you may be pregnant again, see your doctor as soon as possible.

A **heterotopic pregnancy** is a multiple pregnancy in which one twin baby implants normally in the uterus and the other twin implants in the fallopian tube. This is rare, but the physical signs are the same as a single ectopic pregnancy. Treatment involves removing the ectopic pregnancy through a laparoscopy, so the uterine pregnancy is not disturbed and hopefully continues normally.

Emotions: An ectopic pregnancy is traumatic. Losing a baby, undergoing major abdominal surgery and having a fallopian tube removed are all immense issues to deal with. A few women are told they nearly died. Emotions can be conflicting. You may feel grateful to be alive and not in pain, yet saddened by your losses. For some women, fear and anxiety attached to thoughts of a future pregnancy make them decide not to become pregnant again, which can be heartbreaking.

EXCESSIVE VOMITING

Less than 1% of pregnant women with morning sickness experience excessive vomiting (called hyperemesis gravidarum). This is more common for women having their first baby. The main concern is dehydration, if vomiting happens several times a day for many days and the woman can't keep food or fluids down.

Treatment usually involves an intravenous drip in hospital to administer fluids and some caregivers prescribe anti-nausea medications (as an injection or rectal suppository). Treatments may continue for a few days, depending on how unwell you are and how quickly the vomiting settles. However, often resting in hospital becomes a remedy in itself. A few women are in and out of hospital over several weeks, whenever their vomiting becomes severe.

NOTE: *Sometimes excessive vomiting is caused by a virus or food poisoning, totally unrelated to the pregnancy. If your doctor suspects this, you may need tests.*

Retroverted uterus

A retroverted or tipped uterus naturally leans backwards, towards the spine, rather than forwards, to rest above the bladder. This is a normal variation for about 20% of women. It does not generally affect the pregnancy, labour or birth. After 12 weeks the uterus grows up and out of the pelvis and is then positioned in the normal way. In extremely rare cases, the growing uterus is inhibited from moving out of the pelvis by getting 'caught' on the lower spine, or sacrum (incarcerated uterus). This can cause some pain and difficulty passing urine, usually around 12 to 14 weeks. Pelvic rocking on your hands and knees helps release the uterus. If this does not help, a urinary catheter is passed to empty the bladder (in hospital) and is effective within hours or a few days.

whole body (called lanugo). This protects their skin, only being shed a few weeks before their due date. Your baby now explores their own body with their hands. If you are having twins (or more), they may try to locate each other, touching and exploring the body of their brother or sister. There is still plenty of fluid around your baby at this stage, allowing them to turn, twist and change position frequently.

Week 20 – The halfway point. Your baby measures about 22 cm from head to toe and weighs about 340 g (12 oz). Their nails form and fingerprints are now visibly engraved in their fine skin. Their permanent teeth appear behind baby teeth deep within their gums. The bones in their inner ear and their nerve endings are now developed to the point where they can hear sounds (although their ears are not structurally complete until 24 weeks).

Week 22 – Your baby is around 25 cm long and weighs just under 0.5 kg (about 1 lb). You may have felt your baby move, although sensations may still be faint, sporadic and infrequent. Now your baby's nervous system completely connects, as vital links between their brain, spinal cord and nerves mature. Once this happens, your baby recognises warmth, light and sound and senses pain. While primitive brain waves have been detected in unborn babies as early as 7 weeks, it is not until 22 weeks that sustained patterns can definitely be recorded. Their skin becomes increasingly covered with vernix cream and they now have distinct eyelashes and eyebrows. Their eyelids are still fused shut, but their retinas (the back of the eyes that interpret images) are fully developed and their hair follicles now pigment, to give them hair colour. Babies at this stage typically lie transverse, or crossways, in your belly, with their feet and bottom on one side and their head on the other. The placenta is now processing about 1 litre of blood per hour. By 40 weeks this increases to about 12 litres per hour!

Week 24 – Your baby has grown to about 28 cm long and approximately 600 g in weight (1 lb 5 oz). They may now be big enough for your partner (or others) to feel your belly and sense them kicking and stretching. Your baby can rotate their head and may experience hiccups (often sporadic from 12 weeks gestation, but generally stronger and more rhythmic by this stage). They now have sweat glands and a fine layer of fat forms between their muscles and skin, making their complexion look less translucent. A thick layer of white vernix cream covers their body to protect them in their watery environment. The lining of their lungs starts to produce a substance called surfactant, which assists them to breathe after birth. They now have definite sleep and wake patterns (although they usually sleep 95% of the time). Your baby has REM (rapid eye movement), which indicates they may be dreaming! You may notice your baby being noticeably active when you are resting. It is thought that a woman's movements naturally rock her baby to sleep.

Week 26 – Your baby now measures about 33 cm and weighs about 800 g (1 lb 12 oz). They now recognise your voice and are noticeably calmed by it (observed by their heart rate slowing). They may also recognise your partner's voice and different types of music. Your baby's eyelids are no longer fused and they can now open them and even blink and respond to bright light. Newborn babies have vision that is perfectly focused from 20 to 30 cm, about as far away as the face of the person holding them. Their movements are generally more regular now and they may physically respond if you press on parts of their protruding feet, bottom or hands. Their heart beats at around 120 to 160 beats per minute and can be heard using a Pinard's stethoscope.

> **Did you know?**
> Babies have been shown to quieten and listen to songs after birth, if their mother played them regularly during the last three months of her pregnancy. One study showed how a group of babies calmed when they heard the theme song of the TV soap *Neighbours*, presumably because their mother watched it daily!

Week 28 – At this stage an unborn baby is said to be viable, having a good chance of surviving if born after this time. Your baby is about 37 cm long and weighs about 1.1 kg (2 lb 7 oz). Many babies of this gestation like to lie in a breech position (bottom down, head up). Their immune system is now developing, as your natural antibodies pass to them through the placenta. Your baby now starts yawning, sucking, swallowing and drinking the amniotic fluid in preparation for feeding. However, this reflex is not fully mature until 32 to 34 weeks. They may look around and are capable of distinguishing light from dark and tracking movement around them.

Middle pregnancy

Physical changes
The second trimester is often a more comfortable phase of pregnancy. However, it also brings its unique physical changes. A few women find their symptoms linger from the first trimester, and others notice some third trimester changes starting early!

Leaking breasts

Colostrum can leak from the nipples any time after 14 to 16 weeks. This first fluid produced by the breasts is clear, or creamy yellow, and syrupy in consistency. However, not everyone noticeably leaks. Some parents express concerns that there won't be enough for their new baby, but the breasts constantly replenish every three to four hours. A few women breastfeed their older child while pregnant, and occasionally tandem feed after the birth (feeding the older sibling and new baby together).

NOTE: *It is normal for some women to notice a small amount of blood mixed with the colostrum during pregnancy. This comes from within the breast and is caused by the rapid growth of blood vessels in the growing ductal system, in preparation for breastfeeding. Also, drops of blood may be seen on the bra because the sticky colostrum temporarily glues the nipple to the material and a tiny bit of skin can be removed with the bra, which does heal.*

What some women find helpful — Leaking colostrum is normal. If it is frequent and becomes annoying, you may need to wear breast pads inside your bra.

Metallic taste

Having a metallic taste in the mouth is not often formally recognised by caregivers, but natural therapists believe it could be the body releasing toxins through the lymph glands, which transport and produce your body's defence mechanisms against infection. Others believe it is the body's reaction to being run down with stress, or the physical demands of pregnancy. A metallic taste can also be a side effect of some medications, such as the antibiotic Flagyl.

What some women find helpful — Metallic taste sensations are usually relieved by eating and should return to normal after the birth. Homeopaths may suggest remedies such as Cocculus indicus, Cuprum metallicum, Catrum carbonicum, or zinc.

Bleeding gums

The gums have a higher blood supply during pregnancy, making them prone to bleeding and becoming inflamed or infected (called gingivitis), especially with vigorous brushing and flossing. Bleeding gums are normal, and improve after the baby is born.

> **Did you know?**
> There is no truth in the saying 'A tooth is lost for every baby.' If your gums become inflamed and are not treated, it is possible for teeth to loosen. Taking good care of your teeth means you get to keep them all! Also, you do not lose calcium from your teeth during pregnancy. Calcium needed by the baby comes from your diet and stores from within your bones.

What some women find helpful – Keeping your teeth and gums healthy can prevent gingivitis. Use a softer toothbrush and clean your teeth at least twice daily. Take extra care when flossing and visit the dentist at least once during your pregnancy for a routine check. If your gums become inflamed and painful, try regular salt-water rinses to reduce inflammation (a tablespoon of salt dissolved in a cup of warm water to gargle and spit). See your dentist if the condition does not improve. Some herbalists recommend gargling with raspberry leaf (tea or solutions).

Medical treatments – In rare cases, antibiotics may be prescribed (usually penicillin-type, or an alternative if you are allergic to penicillin).

Restless legs

Restless legs can create:
- A sensation that the legs have to move all the time.
- Jittery feelings, or having butterflies in the legs.
- Aching and the need to be constantly walking.

Restless legs can make it difficult to sit for long periods and may prevent you from sleeping well at night. They don't necessarily go hand in hand with varicose veins, or swelling of the legs.

Restless legs are a little recognised condition and we don't really know why they occur. Some theories are a change in the amount of blood circulating in the legs, possibly being anaemic, too much caffeine or a low blood sugar. However, these are all educated guesses. Natural therapists believe they are due to a lack of dietary minerals, especially magnesium.

What some women find helpful:
- Cell salts or magnesium phosphate supplements.
- Massaging the legs with oil, peppermint gel or cream, from the toes upwards before bed.
- A long, warm bath before bed.
- Going for walks, yoga or doing isometric exercises of the calves and thighs (alternating the tightening and releasing of muscles or pointing the toes up and down).
- Acupuncture or acupressure.
- Homeopathic remedies such as Causticum, Zincum metallicum or Sulphur.

Hair changes

Hair growth is often stronger and natural hair loss less, due to increased oestrogen – your hair may be thicker and you may notice more body hair. How oily or dry your hair is depends on your skin changes. If you are sweating more and your oil glands are active, your hair will be oilier. But if your skin is drier, then you may find you don't have to wash your hair as often. A few women experience small amounts of hair loss (alopecia), although this is more common when breastfeeding. Hair changes vary from pregnancy to pregnancy in the same woman, but are not indicative of a boy or girl baby!

What some women find helpful – Wash and use conditioner as often as necessary.

Nails changes

Fingernails may seem stronger, or perhaps more brittle, which is not a sign of lacking calcium. White spots on the nails happen when you knock your nail on something, lifting a small section off the nail bed. This may be more common if pregnancy makes your nails brittle.

Skin changes

Pregnancy changes your skin in many ways, and this may be different for each pregnancy. Again, this has nothing to do with the sex of your baby. Your skin may look healthier and clearer, even glowing, or it may become oily, blotchy and perhaps more blemished.

Heat rashes and itchy skin
These are common complaints, due to hormonal changes and increased sweating. Some women also become more sensitive (or allergic) to skin products, reacting with a rash. Your skin can itch when dry, particularly in the winter months, as it stretches and grows. Rashes may be on small parts of the body, or generalised all over your belly and elsewhere. This is called PUPPS (pruritic urticarial papules and plaques of pregnancy). Tell your caregiver, in case it is caused by other things (scabies, eczema or a fungal infection).
NOTE: Persistent itching after 20 weeks of pregnancy may be a sign of your liver not functioning well (called cholestasis). This is diagnosed with blood tests, which should be done if the itching is constant, especially on your palms and/or soles of your feet.

What some women find helpful – If your skin is oily, try keeping it dry and only using a light moisturiser. For itchy skin try:
- Oatmeal or water dispersible emollients in the bath or shower.
- Replacing soaps and perfumed skin products with sorbelene and glycerine cream.
- Using pawpaw ointment, calendula cream or chickweed ointment.
- Wearing as little underwear as possible.
- Cotton clothes instead of Lycra and synthetics.

- Rolling a hand towel or washer (you may like to wet it) and placing it under your breasts to stop them rubbing on your belly.
- Changing your laundry detergent to one with no dyes or perfumes.
- Calamine lotion.

Did you know?
One woman's caregiver recommended Mylanta antacid liquid on her skin. She swore it was the most effective treatment she had tried. We live and learn!

Medical treatments — Avoid acne medications and creams with vitamin A. If the itch is really unbearable, your caregiver may prescribe antihistamines or steroid creams (to be used sparingly). There is some research claiming that small doses of aspirin can be effective, but this should only be taken if medically prescribed.[1]

Skin darkening

Areas of the skin can become darker or pigmented, usually more so if you have a darker complexion. The anterior pituitary gland in the brain produces more melanocyte-stimulating hormone (MSH), but pigmentation can be made worse by exposing your body to the sun. You may notice changes: On your face (called the mask of pregnancy or chloasma); the nipples and areola; as a line down the middle of your belly (called the linea nigra or black line); in areas under your arms, between your upper legs and around the vaginal area.

What some women find helpful — Darkened skin is natural and generally unavoidable. To minimise excessive darkening:
- Wear sunscreen, put on a hat and keep your skin covered as much as possible.
- Eat foods rich in folic acid.

Some herbalists suggest St John's wort oil (should be avoided before 12 weeks of pregnancy). The pigmentation gradually fades over three to four months after the birth.

Moles

Moles or naevi are dark spots or patches on the skin that can be grey, brown or black in colour. They often become darker, and slightly larger, during pregnancy, and you may develop more of them as the pregnancy progresses.

NOTE: *If a mole changes dramatically, starts bleeding or becomes excessively itchy, you should consult your doctor or a dermatologist, as these could be the early signs of skin cancer.*

Skin tags
Small pieces of skin can overgrow, sometimes looking a little like warts. They occur more frequently during pregnancy, due to an increased metabolism. Skin tags can turn up anywhere on your body, but more commonly in places where the skin rubs (under the arms, breasts and inner thighs). Most skin tags disappear as mysteriously as they came, within months after the baby is born. Some women find them annoying and unsightly, but if you break them off or rub them, they bleed.

Medical treatments – You can ask your doctor or a dermatologist to remove them if they don't go away after the birth, usually by freezing them.

Red spots and spider veins
Spider naevi look like tiny spider leg lines on the skin, sometimes creating intricate patterns or spots. They appear because small blood vessels under the skin break with increased blood circulation, commonly on the chest, upper arms and legs. These are different from the larger, deep-purple blood vessels, known as varicose veins.

Spider veins mostly disappear after the birth. Some women use a homeopathic remedy called Arnica to treat them. Check with your homeopath.

Stretch marks
Stretch marks (striae gravidarum or pregnancy stripes) appear when collagen fibres under the skin break, as the skin rapidly stretches, creating red, pink, purple or brown marks depending on your skin type. During pregnancy, relaxin hormone reduces the amount of collagen fibres in the skin, making them more susceptible to breaking. Stretch marks can appear on your belly as early as 16 weeks and on your breasts, thighs, bottom or upper arms at any time. Putting on weight quickly can make them seem to appear overnight. However, even the normal growth of pregnancy can create them. Stretch marks eventually fade to a silvery-white colour after the birth. If you lose a lot of weight, they may look wrinkled.

What some women find helpful – Generally, there is nothing proven that prevents stretch marks. A well-balanced diet and not overeating fats and sugars, can help keep your weight gain steady, giving your skin more time to stretch, but there are no guarantees. One Spanish study tested Trofolastin cream, containing *Centella asiatica* extract (a plant), alpha tocopherol (vitamin E) and collagen-elastin hydrolysates, applied to the skin daily.[2] It benefited women who had already experienced stretch marks in puberty, stopping them from getting more, but did not benefit women who had never had stretch marks.

NOTE: *Be wary of expensive creams and lotions claiming the impossible. There are many cheap alternatives. If you want to massage creams or oils into your belly, try plain sorbelene and glycerine cream, perhaps with vitamin E and/or collagen; cocoa butter; plain oils, like sweet almond, vitamin B, coconut, apricot, almond or grape seed oil, often mixed in combinations. Aromatherapists may suggest neroli, mandarin or lavender mixed with a cream, gel or carrier oil (such as jojoba, coconut, canola or almond). Essential oils should not be used before 12 weeks of pregnancy. Homeopaths may prescribe Calcarea flourica.*

Nose bleeds

The lining of the nose is very fine and fragile. Increased blood supply during pregnancy makes it more sensitive and produce more mucus. This may cause a constantly blocked (or runny) nose, and/or sudden nose bleeds, as well as a heightened sense of smell.

What some women find helpful – If your nose is prone to bleeding, take care not to blow it too hard if it is blocked, or you have a cold. If it starts bleeding, try pinching the top of your nose near your eyes, and move your head forward (to let the blood drip out) or lean back, to slow the flow and let blood drain into the back of your throat. Some women find applying a cold cloth or some ice to this spot helps stem the bleeding.

Colds, hay fever, sinus

You may find it takes longer to recover from colds, hay fever or sinus problem during pregnancy. **What some women find helpful:**
- Eating nourishing foods and resting as much as possible. Garlic and foods rich in vitamin C can help boost the immune system. Some naturopaths suggest zinc supplements.
- Drinking at least eight glasses of water a day to keep the mucus in your nose runny and easier to clear.
- Using steam to loosen thick mucus. Lean your head over a basin of steaming hot water with a towel covering your head, or a steam vaporiser in the bedroom at night. Aromatherapists may recommend adding a small amount of frankincense or tea tree essential oil to the vaporiser (if more than 12 weeks pregnant).
- Honey and lemon lozenges, or a warm lemon drink with honey for a cough and/or sore throat.
- Salt-water nose drops (normal saline). You can use saline for cleaning contact lenses or make your own with a quarter teaspoon of salt in a cup of water.
- Gargling and spitting a tablespoon of salt dissolved in a cup of warm water for a sore throat.

- Acupuncture or acupressure to help alleviate symptoms and boost the immune system.
- Massaging the skin around the nose and eyes to help loosen mucus and bring relief to aching sinuses.
- Homeopaths may recommend Aconite or Allium cepa.

Medical treatments — If you are feeling unwell, contact your caregiver or hospital. Don't take medications without checking first. Most colds and flus are viral infections, meaning antibiotics won't help. Dealing with them is usually just a matter of putting up with your symptoms until your body recovers. Your caregiver may recommend: anti-decongestant rubbed on a hanky or pillow to breathe in; paracetamol for a fever; or a short course of antihistamines for severe allergy or sinus.

AVOID: Medicated nasal sprays; aspirin, unless prescribed by your doctor; Non-steroidal anti-inflammatory drugs (or NSAIDS), such as naproxen or ibuprofen; cough medicines or cold tablets, which contain a cocktail of medications; and flu vaccines.

Thrush

Pregnancy changes the acidity (or pH) of the vagina, making you five times more likely to experience thrush (candida or monilia). Vaginal thrush usually produces a thick, white discharge that resembles curdled milk and white patches may be seen on the inside of the vaginal skin, with the genitals looking inflamed, dry and red. The vaginal discharge does not smell, but it can feel itchy and sore, and sex can be uncomfortable or painful. If your partner also has thrush, he may experience discomfort when passing urine and rough, dry red skin patches on his penis. Other conditions that encourage thrush to flourish are: taking antibiotics; stress, not sleeping well, a poor diet, and possibly zinc and iron deficiencies; wearing plastic-backed panty liners or sanitary pads; having diabetes.

What some women find helpful – To encourage an acidic environment in the vagina and avoid thrush try:
- Eating well, resting and drinking plenty of fluids.
- Avoiding sweet, yeasty foods, eating live, natural yoghurt with acidophilus, milk culture drinks or lactobacillus capsules or tablets.
- Drinking cranberry juice to acidify the system.
- Taking vitamin C, fresh garlic or garlic capsules and zinc to boost the immune system. (Check with your caregiver.)
- Avoiding vigorous cleansing of the vagina with perfumed soaps. If doing perineal massage, keep oils and creams on the outside skin, not inside the vagina.

- Managing stress with deep breathing, meditation, massage, yoga or relaxation exercises.
- Wearing cotton underwear, (or even no underwear at times, if you feel comfortable with this).
- Avoid tight leggings, stockings etc. for long periods.
- Changing clothes detergent to a non-scented brand.
- Being aware that semen can aggravate thrush (because it is alkaline). Possibly using condoms until it has cleared or avoiding penetrative sex for a while.

To keep mild thrush under control try:
- Using Aci-Jel vaginal gel (available from chemists), until a couple of days after the thrush has cleared.
- Soaking a tampon in one cup of water with one teaspoon of cider or white vinegar, and inserting it into the vagina for 10 minutes, 2 to 3 times per day. Or insert a fresh clove of peeled garlic.
- Putting natural yoghurt with acidophilus into the vagina or acidophilus tablets into the vagina.

NOTE: *Some caregivers advise against putting yoghurt inside the vagina during pregnancy, as it may contain group B strep. There is no evidence to support or reject this claim.*

To relieve itchy soreness of the genitals try:
- Putting plain yoghurt to the outside genital area.
- Applying a poultice of slippery elm bark powder and water, backed with muslin cloth.
- Putting half a cup of cider vinegar or a tablespoon of bicarbonate of soda in the bath.
- Aromatherapists may recommend a few drops of tea tree or bergamot essential oil in a bowel of warm water to sit in (if more than 12 weeks pregnant).
- Homeopathic remedies may include Cocculus indicus, Kali sulphuricum, or Sepia.

NOTE: *Check with your caregiver about these remedies. Do not put anything into the vagina if your waters have broken or you are bleeding.*

If the thrush is severe, or constantly recurring, your caregiver may recommend anti-fungal creams or pessaries (purchased at chemists). As a general rule, Imidazoles tend to be more effective, curing up to 90% of women. However, you may need to treat the thrush again if it returns. There is no evidence that thrush is harmful in any way to your unborn baby, even if present at birth. On very rare occasions, thrush may affect a very premature baby who may be more susceptible to it.

Preparations to avoid – Some caregivers don't recommend vaginal anti-fungal medications during the first 12 weeks of pregnancy. However, others are not that concerned. There is no available research to support or reject the use of anti-fungals during early pregnancy. If you are concerned, you might like to wait a few weeks and put up with it, or try some natural approaches first. Prescribed oral anti-fungal medication tablets are not safe to use in pregnancy.

NOTE: *It is important your partner treats themselves with topical antifungal creams, because they can reinfect you after you have been treated. Some couples use condoms until the medication is finished or the thrush has cleared.*

Gardnerella

Acidic changes in the vagina during pregnancy can make you more susceptible to developing Gardnerella (Haemophilus). Gardnerella is found in about 20% of women, in small quantities, which is normal and does not cause physical signs, nor require any treatments. However, the normal, healthy Lactobacilli bacteria in the vagina can be overgrown with Gardnerella. Other bacteria that can behave in similar ways are Ureaplasma urealyticum and Mycoplasma hominis.

The physical symptoms of Gardnerella include a heavy, watery vaginal discharge that can have a strong, fishy odour and may look greyish, green or brownish yellow. There is usually little, or no vaginal irritation felt, but a few women notice mild itching.

What some women find helpful – Gardnerella may come and go on a regular basis, so you may want to use natural methods (the same as those suggested for thrush) to keep the infection under control, and only antibiotics if it becomes severe. Herbalists may recommend applying St John's wort cream or Yoni powder to the genitals for healing and to combat the odour. Homeopathic remedies may include Borax veneta.

Medical treatments – While many women carry Gardnerella, only a few actually end up needing treatment. Some caregivers like to treat Gardnerella routinely with antibiotics, if a test shows it is present (or other organisms such as Ureaplasma and Mycoplasma). This approach stems from the belief that vaginal infections (vaginosis) may occasionally lead to premature labour. However, research studies to date are inconclusive and treatments may only benefit women who have had a previous premature birth.[3] Therefore, routinely treating all pregnant women with Gardnerella, who have no symptoms, is not generally recommended.

Most Gardnerella infections go away without medical treatments and should not affect the baby if present during a vaginal birth. The most common antibiotic prescribed is metronidazole (Flagyl), taken orally or vaginally. It is advisable that your partner is treated as well, to stop you being reinfected. Studies so far have not found conclusive evidence linking Flagyl to abnormalities in the baby, if given during the first 12 weeks of pregnancy. But many caregivers (and women) like to wait until after this time to treat, if possible. You may be able to utilise natural therapies in the meantime.

ACHES AND PAINS

The growing uterus can cause many strange sensations, some uncomfortable or painful. These unfamiliar feelings can be worrying for a woman because it's hard to know whether they are normal.

Stitch in the groin

The round ligaments supporting the uterus can be strained when walking, coughing, sneezing or exercising, causing sharp groin pains, often on one side. These are sudden and sporadic and may take your breath away slightly, but they soon settle. Rest, heat packs and lying on the affected side (to take the strain off) usually helps. Some homeopaths recommend Bellis perennis. Contact your caregiver if it doesn't ease.

Braxton Hicks contractions

After 20 weeks, Braxton Hicks contractions (or tightenings) can start as the uterus tones the muscles in readiness for labour. These may feel like a hardness, or a tight band pulling across your belly. Many women don't notice them, but others find them quite strong, even labour-like, especially if this is not their first baby.

Braxton Hicks are infrequent and may be shorter (20 to 30 seconds) or longer (90 seconds to 2 minutes), compared to labour pains. Relaxation techniques, acupuncture, homeopathic remedies (Belladonna, Calcarea carbonica or Chamomilla) or herbal preparations (cramp bark, skullcap or raspberry leaf) may help. See your practitioner.

Low, heavy dragging pains

With subsequent pregnancies, feeling heavier, bigger, lower, aching and 'dragging' is common, although often unexpected if previous pregnancies did not involve this. The ligaments and pelvic floor muscles supporting the uterus, being stretched and weakened from previous pregnancies, hold the uterus lower. Doing pelvic floor exercises, yoga, swimming or belly dancing may help. Some women have acupuncture or take homeopathic remedies.

Waist pain

Although not common, pain in the middle back and waist can indicate that a ureter from one of the kidneys is kinked, slowing the flow of urine and causing pain. This usually improves within a week or so, but pelvic rocking on your hands and knees or belly dancing may help. Your caregiver may perform blood or urine tests to check your kidney function and rule out an infection.

Sore hips

Hips can be sore as ligaments over the hip joint loosen with hormonal changes. Sleeping on a hard mattress often aggravates this. Try placing pillows between your legs or a sheepskin under your hip when sleeping. Use heat packs, hip massages, yoga, or sit with your legs apart. A physiotherapist may suggest exercises. A homeopath may prescribe Calcarea phosphorica or Chamomilla.

NOTE: *If you are concerned about any aches and pains, contact your hospital or caregiver. Particularly if you have:*
- *Painful cramping that comes and goes, every 5, 10 or 15 minutes for an hour or more.*
- *Pain associated with bleeding, or a fever.*
- *Severe or constant abdominal pain, or a very tender uterus.*

GROWING BELLY

After 12 weeks the uterus grows up and out of the pelvis, so you can feel the top of it (called the fundus) when touching your lower belly. By 20 weeks this reaches the level of your navel, and by 28 weeks it is close to approaching your ribs!

Having a pregnant belly makes everyone you meet a pregnancy expert. This may make you feel special, or perhaps annoyed at the unwanted attention. You may even feel uncomfortable if people start touching your bump without asking first. The predictable question of 'How many months are you?' is often followed by 'You're so big, small' or even 'You're so fat!' This can erode your confidence, or perhaps make you concerned that something may be wrong. The truth is, not even the most skilled and experienced obstetrician or midwife can tell how pregnant you are just by looking at your belly.

Try to remember that your body is unique in how it responds to pregnancy. It is better to rely on your caregiver's judgment rather than the opinions of well-meaning 'experts'.

> **Did you know?**
> You cannot predict the sex of an unborn baby from the shape of a woman's belly.

Most women produce a baby that is the right size for their body. A few reasons why you may look smaller or larger compared to other pregnant women (even though your baby is a normal size) can include:

- **Whether this is a first or subsequent baby** – When your abdominal muscles stretch for the first time, they are toned and tight, holding your baby close and high, making you look smaller and show later. With subsequent pregnancies, the abdominal muscles are flexible, making you show earlier and look bigger.
- **The position of your baby** – This changes regularly up until 32 to 34 weeks (or later), making your belly look smaller at times and larger at others.
- **Your height** – Tall, long-waisted women have a large space between their hipbone and ribs, providing plenty of room for their baby to grow upwards. Women with a relatively short waist, have less room upwards, so they tend to carry more forward.
- **Your intestines** – Those are often pushed behind the growing uterus, make you look 'all baby'. A few women find their intestines are pushed out to the sides and over the top of their uterus, making their belly bigger, rounder and fuller (but they are less likely to suffer from constipation).

> **Did you know?**
> It is the mother's size at birth, not the father's size (at birth or as an adult) that has a bearing on whether a baby will be big.

MATERNITY CLOTHES

As your waistline thickens, wearing fitted clothing becomes uncomfortable. By 14 to 16 weeks your belly will protrude, but you may still get away with wearing looser or elasticised clothes. From 18 to 22 weeks your belly will definitely 'pop out', and your garments will need to accommodate this.

Maternity wear can be as glamorous, sexy, corporate, formal or casual as you like, and increasingly women are happy to show off their bump. It all comes down to individual taste, work requirements and how you are feeling about your body. Your temperature naturally increases when pregnant, so wear light, breathable clothing (cotton or wool), and possibly a few layers to make it easier to adjust to all conditions.

You don't need to spend a fortune. A few mix-and-match items can provide quality and value. Borrow maternity clothes (or buy 'pre-loved' maternity wear) if you can, especially for one-off formal occasions. Many non-maternity clothes made from stretchy fabric can suffice (or even your partner's clothes). Elasticised inserts are now available to expand the waistline of pants and skirts; however, they may not work with hipsters and can look uneven under tight-fitting T-shirts. Consider stretchy dresses, clothes with elastic or drawstring waists, or wraparounds with adjustable clips. If possible, pick maternity clothes that won't go out of style, so you can use them again (if you plan to have another baby), or lend them to others.

NOTE: *Most women still have a larger than usual tummy for a few weeks after their baby is born, requiring stretchy clothes for comfort, especially if a caesarean was needed. So hold onto your maternity clothes for a while.*

Normal underwear can be worn, but you can buy maternity underwear. These days, there are many choices and innovative designs to help you feel more feminine during pregnancy.

Bras: Your breasts initially enlarge and may do so again after 20 to 24 weeks. If you don't normally wear a bra, you may need to now. Some women find their breasts are very heavy and tender and wear a lightweight bra to bed. It is important you feel supported and comfortable. Sports bras or crop tops are great. Don't use underwire bras as they can injure tender breast tissue.

Maternity bras aren't necessary during pregnancy, but many women do wear them. Generally, the size you are after 24 weeks is the size you will be after the birth. Many breastfeeding women wear their bras day and night to provide support and limit milk leakage. If you plan to wash daily, three bras should do; otherwise buy four to five. When purchasing maternity bras:

- Get measured and fitted professionally (in a department store or specialist lingerie shop). You might buy one bra, then purchase others from a cheaper outlet. Ask about fastening and unfastening the bra cups.
- Choose cotton so your skin can breathe.
- Larger breasts need wide shoulder straps for support and to prevent the straps digging into the shoulders.
- Make sure the band under the cups of the bra is comfortable so it doesn't restrict blood flow to the breasts.

Briefs: You can wear normal briefs that sit under your bump, or oversized underwear that pulls up over your belly (more comfortable after the birth if you have a caesarean scar). Wear cotton underwear (or underwear with cotton gusset) to help prevent thrush.

Pantyhose: Buy pantyhose with a cotton gusset. Maternity pantyhose are available but expensive. You can now get sizes for 'large bellies and thin legs', which aren't necessarily maternity. Full-length support stockings are good if you are on your feet all day.

Socks: Avoid tight socks, or half-leg stockings, which may reduce blood circulation and aggravate swollen feet and varicose veins.

Shoes: Comfortable shoes are a priority. As your belly grows, your centre of gravity changes, making you prone to tripping and falling, so low-heeled shoes are preferable. High heels can also aggravate back pain or leg cramp. Your foot can increase half to one size and may swell further with fluid retention. Backless shoes made of a flexible material can accommodate these changes.

BABY'S MOVEMENTS

At some stage during the second trimester, you will feel your baby move for the first time (called quickening). This may be difficult to distinguish at first, but after a few weeks, those faint, fluttering sensations (or wind feelings) become stronger and more definite movements as your little one wriggles around. Some women describe them as small bubbles popping, a scratching internal feeling, or like involuntary muscle twitching.

Initially you may not feel your baby move every day; within a few weeks, however, the sensations become more frequent as your baby grows bigger and stronger, until you feel them several times a day, every day.

Feeling your baby move is thrilling and exciting. Unborn babies can move from 10 weeks, but they can only be sensed when they place enough pressure on the uterine walls to stimulate nerves in the woman's skin. The timing of quickening is usually between 18 and 22 weeks, but a few women notice vague sensations from 12 weeks, and others don't feel anything definite until 23 to 25 weeks. Your partner and others won't feel anything when touching your belly until 22 to 26 weeks, although most babies stop moving when someone places their hand on the mother to feel the movement. Maybe it is reassuring for them.

NOTE: One way to show others your baby's movements is to put a light object like a paper napkin on your belly while sitting or reclining. As the baby kicks, the object moves, often to the delight and amazement of those watching.

Be aware that:
- Women who have had a previous baby often notice movements earlier and feel their baby is more active. The muscles and ligaments surrounding the uterus are more flexible, allowing more room for the baby to move.

- A placenta implanted at the front of the uterus, close to your belly (anterior), cushions the baby's movements, delaying you feeling them (till about 22 to 24 weeks) and making the baby feel less active.
- Women carrying extra weight may find it more difficult to sense their baby's movements until later in the pregnancy.

Adapting to change

EMOTIONS IN THE MIDDLE MONTHS

The second trimester can seem more emotionally balanced, with a sense of calmness and acceptance of the pregnancy as you start preparing for your baby's arrival.

Emotions for the woman

As the reality sinks in, your thoughts may turn towards making plans for your baby's arrival and reflecting on how you will parent. It can seem that pregnant women and/or new babies are everywhere now, and you may find yourself observing other mothers. Many women imagine (or dream about) what their baby will look like, or have feelings about them being a boy or girl.

> **Did you know?**
>
> An old wives' tale supposed to be able to predict the sex of your baby involves threading a needle or wedding ring, and someone hanging it over your pregnant belly. If it swings from side to side you are having a girl, but if it moves in circles you are having a boy!

Forgetful and vague – Concentration on memory lapses are often put down to 'pregnancy brain' but they have more to do with shifts in your focus as you turn your attention inwards to your baby. For example, you may be acutely aware of your baby moving, while you put the margarine into the oven! It is common to suddenly forget credit card PINs, or go shopping for bread and come home with carrots. Believe it or not, though, pregnant women have sharper reflexes and a better short-term memory, when asked to perform motor tasks or recall exercises.[4]

Mother Nature does slow you down and make you disengage from some aspects of your life, producing subtle changes in your priorities. Often things that used to be very important become less so (job, career, finances) and your baby, relationships, home and family take precedence. This is simply an internal preparation for the exciting lifestyle change to come!

Your relationship with your mother – Becoming a mother can make you think about your own mother more, or see her in a different light. A new grandchild can also make mothers see their daughters differently. Some mother–daughter relationships become closer with the sharing of past experiences and feelings. Others fall apart in the face of painful memories and old hurts. This can feel disappointing and painful for a pregnant woman at this vulnerable time.

Dreams – Vivid dreams are common during pregnancy and can be amazing or scary, especially if they involve losing, neglecting or dropping your baby. Dream analysts believe babies in dreams are symbols of new beginnings, particularly psychological growth and development, rather than a reflection of reality. In some cases, the dream may reflect ambivalence towards nurturing one's own psychological adjustments.

Try not to take your dreams literally. Some women seek homeopathic remedies to help with distressing dreams. If your dreams prevent you from getting back to sleep, try relaxation techniques or positive visualisations.

Emotions for the partner

Most partners connect more with their baby once they see the woman's belly grow, see their baby with ultrasound or feel them kick. You may begin planning (or increasing) your workload to save money or allow for a freer schedule when the baby arrives. If moving house, or renovating, try not to leave this until the final weeks when she is less able to cope.

Becoming a father can be exciting and daunting. You may start seeking the company of other dads if you are a first-time father, or find yourself observing how they interact with their children. Many fathers talk (or sing) to their unborn baby. You can also put your ear on her belly to listen, perhaps detecting the baby's heartbeat (or just getting a jab in the ear!).

> **Did you know?**
> Newborn babies often stop crying and listen intently to their father or mother if they talk to them, relaxing to the familiar sound of their voice.

Feeling protective of your partner and unborn baby is very normal, and you may find yourself questioning things she does, such as climbing ladders to clean light fittings. Discretion can be the better part of valour here. Just being there to make sure she doesn't fall may be better than placing a veto on the activity! Some women enjoy this extra care and attention; others find it patronising and don't react kindly. Finding balance is always hard. Showing that you care but trusting her judgment is a good guide.

New motivations – Impending fatherhood can bring a renewed purpose in life. You may reassess your career, make changes or implement lifestyle or social changes to support your partner (or to just feel healthier).

Your relationship with your father – Having a baby can cause you to reflect on the relationship you have with your own father. Some father–son relationships become closer and involve sharing experiences. If you feel a special connection with your dad, perhaps ask him about his fathering experiences, to nurture positive feelings for your own impending role. However, others find they don't want (or don't have) involvement with their father, which can be disappointing and sad at this time of your life.

BODY IMAGE, SEXUALITY AND LIBIDO

As your body changes, you need to adjust emotionally. Some women like their belly, but others feel unsure or unhappy, seeing themselves as fat or unattractive. Worrying about how your partner feels, and whether they still find you desirable, is also pretty normal. As the partner, it can be difficult to make her feel beautiful, loved and cherished. If you like her body, let her know, because she may need reassurance. Frequent expressions of affection are what most pregnant women want. An impromptu 'I love you', kissing her tenderly, putting your arms around her, holding or stroking her, giving her a foot massage, or telling her how beautiful she is, all help her to feel special and loved.

Many women have a renewed interest in sex once their tiredness, morning sickness and/or fear of miscarriage subsides, pregnancy hormones may also noticeably increase libido. Others feel less sensual as their body changes.

Pregnancy involves changes in a woman's sexuality, as much as it does in her body and emotions. Changes may also be apparent in a partner's sexuality and the way he perceives her body. How you and your partner feel, affects your libido and making love together, as well as your relationship. Depending on your expectations, they may deepen your bond, or perhaps place a strain on it.

Maintaining intimacy, not to mention getting your sexual desire synchronised, is always a challenge. Most sexual frustration comes from different expectations about the frequency of sex, feeling unattractive and/or rejected if advances are not wanted or not made in the first place. Some common sexual attitudes during pregnancy include:
- Loving the look of pregnancy, finding it beautiful, curvaceous, sensual and fascinating.
- Disliking the look and feel of pregnancy, finding the expression of your sexuality difficult.

- Enjoying the spontaneity of sex without concerns of contraception or timing sex for conception.
- Not wanting to have sex in case anything goes wrong.
- Moving from seeing the woman as a sexual being to a sensible mother; feeling uneasy about making love to her.
- Enjoying or disliking her belly or breast changes (especially if there is milk present).
- Feeling special about the miracle of creating a child.
- Feeling envious of the woman's ability to grow and carry a child.

Discuss your cues for sex. If giving a cuddle means 'I want sex', this simple expression of intimacy can be misinterpreted, discouraging (or stopping) advances or possibly provoking feelings of rejection. It is important to be honest about how you are feeling and explain why you are wanting, or not wanting, sex. Then you can work towards how you can best express your love for each other. Look at replacing the sexual act with massage, touching, and caressing without intercourse. The journey of pregnancy to parenthood is easier if you begin by nurturing each other.

As the partner, if you feel uncomfortable with her body and having sex, it is still important to share this, but in a sensitive way. This may not be easy, but she probably senses your reactions anyway. If you don't explain your feelings, she may perceive your disinterest as a personal rejection or that something is wrong in the relationship (such as your being interested in someone else). Continue to give her positive affirmations ('I am so happy we are having our baby') and tell how you feel and why, so you can find other ways to express your love for each other and avoid relationship conflicts.

Concerns about sex

Concerns about hurting the baby during penetrative sex are common, but the woman's cervix is sealed with a thick mucous plug and the amniotic fluid protects the baby. Pressure on the woman's belly should be gauged by her comfort. Braxton Hicks contractions during sex and orgasm are normal and generally subside after a few minutes. They don't trigger labour, unless the body is ready (close to the due date). Some couples feel uneasy about having another 'person' between them. The baby can move during sex, particularly after the woman experiences orgasm. Some may find this fascinating, or a little disconcerting, or perhaps be put off by it. Having sex with vaginal penetration from behind the woman can reduce the awareness of the baby's activity.

As the pregnancy progresses

WHAT TO EXPECT AT YOUR CAREGIVER PREGNANCY VISITS

Pregnancy visits up till 28 weeks are scheduled every four to six weeks, depending on your needs and your caregiver's preferences. If everything is progressing normally, then it is five to six weeks, but if you have a health condition, complications or a multiple pregnancy, you are seen every four weeks (or perhaps every two to three weeks).

You can take your partner, or the person supporting you at the birth. Involving them helps nurture a united approach. Many parents also take their other children to include them in a positive way. They may even hear their little brother or sister's heart beat!

Routine pregnancy visits involve checking your blood pressure, monitoring the growth of your baby and discussing your physical and emotional wellbeing. They also provide opportunities to discuss your birth and any current concerns you have. Write down your questions to take with you. As a guide, you may discuss:

- Physical signs that are concerning you and possible therapies, treatments and support strategies.
- Blood tests, genetic or ultrasound results.
- If and when you sense your baby's movements.
- Things you have read or heard that need explaining or clarification.
- How you are dealing with lifestyle changes, financial, relationship and/or emotional difficulties.
- Aspects of the labour and/or birth.
- What you can expect before the next visit.

Feeling your belly

Your caregiver feels (or palpates) your pregnant belly to ensure the uterus is growing at the expected rate. Your baby is not large enough to detect their position until 24 weeks, when their head and position can be felt. Ask your caregiver to guide your hands, so you can feel your baby's head.

Fundal height – From 16 weeks your caregiver may measure your uterus or fundal height. This aims to detect if the baby is unusually small or large. Research suggests that fundal measurement might be slightly more accurate than palpation alone in detecting very small or large babies.[5] However, caregivers concede they are not reliable and some don't do them.

While lying on your back, the caregiver places the end of a measuring tape on your symphysis pubis bone (just below the pubic-hair line), then up the middle of your belly, to the top of your uterus, giving a height in centimetres. NOTE: *You don't need to take your underpants off to have a fundal height measurement taken.*

Fundal heights have their greatest benefits between 22 and 34 weeks and are not taken after 37 weeks. A textbook fundal height is when the centimetres equal the weeks of pregnancy (20 weeks pregnant = 20 cm). However, it is normal to be 2 to 4 cm higher or lower even though the baby is normal and healthy. This can be caused by:

- The position of the baby. Breech babies may measure higher and babies lying across ways (transverse) measure significantly lower.
- Physical differences between women's bodies (taller, shorter, slimmer, etc).
- First babies tend to be at the expected level. Subsequent babies are often carried lower, measuring less.
- A family history of smaller/larger babies and ethnicity. For example, Asian women tend to have smaller babies compared to Maori women.

Measurements can differ between caregivers, and they may unintentionally accommodate the measure by making it closer to what they are looking for (overstretching or loosening the tape). Some caregivers turn the tape over and measure blindly to try to overcome this.

Listening to your baby

Your caregiver will try to hear your unborn baby's heartbeat. They listen for a few seconds to a minute or so, and possibly time the beats per minute, which can range from 120 to 160.

> **Did you know?**
>
> You cannot predict the sex of an unborn baby by counting their average heart rate. Preterm babies have faster heart rates that progressively slow as they grow, and it is slower when a baby sleeps and faster when they are active.

The heartbeat can sound a little like a horse galloping. Caregivers may use:
- **A Pinard's stethoscope** – This trumpet-type earpiece can only be used after 20 to 24 weeks. When having twins, two caregivers listen to each baby simultaneously, counting their heart rates separately.
- **A Doppler machine** – This emits high-frequency ultrasound waves to create an audible sound. This can detect the baby's heartbeat from 12 to 14 weeks (but definitely by 16 to 18 weeks). When having twins, two machines are used simultaneously.

NOTE: *Some women request their caregiver use only a Pinard's because they prefer their baby not to be exposed to unnecessary ultrasound.*

Irregularities in a baby's heart rate are followed up with continuous monitoring on a CTG machine for 20 minutes or so.

Did you know?
After 30 to 32 weeks, your partner may be able to hear the heart beat by placing their ear directly on your belly, around where the baby's shoulder should be. Have complete quiet in the room and block your other ear with your hand. Using an empty cardboard toilet roll can also do the trick.

Twins, triplets or more

Once more than one baby is discovered, the pregnancy and birth care generally becomes more involved, because it is now classified as higher risk, even though 50% of twin pregnancies progress normally. Higher order multiples (triplets, quads, etc) have an increased chance of complications.

Pregnancy visits are similar to women having one baby, although some caregivers prefer to see you more often. To date there is no research that determines how often pregnancy visits should occur for multiples, so practices between caregivers vary. Discuss the timing of visits with your caregiver to work out what is reasonable medically and what suits you. If it is just a matter of checking your blood pressure, your local doctor may be able to do this between your pregnancy visits. If your caregiver is concerned about complications, or the growth of one (or more) of your babies, then serial ultrasounds at regular intervals may be recommended after 26 weeks.

TESTS YOU MAY BE OFFERED

Routine blood tests are usually scheduled around 28 weeks (ranging from 26 to 30 weeks). If your blood group is Rhesus negative, you will need another antibody screen and may be offered a routine injection of anti-D immunoglobulin to help prevent isoimmunisation.

Full blood count (FBC)

Haemoglobin (Hb) is checked to detect anaemia. It is normal and expected for this to be lower than the first test, due to a natural dilution of blood cells. From 28 weeks your baby stores iron in their liver to meet their needs for the first 6 months after birth. This can decrease your haemoglobin further. Adequate haemoglobin contributes to:
- Supporting your health and how you cope physically and emotionally.

- Supplying your baby with oxygen during the labour, reducing the chances of them becoming distressed.
- Allowing you to tolerate a normal blood loss at birth (or a caesarean) and reducing the chances of requiring a blood transfusion if your blood loss is excessive.
- Assisting your recovery and ability to care for your baby.
- Helping establish your breast milk supply.

Therefore, if your Hb is below 11.0 gm% (110 g/L), your caregiver will talk to you about adjusting your diet and taking daily iron supplements until the birth. If you are already taking iron supplements, you may need to change (or increase) them.

NOTE: Dietary changes and iron supplements take at least 4 to 6 weeks to make any measurable changes in your haemoglobin.

Iron supplements: There are many different brands to choose from, or your caregiver may recommend one. Standard iron supplements (from pharmacies) tend to be slow release tablets or capsules taken once a day and may cause nausea and constipation (or diarrhoea) in some women. Taking the tablet at night, drinking plenty of fluids or changing brands may help. It is normal to have blackish-green bowel motions while taking them.

Natural iron supplements tend to be smaller doses in tablet or liquid. These are taken two to three times a day and can be expensive, but they don't tend to cause side effects. Some women alternate slow release tablets with natural supplements every other day to balance the cost and side effects.

As a guide, you need 30 mg of elemental iron per day every day. On the labels, iron is described as ferrous (Fe) sulphate, fumarate or gluconate or iron aminoates with elemental iron in brackets in mg. For example: Ferrous fumarate 15.3 (5 mg). If written as a percentage, 5% elemental iron in 100 mg equals 5 mg of elemental iron.

To increase iron absorption:
- Take supplements with a drink of pineapple, orange, tomato or blackcurrant juice. Some caregivers recommend a vitamin C supplement. Natural supplements usually have vitamin C added.
- Avoid taking supplements with tea, coffee or wholegrain foods and cereals, which inhibit iron absorption. Taking them before going to bed or mid-morning or afternoon can help.

Iron injections: In the rare circumstance you aren't absorbing the iron supplements, or your anaemia is significantly low, less than 9.0 gm% (90 g/L), your caregiver may prescribe iron injections (and stop iron tablets). These take three to four weeks to fully absorb, with the need for further injections guided by blood tests. However, they may cause a permanent stain to the skin around the injection site, so some caregivers prefer to avoid them unless absolutely essential.

Glucose tolerance test

Glucose tolerance tests (GTTs) aim to detect gestational diabetes, which affects 2.6% of pregnant women. Caregivers and hospitals vary in offering the test routinely. Some places only do them if you have high risk factors, such as:
- A family history of diabetes.
- A previous baby weighing over 4.5 kg.
- Being overweight for your height.
- Being over 35 to 40 years (depending on the policy).
- Having a previous unexplained stillborn baby.

GTTs remain controversial, with some believing they are inaccurate and do not provide any great benefits for women and babies.[6] A few women choose to decline the test.

A short GTT (SGTT) may be offered first (or skipped altogether in favour of a long GTT). This involves having a special sweet drink and a blood test one hour later. The SGTT is a screening test, meaning it only indicates you may be at increased risk of gestational diabetes. If the blood sugar is more than 7.8 to 8.0 mmol/L, you will then have a long GTT. Many women have an abnormally high SGTT, then a normal LGTT, meaning they do not have gestational diabetes.

NOTE: Stress and illness can interfere with your body's metabolism of glucose and cause an abnormally high blood sugar reading. Also, your ability to deal with glucose is better in the mornings, so try to schedule tests earlier in the day.

A long glucose tolerance test (LGTT) may be offered first, or done after an abnormal short GTT. To be of most benefit, a LGTT should be done between 24 and 32 weeks. The test involves having a high carbohydrate diet for three days (breads, rice, pastas, potatoes), then fasting from midnight the night before and not having breakfast. Blood is taken the next morning, before having a special sweet drink, then a second blood test is done one hour after the drink, with a third blood test two hours after the drink. Ideally, the first and third levels should be less than 8.0 mmol/L.

Random BSL is a blood sugar test done at any time, not relating to fasting or eating. These are very unreliable and should not be used to diagnose gestational diabetes.

Post-prandial BSL is a blood sugar test done two hours after eating a large meal (without the sugar drink). The level should be less than 8.0 mmol/L. Some women choose to have this rather than a long or short GTT.

Vaginal swab

It is now fairly routine to offer pregnant women a low vaginal swab test to screen for Group B streptococcus (Strep B), usually around 28 weeks, or delayed till (or repeated at) 34 to 37 weeks. Group B streptococcus naturally occurs in the bowel, bladder and vagina in small quantities. It is not regarded as an infection (nor is it sexually transmitted) and generally does not cause health problems. Between 5 and 30% of all pregnant women test positive for Group B Strep and are not aware they carry the bacteria. Some women tend to test positive, others never test positive, and a few test positive at some times and negative at others.

You can usually perform the swab yourself by placing a sterile cotton bud (provided by your caregiver) about two to three centimetres inside the vagina. Some caregivers prefer to do an anal swab (outside the rectum), instead of (or as well as) a vaginal swab. Results take two to three days, with 'normal vaginal flora' meaning negative and 'GBS positive' meaning you have the bacteria. Some laboratories also comment on 'light', 'moderate' or 'heavy' growth, reflecting the amount of bacteria present. However, this does not affect treatment decisions. If the test is positive, it is recommended you have antibiotics as a tablet once the waters break and/or intravenous antibiotics at six to eight hourly intervals during labour, until the baby is born. While most babies are not affected by GBS, about 1 to 2% become infected during labour or birth. Babies at increased risk are those:

- Born to mothers who had a urine test or vaginal swab showing strep B with this pregnancy, or a previous pregnancy.
- Born prematurely (less than 37 weeks).
- Born after the waters have been broken for more than 18 to 24 hours before the birth.
- Whose mothers developed a fever during labour (above 37.5°C). This is more common with prolonged labours, multiple vaginal examinations during labour and epidurals.

In very rare cases a baby is infected without any of the above risk factors being present. Infected babies usually develop pneumonia symptoms within 7 days of birth, but more commonly within 6 to 24 hours. Physical signs include:

- Breathing rapidly (above 80 breaths per minute, normal is 40 to 60).
- Flaring nostrils; their chest moving noticeably with breathing, making their ribs visible; and sucking in their stomach to take deep breaths.
- Being pale, grey or bluish in colour.
- An abnormally high or low temperature (above 37.5°C or below 36°C).
- An increased heart rate (above 160 to 170 beats per minute).

- Possibly drowsy and lethargic, reluctant to feed, with a weak cry or a stiff posture, screaming inconsolably, being excessively irritable.

GBS can be life-threatening for 15% of infected babies. If your baby has these symptoms, take them to the hospital immediately.

ULTRASOUNDS

The most common routine ultrasound is offered at 18 to 20 weeks. This screens for physical abnormalities in the baby and is called a fetal anomaly or morphology scan. It also locates the position of the placenta. Ultrasounds cannot determine a baby's genetic make-up, so it is important to remember that they cannot exclude every possible problem in an unborn baby nor detect all birth defects.

The baby must be at least 18 weeks gestation to adequately examine all their body systems, although some abnormalities aren't obvious until 22 weeks. If the ultrasonographer suspects a problem, a more detailed 'level 2' ultrasound is scheduled at a later time. The 18 to 20 week timing tries to strike a balance between detecting abnormalities as early as possible, yet hopefully allowing parents more choice in regards to proceeding with the pregnancy if an abnormality is detected.

Pregnancy ultrasounds can be very useful and provide a lot of information, but it is important to know they have limitations. The accuracy of an ultrasound very much depends on the qualifications, skill and experience of the ultrasonographer. However, even the most experienced and skilled pregnancy ultrasonographers with the best equipment can still miss things and misinterpret images.

NOTE: *Ultrasounds have up to a 1 in 10 (10%) 'false positive' rate, meaning they may indicate the baby has a birth defect when in fact they are normal and healthy.*

The baby's sex – By 15 to 16 weeks the baby's genitals become obviously male or female, and can be identified with an ultrasound image. The ultrasonographer looks for a penis. If one is thought to be seen, the baby is said to be a boy. If a penis cannot be identified, the baby is presumed to be a girl. Ultrasounds are about 90% right, with boy babies being more accurately predicted than girl babies. You may want to let the ultrasonographer know before the examination whether or not you wish to find out the sex of your baby.

Photos and videos – Parents now expect a snapshot of their unborn baby as part of their ultrasound. However, ultrasound services are not obliged to provide photos because it is essentially a medical procedure (Medicare and private health insurers don't cover the cost of photos). Some centres ask for a fee to provide a photo or video, or add the cost to their gap fee (or ask you to supply a blank video).

Ultrasonographers are ethically obliged to keep the exposure of unborn babies to 'as low as reasonably achievable' (the ALARA principle), performing everything required in a minimum time. Ultrasounds at 18 to 20 weeks take 30 minutes to 1 hour to complete, so the ultrasonographer may feel it is unnecessary to provide a photo (or even identify the baby's sex), because this means extra time and exposure. Many parents view this attitude as negative and trivial and feel a photo is very important. However, the ultrasonographer may only provide a picture if they have time and/or are willing to please you.

Recently, some commercial businesses have started offering expectant parents 'entertainment ultrasounds' – videos, photos and even voice-over narration for a substantial fee. These have no connection with medical practices or hospitals, do not look for abnormalities and do not take the place of medical ultrasounds. You will need to have additional ultrasounds for any medical reasons.

3D and 4D ultrasounds – Most ultrasounds are the conventional two-dimensional. In recent years, three-dimensional, or ultrasound holographs, have become available. Four-dimensional images are just 3D images seen in real time, so the activity of the baby can be studied. From a medical perspective, 3D/4D ultrasounds are not essential and generally conventional 2D ultrasounds obtain all the information your caregiver needs. Besides, 3D/4D machines are extremely expensive and not widely accessible yet.

Are ultrasounds safe?

At this stage we think so but aren't definitely sure because there is insufficient research to confirm it. Medical ultrasounds work like sonar (used to map the sea bed). During each scan the ultrasound probe (or transducer) generates and receives hundreds of high-frequency sound waves that cannot be heard by the human ear. These are absorbed and bounced back from the baby's and mother's bones, body fluids and tissues (all with different densities) to create black and white images. Frequencies for pregnancy ultrasound waves range from 1.6 to 10 MHz (normally 3 and 7.5 MHz). Diagnostic ultrasounds, which create images, tend to require lower frequencies, which makes them safer than the Doppler ultrasounds used to assess blood flow through the cord and placenta and listening to the baby's heartbeat. The main physical concerns with ultrasound relate to:

- **Heating body tissues** – There is a slight temperature rise, depending on the type of body tissue (highest in bone and lowest in body fluids). Diagnostic ultrasound waves intermittently pulsate to try to reduce

heating, and ultrasonographers aim to keep exposure to a minimum, being conscious of 'dwell times' over specific areas.
- **Cavitation** – The formation of small bubbles in body fluids, due to the heating effect, can potentially cause cell damage, but it is not known what effect this has on a developing baby (if any). It has been questioned that this may cause left-handed tendencies in boys exposed to ultrasound.[7]
- **Streaming** – The level of pressure exerted by ultrasound waves moving through body tissues causes body fluids to flow in the direction of the ultrasound waves. This can potentially work against natural blood flow. At this stage, fluid speeds are thought to be low and unlikely to cause damage to an unborn baby.

Worrying concerns

Parents usually approach their baby's ultrasound with eager anticipation. However, this can quickly turn to anxiety and apprehension if a possible problem is detected. Often this is a minor 'variation of normal', which has no health effects for the baby and is expected to resolve without treatments. However, even the suggestion of a problem leaves parents feeling helpless and concerned for the remainder of the pregnancy, particularly as it can't be treated (or even investigated further) until the baby is born.

The other side of this coin is that ultrasounds can't detect everything, so some problems may be missed, making parents resentful if they felt lulled into a false sense of security.

Sometimes 'soft signs' are found, which are subtle variations of normal that in themselves are not an abnormality but when combined with other soft signs can occasionally indicate a genetic disorder. Usually the baby needs several soft signs to be strongly predictive of a genetic disorder. Up to 90% of babies with soft signs are normal and healthy.

Renal pelvis dilation is where a part of the kidney is enlarged. This occurs with about 2% of babies, but 84% of them don't have a health problem and it generally rights itself by the time the baby is 12 months old.

Choroid plexus cysts are small fluid-filled cysts within the part of the brain that produces cerebral fluid and are found in 2% of normal pregnancies. They are not harmful, don't cause health problems and eventually disappear. However, they are seen as a soft sign for a rare disorder called Edward's syndrome (Trisomy 18), which causes several abnormalities of the limbs, heart, brain, and/or face. The ultrasonographer carefully checks the rest of the baby and if no additional abnormalities are found, the baby is most likely normal and healthy.

Two vessels in the umbilical cord: Most unborn babies have three blood vessels in their cord (two arteries and one vein). Up to 1% of babies (and 5% of twins) have two vessels (one artery and one vein). About 75% of these babies are well and healthy. However, in 25% the presence of only two vessels may be related to a genetic disorder. If the ultrasonographer cannot find other abnormalities, the baby is most likely healthy. Occasionally, a two-vessel cord is associated with the unborn baby not growing as well as expected and further ultrasounds are done to monitor their growth.

Middle pregnancy variations

Women with existing health conditions may require special management to help their pregnancy progress normally. Depending on the condition, a medical specialist may work in partnership with an obstetrician (through the public system or privately) to manage the pregnancy and birth care. You may need to continue seeing the specialist for weeks (or months) after the birth, until the condition stabilises.

HIGH BLOOD PRESSURE

High blood pressure before pregnancy is called essential hypertension. For women with this condition the aim is to control the blood pressure at, or below, 140/90, which may mean starting or changing anti-hypertensive medications. Women with uncomplicated, controlled essential hypertension tend to have similar health outcomes as women with a normal blood pressure (as do their babies). The main concern is the chances of developing pre-eclampsia, which is five times higher than normal.

ASTHMA

Women with mild asthma usually experience uncomplicated pregnancies. However, severe, uncontrolled asthma can increase the risks of premature birth, the baby having a low birth weight; and possibly experiencing high blood pressure during pregnancy. Generally, about one-third of women with asthma find it improves during pregnancy, another third find it worsens and the remaining third don't notice any changes.

Most asthma medications are safe to take during pregnancy but may need adjusting as the pregnancy progresses. Because you are now breathing for two, it is important not to stop medications without your doctor's advice. The best way to control asthma is to avoid allergy triggers, or anything else that tends to bring on an attack. Pregnant women with asthma can exercise under the guidance of their doctor. Influenza vaccines may be recommended after 12 weeks of pregnancy, but are preferable two to three months before conception.

DIABETES

Pre-gestational diabetes mellitus may be insulin dependent, or non-insulin dependent. Pregnancy does not affect the diabetes condition or the woman's health, but blood sugars need to be well controlled (ideally from preconception) to avoid complications. If this can be achieved, it is likely the pregnancy and baby will be normal and healthy. If blood sugars are frequently high, there is an increased chance of:
- Miscarriage.
- The baby developing abnormalities during the first 12 weeks.
- Urine infections and thrush for the woman.
- Pregnancy complications such as pre-eclampsia, making premature birth more likely.
- Too much fluid around the baby.
- Slower growth of the unborn baby, or having an abnormally large baby, which may lead to birth problems (see Chapter 7).
- The baby developing breathing problems at birth, because their lungs take longer to mature (38 to 40 weeks as opposed to 36 to 37 weeks).
- The baby having low blood sugars (hypoglycaemia) soon after birth, requiring intensive care treatments.
- The baby dying in the womb during late pregnancy.[8]

Blood sugars are monitored with finger prick tests three to four times a day. Women taking insulin often find this needs to be decreased during early pregnancy (as their metabolism increases), but they may require more insulin as the pregnancy progresses. Women who control their diabetes with diet alone may start needing insulin at some stage during pregnancy.

Diabetic women without pregnancy complications and relatively good blood sugar control should be allowed to go to 40 weeks of pregnancy before inducing labour is considered. Being diabetic is not a reason in itself for an elective caesarean, as this has more health risks than benefits.[9]

EPILEPSY

Over 90% of women with epilepsy have uncomplicated pregnancies and give birth to healthy babies. Anti-epileptic medications need to be prescribed by a neurologist, who aims to keep doses to a minimum but high enough to prevent seizures. Dosages may need to be slightly increased at the beginning of the pregnancy, then reduced during middle pregnancy and increased again towards the end. Regular blood tests monitor drug levels to make sure they are adequate.

About 40% of women with epilepsy experience fewer seizures during pregnancy; 25% don't experience any changes, and 33% experience more seizures, especially during the first and last trimesters.[10] When a seizure happens, the unborn baby receives less oxygen, possibly making their heart rate slower for up to 20 minutes or so. Most babies tolerate this to a degree, but in rare cases they may suffer various levels of brain damage or die. This is why it is very important *never* to stop taking prescribed medications, as this increases your chances of seizures.

Some anti-epileptic medications reduce vitamin K in the body. Your caregiver may prescribe vitamin K supplements during the last four weeks of pregnancy, to help protect the baby from vitamin K deficiency bleeding (VKDB) after birth. The baby is also given vitamin K at birth.

Heart disease

Up to 1% of pregnant women have heart disease, or a cardiac disorder, usually due to a heart defect present from birth. (Babies born to women with a heart defect have a slightly higher chance of also having a heart defect.) Many women with heart conditions have normal, uncomplicated pregnancies and the pregnancy does not generally affect their long-term health. However, severe heart conditions can complicate pregnancy, in some cases being life-threatening for the woman and her baby.

Pregnancy puts the most strain on the heart from 20 to 34 weeks and bed rest may be needed during this time. If the heart disease is severe, fluid can accumulate in the lungs (pulmonary oedema), which requires hospital admission. Other treatments can include:

- An ultrasound of the heart.
- A halter monitor (a machine worn for 24 hours at home to monitor and record heart beat patterns).
- Planning a diet to support ideal weight gain.
- Preventing anaemia with iron supplements.
- Possibly cardiac medications.
- Intravenous penicillin (or an alternative) during labour.

If the heart condition deteriorates, a decision may be made to deliver the baby prematurely, possibly by caesarean. Otherwise labour may be induced a couple of weeks before the due date and the baby will be continuously monitored. During the second stage of labour, the strain of pushing may further stress the heart. Therefore, forceps may be recommended to deliver the baby. Any anaesthetic given requires much consideration and care. Ideally, your anaesthetist should be experienced in dealing with pregnant women who have heart conditions. After the birth the body excretes excess body fluid (by passing lots of urine), which can also place stress on the heart, requiring a longer hospital stay with closer monitoring. Health risks may persist for several weeks after the birth.

THYROID CONDITIONS

The thyroid gland produces hormones, thyroxine (T4), triiodothyronine (T3) and calcitonin. These stabilise the body's metabolism, temperature, heart rate and blood pressure, and regulate the development of bones and nerves. A normally functioning thyroid is essential for conception, pregnancy and breastfeeding.

Hypothyroidism (myxoedema) is an underactive thyroid, which causes excessive weight gain, intolerance of the cold, an abnormally slow pulse, puffy face and can stop ovulation. Blood tests for T3 and T4 diagnose the condition. Once thyroxine is prescribed, the body usually rights itself, but the drug may need to be continued during pregnancy. Thyroxine does not cross the placenta to the baby.[11]

Hyperthyroidism (thyrotoxicosis or Grave's disease) is due to an overactive thyroid, but is less common. This causes weight loss (despite a good appetite), high blood pressure and a rapid pulse. Blood tests diagnose this. Pregnancy often improves hyperthyroidism, but it may relapse several weeks after the birth. If it is severe, management involves a high-calorie diet and drinking plenty of fluids to avoid dehydration, especially if experiencing diarrhoea. Sometimes anti-thyroid drugs are prescribed. In rare cases, part of the thyroid gland needs to be surgically removed during pregnancy. Being excessively hyperthyroid may lead to poor growth of the unborn baby and premature labour.

BLOOD DISORDERS

Inherited blood disorders can affect your haemoglobin and are thought to affect 7% of the world's population. Genetic counselling may be helpful if you have concerns about the baby inheriting the disorders, which include:
- **Thalassaemia** – This often causes anaemia during pregnancy but is not related to iron deficiency. Folic acid supplements are given instead

of iron to help increase red blood cell production, and sometimes blood transfusions are required.
- **Sickle cell disease** – Here, red blood cells are distorted into a sickle shape, making them unable to carry oxygen and have difficulty passing through tiny blood vessels. This can lead to anaemia and tissue damage in various body organs (sometimes reducing fertility). Iron and folic acid supplements are given during pregnancy and possibly a blood transfusion every six weeks or so. You also need to be mindful of not becoming dehydrated and may require antibiotics, intravenous fluids and extra oxygen during labour.

Urine infection

A urinary tract infection (UTI or cystitis) after 20 weeks of pregnancy may stimulate premature labour. Physical signs can include:
- Passing urine more frequently.
- Burning or stinging when urinating.
- Constant ache in the lower belly.
- Headache, vomiting and/or a fever or chills.

If the infection moves to the kidneys, there may be constant backache and blood in the urine. An infection is confirmed with a urine test and the treatment is antibiotics, which may need to be administered intravenously in hospital if the infection is severe.

To help prevent bladder infections:
- Wipe your genitals from front to back after going to the toilet.
- Wear cotton underwear and avoid synthetic leggings and pantyhose.
- Drink eight glasses of water and one glass of unsweetened cranberry juice (perhaps blended with fresh parsley) or freshly squeezed lemon juice in warm water or barley water.
- Eat garlic and foods with vitamin C and zinc to boost the immune system. Avoid sugary foods to reduce glucose in the urine.
- Some herbalists suggest nettle tea to strengthen the kidneys or dandelion tea (avoid uva ursi, this can irritate the lining of the uterus).
- Homeopaths may suggest Sulphur, Staphysagria, Nux vomica, Mercurius solubilis or Causticum for mild urine infections. See your practitioner.

Antenatal depression

It used to be thought that pregnancy hormones 'protected' against depression. However, it is now known that up to 10% of women experience antenatal depression and are also at increased risk for postnatal depression, although this is not a given. Recognising and acknowledging depression is an important first step. Feelings can seem scary, or wrong, and therefore many women are reluctant to verbalise them to others. However, they are a normal part of a psychological illness, which needs to be dealt with in positive ways and are not reflective of how you are as a person. It is important to tell others about your depression and get help. Symptoms of antenatal depression can be similar to postnatal depression, described in Chapter 14.

Support strategies

- Find support through friends, family, a group environment or professional counselling. Build up a support network and talk to people you trust. Put words to how you are feeling and identify issues affecting you to help make things clearer and your problems more manageable.
- Look after yourself. Eat well and relax. Regular exercise has been shown to reduce depression. Try doing something for yourself each day. Create a quiet space, paint or write, go for a walk, have a massage or long bath.
- Avoid doing too much when you're feeling depressed. Once you achieve something, tell yourself well done. Give yourself positive messages, perhaps record good moments or thoughts in a diary, no matter how small.
- Accept the painful feelings and focus on the good feelings. Be kind to yourself. Avoid being too hard or critical and comparing yourself with others.
- Take one step at a time. It may be a gradual process.
- Allow others in so they can understand your feelings and stop you being isolated. Try doing things with or being around others who make you feel better.
- Make plans for when the baby comes and how you will facilitate support if you experience postnatal depression. Consider setting up emergency contacts with professionals just in case. If you can, organise family help, pre-cooked meals, nappy service and so on to help with the demands of early parenting.

Medications

Anti-depressants are avoided (or changed) during pregnancy if possible. Sometimes the small risks of taking medications are far outweighed by how the depression is affecting the woman's health and wellbeing, making them, on balance, necessary. Discuss your options with a qualified psychiatrist experienced with treating pregnant women.

Partner support
Partners often find themselves out of their depth when the woman is experiencing depression, feeling they are unable to cope with the strains of supporting her, providing financially and preparing for the baby. Support strategies include:
- Reading about and becoming familiar with depression.
- Being patient and working through her emotions. This can take time, involving good days and bad days.
- Listening and not judging her. The signs of depression are symptoms of an illness, not reflective of how she is as a person.
- Not ignoring your own feelings. If you need help, seek it out.
- Journaling your feelings and possibly sharing these with someone you trust.
- Avoiding terms like 'Pull yourself together' or 'What do you want me to do about it?' Her feelings of depression are not logical.
- Letting her catch up on sleep and giving her space. Nurture your relationship whenever possible. Don't force her to venture out if she does not feel like it, although gently encouraging exercise may help.
- Setting up key words, so she can tell you quickly when she is having a bad day.
- Remembering that she is your partner in life, best friend and lover, not just the pregnant mother of your child.

TWIN VARIATIONS
Health variations for multiple babies are similar to those for single babies. However, the chances of complications are often increased (50% of twins and 80% of triplets are premature) and a few rare conditions are unique to identical twins.

Cord entanglement
If identical twins share one amniotic sac, their umbilical cords may become entangled, which can be life-threatening for one or both babies if it leads to a reduction in their blood supply. While there is little anyone can do to prevent cord entanglement, most caregivers recommend regular ultrasounds to monitor the situation. The twins are usually delivered by caesarean, to avoid tension on the cords that may occur with a normal birth.

Twin-to-twin transfusion
Twin-to-twin transfusion syndrome can happen for up to 17% of monochorionic identical twins. Connections form between the deep arteries and veins

in the placenta, causing excessive blood to shunt to one baby, creating a circulation imbalance. In essence, one twin 'donates' some of their blood to the other twin (the recipient) over several weeks; this usually becomes evident by 28 weeks. If the condition becomes severe, it can be life-threatening for both babies, particularly the recipient twin.

Caregivers may try various treatments to prolong the pregnancy (to prevent extreme prematurity) and reduce the effects of the condition. Although, at this stage, there is insufficient research to prove one method is better than another.[12]

BABY DYING DURING PREGNANCY

The shock of finding out that your baby has died is devastating beyond words. If you have just discovered this, we extend our heartfelt sympathy and understand that your journey from here will not be easy. 'Why does this happen?' is the unrelenting question. Sometimes the reason is clear, but often it is never known, leaving parents bewildered. The medical terms given to a baby dying during pregnancy are intrauterine death (IUD) or death in utero (DIU), which can seem very cold when faced with such a loss. Babies lost when less than 20 weeks are referred to as a late miscarriage. The care and management of this is explained in Chapter 2.

Some women notice their baby has not moved for a while. Others feel something is not quite right, or have an intuitive sense of danger or death. Most women are not aware and it comes as a shock. If your baby's heart beat cannot be found, their death is confirmed by an ultrasound.

Choices for birth

It can be hard to make decisions when grief is engulfing you. Give yourself time to absorb what has happened. Ask staff to explain your choices. Some women want whatever is necessary to have their child born immediately. Others need time to think about how they wish to give birth. If you want to go home for a while, do so. This could be for a few hours or a couple of days. If you are carrying twins, and one baby has died, the decisions will be more complicated, and you will need to discuss your options with your caregiver. Other things to consider are discussed in the section on stillbirth in Chapter 7.

Caesarean or labour and birth

Unless there is a medical indication, a normal birth is recommended. Caesarean births have health risks for the mother and avoiding caesarean optimises your chances of a normal pregnancy and birth in the future, if you choose to have another child. Some women find it hard to understand why they should have to endure labour and give birth, but most comment on how important it was to go through the process and to feel involved. Usually labour needs to be induced. However, once the contractions become strong, the progress of dilation and pushing is often very quick, being as little as a few hours or less.

All autumn you danced within me,
Dancing to the music of my soul, I felt the vibrant personality you would be.
Then one day the dancing ceased,
I knew of it before your heartbeat could not be heard.
All my dreams of you, the life that we would share, taken in a day, in a moment.
The dancing has ceased, but my love for you, my precious one, goes on.
Forever a part of me. Forever in my thoughts. Forever in my dreams. I love you.
Anonymous

FAQs

WHAT ABOUT TRAVEL DURING PREGNANCY?

Essentially, travelling during pregnancy is not a problem, but there are a few precautions to be mindful of.

Flying

Concerns about flying are usually related to the small chance that you may have the baby mid-flight, or that a complication might develop, requiring urgent medical attention. Women who have experienced heavy bleeding or threatened premature labour may be advised not to fly, at least until the complication has settled.

Normal commercial aircraft are fine, but non-pressurised planes at high altitude can reduce oxygen to mother and baby and should be avoided (as should visiting places more than 3000 metres above sea level). Potential exposure to cosmic radiation (mainly for pregnant flight crew) is a small theoretical risk that has not been proven.[13]

Domestic flights (less than four hours) generally have no restrictions for pregnant women. Check with your airline.

International flights (or domestic flights longer than 4 hours) generally do not accept pregnant passengers after a certain gestation (from 26 to 36 weeks, possibly earlier with a multiple pregnancy). The airline usually requires a letter from your caregiver stating when the baby is due.

If you plan to visit a country that recommends vaccinations (or anti-malarial medications), discuss this with your doctor. In general, vaccinations are not recommended during pregnancy, but if exposure to certain infectious diseases is considered more risky than the vaccination, it may be considered.

Economy class syndrome can occur after long-haul flights (to people in all classes of plane travel) as well as after long coach, train or car trips, so it is usually called traveller's thrombosis. A blood clot develops in a deep vein of the calf or thigh (deep vein thrombosis), due to not moving around much. Pregnant women are slightly more prone because their blood clotting is more efficient, and being dehydrated also puts you at increased risk. If the clot dislodges, it can move through the bloodstream blocking small blood vessels in the heart, lungs or brain, which is life-threatening. Physical signs may not be evident for up to three days after the flight, often starting with pain or discomfort in one leg. However, not everyone has noticeable symptoms. To avoid thrombosis[14]:

- Move your legs regularly. Get out of your seat every hour or so. When sitting, rotate your ankles and feet occasionally or do isometric exercises (tensing and relaxing your calf and thigh muscles).
- Elevate your legs if you can, for 10 minutes every hour or so.
- Wear full-length support pantyhose. Avoid tight socks and half-leg stockings that may restrict circulation.
- Drink at least a glass of water an hour.
- Avoid sedatives or alcohol (which is advisable when pregnant anyway).
- Some doctors recommend a one-off injection of heparin on the day of the flight to thin the blood (covering for 24 hours) or low dose aspirin. The effectiveness of these has not been researched, but they are generally only advisable for women with other risk factors. The above measures are usually quite adequate.

Cars, buses and trains

When driving during pregnancy, adjust your seat and steering column as needed. An automatic car with power steering generally makes driving easier, especially when your manoeuvrability becomes limited. Pregnant women should always wear seatbelts correctly. The body sash goes between the breasts and over the bump, and the lower sash is positioned over the hips (under the bump), and should not ride up over your belly. If a serious accident occurs, a correctly worn seatbelt makes it less likely you or your baby will be injured.

You are entitled to a seat when travelling on public transport. Take the same precautions for avoiding economy class syndrome when on long car, train and bus trips.

Tips for travelling

- Take your pregnancy record card with you in case medical attention is needed while away from home, as well as your caregiver's (or hospital's) contact numbers.
- When travelling overseas, check your travel insurance. Some only insure until a certain stage of the pregnancy (eg. 24 weeks), and others don't cover overseas births. Australia has reciprocal medical arrangements with Britain, Ireland, New Zealand, Italy, Malta, Finland, Sweden and the Netherlands.
- If possible, don't travel long distances alone.
- It is fairly common to develop swollen, puffy feet. Wear shoes that are loose and/or flexible, or backless slip-ons.
- If you have morning sickness or need to pass urine frequently, ask for an aisle seat close to the toilet.
- If you suffer from restless legs, magnesium phosphate or cell salts (available from health stores) taken an hour before the flight can help. Massage your calves at intervals and stretch and walk when possible.
- Share the driving if you can't be driven all the way. Drink plenty of fluids, have regular snacks and plan plenty of toilet stops. Get out of the car and walk around every one to two hours or so.
- If you have lower back pain, purchase a small circular back pillow for support.

CAN I LIE ON MY BACK?

After 24 to 28 weeks, some women feel light-headed, dizzy and possibly breathless if they lie flat on their back for more than a few minutes. This is caused by the uterus placing pressure on a major blood vessel (vena cava) that lies behind it, reducing blood supply to your heart, brain and the baby. Sleeping on your right or left side, sitting in an upright (or semi-upright) position, avoids vena-caval compression. If you do happen to roll onto your back while sleeping, you will usually wake when feeling the physical effects, so try not to worry about this. It is possible to sleep on your back to some extent, by placing a flattish pillow under the right side of your body to slightly tilt your uterus towards the left, avoiding vena-caval compression.

> **Did you know?**
> When a caesarean is performed, a small wedge-shaped pillow is placed under the woman's right side to allow optimal blood flow to the baby before birth.

What will I do with my belly piercing?

There is no medical reason to take your belly ring or bar out (unless it annoys you), and a few women continue to wear theirs for the entire pregnancy. (Consider taking it out during labour, in case a caesarean is required.) However, if your navel pops out, it may rub on clothing and the jewellery might catch on things more readily.

If you have had your piercing for a long time and the area is fully healed, it will probably remain open after taking your jewellery out. Alternatively, you can run something through the piercing each day to keep it open. One enterprising woman threaded a new piece of fishing line through hers! Another option is to buy a PTFE belly bar. This is made of flexible, plastic-like Polytetrafluoroethylene that fits conventional 1.6 mm threaded accessories.

Be aware that your navel piercing may not heal for several weeks or months (some people find they never really do). Therefore, if your piercing is recent and weeping, red or irritated, you may choose to remove the jewellery and let it heal, perhaps having it repierced after your baby is born.

CHAPTER 4

The final months: 29 weeks till birth

The third trimester is from week 29 until your baby is born. Your belly grows bigger as your baby becomes heavier, ready for life in the outside world.

Your unborn baby's growth and development

Between 28 and 37 weeks, your baby could survive if born, but only with the help of specialised intensive care technology. During the final weeks of pregnancy, your baby's main task is to grow their body systems, build their immunity and put on weight, so by 37 weeks, they are mature enough not to require medical assistance.

Week 30 – Your baby weighs around 1350g (3 lb) and measures 40 cm from head to toe. Their bones start producing blood from the bone marrow, taking over this task from the liver and spleen, and your baby begins storing iron in the liver for after the birth. A special layer of fat called brown adipose tissue begins developing, which will be their main source of heat production after birth (similar to hibernating animals). Your baby's brain is increasing in size and complexity, and the pupils of their eyes now respond to light, allowing them to focus more readily and see dim shapes.

Week 32 – Your baby weighs about 1.7 kg (3 lb 12 oz) and is 43 cm long. They have now put on enough weight to look a little chubby! The fine hair covering their entire body disappears from their face, but remains on their body. They sleep 90% of the time, in between shorts bursts of movement, every 1 to 2 hours. Often being most active in the evenings, when you are trying to sleep, between 9 pm and 1 am! Their lungs continue to mature, producing increasing amounts of surfactant. This is the fatty liquid that lines their lungs to keep them moist and helps the tiny sacs within them to expand efficiently for breathing. Their sucking and swallowing action fully co-ordinates between 32 to 34 weeks, but premature babies of this gestation often require feeding milk through a fine tube inserted in their mouth or nose, because suckling tires them quickly.

Week 34 – Your baby weighs about 2.1 kg (4 lb 10 oz) and is about 45 cm long. They are now fully formed physically and have a firm grasp reflex. During the last six weeks they have built up their immune system from antibodies passed from their mother through the placenta. They can now determine the difference between sweet and sour tastes.

> **Did you know?**
> Unborn babies detect subtle changes in the 'flavour' of amniotic fluid. It is believed this fluid acts as a flavour bridge to their mother's breast milk, which also carries different food flavours from the woman's diet. Up to a litre of amniotic fluid is swallowed each day, being passed as a type of urine through their kidneys and bladder, back into the fluid around them. Most babies assume a head down position around this time, staying this way until birth. You may notice your baby's movements changing to be more stretches and squirms, as they grow larger and there is comparatively less room.

Week 36 – Your baby may weigh around 2.6 kg (5 lb 12 oz), and measure about 47 cm from head to toe. By 36 to 37 weeks their lungs have fully matured. They are now in normal proportion and quite plump. Before 36 weeks their head size is larger than their belly size, but this now equalises. From here on, their belly grows larger than their head, but your baby's overall growth slows considerably. They don't grow as much in length, but gain about 230 g per week (or an ounce a day). Their head may become engaged, but many women don't experience this until closer to their due date.

Week 38 – Your baby may weigh around 3.1 kg (6 lb 13 oz) and measure around 48.5 cm. The proportion of fat on their body has increased, from 30 g at 30 weeks, to around 430 g (approximately 16% of their total body weight). A baby born on time has small pads of breast tissue under their nipples (in both boys and girls) and fingernails reaching the tips of their fingers, often looking manicured. The fine covering of hair has all but disappeared, but they are still covered with vernix. Most baby boys now have descended testes, from their groin into their scrotum. The placenta now covers about a third of the inner surface of the uterus, processing around 12 litres of blood per hour.

Week 40 or 'term' – The average Australian baby weighs 3300g (7 lb 4½ oz), ranging from 2800 to 4500g (6 lb 3 oz to 9 lb 15 oz). The average length is 50 cm, ranging from 46 to 56 cm. Their head circumference averages around 35 cm, but ranges from 33 to 37 cm. By 40 weeks your baby is assumed to be 'cooked' to perfection. Most of the vernix on their skin has gone, but there may be remnants in their armpits and groin. An unborn baby's breathing exercises are believed to naturally stop about 24 to 48 hours before labour commences. The lungs normally hold about 75 to 100 ml of amniotic fluid, and during labour, hormones are released by the mother, triggering the baby's system to absorb most of this fluid into their bloodstream before birth, which is fully absorbed within 24 hours after being born.

Weeks 41 to 42 – Your baby continues to put on a small amount of weight, but if very overdue, they can start to lose weight. Amniotic fluid around your baby gradually reduces and all their vernix cream disappears. Their fingernail tips start to look shrivelled and flaking, and their skin is often dry, peeling and possibly redder in colour. This is why overdue babies are often referred to as being 'overcooked'! However, for a few babies, being born around this time is the right time for them and they are born looking like babies at 40 weeks.

Physical changes in preparation for birth

Each woman's body undergoes many unique physical changes, to carry, grow and nurture her child, then move through labour to give birth.

THE UTERUS

The uterus is made of muscle cells, each growing 10 times in length and 3 times in width during pregnancy. After 24 weeks, the uterus stretches upwards, forming a thick upper segment, leaving a thinner lower segment, which encircles the bottom third of the uterus. The lower segment is fully formed by 36 weeks and takes up, or absorbs, the cervix during labour as the uterine muscle cells progressively shorten with labour contractions. This dilates (or opens) the cervix and pushes the baby down the birth canal.

The pregnant uterus naturally leans towards the woman's right side and is held in place by ligaments attached to her pelvic bones and lower back. These ligaments stretch as the uterus grows, acting like supportive anchors to stabilise it, while facilitating the baby's movements within. Aches and temporary sharp groin pains are common during pregnancy as these ligaments are gently strained.

> **Did you know?**
> The prepregnant uterus is 8 cm long, 5 cm wide and 50 g in weight. By the end of the pregnancy it is 30 cm long, 22 cm wide and weighs 1 kg!

THE CERVIX

The cervix, or neck of the womb, is the entrance to the uterus. It is thick and firm, 2 to 5 cm long, and extends into the top of the vagina at an angle, normally pointing towards your tailbone. The cervix is made of glandular tissue that produces a thick mucus plug during pregnancy, filling the narrow cervical canal to seal the uterus from outside infection, often coming away before, or during, labour as a 'show'.

MEMBRANES AND AMNIOTIC FLUID

Your unborn baby is held within two tough, and slightly elastic membranes (the chorion and amnion), collectively referred to as the sac or bag of waters. This provides a protective layer around your baby and contains the amniotic fluid, which allows your baby to move freely and exercise their limbs. It also acts as a cushion of protection from outside pressure or impact. Amniotic fluid appears as droplets three weeks after conception, accumulating to 20 ml by eight weeks, 400 ml by 20 weeks and 800 to 1000 ml by 36 to 37 weeks, after which time it slightly declines.

THE PLACENTA

The placenta (or afterbirth) grows to a large, flat disc, implanted flat against the wall of the uterus. By the time your baby is due, it is around 2 cm thick and the size of a small dinner plate, looking a little like liver. The placenta acts like a sieve, moving oxygen and nutrients from your body to the baby's, taking carbon dioxide and waste materials from the baby into your body for elimination. The blood vessels of mother and baby are incredibly close together where the placenta is attached but, remarkably, remain completely separate while facilitating this exchange.

THE UMBILICAL CORD

The umbilical cord attaches to the baby's navel at one end and the centre of the placenta at the other. It grows to be 1 to 2 cm thick and approximately 50 cm long, containing 2 arteries and 1 vein, all entwined and enclosed by a protective, gristly substance called Wharton's jelly. This makes the cord slippery and ensures it moves freely around your baby. Blood constantly pulsates through the cord with every beat of your baby's heart.

Did you know?
- The umbilical cord stops growing by 28 weeks.
- Male babies have, on average, a cord 4 to 5 cm longer than female babies.
- About 25% of healthy babies are born with the cord loosely around their necks.

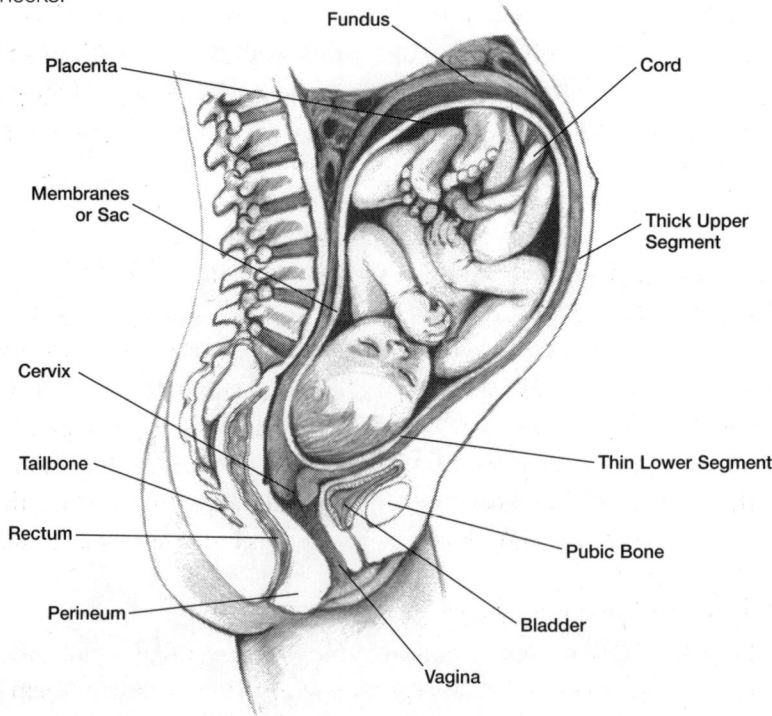

Unborn baby towards the end of pregnancy

THE PELVIS
The pelvis is made of two bones joined by cartilage and ligaments to the lower backbone at the sacroiliac joints and at the front symphysis pubis bone. During late pregnancy, hormones soften and relax these ligaments, making the bones elastic, rather than rigid, so the bones can stretch and open more easily for the birth of the baby.

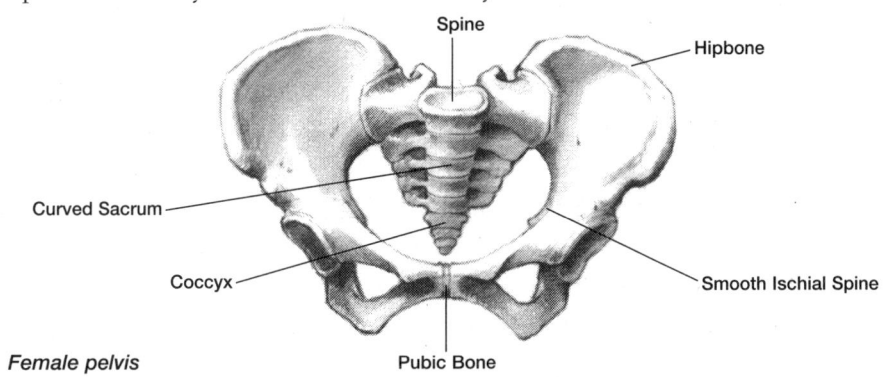

Female pelvis

Some positive thoughts to take with you into labour:
- Your pelvis is not fused and *does* stretch and open, expanding for the amazing process of birth.
- Your baby's skull bones are divided into five plates that cross over during labour, making their head smaller by moulding, to fit the birth canal.
- Your baby has an innate sense of crawling or burrowing, as they move down and out of the uterus and through your pelvis to be born. Gravity helps your pelvis open and aids the descent of your baby.

THE PELVIC FLOOR MUSCLES
The pelvic floor is a strong, layered sheet of muscles that stretches like a hammock from your pubic bone to your tailbone. During pregnancy they support the weight of your uterus and growing baby, and your intestines. During birth they guide your baby through the vagina, helping them negotiate the pelvis. Pregnancy hormones naturally soften the muscles to make them more flexible for the birth. The pelvic floor also helps control the passing of urine, the opening of the bowels and contributes to sexual sensations during intercourse.

Pelvic floor exercise
If the pelvic floor muscles are toned, they recover more rapidly after pregnancy (whether a vaginal or caesarean birth). Exercising them during pregnancy, and after the birth, aids the healing of vaginal tears or stitches and haemorrhoids.

To gain an awareness of your pelvic floor muscles, lie down, or sit comfortably, relaxing your belly, thighs and buttocks. Then concentrate on tightening your anus, as if trying to stop passing wind. These are your pelvic floor muscles tightening. You can also attempt to interrupt the flow of urine before completely emptying your bladder. However, this should be limited to once a week, as it may interfere with the normal functioning of the bladder.

To do pelvic floor exercises:
1. Tighten your anus and vagina. Imagine drawing them up inside you; hold for as long as possible, for up to 10 seconds. Then release the tension.
2. Rest for about 10 seconds.
3. Repeat the squeeze and lift, again for up to 10 seconds, then release.

Aim to work up to 3 sets of 10 squeezes per day. You may initially find you tire quickly, so rest and increase the number you do over time. Quality is better than quantity. You can also try 5 to 10 short, fast, strong contractions as well. Again, doing what you can and increasing over time. When doing pelvic floor exercises, **don't**:
- Tighten your belly, thighs or bottom (although you may feel a slight pulling in the lower stomach or buttocks).
- Hold your breath.
- Push down and out instead of pulling up and in.

Pelvic floor exercises can lay down a body memory for relaxing and letting go, which is needed for pushing your baby out.

THE PERINEUM

The perineum is a strong, flexible muscle between the opening of the vagina and anus. It stretches during a vaginal birth to allow your baby to be born. Since the 1980s, massaging the perineum has been used to try to prevent vaginal tearing. Research indicates this may help to a small degree, but does not guarantee you won't tear.[1] Commercial devices have also been developed to try and mimic perineal massage, although these are quite expensive and not necessarily better, with many women finding them difficult to use.

Perineal massage can allow you time to connect with this part of your body in a way which is neither sexual nor associated with going to the toilet, and it can help you become familiar with the sensation of the perineum stretching and burning during the pushing phase of the labour.

NOTE: There can be emotional and physical benefits from perineal massage, but it is not an essential task, so don't feel pressured or guilty about not doing it. Some women (and their partners) don't particularly like it, or find it a chore. This is fine.

Remember, many women never massage their perineum and don't tear.

You may prefer to do your own perineal massage, or involve your partner. Talk about how you both feel. Most women start after 32 to 34 weeks, massaging once or twice a day (or when convenient). Before starting, make the environment relaxed and private. Turn the phone down and mobile off, have soft lighting, relaxing music, perhaps burn aromatherapy oils (lavender, mandarin, geranium). A warm bath (or warm compress on the perineum) beforehand softens the skin and can also help you relax.

Get comfortable, sit semi-reclining with lots of pillows, or stand with one leg on a small stool, or sit on the toilet. You will need a lubricant (natural oil – almond or vitamin E, or a water-soluble jelly). Whoever does the massage, make sure your hands are clean and nails clipped.

1. Gently rub the oil/lubricant into the external perineal skin until soaked in, taking a minute or two. (Then wipe or wash most of the oil from your hands.)
2. The partner may use their first and second fingers (with one or both hands). The woman uses her thumbs. Place your fingers (or thumbs) shallowly into the lower vaginal opening, just above the perineum, in 3 cm at most.
3. Gently press downwards, towards the anus, and then slowly stretch the skin and muscle towards each side in a downwards and outwards direction until the woman feels a slight burning or tingling sensation. Communicate with each other (if doing this together) to allow her control of the stretch and discomfort level. If using one finger/thumb (or two fingers on one hand), gently stretch down towards the anus, then in a downward sweeping motion from side to side. *Remember, it is only a gentle stretch. It should not be painful.*
4. Hold the stretch for approximately 60 seconds (the average time of a contraction) and then rest for a minute or two, allowing the muscle to recover.

The woman can use her 'out' breath to relax her pelvic floor and perineum, allowing them to 'give'. The partner may breathe with her to help her focus. If doing perineal massage together, the woman may tell her partner to go slower, be softer or apply a little more pressure, and the partner may give feedback to let her know if she is resisting by reminding her to breathe, let go, release. Communicating openly and directly is valuable for giving and receiving support during labour.

NOTE: Don't do perineal massage if you have a vaginal infection or herpes. If using oil, keep most of it on the perineum, rather than inside the vagina, as it can disturb the normal balance of micro-organisms there, making you prone to developing thrush or Gardnerella.

The final weeks

Physical changes
As the pregnancy advances, many women feel heavy and tired. The baby takes up more space, often creating several discomforts. Towards the end, it is normal to feel fed up with being pregnant, just wanting your baby to arrive soon!

Backache and sciatica
Hormones soften and relax the ligaments connecting the pelvis to the lower back, at the sacroiliac joints, making the bones prone to moving out of alignment causing pain. The sciatic nerve may also be pinched, causing shooting pains down the buttock and back of one leg (sciatica). As your belly swells, the centre of gravity shifts, favouring incorrect posture, which doesn't help. Incorrect lifting, sitting, and moving techniques can twist and strain back muscles unnecessarily. After 36 weeks, babies in a posterior position can also cause lower backache. Upper back pain may be felt with desk work, sewing, or holding and feeding a new baby after the birth.

   What some women find helpful:
- **Maintain good posture** – Tuck your bottom under and keep your body straight, to reduce the curve in your lower back. Keep your neck, back and hips in alignment when sitting for long periods. Avoid slumping. Sit well back on the chair with your thighs fully supported and place a pillow in the small of your back. If you can't rest your feet comfortably flat on the floor, use a footrest or phone books, so your knees are at the same level as your hips (or slightly higher). Sleep with pillows between your legs and behind your back.
- **Use proper lifting techniques** – Squat or bend your knees with your feet apart and one foot slightly forward. Don't bend from your waist and hips. Face the object you intend to lift (never twist or turn to pick something up), avoid jerky, sudden movements and hold heavy objects close to your body. If possible, let someone else lift. When picking up a toddler, kneel on one knee and use your free hand to push off from the other knee as you lift.
- **Work at a comfortable height** – If standing, this should be hip to waist level. Kneel to perform tasks at a lower level. When standing for long periods, put one foot up on a footrest to relieve the curve in your lower back, swap feet occasionally. If cleaning, put the vacuum or mop in one hand while putting the opposite leg forward to work, with the forward knee slightly bent.

- **Do pelvic tilt exercises** – Lean your back against a wall, feet slightly apart, with the weight on your heels and knees slightly bent. Breathe in, and on the out breath, tighten your belly muscles and buttocks, flattening the hollow of your lower back against the wall and tilt your pelvis forward and upwards. Hold this for a few seconds. This can also be done lying on your back with your knees bent and feet flat on the floor.
- **Try shoulder rotation exercises** – Place your fingertips of both hands on your shoulders and rotate your elbows in a backward circular motion a few times.
- **Use natural therapies** – Consider chiropractic, osteopathy, Alexander or Bowen techniques; swimming, yoga, massage, shiatsu, acupuncture, herbal liniments or tinctures (St John's wort and skullcap); and homeopathic remedies (Hypericum perfoliatum or Arnica). If you have strained your back, use heat packs on the affected area or have a warm bath. Some women add a few drops of lavender oil to the bath to help with muscle spasm.

Medical treatments: Consult a doctor if your back pain is severe. You may need bed rest until the muscles recover. Avoid painkillers and sedatives unless prescribed by your caregiver. You may be referred to a physiotherapist for exercises and perhaps a pelvic girdle to stabilise the joints (like an elastic corset worn around the hips).

Breathlessness

Breathlessness usually comes and goes, even while sitting and having a normal conversation. During pregnancy, the lungs take deeper breaths, inhaling up to 40% more air to supply extra oxygen for your baby. During middle to late pregnancy, pressure from the baby on the diaphragm can make it difficult for the lungs to expand. Breathlessness sometimes occurs with palpitations (feeling your heart is pounding inside your chest).

NOTE: *Breathlessness that does not go away, or associated with pain in the chest or upper back or sweating and feeling faint, is of concern, requiring urgent medical attention. Contact your caregiver or hospital.*

What some women find helpful: Be patient and don't panic. Breathlessness usually improves after a short period. Sitting upright or sleeping on a couple of pillows may help you catch your breath.

Carpal tunnel syndrome

Carpal tunnel causes a feeling of pins and needles, numbness, stiffness and/or pain in the hands, due to fluid accumulating in the wrists, putting pressure on the median nerve. Slumping your shoulders can also put pressure on the ulnar and median nerves, causing carpal tunnel. Grasping objects can be difficult, especially in the mornings, but it usually improves throughout the day. Discomfort may make it difficult to sleep at night but it generally improves a few weeks after the birth.

What some women find helpful:
- Massaging the wrists with creams or oils (aromatherapists may suggest adding a drop of juniper oil). You (or another person) can massage each side of the wrist using the thumb(s). Start from the middle of the wrist, use a firm but comfortable stroking motion, moving down and straight out the sides, across the base of the wrists.
- Using acupuncture, acupressure or shiatsu massage. The point is located on the fleshy inside pad of the hand, at the base of the thumb. Apply pressure firmly, holding in position for six to eight seconds. Do this two to four times in the morning and repeat as needed throughout the day.
- Physiotherapy splints can be fitted to wear at night, often with your hands elevated on pillows. This may help if it is early in the pregnancy and/or your work is being affected.

Medical treatments: Ultrasound is sometimes used on the wrists to stimulate tissues around the affected nerve. This treatment is not proven and results vary.

Constipation

Constipation can happen with increased progesterone slowing the movement of the gut, and dietary changes and dehydration with morning sickness, as well as direct pressure on the intestines from the growing baby.

What some women find helpful:
- Drink at least eight glasses of water a day and one to two glasses of fruit juice (prune juice is great) and/or fresh vegetable juice. Hot or very cold drinks can stimulate the bowel. Try warm water with a squeeze of lemon first thing in the morning.
- Increase fibre in your diet – cereals, bran, fruit and vegetables, especially dried fruits (prunes, apricots, dates, figs and sultanas). A bit of liquorice may also help.
- Take time to go the toilet. Try not to put off passing motions. Place your feet on a low footstool for support.
- Gentle, daily exercise such as walking, swimming or yoga.
- Change iron supplements to a different brand (check with your caregiver).

- Herbalists may suggest psyllium, flax seeds, liquorice root or sprinkling slippery elm powder onto your cereal or adding a pinch of cayenne to food.
- Aromatherapists might suggest patchouli oil added to carrier oil for a gentle abdominal rub in a clockwise direction, above the level of the uterus (but not before 12 weeks of pregnancy.)
- Homeopathic remedies may include Aesculus hippocastanum.

Medical treatments: Your caregiver may suggest fibre bulking laxatives with plenty of water, or a glycerol suppository inserted into the anus and held for 10 to 20 minutes, to soften bowel motions and make them easier to pass.

AVOID:
- Mineral oils (liquid paraffin), which can be absorbed into the body and interfere with the absorption of vitamins A, D, E and K.
- Oral preparations and suppositories containing stimulants that cause cramping, excess fluid loss and possibly premature labour (castor oil, senna, cascara, bisacodyl, phenolphthalin, danthron or sodium sulphate).
- Salts of magnesium, potassium and sodium, which can be absorbed into the system and interfere with the kidney functioning of the baby.

Haemorrhoids

Haemorrhoids (piles) are essentially varicose veins of the anus due to increased progesterone, making the blood vessels relax. Also, pressure from the baby and uterus on the rectal area makes the blood pool, swelling the veins. Haemorrhoids appear as one (or several) small lumps around the opening of the rectum and are usually painful, itchy and may bleed, especially after a bowel motion. They don't affect the labour and birth, but may be sore for a week or so afterwards, but should eventually go away. For a few women, they decrease in size but remain.

What some women find helpful:
- Avoid constipation. Use the strategies outlined above for this.
- Avoid hot spicy foods (cayenne, black pepper, hot sauces and curries). These can increase congestion in the haemorrhoids and cause them to bleed.
- Try to do at least three sessions of pelvic floor exercises each day. Avoid squatting for prolonged periods, and rest to take the pressure off the area. Perhaps elevate the foot of the bed, or put a small pillow under your bottom when resting. If the haemorrhoid is large, you can replace it back into your bottom with your finger (wearing a glove if you like), to make you feel more comfortable.
- Herbalists may suggest drinking nettle leaf tea, taking bioflavonoids

and vitamin C, or applying witch hazel ointment or pouring liquid witch hazel onto a small gauze pad and applying this to the haemorrhoid. Diluted lemon juice, or apple cider vinegar, are alternatives. (These may sting if the haemorrhoids are bleeding). Ointments with St John's wort flower or calendula may help.
- Aromatherapists may suggest a few drops of geranium oil in a bowl of warm water to sit in, or pouring this over the area with a jug after opening the bowels, or mixing it with K-Y gel and applying this to the area.
- Homoeopaths may prescribe internal or external treatments such as Aesculus hippocastanum or Nux vomica.

Medical treatments: You can use the treatments advised to avoid constipation (above). There are also creams you can buy over the counter from chemists (such as rectinol or anusol). If they are not effective, your doctor may prescribe a stronger cream.

Heartburn

Indigestion or reflux causes burning or discomfort in the chest and throat, usually after eating. Up to 66% of pregnant women experience heartburn, due to increased progesterone relaxing the sphincter muscle at the top of the stomach, allowing food and stomach acids to regurgitate back into the gullet (oesophagus). The muscle sphincter at the bottom of the stomach also relaxes, allowing irritating bile from the bowel to reflux back into the stomach, making heartburn worse. Other contributing factors are nervous tension, stress, smoking, alcohol and caffeine.

What some women find helpful:
- Have small, frequent meals. Eat slowly and chew thoroughly. Try eating at least two hours before bed. Avoid spicy, fatty and rich foods. Yoghurt or chewing slowly on raw almonds may help. Some women avoid bread and foods containing yeast.
- Drink plenty of fluids. Carbonated drinks may be better. Having fluids between meals, instead of with them, may make a difference. Try a glass of milk before going to bed (add honey if you wish).
- Good posture. Your stomach empties towards the right, so sleeping on your right side when first going to bed can help. Some women need to sleep relatively upright on a couple of pillows. Avoid stooping to pick things up. Stay upright and bend the legs.
- Try the flying exercise. Sit cross-legged, arms straight at your sides, raise and lower them quickly, bringing the back of your hands together over your head. Repeat this several times after eating.
- Use relaxation strategies to help with stress.

- Herbal remedies. Slippery elm powder mixed with warm milk, cinnamon and honey or marshmallow root; meadowsweet, fennel, aniseed and peppermint teas; a combination of fennel, anise, cumin and dill seeds chewed before and after meals; a mixture of yoghurt, kefir, warm milk and cinnamon or fresh papaya, papaya tablets or leaves; herbal antacids or peppermint water (available at chemists).
- Acupuncture and acupressure. A point is located in the centre of the breastbone, between the breasts and in line with the base of your cleavage (or nipple line for men). Apply firm pressure for approximately 30 to 45 seconds.
- Aromatherapy. Try burning spearmint oil or putting a couple of drops on a tissue to inhale intermittently (avoid before 12 weeks).
- Homeopathic remedies. These may include Mercurius solubilis or Natrum muriaticum.

Medical treatments: Your caregiver may recommend antacids. Use as little as possible, or as directed. Generally, aluminium, magnesium and calcium types are safest, taken as liquid or tablets. Those based entirely on aluminium salts can cause constipation and interfere with iron absorption. Some doctors prescribe acid-suppressing medications (cimetidine, omeprazole or ranitidine). There is little research to support their safety during pregnancy, but at this stage they are presumed to be safe.

AVOID: Sodium bicarbonate, magnesium carbonate or fizzy antacids, which can cause an imbalance in your blood chemistry. Milk of magnesia can cause diarrhoea and may be absorbed into your system, causing kidney problems in the baby. Avoid preparations containing aspirin (unless prescribed by your caregiver).

Leg cramps

Nearly 50% of pregnant women experience painful spasms in the feet, calves or thighs, usually at night, often jolting her (and her startled partner) awake, adding to the sleep problems. Many causes have been suggested, generally relating to low calcium, magnesium, potassium and/or salt in the body, because these minerals play vital roles in the functioning of muscles. At this stage, it is thought that magnesium supplements are most likely to help and there is some evidence that adequate salt in the diet may be useful. This may be why leg cramps tend to be worse during the hotter months (when you sweat more).

What some women find helpful:
- Use salt to taste. Electrolyte sports drinks or mineral waters may be effective.
- Gentle walking, swimming or yoga can help with blood circulation.

- Avoid pointing your toes. This can trigger a cramp. If stretching in bed, point your toes up towards your body.
- To relieve a cramp, bend your foot back firmly towards your body. You may need your partner to do this if you can't reach. Massage the affected area.
- Try a warm bath (or foot bath) before bed and keeping the legs warm.
- Magnesium phosphate tablets or 'cell salts' (from health stores).
- A full body massage to help blood circulation.
- Homeopathic treatments, such as Magnesia phosphorica.
- Herbalists may recommend raspberry leaf tea or tablets.

Medical treatments: Don't take quinine. There is no clear evidence that it helps, and if taken during pregnancy it can affect the hearing of your baby. Some people drink tonic water, the amount of quinine in this is very low and not thought to be toxic enough to have physical effects on an unborn baby.

Palpitations

Palpitations are a feeling that your heart is racing, or beating strongly and rapidly, in your chest. It is pretty common during pregnancy and may be triggered by stress, anxiety, nervousness, fear, shock or physical exertion and some medications. However, they can also be felt for no apparent reason, often accompanied by breathlessness and usually subsiding after a few minutes.

NOTE: Occasionally palpitations can indicate a heart condition. Your caregiver may suggest wearing a halter monitor at home for 24 hours (a machine that monitors and records your heart beat continuously). If you are feeling unwell, or the palpitations are very frequent, or associated with chest pain, feeling sweaty, faint or nauseated, seek medical attention.

What some women find helpful: Generally resting quietly and taking a few deep breaths is enough. Dealing with stress and using relaxation techniques can be helpful. Some homeopaths recommend Lillium tigrinum. See your homeopath for an assessment.

Swelling

Fluid retention (oedema) affects 65% of healthy pregnant women with a normal blood pressure. It is more common after 20 weeks of pregnancy and usually occurs in the legs, feet and hands, generally more noticeable at the end of the day, on hot days, after a plane trip or after being on your feet for long periods. Rings on the fingers can become tight and you may need to take them off until after the birth.

What some women find helpful:
- Slow down and put your feet up at the end of the day for at least 20 minutes. Rest them on another chair if doing desk work or studying. Wear comfortable flat shoes. Full support stockings may help if you are on your feet all day.
- Try some gentle, regular exercise such as swimming or yoga.
- Cut back on foods with a high salt content (eg. olives, parmesan, ham, bacon, sundried tomatoes, crisps, corn chips, soy sauce).
- Drink at least eight glasses of water a day. Drinking less makes the swelling worse.
- Swimming or having a bath increases urine production, giving short-term relief.
- Acupuncture or Shiatsu massage can help.
- Cell salts with magnesium and phosphorous (from health stores).
- Chiropractic or osteopathy, especially if one leg is more swollen than the other, possibly because your back and pelvis are out of alignment.
- A massage, concentrating on the legs from the feet upwards with a gel, oil or lotion. When massaging the hands, firmly press from the nails to the bases of the fingers. Aromatherapists may suggest adding geranium to massage oils, or a few drops of lemon, neroli, orange or pettigrain to a warm bath. Check with your practitioner.
- Herbalists may recommend dandelion, nettle, or yarrow teas, as well as eating whole grapes, celery, apples and apple juice.
- Homoeopaths may prescribe Natrum muriaticum, Apis mellifica or Phosphorus.

Symphysis pubis pain

The symphysis joint at the front of the pelvis comprises of a small oval disc of cartilage, about three to four centimetres long, held together by ligaments. This feels like a hard bump under the pubic hair, in the middle. Increased progesterone and relaxin hormones soften and relax the symphysis, sometimes causing pain as the pelvis moves. The sensation is felt low, as a twinge, ache, clicking sensation, or sharp debilitating pain, sometimes shooting into the vagina. The position of the baby can sometimes aggravate it, especially if their head is engaged.

AVOID:
- Twisting your body or standing on one leg. Stand with equal weight on both feet.
- Sitting with crossed legs, or on the floor with legs crossed. Sit symmetrically on a chair.

- Lifting and carrying heavy objects or your toddler (if possible).
- Vacuuming the carpet or mopping the floor.
- Squatting; and if swimming, avoid breaststroke.
- Lying on your back for sex. Use alternative positions, such as side-lying.

What some women find helpful:
- Putting a pillow between the knees when turning in bed.
- Adapting your walking stride length to your pain. Walk with very small steps if you have a lot of pain.
- Taking one step at a time on stairs, and doing this sideways.
- When getting in and out of a car, sitting down backwards on the seat and turning around to the front of the car with your knees and ankles together. Do the reverse when getting out. Do not kick open the car door with one foot.
- Using a heat pack, acupuncture, Shiatsu, massage or yoga. A chiropractor or osteopath may be able to do a manipulation. Your herbalist or homoeopath may recommend a remedy.

Medical treatments: Your caregiver may refer you to a physiotherapist for exercises and/or a pelvic girdle (an elastic corset worn around the hips) to stabilise your joints. If it is extremely debilitating you may need a walking frame for a while. Avoid painkillers and sedatives unless prescribed by your caregiver.

Varicose veins

Varicose veins are caused by blood pooling in the legs, making the veins swell into purple/blue bulges. Increased progesterone weakens the valves and walls of the veins, making them less efficient at pumping blood back to the body. Pressure from the growing baby can make them worse. Varicose veins can cause aching, sore legs, especially if bumped or knocked. However, they should improve (or disappear) a few months after the birth. It is possible to have varicose veins surgically removed, but most caregivers advise waiting until after you have had all your children, in case they come back with a subsequent pregnancy.

What some women find helpful:
- Regular, gentle exercise such as swimming, walking or yoga to strengthen muscles surrounding the veins.
- Full-length support stockings if you are on your feet most of the day. Put them on first thing in the morning before getting up. Avoid tight socks and half-leg stockings.

- Moving your feet at frequent intervals, rather than standing in one spot for prolonged periods. Avoid crossing your ankles or legs when sitting. If at a desk, put your feet up on another chair, or flat on a couple of phone books.
- Lie down with your feet elevated for at least 20 minutes at the end of the day.
- Rest as much as possible. Perhaps elevate the foot of the bed to help circulation.
- Naturopaths may suggest bioflavonoids, garlic and vitamin C to strengthen connective tissue around the veins.
- Herbalists may suggest witch hazel ointment or pouring witch hazel or diluted lemon juice, or vinegar, onto a small gauze pad and applying it to the area overnight with a loose bandage, or just cold, wet compresses for temporary relief. Remedies may include nettle, yarrow, St John's wort or Shepard's purse, to help with the blood flow. Homeopathic remedies include Hammamelis or Calcarea fluorica.
- Aromatherapists may suggest a few drops of lemon and/or geranium oil in a bath or diluted and soaked into a gauze pad as a direct compress to the area. Consult your practitioner.

Medical treatments: Some caregivers suggest purchasing medical compression stockings (TED stockings). However, these are thick and some women find them too uncomfortable in summer.

Vulval varicosities

The veins in the outer lips (labia) of the genitals can swell, similar to varicose veins that develop in the legs. Vulval varicosities can feel uncomfortable and make the vulva ache and feel sore. They don't cause any problems for a vaginal birth and should disappear a few days after the baby is born.

What some women find helpful: Pelvic floor exercises are beneficial, to help the blood to circulation and strengthen the supporting tissues around the veins. Try wearing underwear that feels supportive on the vulva, but does not cut into the groin too much. Avoid squatting for prolonged periods and rest as much as possible. Some women elevate their bottom on a small pillow when resting. Avoid straining when going to the toilet. Strategies for constipation and haemorrhoids can help. Natural therapies are similar to those for varicose veins of the legs (discussed above).

Aches and pains
Rib and chest wall pains
The growing baby pushes up under your ribs, moving them slightly outwards (called rib flaring). This may strain the intercostal muscles between the ribs, causing discomfort or pain. Sitting upright and giving your baby a gentle push down with your hand can help.

Splitting, tearing belly pains
Tenderness, tearing or splitting sensations down the centre of your belly can be caused by the two large abdominal muscles stretching and slightly separating to accommodate your baby's growth. This is normal, but not every woman feels this natural separation. Massaging the area, using a heat pack and supporting the belly with a pillow while sleeping may help.

Tender, sore navel
If you have an 'inny' belly button and it pops out, this makes the previously protected skin rub on clothing, feeling raw and tender. Massaging creams, oils or pawpaw ointment can be soothing. Wearing underwear that covers your belly will help protect it. If you have a belly ring, you may want to take it out. Check your belly in the mirror to make sure you haven't scraped it or burnt it while ironing. Easily done!

Bruised sensations or sore spots
Tender or bruised spots on your belly can happen when the baby continually presses on one part of the uterus, making the abdominal muscle over it feel sore. Gently pushing your baby off the tender area with your hand can provide temporary relief. Pelvic rocking on your hands and knees may move your baby off the bruised spot. Homeopaths may suggest Arnica.

Aching thighs and vagina
The weight of your baby (and their head engaging) slows blood flow to the genitals, causing aching in the thighs and vagina. Varicose veins in the legs or vulva can intensify these sensations. Do regular pelvic floor exercises and try to stay off your feet much as possible. Lie down and put your legs up for 10 to 20 minutes each day if at all possible.

Internal vaginal pains
Short, sharp, internal vaginal pains can take you by surprise. They may be experienced as the baby moves and shifts on the softened and more flexible cervix in the final weeks. These sensations are usually sporadic and

unpredictable, settling down quickly. There is not much you can do, except breathe and count to ten. This is *not* how labour feels.

NOTE: *If you are concerned about any aches and pains, contact your hospital or caregiver.*

Your baby's movements

Unborn babies generally sleep for 1 to 2 hours and are then active for 10 to 40 minutes before drifting back to sleep. You won't sense all your baby's movements, and some babies are more active than others. Bear in mind that how your baby 'behaves' in utero does not always reflect what they will be like after birth!

It is normal to have concerns about the frequency of your baby's movements, especially if you haven't noticed any for a while. (A baby moving 'too much' is not a concern.) One common reason for not sensing movements at times is that you become used to them as the pregnancy progresses. After a busy day, you may wonder whether your baby has moved at all. If you are concerned, a few things you can try are:

- **Having a cold drink and something to eat** – Then wait 30 minutes or so. Caffeine (in cola, chocolate or coffee) may encourage movements, but should be limited during pregnancy.
- **Resting and sitting quietly** – Without distractions, focus on your baby's movements. Lying on your side may help, or having a deep bath. Some women notice their baby moves more after exercise (such as a swim or a long walk).
- **Gently massaging your belly** – Try prodding gently with your fingers.
- **Making a loud noise** – Alternatively, get someone to blow a raspberry on your belly.

NOTE: *Making a loud sound occasionally for your baby to respond to is okay. However, unborn babies frequently exposed to loud noises may have disturbed sleep cycles and can exhibit disruptive sleeping behaviours after birth.*[2]

If your baby does not respond after an hour or two, contact your caregiver or hospital. You will probably need a check-up to listen to your baby's heartbeat. Don't hesitate to call. It is better to have peace of mind rather than to worry. A few caregivers provide kick charts to record your baby's daily movements.

Baby hiccups

Some unborn babies hiccup quite frequently. This is normal but it does not happen with all babies and is generally caused by the sudden, irregular contractions of the immature muscle supporting their lungs. You may sense these as small, rhythmic 'jumps' every 10 to 20 seconds or so, for several minutes or longer. A very strange sensation!

Emotions and sex during late pregnancy

It is common to sense a new vulnerability in your relationship, possibly manifesting as wanting your partner close, or having unfounded fears of being left alone or losing them in some way (especially in dreams). This can take you by surprise, possibly making you yearn for frequent expressions of love and caring to reassure you of your bond.

EMOTIONS FOR THE WOMAN
The thought of meeting your baby can bring anticipation and impatience. Some women keep a journal of their feelings, or write a letter to give to their new son or daughter when they are older. As the due date draws nearer it is normal to feel anxious about giving birth and/or parenting, and to feel more vulnerable if you are tired or run-down. Many women lie awake at night wondering how they will make the transition from being pregnant, to being a mother, or coping with an additional child. Concerns may also relate to your health, or your baby's, or feeling nervous about a specific thing, like tearing with the birth. Share your thoughts with someone you trust. If the fear is acknowledged, you may be able to develop some strategies to help deal with it if and when the time comes.

A few women express concerns about dying, which is quite normal. Try relaxation techniques, hypnosis, homeopathy or possibly professional counselling or psychotherapy to help deal with this.

As you move closer to motherhood, you may experience unexpected emotions, perhaps tears. Many women find they are sensitive to what they watch on television, asking themselves what kind of world are they bringing their baby into, and are more selective about the people they wish to be around. Consider visiting a mothers' group, going to pregnancy exercise or yoga classes, or chatting with other pregnant women online, so you can interact with those who understand.

Feeling concerned about whether your baby will be okay is universal, but it can challenge your beliefs about your body's ability to produce a healthy baby. Some women are unable to explain their concerns, others are aware that they come from real issues relating to known health concerns. These emotions are very normal. Thankfully, most babies are born well and healthy.

Many women become anxious about their ability to mother a newborn, especially if they have little or no experience with babies. A new mother's role comes suddenly and with no training, yet women are expected to fulfil it perfectly, cheerfully and effortlessly. If you are a single mother you may worry about how you are going to do it all alone. Try and set up some support networks now. It can be hard giving so much love to your baby when you can't refuel your own body and essence. Let people know you may need to rely on them, at least for the early weeks after the birth.

EMOTIONS FOR THE PARTNER

In recent years, fathers have increasingly provided a more hands-on role with their babies. Some men are eager to find out all they can, while others are happy to learn as they go. You may feel excited and anxious. Both are normal. Perhaps make contact with other fathers through friends, childbirth classes or online.

Your pregnant partner can seem as though she is on an emotional rollercoaster, perhaps crying at the drop of a hat, being more sensitive about your relationship or upset that the house is a wreck. These are normal responses. Try to keep communication open and discuss ways you can deal with her feelings, as well as yours, if you are finding it difficult to cope.

Some men are concerned they will lose the woman they love to the new baby. Others can hardly wait to meet their new son or daughter. The truth is it's a bit of a 'wait and see' situation. Allow your expectations to be open about your new family and parenting.

Partners often take on the provider role when expecting a new baby, working harder and/or taking on renovating or moving house. It is important to take care of yourself leading up to the birth, so you can be refreshed to support her and enjoy the new baby. If you are feeling strained, plan ahead and don't take too much on. Perhaps let go of some commitments and be realistic about what you can achieve. Your baby's birth is more important.

Births, like marriages and the deaths of loved ones, are important events in our lives. We need to make time for them.

A few partners feel they don't want to be present at the birth, or are concerned about coping or fainting (in reality, this rarely happens). It is hard to imagine what the experience will be like. If you are gauging it by watching a birth video, realise that being at your baby's birth is totally different – it's a bit like the difference between watching a surfing movie and actually riding a wave! The exhilaration and emotion will carry you through. Most men are surprised at how emotionally involved they become. Not many regret being part of it.

If you do have concerns, communicate these to your partner and see if you can agree on a compromise. One man felt extremely uncomfortable with the thought of watching the birth. He and his wife agreed he would be there during the labour but leave when the baby was being born, returning soon afterwards. He copped a lot of flack from friends and family, but he was honest enough to take measures to support him and his partner. Be aware that some women are not so accommodating because they feel they don't have a choice.

SEX DURING LATE PREGNANCY

During the final months pregnant women feel big, tired and uncomfortable, which often reduces their interest in sex. However, she still may find love-making enjoyable, although this could involve some inventive positions.

If you are not used to trying different positions for intercourse, then you may need to become more adventurous during pregnancy. As the woman's belly enlarges, the missionary position (partner lying on top of the woman) can be a bit tricky, unless the man holds his weight off her. Even then, some women feel light-headed, breathless or experience heartburn if they lie flat on their back. Using a few pillows to sit a bit more upright can help. Other positions you can try include:
- Lying side by side, with the partner's front against the woman's back and penetrating her vagina from behind. This can also be achieved with the woman on all fours and her partner kneeling behind her.
- The woman sitting or lying on top of her partner, giving her control of penetration and keeping her belly free.

Some couples vaporise essential oils with aphrodisiac properties, such as ginger, sandalwood or ylang ylang.

Close to the due date, the woman's body is more responsive to prostaglandins in the man's semen (and to her orgasm), possibly triggering labour contractions, but only if her body is ready to react in this way. Sex may be useful for starting labour if the pregnancy goes overdue, but this is entirely optional.

NOTE: *Once the waters break, you should not have penetrative sex, but orgasm is okay.*

Sex during late pregnancy may bring up issues for the woman about whether her body will ever be the same again and whether her partner will still find her sexually attractive after watching her give birth, or once she has a caesarean scar. Be prepared to take time to adjust to any changes and keep an open mind. Many women find they have positive changes after giving birth, or at the very least that things are much the same. Talk with your partner and share your concerns to help you both accept any changes.

Monitoring more closely

WHAT TO EXPECT DURING THE REMAINING PREGNANCY VISITS

After 28 weeks, pregnancy visits are scheduled more frequently. However, the timing of these can vary, depending on your needs and your caregiver's preferences. As a guide, they may be every 2 weeks, from 28 to 36 weeks, then every week from 36 weeks until the birth. However, in recent years, research has shown that antenatal visits can be performed less often, if this is acceptable to the woman and the pregnancy is progressing normally.[3] Women with medical conditions, pregnancy complications or multiple pregnancies generally need to be seen this often (or more frequently), depending on the circumstances.

Routine pregnancy visits after 28 weeks are similar to previous visits, involving checking your blood pressure, monitoring the growth of your baby and discussing your physical and emotional wellbeing. During the final weeks, your caregiver will try to determine the position of your baby and when their head engages.

Your pregnancy card records your caregiver's findings, your health history and tests results. This is written in medical jargon, abbreviations and symbols, which can be hard to interpret. Unfortunately, not all caregivers take the time to explain what is written on your card. So ask them if you don't understand. As a guide:

- **Gestational age** is how many weeks pregnant you are. Pregnancy visits halfway between the calculated weeks, say between 32 and 33 weeks, are written as '32+ weeks'.
- **Fundal height** is measured between 16 and 36 weeks in centimetres, generally correlating with the baby's gestation (eg. 32 weeks = 32 cm, plus or minus 2 to 4 cm). Once your baby is 37 weeks, the fundal height is written as 'term' or 'T', meaning the baby feels big enough to be born.
- **The presentation** refers to the part of the baby closest to your cervix and pelvis. Usually this is the crown of the baby's head or vertex

(written 'Vx' or 'V') or, more commonly, Cephalic ('Ceph' or 'C'). If your baby is breech, 'Br' is written. If they are lying across-ways (shoulder down), this is transverse ('trans'). Lying diagonally is 'oblique'.

- **The position** of your baby refers to where their back is lying in relation to your body, specifically your pelvic bones and back. An unborn baby's position is not usually recorded until after 36 weeks, and is written as a 3 letter acronym using:

    L = left side and also 'lateral' (meaning the woman's side)
    R = right side
    A = anterior
    P = posterior
    O = occipito (the occiput is the back of the baby's head)
    S = sacral (the sacrum is the base of the baby's spine; used for breech positions)

For example:
- ROA (right occipito anterior) is when the baby lies on their mother's right side, head down, with their back against the front of her belly.
- LOL (left occipito lateral) is when the baby lies on their mother's left side, head down, with their back against her side.
- LSA (left sacral anterior) is when the baby is breech, lying on their mother's left side, with their back towards the front of her belly.

Your caregiver may also use small drawings that look like tadpoles to illustrate the baby's position. For example, a 6 if your baby is head down on your right side, or a 9 if your baby is breech on your left side.

- **Engagement and station** – About one to four weeks before the birth, the baby's head lowers into the pelvis or engages. A breech baby's bottom can also engage. This is often measured in how many fifths the caregiver can feel or palpate, roughly based on the baby's head being about the width of an adult hand, or five fingers. Therefore, if they can feel:
    - 5 finger widths, it is written as '5/5 palpable' or 'unengaged'.
    - 3 finger widths = '3/5 palpable', or '2/5 engaged'.
    - 1 finger width = '1/5 palpable' or '4/5 engaged'.

If your baby's head cannot be felt at all, it is 'fully engaged' or 'not palpable'. Some caregivers don't record fifths, just write 'engaged' or 'unengaged'. Other terms are 'free' (unengaged) or 'fixed' (engaged), relating to whether the baby's head can be moved. Just before engagement the baby's head starts to settle into the top of the pelvis, but is not yet engaged, often recorded as 'at the brim'.

Most babies become ⅖ or ⅗ engaged before labour commences, then fully engage during labour. If your baby is very active during pregnancy, they can move in and out of different levels of engagement, especially if this is not your first baby. A few babies don't engage until labour starts.
- **Baby's movements** are usually recorded as 'fetal movements felt' ('FMF', 'FM+', or 'FM √').
- **The baby's heartbeat** is recorded as 'fetal heart sounds heard', ('FHS', 'FHH' or 'FH+'). If your caregiver uses a Doppler to listen to the heart beat, they may write 'Doppler+' or 'D+'.

Talking about the birth
As the due date draws nearer, pregnancy visits focus more on the birth and you may discuss:
- A birth plan.
- What you need to pack.
- Your labour support plans and perhaps the involvement of other children.
- Issues around managing labour and pain relief options.
- When you should contact your caregiver, delivery suite or birth centre.
- The possibility of interventions (eg. induction, caesarean birth, vitamin K for the baby), or the need for your baby to go to intensive care.

These are covered in childbirth classes or books, but practices and policies vary and it is important to gain an understanding of your caregiver's (or birthplace's) approach, and what you can expect in various circumstances.

Tests you may be offered
Most women don't require further tests after 28 weeks unless they have health conditions or complications. However, if your blood group is Rhesus negative, you will need another antibody screen at about 36 weeks.

Full blood count (FBC) – If your haemoglobin was low at 28 weeks, another full blood count is done at around 36 weeks to see if the level has improved. If not, your caregiver may discuss adjusting your iron supplements.

Ultrasounds – These are only done if there is a medical reason, such as:
- Seeing whether a previously low-lying placenta has moved up and away from the cervix (done at 34 to 36 weeks). Most placentas do move.
- Measuring the growth of the baby if there are concerns.
- Monitoring a multiple pregnancy.

- Checking the baby's position, if thought to be breech.
- Finding a cause for vaginal bleeding.
- Checking the amount of amniotic fluid, or blood flow through the baby's cord (especially if more than one week overdue).

Kick charts – A few caregivers recommend kick charts after 26 to 28 weeks, to record and monitor your baby's movements. These are not routine, but may be suggested if you have a health condition or pregnancy complications, or express concerns about the frequency of your baby's movements. Kick charts can only provide a general guideline as there are no standard criterion that defines what sufficient (or insufficient) movement is. Some women find them reassuring, but others feel they are time-consuming, obsessive or stressful.

Kick charts aim to record all types of movements. So flutters, elbows, rolls, pushes, jabs and stretches all count. If your baby has a run of rigorous movements – kick, kick, kick – this is three movements not one.

The Cardiff count to ten method requires your baby to have 10 movements within an 8 to 12 hour period. You start your timing at around the same time each day. The first movement you feel is recorded with the time. When you feel the tenth movement, record the time again. Then stop counting till the next day.

The 1 to 2 hour method involves lying quietly on your left side for about 30 minutes (usually after eating and without distractions). Your baby should move 3 to 5 times within 60 to 75 minutes or 10 times in 2 hours.

Getting ready for baby

FEEDING YOUR NEW BABY
In an ideal world every newborn baby would have their mother's breast milk as their only source of nutrition for six months, and continue being breast-fed as a complement to solid food until one to two years.[4] However, this is not always achievable (or possible) and some women choose not to breast-feed, or wean their baby earlier than recommended, for various reasons. In these circumstances young babies need a specially designed milk formula, until they are 12 months old.

Breastfeeding
'Breast is best' for baby and mother, and breast milk cannot be replicated. It changes in composition during each feed and adapts over time to accommodate

each baby's nutritional needs, with anti-infective and anti-allergenic properties, making it far superior to artificial formula. This is why the Baby Friendly Hospital Initiative (BFHI) was developed by the World Health Organisation and UNICEF. BHFI aims to educate caregivers and create healthcare environments in which breastfeeding is perceived as the norm. Hospitals abiding by the initiative agree to implement a range of policies and practices to support and encourage breastfeeding; for example:

- Informing all pregnant women of the benefits of breastfeeding.
- Helping mothers initiate breastfeeding within an hour of birth.
- Showing mothers how to breastfeed and maintain lactation, even if separated from their infants.
- Not giving newborns additional drinks, other than breast milk, unless medically indicated.
- Encouraging mothers and babies to room-in together 24 hours a day.
- Encouraging breastfeeding on demand.
- Not giving a dummy.

Ask your caregiver if your maternity hospital is BFHI accredited.

Breastfeeding rates during the first week after birth in Australia are relatively high (around 87%). However, by the time babies are 6 to 12 weeks old, many mothers have introduced formula and/or ceased breastfeeding.

Many women take it for granted they will breastfeed, but others are not so sure, or perhaps have definite reasons for wanting to bottle-feed. A woman's decision to breastfeed is based on many complex factors.

Age, education and financial status: Women over 25 years, with a higher education and who are financially better off, are more likely to breastfeed. This brings up concerns that the high cost of buying artificial formula, bottles, teats and sterilising equipment contributes to many women's financial disadvantage.

Cultural background and local community: Women migrants may choose not to breastfeed (or only do so for a short period) because of less practical and emotional support from extended family, and increased pressure to return to work. Some migrant women also have a false perception that Australian women don't breastfeed, because they rarely see women breastfeeding in public.

Support from significant others: How a woman feels about her breastfeeding and the level of positive emotional and practical support she receives is crucial. Partners are now recognised as playing an essential role. If they agree with, and encourage, breastfeeding, the woman is more likely to continue breastfeeding for longer. It is important to discuss ways your partner can provide practical support, so you can take the time you need to breastfeed.

A woman's intention to breastfeed for a specific period of time is a strong predictor of how long she actually feeds for. However, some women who expect their breastfeeding experience to be negative are pleasantly surprised, continuing to feed for much longer than they intended.

Sexuality: Western cultures emphasise breasts as sexual objects, bringing up conflicting feelings for women and their partners. Issues can include:
- Feeling uncomfortable about breastfeeding in front of family, friends and in social situations. Or being made to feel uncomfortable when trying to breastfeed in public.
- The partner feeling jealous, or having issues about the baby suckling on his partner's breasts.
- The woman having issues about the baby's sex in relation to breastfeeding or not feeling comfortable with touching her own breasts.
- Worried that breastfeeding will change the appearance and attractiveness of her breasts (although this is more determined by genetic make-up, age and the physical changes of pregnancy).

If you are experiencing these feelings, it is important to make them known to your partner (or someone you trust), to help work through them, and possibly develop ways to deal with them.

Society's perceptions: Women often have little contact with female relatives and friends who openly breastfeed, meaning they are less likely to have a positive role model. Some argue that girls are given subliminal messages from a young age, often being given dolls with bottles. However, social attitudes are gradually changing to see breastfeeding as the norm.

Confidence in ability to breastfeed: Breastfeeding has become a learnt skill, requiring a degree of patience and perseverance, as well as ongoing positive support. Some women question their ability to breastfeed if their mother or sister had difficulties. This can create a loss of trust in your body's ability to make milk and breastfeed your baby, perhaps setting you up for failure even before you begin. Attending breastfeeding education classes during pregnancy has been shown to increase confidence levels associated with breastfeeding, helping women breastfeed longer. Also, bear in mind that each breastfeeding experience is unique (as is each birth) and women tend to have fewer breastfeeding difficulties with subsequent children, producing more milk and spending less time feeding, because their milk transfer is more efficient.

Did you know?

Outdated practices and inappropriate advice from health professionals in the past often developed attitudes that breastfeeding was difficult and problematic and could only be achieved with expert help. Other unhelpful approaches were:

- Strict four-hourly feeds (whether the baby was hungry or not).
- The baby not sharing the room with their mother in hospital.
- Limiting the time the baby was allowed to feed at each breast (eg. five minutes each side).
- Test weighing babies on scales before and after breastfeeds, to see if they were getting enough milk.
- Suggesting the early introduction of solids (two to three months) with the unsupported belief that the baby would sleep through the night.
- Telling women they had lost their milk when babies went through normal growth spurts and typically wanted to feed more often (at six weeks and three months).

Conflicting advice from health professionals has also been a common problem, frustrating new parents trying to get breastfeeding right. Efforts are now being made to make breastfeeding information more consistent.

Breastfeeding myths

There are many urban myths that are thought to affect breastfeeding, but actually don't. These include:

Flat and inverted nipples (where the nipple turns inwards) are normal for 10% of women and do not prevent successful breastfeeding. Extra care may be needed to make sure the baby is latched on correctly during the early days, but this is the case for every woman. Past outdated practices included:

- Repeatedly squeezing the areola to encourage the nipple to pop out.
- Wearing plastic covers or shields inside a bra (and over the nipples) to encourage them to poke out.
- Using devices to pull out the nipple.

These should be avoided as they can bruise and damage the nipples.

Skin type has nothing to do with the cause of sore nipples. Nipple damage is solely the result of the way the baby is attached or positioned on the breast. Some women express concerns that eczema or dermatitis may affect their breastfeeding. However, it can be painlessly achieved if the baby is attached correctly.

NOTE: *You do not need to do anything to prepare your nipples for breastfeeding. The only way to prevent sore nipples is to ensure your baby is correctly latched on the breast for each feed. The nipples naturally manufacture small amounts of oils to keep them supple and moist. Therefore, don't vigorously wash them with soapy products, as this can make them dry and itchy. Plain water is generally adequate for cleansing, or use sorbelene cream.*

Breast size does not affect breast milk production. The amount of milk is related to how often and how long the baby suckles for.

Breast implants are normally inserted under milk production sacs and ducts and do not tend to interfere with breastfeeding.

Breast reductions in which the nipples were surgically removed and restitched can interfere with the nerve supply and milk ducts. This does not mean you cannot breastfeed, but it may make breastfeeding less likely to succeed. Consult the lactation consultant at your hospital.

Breast cancer, or specifically needle biopsies of breast lumps, or the removal of a breast lump, should not affect breastfeeding. The removal of a whole breast means breastfeeding from one side, which is not a problem. Radiation therapy may damage the glandular tissue that produces breast milk and could affect milk supply. Discuss your individual circumstances with a lactation consultant.

Being a smoker should not discourage you from breastfeeding, but always smoke outside the house or car, away from your baby. Cut down to as few cigarettes as possible and try not to smoke at least an hour before breastfeeding, to help your milk supply (although this can be hard to predict at times). Women who smoke heavily can sometimes find their milk supply slowly declines after a few months.

Help and support – Research shows that many mothers require ongoing support and appropriate advice to assist them in establishing and continuing their breastfeeding. Experiencing sore or cracked nipples, problems attaching the baby or having issues about your milk supply can usually be overcome with sufficient support and appropriate advice, especially during the early weeks. Volunteer breastfeeding counsellors are available throughout Australia; see the resources section for details.

Bottle feeding

When breastfeeding is not possible, or desirable, bottle feeding is the alternative. This may be an easy, clear-cut decision for some women, based on an informed choice they feel very comfortable with, or something that just slowly eventuates. If breastfeeding ends up becoming very difficult and/or there is little help or support available, then bottle feeding may feel like a positive step. Sometimes breastfeeding is combined with bottle feeding for various reasons.

Safe formula feeding for newborn babies is essentially based on:
- Having accurate and understandable information about formula feeding and correct formula preparation.

- Being able to access a continual, clean water supply.
- Being able to prepare formula and sterilise equipment in a clean environment.
- Being able to store prepared formula milk in a refrigerator.
- Being able to afford the cost of purchasing specially designed formula milk for the first 12 months of the baby's life.

Further information on preparing formula and bottles is in Chapter 13.

Companies who manufacture infant formulas have to carefully modify cow's milk and soy bean products so they come as close as possible to what a baby would drink, if having breast milk. The infant formula must comply with Australian quality control standards and are labelled as 'suitable from birth' for babies up to 12 months old. There are many brands available and the costs vary, but do not reflect their quality. Also, buying at the supermarket is often cheaper than at a pharmacy, so shop around. Changing brands is not an issue for your baby and rarely 'cures' an unsettled or colicky baby.

NOTE: *Cow's, goat's milk or soy substitutes and regular powdered or condensed milk, are **not** suitable for babies under 12 months. Australia abides by the International Code of Marketing of Breast-milk Substitutes by the World Health Assembly. This means there are restrictions in the way formula is marketed, so that it is less likely to be seen as better than breastfeeding. For example:*

- *Formula cannot be openly displayed or promoted in hospitals, or included in hospital gift bags.*
- *Health professionals cannot actively promote formula milks or certain brands of formula over other brands.*
- *Parents wishing to artificially feed from birth are often advised to purchase their own formula and bring it with them to hospital.*

Cow's milk formula is the main type recommended by caregivers. It is made from skimmed cow's milk, with casein protein replaced by whey protein, lactose added, salt reduced and some of the milk fat replaced by vegetable fats. Iron and vitamins and minerals are also supplemented.

Soybean formulas are only recommended if the baby has a metabolic disorder, such as galactosaemia, or is truly cow's milk intolerant (only 1.8 to 3.4% of babies). These are protein soy extracts with specific amino acids added, vegetable oils fats, cornstarch and sucrose. Iron and vitamins and minerals are also supplemented.

NOTE: *Some babies are allergic to soymilk formula (0.5% to 1.1%) and both cow's and soymilk formula can cause bowel irritations.*

Soy-based formulas are high in aluminium, which competes with calcium in the body, affecting bone growth and density. Babies born at term do not appear to be affected by this, but very premature babies can have less weight gain and growth, so it is not generally recommended.

Extensively hydrolysed formulas aim to help prevent allergies in babies who are unable to breastfeed, especially if their parents have specific allergies or a food intolerance. The proteins are broken into smaller parts to reduce allergic reactions. These are relatively new, not widely available and cost about twice as much as standard formula. So it is ultimately your decision as to whether you can afford to give them to your baby.

Specialised formulas for babies with nutritional and/or health problems are usually prescribed by a paediatric doctor.

Goat's milk formulas may be used as an alternative for babies allergic to cow's or soybean formulas.

Many women express concerns about feeling alienated or unaccepted by other mothers who breastfeed. This may come from friends or relatives, or perhaps something they just feel personally. The promotion of breastfeeding by health professionals can compound these feelings and some advocates of breastfeeding can seem very unsupportive.

Sleeping arrangements

Where your newborn baby sleeps is a very personal choice. Try to stay flexible and to avoid being pressured by family and friends. If your baby's sleeping arrangements are not working at any time, you can always change them, provided you have the space and relevant equipment available. Arrangements can also change each night, and at different times of the night, depending on what is working for everyone, including the baby's siblings.

Sharing your bed

Bed-sharing is normal in many parts of the world, but remains controversial in western countries, often being seen as nurturing a habit that may be hard to alter later on. Regarding SIDS, at this stage most studies suggest there is no increased risk, unless the parents are smokers.[5] However, bed-sharing is unsafe if the baby:

- Slips under the bedding or into pillows.
- Becomes trapped between a parent and the bed or wall, or falls out of bed.
- Becomes hot, from too much bedding, or is rolled on (usually if the parent is affected by alcohol or sedative drugs).

Ways of addressing these concerns are:
- Wrapping your baby independently from your own bed-coverings.

- Not overdressing your baby in the warmer months. Remember, your baby will receive some warmth from your body.
- Placing a pillow below the baby's feet to stop them moving under the bedcovers.
- Keeping pillows clear of your baby's face.
- Placing them where they will not fall out.

NOTE: *Never sleep with your baby on a couch. Babies have died from being trapped, face-down, in a space between the parent and the back of a couch. Bed-sharing is also not recommended if you have a waterbed.*

Bed-sharing may be a starting point before progressing to independent sleeping when everyone feels ready. Often if the move is made by three or four months of age, the transition is easier than if left until later. However, this may not work for all babies (or all parents!).

Some considerations:

- Bed-sharing can make breastfeeding easier, and often the baby settles back to sleep relatively quickly. Some babies want to breastfeed more often.
- Most babies are noisy sleepers. They snuffle, grunt, hiccup and pass wind (at times loudly!). You may feel they frequently interrupt your sleep as you anticipate their needs.
- You may need to be sexually inventive with your partner, using other places for intimacy (when you are both feeling ready).
- Probably not a reasonable option if you have twins or more.

Same room, separate bed

Your baby may sleep in their own bed but in your room. This arrangement suits many parents because they can maintain their sleeping space, while feeling reassured by being close to their baby. Research indicates that babies who sleep this way for the first 6 to 12 months may be protected to a degree against SIDS, possibly because parents can see their baby and easily check them. This does not work if the baby shares their room with other children, probably because they don't know whether a baby is safe or not.[6]

Separate bed, different room

You may prefer your baby to sleep in their own room (or with siblings). However, if their room is positioned far away from yours, consider getting an audio speaker system so you can hear your baby cry. This arrangement means you are not disturbed by your baby's noises (until they cry loudly), but you have to get up for feeding. A few parents also worry about their baby's wellbeing and frequently get up to check them.

The needs and reactions of your other children
Negative reactions from siblings may be heightened if the new baby's arrival coincides with a change in their sleeping arrangements. Try to make changes a few months before the birth, but expect a regression once the baby arrives. Some parents set up a single bed or mattress bedside their bed (if they have the room), to make this process less disruptive.

BUYING FOR BABY
Buying for your baby is exciting, but with seemingly endless products to choose from, it can quickly feel overwhelming and confusing. Budget constraints usually mean you have to work out what you really need and can afford, and to resist buying every conceivable gadget or cute outfit. If you intend to keep your purchases for the next baby, quality is fairly important. Ask other parents what they found useful and reliable. Shop around. Make notes of model and serial numbers and then use the telephone and/or Internet to compare prices. Consider delivery costs if mail-ordering.

Product safety
Up to 20% of injuries to children in their first year of life are caused by unsafe nursery furniture.[7] Sadly, most of these are preventable. Some items, such as cots and baby car seats, have mandatory safety regulations. Look for the Australian Standards Mark or Safebaby logo on products. The Australian Consumers Association's *CHOICE Guide to Baby Products* book can also be invaluable.

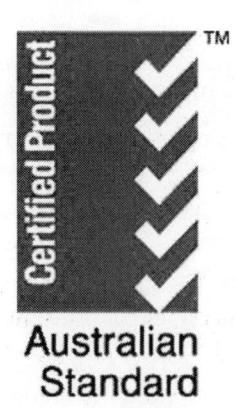

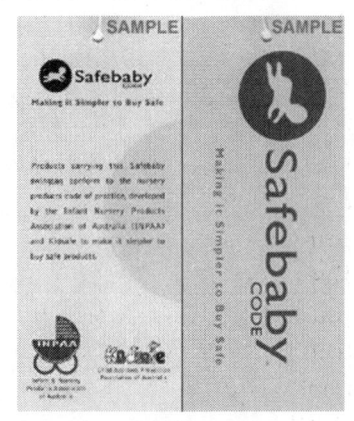

Australian Standards Mark   Safe Baby logo

Equipment check list
When purchasing, keep in mind that you will probably receive gifts from family and friends (soft toys, mobiles, bibs, outfits, hats and booties). Consider

borrowing some items or buying them second-hand. Just make sure they are in good order and comply with safety guidelines (if appropriate).

Before the birth:
- Baby car restraint.
- Cot, bassinet and/or cradle.
- A mosquito net.
- Sheets, blankets, mattress protector (no pillows or bumpers, as per SIDS safe-sleeping recommendations).
- Stroller or pram.
- Baby sling or backpack.
- A baby bag with change mat for outings.
- 2 soft bath towels.
- **Cloth nappies** – 2 to 3 dozen, fasteners, waterproof pilchers and possibly liners; 1 to 2 buckets with lids and sterilising powder for presoaking.
  or
- **Disposable nappies** – 60 to 80 newborn-sized for the first week.
- Baby wipes or 6 washable facecloths (or cotton balls or pads) for wiping their bottom.
- Sorbelene cream for cleansing and moisturising. A fine-tooth hair comb.
- 6 to 8 singlets or body suits. A few 000 newborn, and a few 00 size (6 weeks to 6 months).
- 6 to 8 nighties or jumpsuits.
- 4 to 6 bibs.
- **Winter** – 2 to 4 cardigans, jackets or jumpers, with a neck that stretches over your baby's head; 2 to 3 woollen hats; 4 pairs of socks, booties and/or tights (try same coloured socks for when you lose one); 6 to 8 brushed flannelette wraps. A shawl or sleeping bag for outings.
- **Summer** – 2 to 3 sunhats; 6 to 8 muslin, cotton or gauze wraps.
- **Breastfeeding** – Breast pads. If you choose to express and store milk you may also need a breast pump, 2 to 3 plastic bottles and newborn teats, a bottle cleaner and sterilising kit, and cooling bag for transporting milk.
- **Bottle-feeding** – 6 to 8 plastic bottles and newborn teats; bottle cleaner and sterilising kit; formula powder (check use-by date). Cooling bag for transporting milk and/or a thermos for warm water to make up formula when out.

Optional items:
- Change table or change mat on a chest of drawers (consider the height for your back).
- Baby bath.
- Dummies.
- Auditory monitor.
- Portable cot.
- Bouncer or cradle chair.
- Toys, mobiles, music tapes, play mat, playpen.
- High chair (6 months+).

Cloth or disposable nappies

Newborn babies go through 60 to 80 nappies a week. When choosing cloth or disposables, it usually comes down to cost and convenience. Environmentally:
- Disposables (plus plastic bag to wrap soiled ones in), produce 4 times more solid waste (0.2% of landfill) and are made of pulped wood and synthetics.
- Cleaning cloth nappies produces four times more water-borne waste and uses detergents, large amounts of water and electricity.

Many parents combine both, for various reasons. Maternity hospitals supply one or the other, so check with your caregiver.

Cloth nappies

Cloth nappies are traditionally white squares of towelling material folded into various shapes to fit your baby snugly. Tailored cloth nappies come pre-folded, often with inbuilt fasteners. Many new parents balk at the task of using cloth nappies, but your baby needs changing 10 times a day, so it won't be long before you're an expert!

Advantages:
- Least expensive in the long run, even after the initial outlay, extras (fasteners, pilchers, liners) and ongoing laundering costs. Top-quality nappies last two to three years and are a good investment.
- Made from natural fibres and can be folded in different ways to fit your baby as they grow.
- Nappy service is about equivalent to the cost of disposable nappies.

Disadvantages:
- More time and domestic duties required for soaking, washing and drying.
- Drying during winter months can be a problem (or extra cost for a dryer).

- Holidays or weekends away may create issues with soaking and washing (or storing dirty ones till you get home).

Tips for cloth nappies:
- Prewash them before your baby is born.
- Consider investing in a high-quality washing machine (if you don't have one).
- Buy spare pins or fasteners as they always go missing.

Disposable nappies

Disposable nappies are convenient, easy to use and don't require laundering. They are an all-in-one solution with inbuilt plastic coverings, liners and fasteners, being thrown away after use. Disposable nappies come in different sizes, depending on your baby's age and weight. Most babies start in 'newborn', but rapidly grow into 5 to 6 kg sizes after 4 to 6 weeks. There are also sex-specific brands that have extra padding in various areas, where boy and girl babies tend to wet.

Advantages:
- Portable while out and on holidays.
- Very absorbent and less likely to leak. Good for overnight nappies as your baby gets older.
- May help prevent nappy rash (although not always the case).

Disadvantages:
- An expensive, ongoing cost for two or more years.
- Contain chemical agents that may irritate the sensitive skin of a few babies.
- Some brands fit better than others. Not all nappies suit all babies.
- Cheaper brands have sticky tabs instead of reusable velcro, which don't stick if your hands are wet or greasy.

Tips for disposables:
- Try a few different brands until you find one that suits your baby. Don't bulk buy before the birth.
- The cost can vary significantly, so shop around.

Planning childcare arrangements

If you think you may need childcare before your baby's first birthday, you need to plan ahead. Don't underestimate the task of organising this, as leaving it too late can mean missing out. The main considerations are:

- Finding out what is available.
- Booking into several day-care centres (near home or work) during the pregnancy. Many have long waiting lists.
- Having back-up arrangements if your preferred childcare doesn't work out, or when family carers are sick or go on holidays.
- The cost. Returning to work may not be financially viable.

In Australia, the Commonwealth Department of Family and Community Services Childcare Program provides a booklet, *Your Guide to Childcare*.

It is very natural to feel unsure, guilty and/or anxious about the prospect of leaving your child in someone else's care. Little wonder this decision is often ignored or delayed. However, researching all your available options makes it more likely your baby will end up in the hands of someone you feel comfortable with, which helps you feel more relaxed about leaving them when the time comes.

Late pregnancy variations

A few women experience health variations towards the end of their pregnancy, provoking a great deal of anxiety. Depending on what is happening, your caregiver may recommend inducing labour or performing an elective caesarean before the due date, weighing up the risks of delivering a premature baby. This decision essentially comes down to whether the baby (or babies) is better off remaining in utero to grow and mature further, or whether the risks to mother and/or baby are too great to let the pregnancy continue.

PREMATURE BABY

About 6 to 8% of babies are born premature or preterm, between 20 and 37 weeks of pregnancy.[8] Babies born:
- **32 to 37 weeks** are 'mildly preterm' (80% of preterm babies) and normally do very well, but may require some time in the intensive care nursery.
- **28 to 31 weeks** are 'moderately preterm' (11%). These babies often need help to breathe and many medical treatments.
- **24 to 28 weeks** are 'extremely preterm' (9%) and need advanced life support. These babies are at increased risk of developing complications and having long-term health problems.[8]

Did you know?
A premature baby has two ages:
1. Their actual or chronological age that starts from birth.
2. Their adjusted age, or the age they would have been had they been born on time. For example, a baby born two months premature who is six months old (their actual age) has a corrected age of four months to help track their developmental milestones.

Causes of premature birth

While preventing preterm birth remains elusive, we do know that certain factors can contribute to babies being born prematurely.
- Premature ruptures of membranes (waters breaking early).
- Severe urine and kidney infections.
- Multiple pregnancies (50% of twins and 80 to 95% of triplets are preterm).
- IVF and assisted reproductive techniques (15% chance, compared to 6% for natural conceptions).
- A previous spontaneous preterm birth (not an induced or elective preterm caesarean and not a previous multiple pregnancy). For one previous premature birth the risk is 15% for the next pregnancy; for two preterm births it is 30%, and 50% for three or more.
- Cervix opening unexpectedly (incompetent cervix).[9]
- Pregnancy complications (heavy vaginal bleeding).
- A severe fall or a car accident.
- Excessive workloads (heavy lifting, excessive noise, standing for long hours or work causing extreme tiredness). Most normal paid jobs and caring for children are not linked with premature labour.
- Excessive alcohol, smoking narcotics and other addictive substances.
- Single highly stressful events. This is inconclusive.[10] Everyday stresses do not cause preterm births.
- Domestic violence. If you are dealing with this, speak with your caregiver or hospital social worker to obtain support and advice.

Many parents feel responsible or guilty if their baby is born premature. However, in many cases there is nothing you could have done to prevent it and it is unlikely you caused it. So try not to blame yourself. Previous factors that are now known *not to cause* premature labour include:
- Sex during pregnancy.
- Normal exercise. (Strenuous exercise or lifting heavy weights may.)

- Travelling or flying.
- Past terminations of pregnancy before 12 weeks. It is unclear whether multiple terminations after 12 weeks can increase the risk.

Previous factors that are now known *not to prevent* premature birth include:
- Routine bed rest (for single or multiple pregnancies).
- Diet, although magnesium, zinc and calcium supplements may be beneficial.[11]

Threatened premature labour

Threatened premature labour (or TPL) is when labour starts before 37 weeks. Physical signs are very similar to labour at term, but often not as painful. If you suspect you might be experiencing regular contractions, or your waters may have broken, trust your instincts and contact your caregiver or hospital. Preterm contractions are usually cramps or aches in the lower belly or back that come and go every 5, 10, 15 or 20 minutes, lasting 40 seconds or more, for at least 1 hour. Additional signs can be vaginal bleeding or a thick mucus show.

If you are showing signs of premature labour you will be admitted to hospital for observation until the contractions settle down. If the baby is less than 34 weeks, and the labour appears to be intensifying, you may need to transfer to a major public maternity hospital with a level 3 intensive care nursery (unless already there). In most cases labour stops and the baby is born on time (or even frustratingly overdue!). Women who experience several episodes of threatened premature labour are said to have an 'irritable uterus'. As a guide:
- 60% of women stop labouring without medical treatments.
- 25% have their baby(s) within 48 hours, regardless of medical attempts to slow or stop the labour.
- 13% continue the pregnancy because they were (rightly or wrongly) given medications to suppress the contractions.

When premature labour is happening, it can be difficult for caregivers (and the woman) to know whether it is just a threat, or will definitely increase and intensify, resulting in a premature birth.

To try to decide whether the contractions are working towards a preterm birth, the caregiver will look at the cervix with a speculum to see if it is thinning and dilating (this may also be done using ultrasound). A vaginal swab and urine test may also be taken to check for infection. Depending on the circumstances, labour may be allowed to continue and the baby born, but if

the baby is very premature, attempts may be made to try and stop, or delay, the labour, by giving:
- Antibiotics, if the waters have broken.
- Steroid injections, to help mature the baby's lungs and reduce breathing difficulties after the birth.[12]
- Medications to suppress contractions, given only if the cervix is less than 4 cm dilated, to allow more time for the baby to grow and mature and/or delay labour for at least 24 to 48 hours, until the steroid injections are effective.

Threatened preterm labour can be frightening, upsetting and frustrating, and if transfer to another hospital is necessary, this can be very lonely, as well as disruptive. Once the birth becomes inevitable, most parents feel vulnerable, guilty and concerned that their baby will be all right. Even after birth, the unpredictable recovery of premature babies means their health expectations may not be clear for days, weeks or even months.

If you have more than one preterm baby, it can feel as though you are being torn apart trying to focus on, and be with, both (or more) babies. Going home and leaving your baby(s) in the nursery is also very sad and lonely. Parents often find it hard to relax until their baby(s) is home, and even then the worry continues. Try to take one step at a time and keep communicating with your baby's caregivers, who will guide you through this difficult experience.

BREECH BABY

When an unborn baby's bottom is positioned down, close to the woman's cervix, it is in a breech position. This is normal from 20 to 35 weeks of pregnancy, but the baby should turn head down by 37 weeks, in readiness for the birth. About 3% of babies remain breech. Occasionally there is a physical reason that makes this more likely, including:
- A premature baby.
- Low amniotic fluid, often associated with small babies.
- Placenta previa.
- Twins or more (40% of twins have one breech baby).
- Bicornuate uterus with a septum inside the uterus.
- A very large fibroid low in the uterus.
- The baby having a physical abnormality.

Your caregiver may suspect a breech position by feeling your belly during a routine pregnancy visit. This is checked with an ultrasound to rule out

physical complications and confirm the type of breech, which may be:
- **Frank breech** – The baby's feet are up near their ears.
- **Complete breech** – Where the baby is sitting with their legs crossed.
- **Footling breech** – Where one of the baby's feet or knees 'leads the way' down the birth canal.
- **Stargazer** – Where the baby's neck is fully extended, so they are 'looking up to the stars'.

NOTE: *Even the most experienced caregivers can miss a breech baby until labour is well advanced.*

External cephalic version

You may consider an external cephalic version (ECV) to turn your baby into a head down position. The caregiver manipulates the baby from the outside of your belly, usually between 35 to 37 weeks. An ECV tends to be more successful for subsequent babies (50 to 85%), compared to first babies (25 to 50%). The likelihood of success depends on the skill and experience of the caregiver, the size of the baby (2 kg to 4.5 kg) and the amount of amniotic fluid. Drink 8 to 10 glasses of water a day, or more, for a few days beforehand to increase the amniotic fluid.[13]

An ECV is not done if there are physical complications or the baby is a stargazer. Some caregivers won't perform an ECV if you have had a previous caesarean. Complications of an ECV are rare, but may include entanglement of the umbilical cord, the baby becoming distressed (with a prolonged low heart rate), the waters breaking within 24 to 48 hours, or rarely, a placental abruption due to tension on the cord, which may require an emergency caesarean.

Some women try to turn their own baby with exercises and/or natural therapies. You should refrain from using these until 34 weeks, as your baby may turn anyway. Some caregivers also advise an ultrasound first, to rule out physical complications and confirm the baby is indeed breech. Some popular methods include:
- A knee–chest position (on hands and knees, legs apart, head down, bottom up and pelvic rocking); or an Indian bridge position (lying on your back, knees bent, bottom raised on pillows about 30 cm high).
- Acupuncture, acupressure or moxibustion on the little toe point. (See acupressure appendix.)
- Massaging your belly gently in a circular motion, so the baby 'follows their nose'.
- Homeopathy – Pulsatilla nigricans.
- Playing relaxing music close to your lower belly, talking to the woman's

lower belly in an encouraging voice, or shining a torch on her lower belly (unborn babies are thought to be attracted to light).
- Swimming or yoga positions to relax the abdominal muscles.
- Chiropractic or osteopathy to bring the pelvis and spine into alignment.
- A macrobiotic diet to create a 'yang state'; eating meat, fish, chicken, eggs and dairy products (foods that warm the body).
- Visualisation and hypnosis, such as looking at pictures of babies in head down positions.

NOTE: *If you think your baby has moved, see your caregiver so you can stop your baby-turning therapies.*

Some believe that a woman's emotional state may influence the position of her baby, as the baby stays close to their mother's heart for attention and love, moving head down once their mother reconnects with them or works through personal issues. There is no evidence to support this, so don't feel your baby being breech is in any way your fault. However, if you feel your emotions could be involved, talking to your baby and giving them permission to move head down (and forgiving them if they don't!) may help.

Vaginal or caesarean breech birth

Until recently vaginal breech births were offered to women as an option if their ECV was unsuccessful (or not chosen). Criteria included the baby estimating to be between 2.5 and 4 kg and not a footling breech or stargazer. About 55% of women who plan a vaginal breech birth achieve it (more likely if you have had a vaginal birth before) and 45% require a caesarean, usually because their labour does not progress.

In October 2000, however, the Term Breech Trial showed a two-thirds reduction in babies being injured if the woman had a planned caesarean (1.6%), compared to women who had a vaginal breech birth (5%).[14] This has made many caregivers swing towards elective caesarean as the only option for a breech birth, often because they are fearful of being seen as negligent practitioners by their peers and/or are concerned about the threat of litigation.

A few caregivers still offer vaginal breech birth after informing the woman of the risks and benefits. It can be explained that 98.4% of babies are uninjured with a caesarean, compared to 95% of babies born vaginally in a breech position, but on the other hand the health risks for the woman are significantly increased with a caesarean.[15]

The main health concerns for babies in a breech position born vaginally are:
- The baby's head being unable to be born (0.9%).

- Reduced oxygen to the baby, if the birth of their head is delayed more than five to eight minutes.
- Increased chance of cord prolapse (with a complete or footling breech).
- Injury to the baby, from the caregiver's efforts to help the baby to be born.

If a woman's baby is breech, she faces a great deal of pressure to have a caesarean. This may be her preferred option, or something she finds upsetting and disappointing. The negative attitudes of others can erode a woman's innate confidence in her ability to have a vaginal breech birth. Therefore it is usually only the most determined, motivated and committed women who persevere to seek out a supportive caregiver so they can avoid a caesarean.

Vaginal breech labours

Vaginal breech labours progress similar to normal labours. Just the baby's bottom first, then legs, arms and head last. Pressure on the baby's buttocks and abdomen from the woman's birth canal often makes them pass a thick blob of meconium during the pushing phase, which is normal and does not indicate distress. Reasonable progress for a breech labour is the cervix dilating at least 0.5 cm per hour during first stage, and 2 hours of second stage, with at least 1 hour of active pushing.

During the birth the baby usually delivers themselves. Experienced caregivers try to abide by the rule 'Hands off the breech', unless the baby obviously needs assistance. Once the baby's entire body leaves the mother, this is documented as the time of birth.

As a guide:
- Medications to induce or augment contractions are controversial because they can mask possible difficulties with the baby negotiating the birth canal. They should be used with caution (if at all).
- Epidurals should not be routine. Some caregivers insist on them to reduce an early urge to push (and possibly make the use of forceps an easy option, if needed). However, epidurals relax the pelvic floor muscles, which can interfere with guiding the baby efficiently down the birth canal and the woman pushing effectively.
- Forceps and episiotomy should not be routine.
- Lying on your back with stirrups supporting your legs should not be routine. A few caregivers allow women to give birth in the position of their choice.

SMALL BABY

When unborn babies grow slowly, they are called 'small for gestational age' (SGA). (Other terms are 'small for dates' or 'intrauterine growth retardation or restriction'.) These babies are in the lowest 10% of average birth weights for their gestation, at 40 weeks this is less than 2800 g. Reasons for being small can include:
- The woman's diet having insufficient carbohydrates and proteins.
- Smoking, creating placental insufficiency (less nutrients and oxygen to the baby).
- Multiple pregnancies.
- High blood pressure or placenta previa.
- A viral infection (rubella).
- The baby having a genetic disorder.

Some babies are naturally small, despite being very healthy, because their family members are genetically small, meaning there is no cause for concern. However, if health conditions are involved, the baby might:
- Become distressed during labour.
- Require resuscitation at birth and be susceptible to infections.
- Have low blood sugars and/or a low temperature soon after birth.
- Have a physical abnormality detected, or possibly die before, or soon after birth.[16]

Many SGA babies need to spend some time in the intensive care nursery. Methods used to detect whether a baby is abnormally small (after 28 to 30 weeks) include:
- Examining your belly and measuring the fundal height.
- Ordering regular CTG monitoring of the baby's heart rate.
- Ordering serial ultrasounds (consecutive ultrasounds weeks apart). A one-off ultrasound is of limited value. The ultrasonographer measures blood flow through the umbilical cord and the amount of amniotic fluid, as well as the baby's head circumference and abdominal circumference. SGA babies tend to grow out of proportion, channelling most of their nutrients to their brain, at the expense of their body.[17]

However, these methods are a guide only and in many cases it is hard to tell whether the baby has a problem or not. Many babies are suspected of being abnormally small but are actually healthy and normal.

Care usually involves closer monitoring while you wait and see what happens. Your caregiver may suggest inducing labour (or performing a caesarean), if tests indicate the baby is not coping well. Other treatments may include low dose daily aspirin, bed rest in hospital, energy and protein supplements, giving up smoking, and possibly relaxation strategies to deal with stress.

TOO MUCH OR TOO LITTLE FLUID AROUND THE BABY

Amniotic fluid is constantly circulated and renewed, swallowed by your unborn baby and excreted through their kidneys, as well as being produced by the amniotic sac. How its volume is regulated is not really known, but it is thought that prolactin and prostaglandin hormones work together to maintain the balance.[18]

Polyhydramnios

Polyhydramnios is when there is too much fluid around the baby, usually increasing slowly after 28 to 30 weeks and eventually exceeding 2000 ml (double the normal amount). Very rarely, it can happen suddenly at around 20 weeks, reaching abnormally high levels in just 4 days. Your caregiver may suspect polyhydramnios when feeling your belly at a routine pregnancy visit. This is confirmed with an ultrasound.

For about 65% of women, the cause remains unknown; 18% are due to the baby (genetic disorders, physical abnormalities or identical twins); 15% are due to health conditions for the woman (eg. diabetes, isoimmunisation); and less than 1% are due to an abnormally developed placenta. Health concerns include premature labour, an umbilical cord prolapse or, very rarely, placental abruption.

Treatments depend on how much fluid is present and how quickly it is increasing, but can include:
- Bed rest (sitting upright for comfort).
- A needle inserted to remove some amniotic fluid (500 ml at a time), repeated as often as necessary. This carries small risks of infection and premature labour.
- Prescribing medications aimed at inhibiting prostaglandin production.[19]

Oligohydramnios

Oligohydramnios is when the amount of amniotic fluid around the baby is abnormally low (less than 500 ml at 40 weeks). The most common causes for this include:
- Being overdue.
- Waters breaking prematurely.
- Baby being small for gestational age.

- The baby's kidneys not functioning well.
- The baby having a genetic disorder or abnormality.

Oligohydramnios is detected in the same way as polyhydramnios. Treatments depend on how severe the condition is and how much longer the pregnancy has to go, but usually involve just waiting and seeing, with rest, closer monitoring and the woman drinking plenty of water to increase amniotic fluid. Occasionally, amnio-infusion is tried (putting warmed, sterile saline water into the uterus via a needle). However, this is controversial and is probably not beneficial.[20]

PRE-ECLAMPSIA

Pre-eclampsia – also known as pregnancy induced hypertension (PIH), hypertensive disease of pregnancy (HDP) and pre-eclamptic toxaemia (PET) – is high blood pressure developing after 20 weeks of pregnancy. The precise cause is not clear, but it tends to be more common for women:

- Having their first baby or another baby with a new partner.
- Under 20 or over 35 years.
- With a family history of pre-eclampsia (mother or sister).
- With diabetes or a multiple pregnancy.
- Who experienced pre-eclampsia with a previous pregnancy (50% chance, but often milder).

Mild to moderate pre-eclampsia is often not noticed and many women feel well. Sudden swelling of the face, hands and feet may occur, but not always. If it does, it is often worse in the mornings, rather than at the end of the day, or in hot weather. A urine test for protein shows 2+ or more. The blood pressure may be 130/90 or above, increasing over days or weeks. If it reaches 160/100 (or higher), there may be more serious physical symptoms, such as:

- Headaches across the forehead; possibly feeling drowsy.
- Blurred or tunnel vision; seeing stars in front of your eyes.
- Constant pain at the base of the chest.
- Overreactive reflexes, muscles being jittery.
- Possibly feeling unwell, irritable, shaking, feverish and/or vomiting.
- Poor kidney and liver function and low platelet blood cells (referred to as HELLP syndrome).

Problems for the unborn baby can include poor growth, premature labour or a placental abruption. Thankfully, only 5% of women experience severe pre-eclampsia, but there is no reliable way of predicting which women will do this.

You will need more regular blood pressure checks (with your caregiver or GP). If the blood pressure continues to remain high, antihypertensive medications are prescribed. Depending on how severe it becomes, you may require admission to hospital. Blood tests are done to monitor your kidneys and liver, and the baby's heart rate is regularly checked with a CTG machine. If the condition worsens, despite medications, labour is induced, or an elective caesarean performed. During labour an epidural is often recommended because this is the most effective way to lower the blood pressure.

Pre-eclampsia normally improves within a week of having the baby, with a complete recovery within a month. Antihypertensive medications may need to be slowly weaned over several days or weeks.

You may wish to try managing your blood pressure naturally, particularly if the pre-eclampsia is mild. Methods may include:

- Eating lots of fresh fruit and vegetables (eg. cucumbers, grapes, celery and apples), and plenty of protein, carbohydrates and foods rich in potassium, magnesium and calcium.
- Drinking eight glasses of water a day (this also improves swelling).
- Supplementing with vitamins E, B6, magnesium, calcium, potassium and/or zinc. Check with your caregiver.
- Resting, stopping work or getting help to look after other children. This is **essential**. You may use relaxation techniques and massage to reduce stress and anxiety.
- Herbal remedies include chamomile, nettle, lime flower, raspberry leaf or dandelion teas, tinctures with cramp bark, black haw and nettle. Eating flaxseed or deep-sea fish oils. Consult your herbalist.
- Homeopathic or Bach flower remedies.

When pre-eclampsia becomes eclampsia

Eclampsia is rarely seen these days because of early treatments and actions taken by caregivers, but it can occur if the blood pressure becomes uncontrollably high, to the point where it is life-threatening for the woman and her baby. The main health effects for the woman are:

- Liver and kidney dysfunction or failure.
- Fluid on the lungs, straining the heart.
- Abnormal blood clotting.
- Fits or seizures (which can reduce oxygen to the baby).

Treatments include intravenous magnesium sulphate, sedatives, oxygen and delivering the baby once the woman is stable. Eclampsia is possible for up to five days after the birth.

GESTATIONAL DIABETES

Pregnancy can sometimes involve a temporary diabetic condition called gestational diabetes. This develops after 20 to 24 weeks and lasts until 24 hours after the baby is born. Gestational diabetes is detected with a long glucose tolerance test (LGTT) at about 28 weeks. The baby is not born with diabetes but has a higher chance of developing it later in life.

Most women are not aware that they have gestational diabetes. The main health concern is having an abnormally large baby (over 4.5 kg or 10 lb), which can increase the chances of:
- Requiring an induction of labour, a forceps delivery or caesarean birth.
- Shoulder dystocia.
- The baby having low blood sugars soon after the birth.

If your blood sugars are kept within normal limits, all these risks are similar to those for women who do not have diabetes.

Gestational diabetes is usually managed by changing your diet. The dietician at the hospital can help you plan this. You need to do finger prick blood tests up to four times a day and record the results. Blood sugars should be kept below 8 mmol/L. However, a few women require insulin injections because their new diet is not able to keep their blood sugars low.

BLEEDING DURING LATE PREGNANCY

Significant bleeding after 20 weeks is called an antepartum haemorrhage. This can be caused by similar factors to those for bleeding during early pregnancy (50 to 60% of cases; see Chapter 2), or by placenta previa (20 to 25%) or placental abruption (20 to 25%).

Placenta previa

If the placenta implants low in the uterus, close to the cervix, this is placenta previa. (About 5% of ultrasounds at 18 to 20 weeks indicate the placenta is low, but more than 95% of these move up by 34 weeks of pregnancy.)

Vaginal bleeding is normally painless and bright red, happening on and off from 28 to 30 weeks. It may start as spotting but become a little heavier with each bleed as the baby grows. An ultrasound can estimate how far the placenta is away from the cervix.
- Grade 1 = more than 5 cm.
- Grade 2 = the edge of the placenta touches the cervical opening.
- Grade 3 = the placenta covers some of the cervix.
- Grade 4 = the placenta covers the cervix altogether.

Sometimes a small section of the placenta (succenturiate lobe) implants away from the main placenta, near the cervix. A normal birth is possible with grades 1 and 2, if the bleeding does not become too heavy before the baby is born. A caesarean is required for grades 3 and 4.

Placental abruption

If the placenta unexpectedly lifts off the wall of the uterus, this is an abruption. Blood pools and clots behind it, causing moderate to severe constant pain in the belly and/or back and some bright vaginal bleeding. The cause may not be known, but can be associated with:
- Severe pre-eclampsia or eclampsia.
- Smoking.
- Polyhydramnios.

Depending on the size of the blood clot and whether the bleeding continues, care may include:
- Observation with ultrasounds.
- Allowing labour to continue if contractions start, breaking the waters broken to release pressure and the baby's heart rate being continuously monitored.

If the abruption is severe, the woman may need oxygen, a narcotic injection for pain relief, an intravenous drip and possibly a blood transfusion. The baby is delivered as soon as possible as this condition can be life-threatening for them.

Isoimmunisation

Isoimmunisation, or being 'sensitised', is fairly rare these days, but can occur when a woman with a Rhesus negative blood group develops antibodies to Rhesus positive blood from her baby. Anti-D is the most common. Other rare red cell antibodies include anti-C, anti-K or anti-E.

It can sometimes be hard to know when or how a woman has become sensitised. About 50% are caused by a previous blood transfusion and 50% are thought to be due to an exposure with a previous pregnancy (at birth or through miscarriage, bleeding or an amniocentesis or CVS procedures). Antibodies do not affect the woman's health but stay dormant in her system until there are further foreign red blood cells present, which can occur with a future pregnancy if the baby is Rhesus positive. When this happens, the woman's antibodies cross the placenta and start attaching themselves to the new baby's red blood cells, breaking them down and causing a degree of jaundice and/or anaemia, called haemolytic disease of the newborn (HDN).

Isoimmunisation can have a range of effects for the baby, from nothing at all to quite severe. It is hard to predict what will happen and it is very much a wait and see situation. Frequent blood tests every two to four weeks for antibody titres, can be a guide to when the baby may be affected: 1 in 8 or less is interpreted as the baby not being affected, and 1 in 16 or 1 in 32 may mean the baby is affected. The accuracy of critical titres is questionable;[21] and sometimes more complex blood tests are performed.

A high titre may prompt the caregiver to recommend an amniocentesis to see whether the baby is jaundiced. Depending on the severity, the baby may be given a blood transfusion inside the womb (if very premature) or delivered prematurely (by induction or caesarean). After birth, the baby may require phototherapy for jaundice and/or a blood transfusion. Generally, 50% of babies don't need treatments or just have phototherapy, and 50% need a blood transfusion before or after the birth.

A baby dying from this condition is now quite rare, but it is possible. Also, amniocentesis and intrauterine blood transfusions hold their own small risks. However, only a few babies have HDN severely enough for it to be life-threatening, and in most cases it is treatable and/or the baby is delivered before becoming too ill.

Preventing Rhesus isoimmunisation

Rhesus negative women need an injection of anti-D within 72 hours of having their baby, to reduce the chances of forming antibodies (from 10–20% to 0.2–1.5%). In the past, anti-D injections were also routinely given at 28 weeks of pregnancy (and sometimes 34 weeks as well) to further reduce the chances from 0.2 to 0.06%. However, anti-D is a blood product and stocks have become scarce worldwide (and at times unavailable in Australia). Plans are underway to reintroduce the administration of anti-D during pregnancy and should be fully available by 2004–2005.

CHOLESTASIS

Cholestasis of pregnancy is a liver disorder, usually occurring after 20 weeks. It is thought to be caused by oestrogen hormones interacting with the liver, causing a build-up of toxins (liver enzymes, bilirubin and bile acids) in the woman's blood stream. It is detected with blood tests for liver function and bile acids. Cholestasis may be hereditary and up to 40% of women who experience it will do so again with a subsequent pregnancy. If cholestasis is diagnosed, the main health concerns are for the baby, including:
- Premature birth.

- Becoming distressed during labour.
- Jaundice.
- Stillbirth (about five times more likely).

The main health concern for the woman is excessive bleeding during labour (or after the birth), because her blood clotting is disrupted. However, in most cases the baby is born well and the woman recovers within four weeks after the birth.

The most common physical sign is itching, especially the hands and feet, sometimes extending to the rest of the body. It is usually worse at night, contributing to insomnia and tiredness. There are often no obvious signs of a rash and the skin feels heated. Some women feel nauseated and can vomit intermittently. About 20% of women become mildly jaundiced, and possibly experience darkened urine and pale bowel motions, perhaps with recurrent urine infections.

Care involves close monitoring for the remainder of the pregnancy, doing regular blood tests and perhaps ultrasounds, and CTG monitoring of the baby. If the condition becomes severe, the labour is induced, even if the baby is premature. It is generally recommended that the pregnancy does not progress past 39 weeks, to reduce the chances of stillbirth. The baby's heart rate is continuously monitored during labour to check for distress.

Treatments for cholestasis can vary, and there is much debate about their efficacy and safety. Medications may include antihistamines and tranquillisers (to make the woman more comfortable), but these can further affect the liver. Some caregivers prescribe ursodeoxycholic acid, although its effects on the baby and woman are unknown.[22] Guar gum (a gel-forming fibre taken orally to eliminate bile acids from the bowel) may stabilise cholestasis, but this is not confirmed.[23]

Natural therapies to help reduce stress on the liver include:
- Rest and relaxation strategies.
- Drinking 8 to 10 glasses of water a day and avoiding fatty foods.
- Acupuncture or acupressure.
- Herbal remedies with dandelion, alfalfa, burdock or yellow dock.
- Homeopathic remedies such as Chelidonium majus or China officinalis.

FAQs

WHEN SHOULD I STOP WORK?
Modern life has created increasing pressure on pregnant women to continue to work closer to their due date and to continue to work full, or part-time

after their baby is born. Single women particularly need to plan their income carefully, so they can financially support themselves.

As far as an ideal time to stop work, there are no specific rules. If you are feeling well and coping (or even thriving), and your pregnancy is progressing normally, it is your own personal choice. However, remain flexible. Babies come when *they* are ready. Some women are forced to finish work earlier because of health concerns. Also, your planned two weeks off may turn out to be a couple of days if your baby comes at 38 weeks!

As a guide, most women find they can cope physically until 32 to 34 weeks. After this, achieving normal tasks often feels harder and involves substantially more effort. It is reasonable to finish paid work at around 34 to 36 weeks, but if you and your baby are well, you may choose to work later than this. Women expecting twins or more are often advised to stop work earlier. Keep in mind that the tiring demands of early parenting make many women regret not having a holiday before their next 'job' started.

Do I need raspberry leaf?

Raspberry leaf (*Rubus idaeus*) is a traditional herb made into a tea, tablet or tincture. It is often taken during pregnancy as a uterine tonic for childbirth, and it contains high concentrations of fragarine and flavonoids, which are believed to strengthen, tone and relax the uterus and pelvic muscles. It also contains calcium, iron, zinc, magnesium and vitamins B and E, making it a nutritive tonic.

Raspberry leaf may be prescribed by natural therapists and maternity caregivers for a variety of reasons, including anaemia, balancing the menstrual cycle, enhancing fertility, preventing miscarriage, easing morning sickness, helping leg cramps or bleeding gums, and relieving painful Braxton Hicks contractions, or afterpains.

Raspberry leaf is currently regarded as safe to use after 34 weeks of pregnancy, but there is little research to support its many claimed benefits. Two studies looking at the effects of raspberry leaf tea found:
- It may help prevent premature or overdue babies and may lessen the need for a caregiver to break the waters during labour or perform a caesarean, forceps delivery or vacuum birth.[24]
- It did not shorten the first stage of labour, but slightly shortened the pushing phase by about 10 minutes.[25]

At present there are no clear guidelines for the safe use of raspberry leaf tea, especially during the first 12 weeks of pregnancy. If you do want to take it, check with your caregiver, as recommendations vary. When taking raspberry

leaf, do so after food, as it can drop your blood glucose level. As a guide for use during pregnancy:
- **Tablets** – 2400 mg a day from 32 weeks.
- **Tea** – 1 teaspoon per cup; 1 cup per day during early pregnancy, increasing to 3 to 4 cups from 32 weeks. Add honey or sugar to taste or mix with peppermint or spearmint tea.
- **Tincture** – 1 teaspoon a day (depending on the concentration).

Raspberry leaf can increase colostrum production, but may decrease milk supply, so you should stop taking it three days after the birth. Some women experience diarrhoea when taking raspberry leaf.

What about clicking or popping noises?

A few pregnant women describe clicking or popping noises from inside their belly, usually when their baby moves. It is difficult to know exactly what causes this. One plausible explanation may be the baby's joints rubbing. In our experience, women who have noticed this have gone on to have healthy, normal babies.

Should I be concerned about my belly feeling cold?

Many women (and their partners) notice that their belly (and possibly the outside of their thighs) feels ice cold at times. This may be due to less blood circulating through fat tissue in these areas, as blood flow to other areas of the body increases. This mystery is not a problem, just a fascinating change!

CHAPTER 5

Preparing for birth

How you prepare for your baby's birth depends on your personal circumstances. This may be your first baby, or perhaps your third. You may be planning a natural birth or be scheduled for a caesarean. Some parents have detailed plans, while others choose to wing it on the day. A few don't get a chance to prepare because their baby is born well before their due date!

CHILDBIRTH CLASSES

Prospective parents seek childbirth classes for information and education, and possibly to meet other couples to continue supportive relationships after the birth. Childbirth classes are conducted through maternity hospitals (public and private), as well as by independent educators in the community. Fees are usually charged, but some public hospitals provide them for free.

Types of classes

Most childbirth classes aim to provide comprehensive information on labour and birth and how to prepare for this. The classes generally run as a series. This involves the same group of women and their partners/support people meeting with the educator each week for a two-hour session, for five to eight weeks (or more). A series is timed to start around 28 to 34 weeks of pregnancy, so it is completed before your baby is due. Other options are intensive courses (run over one or two days), refresher courses for women who already have children, and private sessions in your home, offered by many independent educators. Classes can also be taken online, either replacing face-to-face classes or complementing them.

Separate classes which may also be locally available are:
- Early pregnancy (diet, choosing a caregiver).
- Breastfeeding.
- Parenting skills (changing, bathing).
- Fathering groups.

- Infant massage.
- Settling techniques for crying babies.

Often elements of these are included in topics covered by a standard series of childbirth classes. Postnatal groups are also becoming popular, either as a one-off reunion with your pregnancy childbirth class or as an open group for new parents to meet regularly for support and education.

When enquiring about classes try to think about what is important for you and how you prefer to learn. Individual educators have their own style of teaching, which will affect the class structure, content and how they are presented. To help you choose, perhaps ask about the:

- Course length, times, location and cost.
- Number of people in each class.
- Course format (lectures, discussion groups, use of videos, etc).
- Topics covered – natural birth, caesarean, pain relief, emotional reactions, relaxation, breathing techniques, labour and birth positions, support strategies, unexpected outcomes, and extras such as birth plans, parenting issues, breastfeeding or sibling preparation. Perhaps ask for a weekly syllabus.

Childbirth preparation classes can fill up quickly and most caregivers recommend you book in by 20 to 24 weeks, even though they won't start until several weeks later. Waiting until the last few weeks of pregnancy may mean missing out.

Do I need a support person?

Every woman needs a support person during labour. Being on your own can be very isolating and scary. Having someone you know and trust, such as your partner, a close friend, a relative (or all of the above), can help make the experience a more positive one. Some women employ a professional support person (or doula – Greek for 'women who serve').

Research shows that if a woman has continuous hands-on nurturing and encouragement from a sympathetic companion throughout her labour she is *less* likely to:

- Need medical pain relief.
- Need an operative delivery (ie. forceps, ventouse or caesarean).
- Have her baby become distressed during labour, or need medical assistance after birth.

and *more* likely to:

- Have a spontaneous vaginal birth.
- Be satisfied with her birth experience and feel she was more in control.[1]

Some birthplaces restrict the number of support people you can have and you may need to seek permission if you wish to have more than one or two people, or have your child(ren) present.

Staffing levels (in both public and private hospitals) make it difficult for the midwife to provide constant support. Often one midwife will care for two or three labouring women at a time. If you have your own obstetrician, they are present for the birth but not the hours of labour. Midwives also work shifts and you may have two (or three) during the course of your labour. This can be disappointing if you establish a good relationship with one, or perhaps helpful if you don't. Some women employ their own private midwife to provide continuous care throughout their entire labour.

Often partners need an extra support person to help them and give them occasional breaks, especially if the labour is long. This may also help if you feel your partner may not be able to meet all your practical needs, such as massage and emotional encouragement.

Choosing a support person

The person you choose should be unconditionally supportive, on both emotional and physical levels. Many women feel a female support person is important, especially if they are also a mother, or experienced in being with women during labour. If your support person has no experience of birth, they should consider reading or doing some preparation with you. If you employ a doula, meet them during the pregnancy (perhaps more than once) to make sure you connect. Get to know them, share your birth plans and explain what you expect from them.

As a guide, you should aim to choose someone who:
- You feel totally comfortable with, even if you are naked, screaming or crying.
- Your partner gets on with and can work with. As the partner, discuss how their role can fit in with yours, so you're not made to feel redundant.
- Is a real support for you, not there for the show. Don't feel pressured to invite anyone (including your mother).
- Is available 24 hours a day around your due date.
- Is supportive of your birth choices and will not pressure you into making decisions. For example, talking you into pain relief because they feel uncomfortable seeing you in pain, or pushing you into not accepting pain relief, because they want you to achieve a natural birth.
- Is open-minded and relaxed about birth. If this person is a mother, will they bring prejudices or unresolved fears?

- Feels okay if you decide not to call them and happy to leave the room if you need them to. Open communication is important.

NOTE: *If English is your second language, consider, if possible, having someone who speaks your mother tongue. Women unconsciously use their first language when in strong labour and your bilingual support person can communicate with you and perhaps relay your requests to your caregiver.*

Preparing your other children

The birth of a new brother or sister (or both!) is a major life event for a child. Deciding whether your child(ren) will be at the birth and how to introduce the new baby, are important issues.

There are many ways to prepare your child for the birth, whether they will be present or not. If you plan to leave them with someone else, let them know that you are going to the hospital and what the arrangements will be, including the fact that this might be while they are sleeping. If they have to be taken elsewhere, arrange an occasional stay-over before the birth.

When you leave your child, say goodbye (if awake) and perhaps give them something special to mind until you see them again. Try to see them within 24 hours after the birth (or organise early discharge, if you want this). Have daily contact, even if it is just a phone call. Bear in mind that even if you have no intention of bringing them to the birth, unforseen events (eg. sick childminder, fast labour) can sometimes mean you need to take them with you, so prepare them for this.

Having your child at the birth

Involving your child with the birth of their sibling will depend on their age, personality and how you feel about it. You know them best. Some parents view birth as a family event and feel comfortable having their child present (or in close proximity). Others see it as an adult event, not suitable for children. However, children usually find birth fascinating and generally approach it very casually, to everyone's surprise. If others around them are calm, relaxed and accepting of the process, the child picks up on this and reacts accordingly.

Research shows there is no difference in the levels of sibling rivalry whether an older child is at the birth or not,[2] and there are no short-term adverse effects on preschoolers who attend the birth of siblings, provided they were well prepared and familiar with the environment.[3] Preparing your child for what they may see and hear minimises any negative responses (which in our experience is very rare). Be aware of your own feelings or fears and take care not to pre-empt your concerns for them.

Common issues that come up when deciding include:

- Excluding children if scheduled for a caesarean. This can be worked around by having them wait close by and be with you and the baby soon afterwards.
- Feeling nervous about how they may react to seeing and hearing you in pain, watching the birth or seeing blood. Give your child the flexibility to leave the birth room when they want, to provide acceptable comfort zones. Don't force them to be present. If they are old enough, talk to them about having this choice. Whether they actually witness the birth is probably not as important as them being in close proximity to you and your partner.
- Feeling torn between not really wanting your child around but feeling you can't be apart, particularly if they are not used to extended periods of separation. You may be able to organise well-timed visits, although repeated separations can also be distressing.

If you and your partner disagree as parents, then you will need to come to some sort of compromise. If you have no extended support from family or friends, your options may be limited and you may need to bring your other children with you.

Preparing your child for the birth

When preparing your child, try not to bombard them with information. Allow their natural curiosity to bring up issues, or address them yourself at appropriate times. Try to answer their questions simply and honestly, using the correct terms. Talk about the possible sequence of events and reinforce the role of their chosen support person. You can also explore their role – perhaps give them a special job, like wiping your face during labour, or announcing the baby's sex after the birth. Other things you can do include:

- Showing them books or videos about births, and photos of their own birth (if you have them).
- Play-acting the birth with them, perhaps using a doll or drawing activities.
- Making loud birth noises and talking about the hard work involved in having the baby.
- Bringing the birth experience back to them, to emphasise it as normal: 'It was hard work having you, I had to make lots of noise' or 'There is a little blood but Mummy will be okay. That happened when you were born.'

- Preparing them for seeing you naked, the presence of blood, the baby being wet, naked, slippery and crying. Liken cutting the cord with cutting your fingernails or your hair, emphasising it does not hurt.
- Familiarising your child with your birthplace and caregiver. Take them to some pregnancy visits if possible.

Choosing your child's support person

Your child will need a support person to talk with them and see to their needs. This helps prevent you from being distracted and frees your partner to support you. If you are unable to find an extra support person, you may feel comfortable having your partner support them, depending on their age and the polices of your birthplace. Discuss this with your caregiver as their main concern is looking after you and not being caught up in dealing with a demanding toddler. Whatever you decide, you need to take responsibility for your child. This may mean your partner needing to take them out, leaving you to manage without them for a while.

When choosing your child's support person, consider someone who:
- Is aware of their important role, being there wholly for your child.
- Your child trusts and who can care for your child in a way you feel comfortable with.
- Is tolerant of, and has realistic expectations about, your child's behaviour. Children don't change just because they are at a birth.
- Is freely available around the time of the birth (remember, your baby may come early, or arrive later than expected). Consider contingency plans if they, or your child, are ill.
- You and your partner feel comfortable with being present at the birth.
- Feels comfortable with witnessing childbirth, and who will be calm and composed.
- Feels comfortable about missing the birth if your child needs to leave the room.
- Can listen to your child's questions and give simple explanations as the birth is happening. Discuss this during the pregnancy, so you are happy with what your child is being told.

Facilitating the labour with your children present

You need to be free to focus on your labour, so it can establish and progress. During prelabour and early labour it can help if your child is occupied so you can concentrate on the task at hand. This is why many women find they start labouring once older children are asleep.

Once the contractions are strong, others around you become less important.

However, vocalising is an important part of letting go, so if you feel you are holding back, you may need to reconsider your child's presence. In reality, most children find the noise quite entertaining. Sometimes a woman labours better with her children around, because she knows where they are; she can usually ignore their activities because she is so used to their behaviour.

What if . . .

The labour is long? Children have a limited attention span. Even a two-hour labour is a long time for a toddler. Pack a bag with activities, change of clothes, snacks, drinks, bottles, dummies, their favourite comforter and possibly a new toy. Include a pillow and blankets in case they need to sleep. If you leave at night, their support person may be able to bring the children when they wake or when the birth is near.

It happens at night? All these scenarios need contingency plans. However, it is rare to start labouring until things are in place. Some people advise not waking children for births, but mostly they are fine. If they are old enough, perhaps ask them whether they want to be woken. When waking them, do this gently, but if they don't feel like stirring, let them sleep. Try to time waking them for about half an hour before the birth, to give them a chance to adjust. Many children naturally wake if they are close by. Perhaps the escalation of sound contributes to this, or they just have an innate sense that their sibling is about to arrive!

Your child's support person is ill or unavailable, or your child is ill? Again, some contingency plans are needed here. Explain any alternate plans to your child.

Your child does not wish to be there? This may hurt you, but it is something you have to accept. Forcing your child to attend a birth could be traumatic. Children are amazingly honest and seem to know whether they will cope. They also change their minds frequently and need flexibility to do this.

You need to ask your child to leave? This may occur and could be an issue if your child does not want to go. This may affect your decision to include them in the labour and birth altogether. Discuss this with them as part of their preparation.

There are complications? You may need to consider taking your child out of the room. If you need transfer (or a caesarean), make plans for your child.

Some parents shield their child from certain procedures (internal examinations, epidural insertion or an episiotomy). This is at your discretion, and possibly the choice of your child.

NOTE: *Bear in mind that some children feel stressed or traumatised if they witness complications, or hear conversations that relate to the health of their mother and/or sibling. Debriefing them after the birth is important. You can encourage them to share and express their feelings (if they can verbalise them) or draw pictures to tell you how it was from their perspective. If you are concerned about their reactions and behaviour, seek the services of a qualified counsellor experienced in dealing with children.*

Your birthplace's attitudes

Your birthplace should always accommodate your child's involvement. Unfortunately, some institutions (and caregivers) are still reluctant to do this. You may be required to write a letter of request to the nurse unit manager of the delivery suite, or the hospital administrator. This request is rarely denied, but it creates a formal hurdle to jump. Conditions may be attached to their consent, such as having an extra support person (which is advisable anyway) or taking your child out in the event of complications. However, you have the right to question anything you feel is unreasonable. There is no medical reason to restrict the number of support people present and you are within your rights to challenge this to satisfy your child (or yourself for that matter). Hopefully in the years to come, children at births will be as accepted as fathers are today.

WHEN CONSIDERING A WATER BIRTH

Using a bath for pain relief during labour is now more common, and in some cases this leads to a water birth. Ask your caregiver or childbirth educator if your birthplace facilitates water births (or if your caregiver is likely to get you out of the bath). Some birth centres have a 25 to 30% water birth rate, while other birthplaces have the odd one or two. This can give you an idea as to how supported water birth is.

If planning a water birth, it is important to be open and flexible. Many women end up getting out of the bath for the birth (for gravity to push, or just because they feel waterlogged). Others have no intention of having a water birth but don't want to move from the bath once the birth is imminent. The bath can provide relaxation, pain relief and feel very comfortable, but there is no evidence that water births are better for babies.[4]

Many people express concerns about the safety of water births, particularly for the baby. The main issues are:

What if the baby breathes in water? – Newborn babies have a natural dive reflex which is activated once their head is born. Their larynx (the opening to their lungs) closes over and automatically stops their desire to breathe. Once their body is born, they are brought straight to the surface (within 5 to 10 seconds) to take a breath. Air on the baby's face prompts them to breathe. So if you stand and lift the baby's face from the water, you can't resubmerge. The whole birth must happen below the water or be completed above it.

Bear in mind that the baby's head can be underwater for three to five minutes, until the next contraction and their body is born which is acceptable, but may make you feel nervous. During this time they still receive oxygen from you through the umbilical cord. In some cases the baby's dive reflex can be inhibited and a water birth is not to be recommended. These include:
– The baby being distressed (low heart rate or meconium stained amniotic fluid).
– The woman is taking beta blocker medications for high blood pressure.[5]

What about infection? – Women and babies are not at any higher risk of developing an infection, and the baby does not have more breathing difficulties after being born in water.

Generally, using the bath for pain relief, or a water birth, is not advisable for women or babies who are unwell, for premature babies, or for twins or breech births (although there are documented cases of twins and breeches being born into water, usually with homebirths).

WHAT TO PACK FOR THE BIRTH

In the final weeks of pregnancy (or prelabour) it is a good idea to put together what you might need for the birth. The following is a suggested list which can be adjusted to suit your individual circumstances. Ask your caregiver or childbirth educator whether you need anything specific and what your hospital or birth centre provides. Remember that your partner or support team also need supplies to keep pace with you during the hours of labour, so much of what you pack will be for them.

Delivery suite or birth centre
Personal items for the woman and partner:
- 2 comfortable T-shirts, pyjamas, dresses or sarongs to labour in.
- A dressing-gown or housecoat.

- 2 pairs of warm socks (labouring women get cold feet – literally!).
- Comfortable clothes and flat comfy shoes to wear in hospital and to go home in.
- 6 pairs of underpants (old ones or disposables).
- 2 packs of large maternity sanitary pads.
- Toiletries a box of tissues a roll of super soft toilet paper (for after the birth).
- Clips or bands to keep the hair off your face.
- Personal belongings to create your own labouring atmosphere (eg. pillows doona photos).
- 2 to 3 maternity bras.
- A box of breast pads.
- A set of clothes for your baby to go home in.
- For the partner – toiletries (to shower and clean teeth) a change of clothes comfortable shoes swimmers and a towel (in case they are with you in the shower or bath).
- If you intend to bottle feed – bottles equipment and formula (find out if you need to supply these). Most hospitals supply sterilising equipment.

Drinks and snacks:
- Nonacidic juices (apple or pear) herbal teas mineral waters PowerAde or homemade Labourade (see recipe). Tea/coffee for support people.
- Flavoured ice blocks (you may need an esky).
- Bendable straws.
- Hard lollies (eg. barley sugars or lollipops).
- Fresh fruit yoghurt soups chocolate muesli bars dried fruit or nuts.
- Food for your partner or support people (or a pizza delivery number).

Labourade recipe

$1/4$ cup of honey

$1/2$ teaspoon of salt

$1/3$ cup of lemon juice

1 calcium tablet and 1 magnesium tablet – crushed

Mix ingredients and add about 1 litre of cool water.

Massage and support tools:
- Massage oil (in squirt bottles if possible) gels or heat rubs.
- Massage implements compresses.
- 2 face washers water spray bottle lip balm.
- Music tapes or CDs. Check whether your birthplace supplies players.

- Heat packs. (Perhaps a hollow, plastic rolling pin that can be filled with warm or cold water to roll over the lower back.)

NOTE: *Check with your birthplace about their heat pack policy. Some restrict the type you can use in case the woman is inadvertently burnt, or because the way they are heated is considered a fire hazard (eg. wheat packs in microwaves can set alight).*

Other helpful items:
- Pregnancy card, Medicare card, private health insurance details (if applicable).
- Labour support guide (at the end of the book).
- Camera and film, or digital camera. If you don't want to use a flash, have 400 to 1000 ASA film or an infrared flash. Pack extra batteries.
- Video recorder and tripod (if you're really serious).
- Phone card, coins for public phone, phone numbers. (Mobiles can't be turned on in hospitals.)
- Champagne, a birthday cake?
- Baby car seat.

Natural therapies:
- Bach or bush flower essences, homeopathic remedies, herbal tinctures.
- Aromatherapy oils for massage, compresses or burners (electric burners only in hospitals).
- Visualisation tapes or scripts.

Additional preparations for a homebirth

In addition to the above list you will need to make extra preparations. Check with your caregiver.

Household and personal items:
- Lots of clean towels and face flannels.
- Old clean sheets and a plastic drop sheet to give birth on.
- 2 to 3 large garbage bags to put soiled linen into.
- A largish mirror, if you wish to watch yourself give birth.
- A mattress, pillows or futon for kneeling on the floor.
- A birth pool, or your own bath (if big enough), or hire/buy an inflatable pool.
- 1 to 2 buckets to empty the pool and top it up with warm water. A bucket or bowl for any unpredictable vomits.
- A 'poo scoop' (or sieve) for a water birth.
- Large incontinence sanitary pads to save soiling bed linen after the birth.

- A fan or heater to keep the room at a comfortable temperature, depending on the season.
- Candles and holders, matches/lighter.

NOTE: *Have all your birth equipment in one place, so your midwife and support team can find things easily.*

Items for the baby:
- Flannelette baby blankets to cover them at birth (warmed if possible). A bonnet to put on their head.
- Clothes to dress your baby in.
- Nappies (at least 2 dozen prewashed cloth, or 60 to 70 disposable – 1 week's worth). Pins or clips for cloth nappies.
- A couple of packets of cotton balls/pads (or face washers) to clean your baby's bottom and plain sorbelene cream for bathing.

Drinks and snacks

Keep nonperishable labour food separate, so if you are due to shop when labour starts, you still have things available. Make sure there are plenty of ice cubes in the freezer. Have easy-to-eat food available for support people (precooked and frozen meals can be handy).

Birth tips
- **Water supply** – Hot water is needed for heat packs, baths and showers. Your electricity company may be able to turn your off-peak system to on-peak for the month you are due. You can hire water urns, or a water heater for the birth pool. Purchase or borrow a few large pots to boil water on the stove.
- **Other children** – Set up a room or play area for siblings with activities and/or a TV/video. Your support person might be able to help them bake a birthday cake for the baby. Consider purchasing a present for them 'from the baby'.
- **Extra helpers** – They can organise meals, clean or care for your other children in the week or two after the birth. Consider asking visitors to bring food rather than flowers, or taking a load of washing!
- **Transfer to hospital** – To make this transition a smooth one, be prepared. Pack a bag for hospital using the list above. Have petrol in the car. Know the way to the hospital. Consider who will lock the house and what will happen with your other children and pets. Type a list of phone numbers and place them beside the phone (caregiver, support people, delivery suite or birth centre, ambulance – 000 in

Australia). Write out your full address and nearest crossroad for the ambulance. Note any unusual access tips for your property and give them a mobile number just in case.

How to make up heat packs

Traditional hot packs require cloth nappies, a bucket of very hot water and a pair of thick rubber gloves (to wring out excess water). Pros: the wet heat feels great. Cons: a work-intensive method, taking the entire time of a support person; nappies need replenishing every contraction or so; can also be a bit wet and messy.

Blue gel in plastic (sports packs) are soaked in very hot (close to boiling) water for 10 to 15 minutes, or microwaved. If using water, you need four, so that two can soak while the others are in use. Pros: effective, lasting for an hour or more; can be moulded to shape where needed. Cons: slightly expensive and need time to reheat. Take care if using a microwave; they can burst if overheated.

Hot water bottles should preferably have a cover. Pros: cheap and easy to refill; can be used in the shower or bath during labour; great for back pain and afterpains. Cons: standard sizes are too large to fit snugly under your belly; can be difficult to hold in place if leaning forward or on all fours; some birthplaces don't allow them.

Microwave nappies involve cloth nappies or hand towels moistened with water and wrung out before folding (a flat square about 30 by 15 cm), then placed in a thick, plastic bag and taped with masking or gaffer tape. (Remove most of the air from the bag before taping.) Double-bagging the nappy helps stop leaking. Place in the microwave on high for three to four minutes (about one minute for reheating). Wrap in a pillowcase or towel before use. Pros: cheap, easy and effective, providing good pain relief for up to an hour or more. Cons: you need a microwave, but most hospitals have these; they can become extremely hot, so take care.

Wheat packs are commercially made and consist of raw wheat grains encased in cloth, often scented with lavender or other herbs. They are heated in a microwave or oven (if at home). Pros: soft, warm and pleasantly scented, able to mould to your shape. Cons: expensive; cannot be used in the shower or bath; most hospitals don't permit them (they can set alight if overheated), but may be used at home for early labour or for a homebirth.

NOTE: Occasionally women are burnt from heat packs. Support people should feel the pack to gauge the heat and check the woman's skin for redness, perhaps removing the pack between contractions. Don't use heat packs if she has an epidural (she can't feel them anyway!).

WRITING A BIRTH PLAN

A birth plan is a written plan or verbal agreement outlining your preferences for labour and birth. It can range from a few ideas to an extensive preparation, covering many contingencies. It is also a way to make special requests known to your caregiver, especially if you have not met them beforehand. A caesarean birth plan can also be done, to discuss your preferences and needs with your caregiver and help make it a positive experience. (This is included in our sample birth plan at the back of the book.)

Labour brings many unknowns and your circumstances can change rapidly, making your preferred choices no longer feasible. So, having some knowledge about your options can help make your birth plan workable and accommodate events as they unfold. If you have specific issues that are not negotiable, clarify these with your caregiver or childbirth educator during the pregnancy, in case there are circumstances you are unaware of that could make them unworkable. Your plan can also state whether you are open (or not) to suggestions from your caregiver.

A birth plan can be for:

- The woman giving birth to identify needs and preferences, and prompt questions for her caregiver and/or birthplace.
- The partner and/or support person, to help them fully understand what is important for the woman and what is expected of them.
- Your private caregiver, to clarify your choices and let them know your preferred approach. It is better to negotiate this prior to the labour rather than during it. Sometimes issues are raised making you reconsider your choice of caregiver (or birthplace). It can also act as a reminder for them, in case they are busy and cannot recall what was discussed during the pregnancy.
- Your delivery suite or birth centre midwife. It is likely you will not have met them before labour and a plan can let them know your wishes and their expected role, so you don't have to explain these during labour.

Some people argue against doing birth plans, claiming:
- They can create a defensive environment.
- They may set you up for feelings of failure.
- That birth cannot be planned for and it is important to be open in your approach, trusting your body as it happens.
- They may stop you from exploring the extent of your personal coping resources.
- 'All birth plans are the same' and some caregivers don't respect them.

People need different tools to assist them in their journey to birth. A birth plan can be useful, or inhibiting. However, working on one does tend to motivate women and their partners to learn about the various interventions they may be confronted with, and how they might deal with them, as well as exploring the approaches of their caregiver or birthplace. If a birth plan achieves this, it has been a useful exercise, even if it never sees the light of day.

Writing your birth plan

You can write your birth plan alone or with your partner or support person. Some couples write separate notes, and then make necessary changes before writing a united plan. Simple and flexible is a good approach; take your time to let it grow. Possibly start with a list on the fridge, then add and delete as your knowledge and preferences develop.

Your final draft should be typed (if possible) and done in point form, no longer than a couple of pages. Open with a short introduction and use statements like, 'I would prefer' and 'If it is not an emergency, we would like options A, B and C discussed.' If you feel strongly about certain procedures you can write something like: 'I do not wish to be offered pain relief at any time. I will let you know if and when I need it.'

You can give copies to your support people and caregivers during pregnancy and hand one to the midwife on arrival at your birthplace when in labour.

Prelabour

The prelabour phase is when physical signs are felt, which will at some stage change to become active or established labour (the first stage). Prelabour can be experienced for hours, days or even weeks before labour starts, often coming and going unpredictably. Caregivers refer to this as false or spurious labour, and don't count it as actual labour. This is why a three-day labour can be turned into eight hours on the hospital paperwork!

Most women experience some form of prelabour. Sometimes this is only acknowledged in hindsight, because the physical signs were vague (slight backache or cramping). A few women start established labour without any obvious prelabour.

If you have to ask, 'Is this labour?', then it's not! However, each woman's body differs and yours may not always behave in a textbook manner. Prelabour contractions vary considerably but are usually further apart,

shorter (or longer) in length, and more erratic than first stage contractions. But they are usually not strong enough to stop you talking or doing normal tasks. As a guide they may be one of the following:
- Regular, mild or strong, coming every 5, 7, 10 or 15 minutes apart, lasting approximately 20 to 40 seconds.
- A dull ache in the lower belly, upper thighs and/or lower back, perhaps with period-like cramping.
- Erratic or irregular, with no rhythm developing, making it difficult to rest or sleep.
- Not start at all, because you don't have a prelabour!

There is no need to time all the contractions during prelabour. This is tiresome and places pressure on the woman to get into active labour. Just time a few every hour or so, or if they seem to be intensifying. Contact the hospital or birth centre if you need to clarify what is happening.

NOTE: *If you are less than 37 weeks pregnant and are experiencing painful contractions or cramping sensations every 15 minutes or less, contact your caregiver in case it is premature labour.*

Coping with prelabour contractions

Prelabour can be frustrating and disheartening, especially if prolonged. If you've never had a baby before, it can be hard to know whether this is the real thing; it can be distressing being in pain but not yet in established labour.

After several hours (or days) of pain, tiredness can ensue (often for the partner as well) and may lead to you requesting pain relief sooner or accepting interventions to speed the progress of labour. If you and your caregiver feel this is the right decision for you, then use the options you are most comfortable with. However, if you wish to avoid interventions unless necessary, you may take comfort in knowing that once labour establishes, the progress is often comparatively quick. For example, it may take 2 to 3 days to get to 3 cm dilation with prelabour, but only 2 to 8 hours for the baby to be born once established labour starts.

Physical signs of prelabour

Cervix ripening, thinning, opening. The cervix is normally 3 to 5 cm long, but becomes paper thin during prelabour (called effacement). This is measured in percentages. A long, or uneffaced, cervix is 0%, and a paper-thin cervix is fully effaced, or 100%. Effacement indicates that the cervix has been partially pulled up (or absorbed) into the lower segment of the uterine walls.

The opening, thinning and pulling up of the cervix happens simultaneously. The cervix cannot open (or dilate) beyond 3 or 4 cm until it is fully effaced (100%), and it cannot shorten and thin without opening (or dilating). When the cervix is thin, but less than 3 to 4 cm dilation, this is regarded as prelabour.

NOTE: *During the final weeks of pregnancy pressure from the baby's head engaging can dilate the cervix 1 to 3 cm (especially if this is not your first baby), but it remains thick. This does not indicate labour will happen soon.*

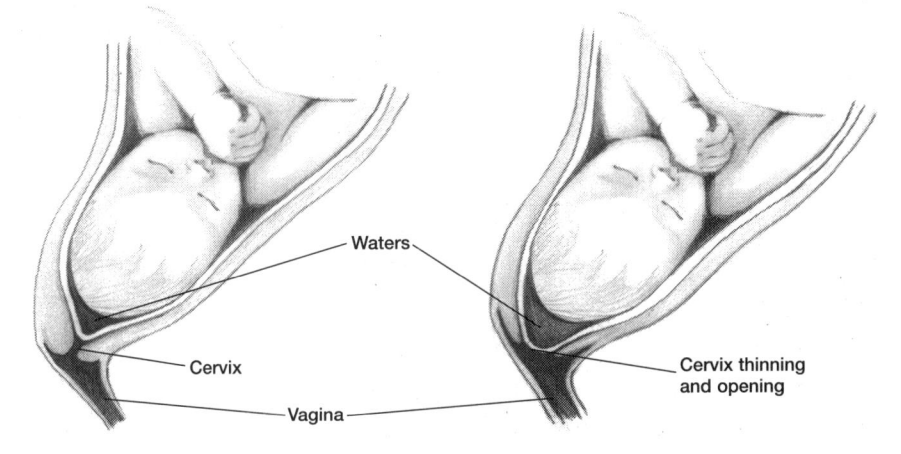

Cervix thinning and opening during first stage

Backache and/or period pain can come and go, or may be constant. This happens as the cervix softens and ripens and/or the baby's head engages.

Vomiting and feeling nauseous is common, but is generally more likely when the labour intensifies.

Diarrhoea is a classic sign of prelabour. The bowel is stimulated as the woman's cervix changes and ripens, but the diarrhoea can be made worse by some natural induction methods (eating a strong curry or taking castor oil). Diarrhoea usually settles once established labour is in progress.

A mucus plug or show can come away as the cervix thins and softens. This may be clear, or yellow and creamy, or have streaks of red, pink or brown blood in it. The show can be a large blob, enough to fill your hand, or a neat plug (similar to a tampon), or just a thick vaginal discharge over several days, noticed when wiping yourself after going to the toilet. A show may be noticed days or weeks before labour begins.

The bag of waters breaking (amniotic fluid) around your baby can rupture at any time during labour, or before contractions start. They should be clear, or pink, in colour (green indicates meconium staining) and you should definitely let the hospital or birth centre know.

Did you know?
In past generations, women were warned not to have their waters broken, as it would make for a 'dry birth'. In reality, the amniotic membrane continues to produce fluid. If your waters are broken, the contractions may intensify but the birth itself will not be any harder than if the waters were left intact.

SUPPORT STRATEGIES

A summary of labour support strategies is provided as a labour guide at the back of the book, for quick reference during labour. The most important thing to remember is that this is just the beginning. So try to stay calm and carry on as normal as possible to conserve your energy.

Support strategies for the woman

Ignore your prelabour until it becomes too strong to disregard. You may feel like going for a walk, or staying close to home. You can pack your bag, if you haven't already done this. If the prelabour is relentless and fairly strong, you may need to go in for a check-up, and then return home again until labour steps up. Other support strategies include:

- **Not phoning everyone to let them know** – Friends and family mean well, but if they start ringing constantly, it can put pressure on you to perform. Turn the answering machine on or disconnect the phone. Only contact support people if they need to travel or make arrangements.
- **Following your body's needs** – There is a fine line between being active to stimulate contractions and exhausting yourself before labour starts. Try to sleep or rest. Make up a heat pack and return to bed. If you can't sleep, have a long, warm bath (if your waters have not broken) or shower, and then rest in a comfortable position. Only go walking if you feel energetic.
- **Eating and drinking as much as you can tolerate** – The uterus is a muscle and it needs energy to function. Sips of watered-down pear or apple juice (50/50) or mineral water, as well as soups, yoghurt, fruit, toast, chocolate or muesli bars can help you keep energised and hydrated. Once you are in strong labour you usually don't feel like anything but fluids and ice. If you vomit, don't stop drinking. Sips of fluid will still be absorbed.
- **Keeping your bladder empty** – Try to pass urine at least every couple of hours (if awake).

- **Using natural therapies** such as:
  - Acupuncture or acupressure to stimulate contractions, or tone things down if tired.
  - Massage and visualisation techniques (see visualisation appendix).
  - Aromatherapy, such as lavender to calm or clary sage to stimulate the labour.
  - Homeopathy (Caulophyllum) or herbal tinctures (blue cohosh) to help labour progress. Try to organise a birth kit during the pregnancy.

Support strategies for the partner/support person

- **Be prepared, in case active labour starts** – Pack your bag (see the check list), organise time off work, put petrol in the car, have money for parking at the hospital. Be aware of organised street events or peak-hour traffic times, as these may influence the timing of you leaving or the best way to get there.
- **Support her in what she feels like doing** – Don't force her to walk if she is tired, or to rest if she wants to pace. Don't rush her into going to hospital if she is not ready and don't convince her to stay at home if she is uncomfortable with this. Contact her caregiver if you need guidance.
- **Communicate how you are both feeling** – Nervous, excited, scared or glad, the day/night has finally arrived.
- **Try going back to sleep** – This mean both of you. If it is daytime, hire a video or go see a film (if she feels up to it). Arrange a massage for her or give her one yourself.
- **Start supporting her** – Find the heat packs, play some music, burn some aromatherapy oils (ask her what she wants). Remind her to keep eating and drinking, and to pass urine every couple of hours. Don't forget to eat and drink yourself.

EMOTIONS
Emotions for the woman

You may feel relieved because you have had enough of being pregnant or unsure about moving forward into the labour and birth. It is normal to have questions and concerns about the unknown path ahead, or to be worried about becoming exhausted because you don't know how long it will last. Try to stay positive. Take one step at a time.

We are taught from an early age to control our bodies and behaviours. Yet labouring and giving birth is a primitive, uncontrollable process. Trying to hold it together can be exhausting, often prolonging labour. Your mind and body need to work together to facilitate it. Often the body will let go if the mind is willing to let it. During pregnancy, focus on letting go and losing these inhibitions. It might help to discuss with your caregiver or support person any fears you may have of losing control.

It can be hard to believe you will endure labour, especially if you have a long and tiring prelabour phase. However, many women are surprised with their ability to deal with it. Positive thoughts that can help include:
- I am bringing my baby into the world.
- Nature will not send me anything my body is not capable of dealing with.
- I am made to give birth. Millions of women have done this before me.
- There are breaks between the contractions, with periods of difficulty and periods of ease. Take it as it comes.
- Labour is a healthy pain, not an injury.

A few women are shocked by the unexpected intensity of their labour, feeling nothing could have prepared them for it. However, rather than worry whether this will be the case, try to be open, because until you are in it, you won't really know.

If you are worried what your partner will think if you 'can't do it', communicate this to them. Try not to think of it in terms of success or failure, but as one day in the long process of parenting.

Emotions for the partner/support person

What if she can't contact me when it starts? Leave a number where you can be contacted each day. Don't plan trips away two weeks either side of the due date. If you have a mobile, don't leave it turned off for long periods; check your voicemail frequently. (Consider hiring a mobile or pager for a month if you need to.) Have call waiting on your phone if you don't have PABX at work. If there is a chance you can't be contacted, organise another support person and a contingency plan for everyone to get to the hospital.

How will I cope if the labour is long? No one can tell you how long your partner's labour will be. The average time for first babies is 12 to 14 hours but it could range from 5 to 30 hours, with several hours (or days) of prelabour preceding this. This is why it is important to rest, sleep and conserve your energy for when it is really needed.

How will I feel seeing her in pain? It can be distressing seeing your wife/lover/friend in pain. She will be working hard and using every ounce of her being to deal with her labour and will not be able to comfort or support you. If she senses your anxiety, her focus will shift from her labour to you, which can impact on her progress.

To prepare yourself, talk about different labour scenarios together (fast and furious, prolonged and tiring, or intense and not progressing). You may get a chance to talk to other partners during the pregnancy, to find out what helped them. Organise an extra support person if you think this may be useful. Arrange to have someone to talk to after the birth, as you may need to debrief.

Will I know enough to support her? Labour support often means just being there. You know your partner best and even if you know nothing of labour, no one else can help her like you can. Your love and reassurance can reduce her fear and tension, inspire confidence in her and give her the strength to persevere.

Become informed. Knowledge is a powerful tool. Keep an open mind and be flexible to changes along the way. Always ask for reasons behind suggested medical interventions, the advantages and disadvantages for mother and baby, and whether there are alternatives. Discuss these with your partner (in private if possible), so you can make your own decisions.

Are my expectations reasonable? Your partner can only labour and birth the best way she is able. Sometimes this is not the way you would prefer. Consider your own expectations. You may not want her to have pain relief, or may think this is best (perhaps because it makes your job a whole lot easier!). Be aware that this decision is out of your control.

When supporting her, try to accept how she labours and don't override her decisions, even if they don't follow your agreed birth plan. Talk to each other about your expectations and be realistic about the choices she makes. If unexpected things occur, she may feel she has failed and needs to grieve for her birth experience. It is important she knows you support her and that you are not judging her in any way. Listen and be aware of how she is feeling. Be prepared to help her and organise professional help if she wants it.

WHAT TO EXPECT FROM YOUR CAREGIVER DURING PRELABOUR

During prelabour, contact with caregivers is primarily over the phone. The caregiver usually prefers to speak with the woman (if the partner rings), to listen to her sounds and the depth of her breathing with a contraction. This gives them feedback about their intensity and the possible stage of labour. Questions they may ask include:

- Your due date; if this is your first or second baby (or more); if you're having twins or a breech baby, or have had any pregnancy complications.

- How frequent, long and intense the contractions feel.
- Whether there is any vaginal discharge or the waters have broken; if so, what colour is this?
- Whether you have felt your baby move recently.
- Whether you are eating, drinking, resting and passing urine.

Depending on what is happening, they may discuss your staying at home a bit longer, or suggest you come in for a check-up. In most cases, encouragement and reassurance is all that is needed.

Admission to the delivery suite or birth centre

You do not normally go to the hospital or birth centre during prelabour (unless your caregiver recommends this). However, some women do arrive there during this time, even though their labour has not yet started in earnest. The following is a guide to what might happen, and the level of attention you are likely to receive. Ask your caregiver or childbirth educator about the routine admission procedure, so you know what to expect.

Always ring the delivery suite or birth centre before leaving home, to make sure a room is made available and staff are prepared to provide the care you will need. This also helps confirm the stage of labour you are in. If you have a private midwife, contact her and she will contact your birthplace, or come to you for a home visit.

Coming in

If you have a long distance to travel, let the staff know so they can accommodate this, possibly by accepting you earlier than they would normally. In the event that prelabour goes on for a while, make plans to stay at a friend's or relative's home close by, or rent a hotel room.

When coming in:
- **Make the car comfortable** – Take a couple of pillows, put the baby capsule in the boot and let the woman lie or kneel on the back seat, or recline the front seat back. Take a container in case she needs to vomit, and put a towel on the car seat in case her waters break.
- **Drive carefully** – Don't speed or run red lights. An accident on the way is the last thing you need.
- **Know where to park** – Most birthplaces have an emergency drop-off that can be used for 15 minutes while you get her settled before reparking the car.

Public transport: It is possible to use public transport if you are not in strong labour, but not ideal if you are looking as though you will give birth any minute! Some taxi drivers won't transport a woman in labour, but ambulances should only be used for emergencies. (Check ambulance insurance, as this option is expensive.) Be aware that ambulance officers may only take you to the closest maternity hospital, not necessarily the one you are booked into.

RFDS: If you live in an isolated rural area, you may rely on the Royal Flying Doctor Service. Check the normal procedure with your caregiver. A few women organise moving closer to a city or town for the last couple of weeks of pregnancy, which is difficult if you have other children or cultural reasons for staying close to home. Have contingency plans for floods or bushfires which could leave you cut off from your birthplace.

On arrival

On arrival at your birthplace, your first point of contact will be the reception or admission desk, where your paperwork is issued. This is normally brief, but in an emergency you can go straight to your birthplace. On arrival at the delivery suite or birth centre, the midwife takes your paperwork and shows you to a room. This could be a temporary assessment room or the place you will eventually give birth in.

The midwife performs some routine observations to assess how your labour is proceeding and to check you and your baby. These usually consist of:

- Taking your blood pressure, temperature and pulse. Perhaps asking for a urine specimen to test (not routine in all birthplaces).
- Observing the intensity and frequency of the contractions and how you are reacting to them.
- Palpating your belly, to feel the position and engagement of your baby.
- Noting the colour and amount of any vaginal loss. (Try to wear white sanitary pads rather than coloured ones, to make this easier.)
- Checking your baby's heart rate. Some hospitals routinely perform a 20 minute CTG to continuously trace the baby's heart rate.

If you have your own obstetrician, the midwife notifies them of your arrival and the progress of your labour. It is unlikely you will see them at this stage, unless they happen to be in the hospital at the time.

Vaginal examinations

A vaginal examination is usually offered as part of your admission observations, to assess whether you are in prelabour or established labour. Although your caregiver can visually assess this, by observing your contractions and how you are reacting to them, these observations are not always reflective of the typical stage of labour – a few women appear to be in prelabour when they are in fact more advanced, and vice versa.

Not all women require routine vaginal examinations. However, most caregivers prefer to do them so they know where the woman is at in her labour. If you feel your body is giving you enough information, and there are no complications, then you may decline or ask the midwife to wait until you feel you would like one. (A vaginal examination is necessary if a decision is made to break the waters to speed up the labour.) Vaginal examinations can be encouraging if the cervix is dilating and do help some women pace their labour, but they can be very disheartening if you feel you have done a lot of work but discover you are only 1 cm dilated. So consider your possible reactions when deciding to accept or decline this procedure.

How is it done? The caregiver puts a small amount of white antiseptic cream or K-Y gel on their gloved fingers and places their first two fingers inside the vagina until they can feel the opening of the cervix. This should be done in between contractions, when you are most comfortable and relaxed.

Ideally, vaginal examinations should be limited to four hours apart, or less often than this, especially if the waters have broken. This reduces the chances of infection. They may be done more often if there are complications, or decisions need to be made about pain relief or interventions.

SHOULD I STAY OR SHOULD I GO?

When in prelabour (or very early labour), your caregiver may offer you the option to go home to see whether the pattern of contractions changes or intensifies. Alternatively, you may remain in an assessment room or be moved to the antenatal ward until labour establishes itself.

See how you feel. Some women find their established labour unfolds if they stay for an hour or two, because they are more relaxed about being in the place they intend to give birth. (If planning a homebirth, this may also occur once your midwife arrives.) Perhaps go for a walk, or have a meal out, to help pass the time. It is also normal and natural for labour to temporarily stop or slow when moving from home to your birthplace (just as animals stop labouring when moved). If your contractions felt more intense at home, then stay a while to see whether the stronger contractions return. If your labour does not change after a while, then it may be a good idea to go home, as disheartening as this can be – it may make you feel less tense.

If you stay at your birthplace, contact with caregivers will probably be minimal. Generally, they will do observations every four hours and not remain with you in between these observations. If planning a homebirth, your caregiver will visit you at home as needed (perhaps once a day), but not remain with you unless labour looks as if it is intensifying.

Your caregiver may offer interventions to bring on the established labour at some stage (called augmentation). This could be breaking the waters, or starting an intravenous Syntocinon drip (discussed in detail in Chapter 10).

Variations for prelabour

Health variations experienced during prelabour may require some medical interventions.

WATERS BREAKING, NO CONTRACTIONS

For about 13% of women, their waters break before contractions start, or only mild, prelabour cramping is felt. This is called prelabour rupture of the membranes. The waters breaking may present as:

- **A slow leak or trickle**, if the amniotic sac develops a small opening that allows fluid to trickle away, usually dribbling intermittently when you or your baby move (or with a contraction). This is common if the baby is very engaged, because it sits snugly over the cervix, plugging the opening; and it is more common for first babies.
- **A big gush of fluid**, if the bag of waters suddenly breaks. This is more common if the baby's head is not fully engaged. For example, with second or subsequent babies, posterior or breech babies.

NOTE: *If the waters come away as a trickle, it can be difficult to know whether it is amniotic fluid or urine, although amniotic fluid will continue to drain away in the coming hours. To help you know, go to the toilet and empty your bladder, then put on a pad and see if any more comes away. Also, amniotic fluid does not smell acidic like urine. It has a more alkaline aroma, smelling like almonds or semen (this can make it more difficult to tell, if you have just had intercourse). It can also feel thicker, or even slimy.*

If you think your waters have broken, contact your caregiver. Keep any pads or underwear and take them with you to the hospital or birth centre. If there are doubts as to whether your waters have broken, your caregiver may try to determine whether they have by:

- Placing a speculum into your vagina, to see whether water comes away from the cervix or pools on the speculum. Sometimes a swab test is done (with a sterile cotton bud), to check for infection.

- Using an amnicator. This is a long, orange coloured cotton bud which changes colour to navy blue if it comes in contact with alkaline amniotic fluid (like a pH indicator).

Sometimes neither of these methods can confirm whether the waters have broken and even the most experienced caregivers can find it difficult to know. If this is the case, the most common approach is to wait and see by allowing you to go home until something more happens.

If your waters have broken, what happens next will usually depend on your birthplace's policy, and your preference and your caregiver's. You may be required to go into your birthplace, and perhaps be induced within 12 to 48 hours if the labour does not start. This aims to reduce the chance of infection. Statistically, the chances of infection are slightly reduced if labour is induced within 32 hours of the waters breaking, when compared with waiting longer (expectant management).[6] However, many caregivers and birthplaces (especially birth centres) are becoming increasingly flexible, allowing women to stay at home for 12 to 24 hours, before coming in for their first check-up (if the water is not meconium stained and the baby is felt to be moving), then waiting up to 2 to 3 days (or more), with daily CTG monitoring, until labour starts (taking antibiotics if the vaginal swab test during pregnancy was positive for group B strep). Up to 80% of women spontaneously go into labour within 48 hours of the waters breaking and up to 93% by 5 to 7 days (if you wait this long). This is something you need to weigh up and discuss with your caregiver.

NOTE: Be aware that if you are given an unrealistic time frame to start labouring (6 to 12 hours), this can put enormous pressure on you to perform, making it more difficult to labour naturally. Therefore, consider going home between your check-ups.

If your waters break, you need to be aware of not introducing infection, because the membranes are no longer acting as a protective barrier for your baby. You should not have sex or swim and you should avoid baths until the strong labour starts (because you are then 'on your way'). If staying at home, check your temperature twice a day (if possible). If it is above 38°C, contact your birthplace. Rest and eat well. Garlic, ginger, vitamin C, zinc and echinacea can help boost your immune system. Check with your caregiver or practitioner.

Signs of infection can include:
- A temperature above 38°C.
- The fluid or vaginal discharge smelling offensive.
- Pain in the lower belly.

In the case of infection, antibiotics are prescribed and the labour is induced, with the baby's heart rate being continuously monitored with a CTG machine until the birth. Sometimes it is hard to know whether the infection developed after the waters broke or whether the waters broke because an infection of the amniotic sac weakened the membrane.

If the waters are meconium stained, having a yellow, green or brown discolouration, contact the delivery suite or birth centre straightaway and prepare to go in. Meconium is the first bowel motion your baby passes and meconium-stained waters may indicate your baby is distressed or has been stressed at some time previously. If the discolouration is faint, it may not be of great concern, but if it is heavy (a pea soup consistency), it can be more serious. Keep any tissues, underwear or sanitary pads with fluid on them to show your caregiver.

Generally the baby's heart rate is continuously monitored with a CTG machine and the labour is induced. If you are booked into a birth centre, or planning a homebirth, thick meconium staining usually requires you to be transferred to the hospital delivery suite.

Dehydration and ketosis

If you become dehydrated, ketosis may occur. This is when the body breaks down fat stores for energy, causing an abnormal accumulation of ketone bodies in the blood, body tissues and urine. Excessive ketosis can cause:
- A mild fever, fast pulse and lowered blood pressure.
- Weakness and reduced muscle function.
- A slowing or stopping of contractions, or making them irregular and ineffective.

A quick dipstick urine test will show whether ketones are present.

Interventions include rehydration with an intravenous drip and possibly augmenting the labour by breaking the waters and/or adding another drip with Syntocinon to speed up, strengthen and coordinate the contractions.

NOTE: If you are planning to have your baby in a birth centre or at home, you may try to drink plenty of sports drinks to reverse the dehydration and use natural therapies (acupressure, acupuncture, herbs, homeopathy or nipple stimulation) to stimulate contractions and so avoid transfer to the delivery suite for a drip.

CHAPTER 6

First stage of labour

The first stage of labour starts when active labour begins, and ends when the cervix is fully open (10 cm dilated). Each contraction makes the uterus tilt forward and downwards, helping your baby's head place pressure on the cervix to open. Contractions also make the uterine muscles retract, so the womb becomes smaller and pushes your baby down in readiness for the birthing phase. Strong contractions flex the baby's head, bringing their chin to rest on their chest, so the crown of their head, which presents the smallest circumference of their skull, leads the way.

The first stage of labour is divided into three different phases, although not every woman distinctly shows signs of all three. These are:

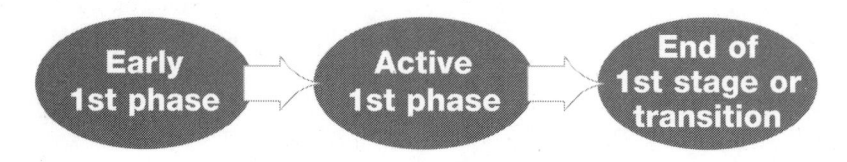

Early 1st phase → Active 1st phase → End of 1st stage or transition

EARLY FIRST PHASE

The cervix is very thin and opens (dilates) to about 3 to 4 cm.

Once a woman appears to be in the early phase of first stage, the caregiver records this as the starting time of labour.

If this is your **first baby**, you usually spend this stage at home, letting your caregiver or hospital know you have started. Contact support people when you need to, giving them time to make any arrangements to be with you.

If this is your **second or subsequent baby**, you will probably need to organise your other child(ren) and contact your caregiver to move to your birthplace soon, before the contractions become too painful.

Contractions

Contractions during early first phase can present in a wide range of strengths and patterns. They may:

- Become more definite pains that build up to a peak and then fade away being 3 to 7 minutes apart, lasting 40 to 60 seconds.
- Be mild (or painful) and irregular, then become more regular, lasting longer and coming more frequently.
- Be strong from the very beginning, or stronger once the waters break.
- Not eventuate – that is, prelabour stops! This is not uncommon and it could be hours or days before labour returns. Rest, sleep, eat and drink. If the house is full of visitors, maybe it is time for them to leave. A watched kettle never boils!

NOTE: To time contractions you will need a clock with a second hand and a labouring woman! Time the contractions from the beginning of one contraction to the beginning of the next one. For example, if a contraction starts at 6 pm, and lasts for 60 seconds, and the next one starts at 6.05 pm, they are 5 minutes apart (not 4 minutes apart).

Emotions

As **the woman** you may feel:

- Excited.
- Nervous.
- Tired.
- Worried, anxious or confused.
- Relaxed and simply dealing with one contraction at a time.

As **the partner or support person** you may feel:

- Excited.
- Relieved and relaxed.
- Worried, about how she (or you) will cope with the labour ahead.
- Tired, if the prelabour was very long.
- Nervous and thinking you should be at the hospital by now.
- You didn't really notice an early phase.

ACTIVE FIRST PHASE

The cervix opens from 3 to 4 cm to around 7 to 8 cm.

As the cervix dilates, labour changes again, moving into what caregivers call strong established labour or active labour. The woman's body is working very hard now. Remember, the contractions need to be strong and close together to bring your baby down to be born.

Contractions

The contractions of active first phase usually step up, becoming stronger and closer together, possibly lasting longer, or staying similar to early first phase contractions but more intense. They may:
- Come every 2, 3 or 4 minutes and last 45 to 70 seconds.
- Be mixed, with every second contraction feeling strong and milder ones in between.
- Be very painful, demanding the woman's full attention, so she is unable to talk during each contraction.
- Stop, or slow down for a period, when you move from home to your birthplace.

If this is your **first baby**, contact the hospital or birth centre now. Let them know the frequency and length of the contractions. This is usually the time you would consider moving to your birthplace, or calling your midwife to come for a homebirth.

If this is your **second or subsequent baby**, you should already be at your birthplace. If not, get there as soon as possible.

Emotions

A woman's focus naturally turns inward and she becomes less aware of what is happening around her.

As **the woman** you may feel:
- Restless and wanting to be at your birthplace (if not already there).
- Tired.
- Centred and focused.
- Frustrated that the labour is taking so long.
- Overwhelmed with pain and/or fatigue.
- Confused or disappointed, because you thought your labour would be different.
- Positive about what is happening.
- Calm and accepting.
- Concerned about what may lie ahead.

As **the partner or support person** you may feel:
- Relieved that you have arrived at your birthplace.
- Excited that labour is progressing well.
- Vulnerable and unsure.

- Shocked, unprepared for the intensity of active labour.
- Frustrated with caregivers if they are not communicating with you.
- Torn between wanting to take the pain away from her but knowing her labour is necessary.
- Uncomfortable with the sounds she is making.
- Tired and/or hungry.
- Proud of her.

END OF FIRST STAGE OR TRANSITION

The cervix opens from 7 to 8 cm to 10 cm (fully dilated).

Transition precedes the pushing phase (or second stage) of labour and normally generates definite changes in the labour's pattern and/or the woman's behaviour (whether this is her first or subsequent baby). If she has had pain relief (such as an epidural), this can mask many of these typical signs. Transition may be brief (one to two contractions) or last up to an hour or more. Some women don't notice a definite transition.

Contractions

Contractions during transition often step up in intensity again. However, the woman's body releases endorphins to help her cope. Contractions may:
- Be 1 to 3 minutes apart, lasting 50 to 70 seconds.
- Have little or no rest in between them.
- Feel like one continuous contraction.
- Bring an occasional urge to push during some (or all) contractions.

Transition is a challenging phase for most women. At times it can take immense effort to change positions, or even talk. The woman's support team become crucial at this point. Many caregivers view transition as the hardest time of the labour, but some women find it motivating because they feel they are getting close.

Emotions

The woman can appear lost, unaware or unresponsive. People around her can find her hard to reach, because she is absorbed in her own world. It may seem she is no longer aware of her surroundings (or no longer cares what is happening), but often she is acutely aware of everything, just unable to respond to it. Many women speak of having endless thoughts running through their minds at this time, but not verbally expressing them.

As **the woman** you may feel:
- Irritable, you've had enough and want to go home.
- Frightened, wondering how much longer it will take.
- Angry or snappy, not wanting anyone to touch you or talk to you.
- Out of control.
- Considering pain relief.
- Very tired, wanting to sleep.
- Restless, needing to move or wriggle, unable to get comfortable in any position.
- Lost and disorientated.
- Like you don't want to continue.
- Upset, because you wanted a natural birth and feel you can't do it, or medical interventions are needed, or you wanted drugs but others aren't listening to you or are telling you it is too late to have them.

As **the partner or support person** you may feel:
- Excited, because you know she has progressed.
- Overwhelmed by her reactions and noises.
- Frightened by the sheer intensity of her labour.
- Confused by her irrational and conflicting demands.
- Worried, out of your depth, wondering if what she is doing is normal.
- Calm and accepting.
- Helpless.
- Embarrassed or shocked by her behaviour.
- Upset if you'd planned a natural birth and she wants pain relief, or needs medical interventions, or is unable to have pain relief.
- Relieved that it is her and not you!

Transition is a demanding time, with partners and support people often bearing the brunt of the woman's demands and grievances. Some partners are shocked when their polite, mild-mannered lover starts tearing all their clothes off, screaming profanities, even hitting or kicking. The following are some exclamations from many labouring women in transition:
- 'Your breath smells, I can smell cigarettes, I'm going to be sick!'
- 'Don't leave me. No, you can't go to the toilet!'
- 'Look what you've done to me! I never want you to touch me again!'
- 'I can't stand it. I want a caesarean/an episiotomy/a gun!' (Hopefully no one will meet any of these requests unnecessarily!)

- 'I'm cold. No, get that blanket off. Turn the fan on. The heat pack's not hot enough. I'm shaking.'
- 'Don't tell me what I need!'
- 'What would *you* know? Have you ever had a baby?'
- 'I don't care what the birth plan says!'

Like the noises of labour, these exclamations are usually forms of release and most women describe it as just needing to whinge, and perhaps feel a little embarrassed after the birth. Don't worry about what your caregiver thinks. They take these comments with a grain of salt. This is what labouring women do.

If, as the pregnant woman, you are concerned about what your partner or support person's reactions will be, discuss this during the pregnancy and prepare yourselves for this possibly awkward time. You may even need to rethink your choice of support people, if you feel this is going to be a problem, or negotiate for them to leave for a while. If you are worried about losing it, try to accept that it may be a necessity for you to progress well and give birth to your baby. Trying to remain nice and polite can slow the labour.

Physical signs

Some physical signs associated with the different phases of the first stage can include:

- **Waters breaking** – Also referred to as the membranes rupturing, this can happen at any time during the labour process, even just as the baby is being born. If they have not broken during prelabour, they are more likely to during the first stage for about 75% of women.
- **Pink or bloodstained vaginal loss** – This happens as the cervix opens and bleeds a little. If the waters have broken, it is diluted with amniotic fluid, making it look pink. Blood can also be mixed with a mucus show and may slightly increase after the caregiver performs an internal vaginal examination.

The amount of blood loss can be light, or like a normal menstrual period. During transition, a moderate trickle of fresh, bright blood often comes away, perhaps mixed with the show. This is a classic sign of the cervix reaching full dilation, before the pushing starts. A few women have a bloodless labour, losing nothing until the baby is born and the placenta separates.

Moving from the dilating phase of the first stage to the pushing phase of the second stage brings some dramatic physical changes unique to transition. You are possibly feeling:

- Exhausted, as the body releases endorphins.

- Hot and cold at different times.
- Involuntarily shaking.
- Nausea and/or vomiting.
- Pressure in the bowel and/or an overwhelming feeling to open the bowels.
- The need to release sounds (groan or yell) and breathe more heavily.

Support strategies

Women differ in the support they require. This can range from lots of massage and touch, to just verbal support or nothing but your silent presence. Often it's a combination of these, changing as the labour progresses. Keep in mind support strategies described in Chapter 5 for prelabour and Chapter 9 for pain relief, as well as the following.

A safe and private environment
Labouring and giving birth is a very intimate and private process. This does not mean being alone, but it does mean feeling comfortable with those around you and having as few strangers as possible present. Allow only necessary staff in the room: an audience can inhibit labour. If all is going normally, you should only need one midwife, with possibly a student midwife (a registered nurse doing her midwifery training). When the birth is imminent, then your doctor (if you have one) will also be present. Other staff may need to enter, depending on the circumstances, but ideally, the fewer the better. Trust your instincts and request more privacy if you need it.

Think about the type of atmosphere you would like to create for your baby's arrival. Depending on your chosen birthplace, you may:
- Dim the lights.
- Use fans or heaters to maintain a comfortable temperature.
- Burn selected aromatherapy oils (electric burners only).
- Play music and keep noise and conversation to a minimum.
- Bring personal effects (eg. photos, your own pillow).
- Wear your own clothes, rather than a hospital gown.
- Ask staff to place mats on the floor and provide beanbags. Arrange them so you feel comfortable.

Food and fluids
Your body needs food and fluids for energy during labour to prevent dehydration and ketosis. Some hospitals still restrict women from eating (and

even drinking) during labour, in case a general anaesthetic is required. This is aimed at preventing a rare complication called aspiration (breathing in stomach contents). Restricting eating and drinking is controversial, and you may wish to negotiate this with your caregiver. As a guide:

- There is no evidence that restricting food and fluids during labour actually protects against aspiration.[1]
- The main reason aspiration occurs is because of a failure to apply proper anesthetic techniques. Trying to reduce stomach contents does not make a difference if the anaesthetic technique is inadequate.[2]
- The risk of aspiration is related to a general anaesthetic, which is not commonly used in childbirth because of the widespread use of epidurals and spinals.
- Having intravenous fluids, in place of eating and drinking, may create chemical and fluid imbalances in the woman's blood, causing problems for mother and baby.[3]
- Medications to reduce stomach acidity do not prevent aspiration, or reduce its severity.[4]

It is generally recommended that women eat and drink as desired. Most women find that as their labour progresses, their appetite wanes anyway; they generally rely on sips of fluids, or sucking on ice chips or lollies. This is something your partner/support person will need to remind you to do.

Support strategies for the woman
Movement and positions

Moving and changing positions helps enormously and can greatly assist the labour's progress, as well as help you deal more effectively with the pain. Using movement during labour is explored in Chapter 9. Women often forget to change positions, so support people or caregivers may need to suggest this occasionally. However, if you feel relatively comfortable, stay where you are. Positions for birth are shown in Chapter 7.

Resting between contractions

As the labour intensifies, your body releases endorphins, making you feel tired. It is important to rest and relax to gather your strength in between contractions, possibly dozing for two to four minutes.

Part of resting is releasing tension. Most women tense their muscles during labour. Your support person may need to do a body check exercise, in which they guide you to relax, perhaps saying 'Soften your hands' or 'Let all your muscles flop.' Many people habitually use the word 'relax', but often women feel they can't relax because labour is not relaxing, but they can 'let go', 'release' or 'come down'. It requires a lot of energy to tighten and flex muscles, energy that is needed elsewhere during your labour.

A bath

The bath can provide privacy, pain relief, buoyancy and help you change positions. It can lower your blood pressure slightly and relieve anxiety. Baths tend to speed up labour, especially if used during the active and transitional phases of the first stage, but it may slow contractions if used during prelabour or early first stage. Try leaving the bath until labour is strong and established. Some women don't like being in the bath for too long, while others stay in for hours. Using water as a natural method for pain relief is further explored in Chapter 9.

Letting go of time

It is common to become frustrated or overwhelmed if labour goes for longer than expected. You can't control labour, and neither can anyone else. No one knows how long your labour will be. It is important to be patient and not aim for a specific time frame. The intensity of labour does ebb and flow, so don't panic if you feel you aren't coping at 3 to 4 cm dilation, because this doesn't mean you won't cope at 8 to 9 cm. Some contractions feel unbearably intense, but the few that follow may be more tolerable. Try to stay with the here and now and not focus on how it may be in a couple of hours time. Take one contraction at a time. Cover up the clocks, take your watch off and let go of time.

Working with the labour you are having

Labour will always be different from your expectations. It helps to think 'Whatever will be, will be', rather than struggle to have things go the way you intend. At some stage you will need to come to terms with how your labour actually *is* and begin working with it, rather than against it. If you approach your labour with an open mind, this can make the birth easier to accept, whatever that outcome may be.

SUPPORT STRATEGIES FOR THE PARTNER/SUPPORT PERSON

As the woman moves into established labour, you will need to be sensitive to her needs. Trust your instincts and be guided by her.

Close physical contact
Close contact can make her feel safe. Have your hand available to squeeze during a contraction. Tie her hair off her face, if she is happy to have this done. Obtain eye contact if you feel she is looking lost or overwhelmed. Communicate and encourage her, unless told to stop. Kiss her, tell her you love her and how proud you are of her. Wipe her brow, and stroke her arm. These simple gestures are often enough to motivate her to persevere.

Some women don't like people being close, finding it claustrophobic. This does not mean she wants you out of the room. It may be that she does not want you to do or say anything in particular, just to be there for her and to listen.

Breathing with her
Most women breathe the way they need to when dealing with contractions. However, if they are very intense (or she is hyperventilating), your assistance may be needed to help her breathe more deeply. Make yourself familiar with 'Breathing and birth noises' in Chapter 9, so you can support and guide your partner effectively.

Communication
Communicate with her throughout the labour. Listen to her and support her choices. Be open to your plans changing as the labour unfolds. Liaise with your caregiver(s), as needed. Let staff know if you have particular needs that are important to you both. If decisions need to be made, communicate with (and for) your partner to assist joint decision-making.

Many partners and support people feel they need to take on the role of negotiator, especially if things are not going to plan and intervention is required. This can sometimes feel disempowering, because you are relying on information and recommendations from professional caregivers. Most partners instinctively want to protect the woman and feel distressed if they are unable to. If you don't have enough information, or don't understand, ask the caregiver to explain fully, in simple terms. Sometimes a caregiver's suggestions are welcome, and if it is an emergency situation, you generally won't have an opportunity to negotiate. Just trust in your caregiver's actions and judgments.

Staying calm
If you start feeling anxious or nervous, take a short breather, perhaps debriefing with the caregiver, or try some deep breathing to ground yourself. Your uneasiness can be sensed by your partner and may distract her.

Avoid unnecessary conflict with staff and other support people if possible.

If conflict does arise, deal with it and defuse it – it is not worth disturbing her rhythm.

If things start getting out of your control, with regards to emergency medical interventions, stay close to her, speak with her and talk her through it. You may be nervous but she will probably be feeling worse. She needs you to be stable through this. Try to hold it together until the crisis has subsided. Ask your caregivers to explain what is happening. You may need to debrief with staff after things have calmed down.

Being sensitive to her needs

She now needs you to be there for her unequivocally. Your own pressures, tiredness, aches, pains or illnesses need to take a back seat. If you really are unwell and not up to the job, consider calling an extra support person to help support you.

Remind her that there is purpose in the pain. Let her express her pain by moaning, complaining and whinging. She is not necessarily asking for help, or pain relief to fix it; she usually just needs someone to listen. Reassurances and words of encouragement can be 'That's good', 'Keep breathing' or 'This one is nearly finished.' One golden rule is: **Don't talk during a contraction**. Leave conversation for when the pain has gone. Avoid idle chat with her caregiver or others. Many women say how annoying and distracting this can be.

Expectations for care

Once you are in established labour, you need to be in your birthplace. If:
- You are already at the hospital, you may be moved to a labour and birth room.
- You are planning a homebirth, your caregiver should be with you now.
- Your primary caregiver is an obstetrician, the midwife will notify them of your arrival and progress. They will come when the birth appears imminent (or if complications arise).

WHAT TO EXPECT FROM YOUR CAREGIVER

Routine observations of you and your baby become more frequent in active first stage, usually involving:
- Listening to your baby's heart rate every half an hour (possibly with a CTG if you are in the delivery suite).

- Checking the amount and colour of any vaginal loss and observing the frequency and intensity of the contractions every half-hour.
- Taking your blood pressure, pulse and temperature every two to four hours (more often if you have high blood pressure or a fever).
- Possibly checking dilation of the cervix with a vaginal examination every four hours (if you want this).

Some caregivers ask you to provide a specimen of urine to test. You may also be offered pain relief (natural and/or medical). In birth centres and during a homebirth the caregiver does not generally suggest medical forms of pain relief unless the woman asks first.

An experienced and intuitive caregiver allows the woman space to labour as she needs to, sensing when to come and go, when to guide her and when to simply observe. Sometimes your caregiver will look to you for guidance if they are unsure how you are coping. A woman needs time to adjust and work with the rhythm of her labour. This rhythm can be very fragile and easily lost, especially if the caregiver feels they need to control the labour instead of tuning in to the woman's rhythm.

If you feel your caregiver is offering you things you are not ready for, and you and the baby are well, let them know you will ask for them when needed or for advice if you are not coping. This can communicate your need for more space, although sometimes you need to ask for this directly.

Continuous monitoring

Your baby's heart rate may be continuously monitored during labour using a cardiotocograph machine or CTG (also called electronic fetal monitoring or EFM). The baby's heart rate is recorded on a piece of paper (a trace). Continuous monitoring is used any time there are health concerns for the woman and/or her baby. However, many hospitals routinely perform a 20 to 30 minute trace for all women on arrival at the delivery suite.

Continuous monitoring of the baby's heart rate can be done:
- **Externally** – Leads from the machine are strapped to the woman's belly. One lead records the baby's heart rate in beats per minute (bpm) and the other detects contractions.
- **Internally** – With a wire placed inside the woman's vagina, a circular needle is gently rotated into the baby's skin (called a fetal scalp clip or electrode). The wire leads to a small conducting device (about the size of a matchbox), which is strapped to the woman's thigh, then on to the CTG machine. Internal monitoring is suggested if the caregiver feels the baby will need to be continuously monitored until birth because

there are health concerns. The waters need to be broken to perform internal monitoring.

NOTE: *Piercing the baby's skin may lead to an infection at the site of the piercing. Women who carry herpes, hepatitis B or C, or HIV/AIDS viruses are generally not given internal monitoring because it can increase their baby's chances of becoming infected with these viruses.*

Both monitoring methods produce readouts on the machine, as well as a printed record on a strip of paper. The caregiver interprets the pattern of the baby's heart rate in relation to the contractions to help make judgments about the wellbeing of the baby and decide whether interventions may be needed. Caregivers look for patterns in the trace, these being:

- **Variability** – how the heart rate fluctuates.
- **Reactivity** – how the heart rate 'reacts' to the baby moving, or to a contraction.
- **Decelerations** – if the heart rate slows or dips.

If you are being monitored, ask your caregiver to explain your baby's trace in more detail.

NOTE: *Sometimes the machine can inaccurately record the baby's heart rate, especially if the mother (or baby) moves. The external lead may need to be manually adjusted (a few times). However, if this continues, your caregiver may suggest internal monitoring. Many women prefer not to accept internal monitoring unless their baby is considered quite distressed. Try getting your partner or support person to hold the lead in place and adjust it accordingly. Ask your caregiver to show you how to do this.*

Continuous monitoring was adopted long before any research was done to evaluate its effectiveness. While it remains widely used in Australia (up to 75% of women have it), extensive research has not been able to prove any real benefits for babies, compared to babies who are monitored intermittently in normal labours.[5] (Intermittent monitoring is when the heart rate is listened to straight after a contraction, every half an hour in the first stage of labour and every 5 to 10 minutes during second stage.) The main issues surrounding continuous monitoring include:

- Experienced caregivers frequently disagreeing about the meaning of a trace (agreeing on only 42% of traces).[6]
- Readings tending to be biased towards the baby having a problem when one does not exist.[7]
- Studies showing CTGs don't save the lives of babies or prevent cerebral palsy.
- Overusing monitoring for women experiencing a normal labour sometimes leading to unnecessary caesareans and forceps.

Despite this evidence, the reality is that nearly all caregivers rely heavily on this technology, possibly aiming to avoid litigation. If you feel this is fair and can accept the inaccuracies of CTGs (and the possible increase in unnecessary interventions), then having your baby monitored may not be an issue. However, if you prefer to avoid unnecessary monitoring and interventions, you may negotiate its use and possibly decline it.

If a routine 20 minute CTG indicates a possible problem and continuous monitoring is being suggested for the rest of the labour, you may request a compromise of having a 20 minute trace every hour or so (instead of the monitor on for the whole labour). However, if there are complications (such as heavy meconium-stained amniotic fluid), then continuous monitoring is probably a reasonable intervention.

Many women dislike continuous monitoring because it restricts their movement, potentially increasing their need for pain relief. It also rules out the options of using the bath or shower. A common complaint is that it also reduces personal attention, with caregivers and support people paying more attention to the monitor than the woman. However, a few women like monitoring and find the continual sound of their baby's heartbeat very reassuring.

A recent development in continuous monitoring is fetal electrocardiographic (ECG) waveform, which measures the electrical impulse in the baby's heart muscles (similar to ECG machines used to monitor adults). ECG waveform uses a scalp clip attached to the baby's head (as with internal monitoring), but it is easier to interpret than a CTG, reducing the chances of conflicting interpretations between caregivers and unnecessary interventions. At present this technology is not widely available, but it is recommended for use (if available) when an external CTG indicates the baby may be not coping with labour.[8]

Variations for the first stage

Sometimes the first stage of labour varies from the norm. Having some knowledge of these possibilities can prepare you and help you make informed decisions if they eventuate.

Continual vomiting
It is normal to vomit at some point during labour, but a few women vomit continually, possibly leading to exhaustion, dehydration and ketosis. Continual

vomiting can be uncomfortable, frustrating and demoralising, having a direct impact on how you cope with your labour.

Continually vomiting can be caused by medications given during labour, but it has also been linked with women who have experienced eating disorders in the past (anorexia or bulimia).[9] Sometimes it is connected with anxieties about the labour and birth, and sometimes it just happens for no obvious reason.

Many caregivers suggest anti-emetic medications to relieve nausea and vomiting and prevent dehydration. These are usually given as an injection, but may be given as a suppository. (Tablets can be vomited up.) The types of anti-emetics used can vary, having different effects and side effects. Discuss these with your caregiver.

Some women try natural therapies such as:

- **Acupressure** to the wrist point (see acupressure appendix). Firm pressure is placed on the point until the woman feels relief. This may take up to five minutes. Pressure can be repeated when necessary, to one or both wrists. Wristbands for seasickness (or morning sickness) can be worn. These can be purchased from chemists.
- **Homeopathic remedies** such as Ipecacuanna, Nux vomica, Sepia or Pulsatilla. Read the directions provided by your practitioner, as remedies often depend on how you are feeling emotionally.
- **Working through it**, as the vomiting may be reflective of unresolved fears and concerns. If you can identify and acknowledge these, and work through them before labour, this is ideal. Consider sharing with your partner and/or caregiver to help them provide you with some emotional reassurance and support during labour.

Fever

A fever above 38°C during labour may indicate an infection. Other signs can include a rapid pulse (over 100 beats per minute) and the unborn baby having a rapid heart rate (above 170 beats per minute). Infections during labour are normally of the uterus, but could be related to:

- The waters being broken for a prolonged period of time (24 to 36 hours or more), and/or having several internal vaginal examinations if the labour is prolonged.
- A urine infection.
- An illness, such as the flu or a viral infection.

Be aware that having an epidural for more than four or five hours can lead to a fever that is not related to an infection but which may still be treated with antibiotics just in case.

NOTE: *The hard work of labour naturally increases a woman's temperature slightly, even more so if she is dehydrated. Extra fluids and cool face washers may be all that is needed.*

> **Did you know?**
> In the past, hospital rooms were tiled; caregivers 'scrubbed up' and wore surgical gowns, caps and masks; and the women's legs were draped with sterile sheeting, so only her vagina was visible, and her vulva was routinely shaved and washed down with antiseptic solution. Birth is not a sterile event and there is no evidence that any of these procedures prevents infection. Although caregivers still wear masks, gowns and plastic glasses, it is to protect themselves from blood splashes, rather than to protect the woman or her baby from infection.

A fever does not usually affect labour. However, if the temperature is high, the baby may become distressed, which can have short-term effects on their health, such as having less muscle tone or requiring oxygen and resuscitation at birth, possibly needing transfer to the intensive care nursery. If the woman's uterus and amniotic fluid are infected, the baby can be quite unwell, with breathing difficulties due to pneumonia. In some cases this can be life-threatening for them. The main concern for the woman is an infection of her uterus after the birth.

Antibiotics are normally prescribed intravenously during labour. Swab tests of the woman's vagina may also be taken. Continuous monitoring of the baby's heart rate with a CTG machine is often recommended. After the birth, the baby's temperature, colour and breathing are checked every few hours for 24 to 48 hours. Caregivers also check the baby's feeding and how alert they are.

Some hospitals routinely take swab tests of the baby's skin and perform a 'septic work-up' in the belief that infected babies can become ill quite quickly and it can be hard to predict which babies will do this. However, this subjects a large number of babies to unnecessary tests, antibiotics and separation from their mother, just in case. Unnecessary antibiotics can lower a newborn's resistance to other infections; besides, it will not be clear that an infection actually caused the woman's fever until tests results are available one to two days later. It can be hard to know what to do in this situation. Many parents are happy to take every precaution, but some are angry if all the tests come back clear. A few parents decline the septic work-up unless their baby is showing signs of becoming unwell. Discuss this with your caregiver.

Difficulty urinating

It is possible to have difficulty urinating during labour, usually if the baby's head puts pressure on the urethra, closing off the exit of urine, or an epidural reduces feeling in the area. An overfull bladder can cause constant pain or tenderness around the lower belly felt in between the contractions, and can, in some cases, literally stop the baby from descending down the birth canal and inhibit effective contractions.

Try emptying your bladder every two to three hours. Your partner, support person and caregiver should occasionally remind you to do this. If you are having difficulty urinating, try:

- Having a drink of water; turning a tap on.
- Visualising a waterfall or running water.
- Getting into the shower or bath to urinate (if you don't have an epidural).
- Having your partner or caregiver gently trickle a small amount of cool water down your lower back.

If the previous methods fail to help, your caregiver will need to insert a catheter to empty the bladder. Depending on the hospital's policy, or your caregiver's preferences, this may be a short tube inserted into the bladder until it is emptied and then removed (an in-and-out catheter), or a longer tube which is left in and drains into a bag (an indwelling catheter).

Leaving the catheter in may be embarrassing or inhibiting if you are trying to have an active birth. However, the in-and-out catheter may need to be repeated, increasing your chances of developing a urine infection. (Catheters can be inserted in birth centres or for a homebirth. Caregivers tend to use the in-and-out type.)

One controversial aspect is whether to leave a catheter in the bladder during the pushing phase. Some argue that the tube may injure the bladder and urethra. Others believe it is better to have an empty bladder to decrease the chances of the woman bleeding after the birth (which is more likely with a full bladder) and negate the need to reinsert it if forceps or a ventouse is needed. You may wish to exercise your choice in this respect.

Posterior labour

A few babies start labour in a posterior position, with their back against the woman's back. This is a variation of normal, not a complication. About 90% of posterior babies turn to an anterior position during labour, and the remaining 10% come down the birth canal, still in the posterior position, and are born looking up at their mother's belly (instead of looking down towards her bottom).

Posterior labours increase the chance of:
- A longer prelabour and first stage.
- More back pain, rather than pain at the front.
- The baby's head being deflexed rather than flexed, meaning their head may take longer to fully engage.
- A longer pushing phase if the baby's head hasn't fully rotated by second stage.

However, none of this is guaranteed. Most babies do turn and posterior labours can progress just as efficiently as anterior labours, especially if the woman has good contractions. It helps to use active birth positions and maintain a positive attitude.

Some caregivers pre-empt problems with posterior babies, assuming the labour will be long and difficult. Unfortunately, women who are told that their babies are posterior start receiving negative messages, which may reduce their confidence, making them anxious and pessimistic about labour and/or accepting of interventions earlier than needed, possibly even before labour begins! Anxiety about labour can release adrenaline, inhibiting the contractions and distressing the baby, turning these negative predictions into a self-fulfilling prophecy.

It appears that the incidence of posterior babies is increasing because we now lead more sedentary lifestyles. However, even very active women have posterior babies. Strategies which may help include:

- **Encouraging your baby to turn to an anterior position** – Practise for this by using pelvic rocking or crawling on your hands and knees for 10 minutes twice a day. Alternatively, you can hire or buy pelvic rocker chairs. Research has shown that these interventions can have a temporary effect on the baby's position but are not guaranteed of success.[10]

  You can also try sleeping on the opposite side your baby is lying on (for example, the left side if they are right posterior) and swimming freestyle, or with a kickboard, during late pregnancy.

- **Natural therapies** – These can include the homeopathic remedy Pulsatilla for the final weeks of pregnancy and/or acupuncture or acupressure to the toe points and/or lower spine point (see acupressure appendix), applying firm pressure during the contractions.

  During labour try:
  - Kneeling or leaning forward on all fours.
  - Sitting on the toilet or birth stool towards the end of the first stage to help the pelvic floor muscles let go and give your baby more room to rotate and move down.

- The 'double hip squeeze' during contractions when pushing. The support person or caregiver places their hands firmly on both of the woman's hipbones (from behind), pressing them firmly in towards her waist, aiming to flare the pelvis slightly and allow the baby more room to move down and around to an anterior position.
- Using heat packs or pressured massage on the lower back for pain relief. Occasionally deep-heat sports rubs or a compress with black pepper aromatherapy oil helps.
- **Dealing with the labour you have** – Try to stay positive. This is just an individual difference. Other women are faced with different challenges. Your body is designed to give birth. Have faith in this.
- **Pain relief** – If the labour is prolonged and tiring, you may wish to consider medical forms of pain relief, such as epidural. However, be aware that epidurals relax the pelvic floor muscles and discourage the baby from turning, possibly prolonging the second stage of labour and increasing the chances of needing a forceps or ventouse delivery.

SLOW PROGRESS

Time limits on labour are increasingly becoming an issue. Where once an 18 hour labour was considered normal, it is now more like 12 to 15 hours. Once labour becomes established, caregivers tend to focus on how quickly the woman is progressing.

The medical definition of 'reasonable progress' for first babies is if the cervix dilates at about 1 cm per hour (or dilates to some degree every 4 hours). With second or subsequent babies, progress is expected more quickly. However, the World Health Organisation recommends this as a guide only, to evaluate the labour not necessarily to intervene in it.[11]

Different hospitals and caregivers have their own interpretation of what constitutes a slow labour, some are flexible in accommodating individual differences, such as natural lulls in the contractions, but many caregivers want to intervene once the labour deviates from the textbook norm. Few women get to birth in their own time. The labour is often hastened by breaking the waters, or using a Syntocinon drip, and if not enough time is allowed for these methods to work, a caesarean is performed. Consider discussing these issues with your caregiver during pregnancy. When in labour and negotiating these interventions remember that if you and your baby are well, time is on your side.

BABY DISTRESSED

Sometimes an unborn baby shows signs they may not be coping with the labour (called 'fetal distress'). This can be an abnormally high or low heartbeat or meconium-stained amniotic fluid. The most common reason for fetal distress is the baby not receiving enough oxygen because there is inadequate blood flow through the placenta and cord. This can be caused by one of the following:

- The placenta not functioning well due to health conditions such as high blood pressure.
- Overstimulation of the uterus due to induction or augmentation medications.
- A sharp drop in the woman's blood pressure due to an epidural, spinal block, heavy bleeding or lying for a prolonged period flat on her back during labour.
- Cord compression, a cord prolapse, or the cord being wrapped several times around the baby's neck and/or body.
- Placental abruption.
- Identical twins sharing a single placenta (twin-to-twin transfusion).
- The mother or baby being unwell due to pre-existing health conditions or a pregnancy complication.

If fetal distress is suspected, the caregiver usually monitors the baby's heart rate with a CTG machine. If it appears the baby may be severely distressed, a fetal blood sample is performed. A sample of blood is taken from the baby's scalp (through a vaginal examination for the woman) and is tested for oxygen, carbon dioxide and chemistry levels to determine whether the baby is in fact distressed. Fetal blood sampling can reduce unnecessary caesareans caused by a misinterpretation of the CTG trace. However, not all birthplaces offer this fetal blood sampling. As an alternative, some caregivers try stimulating the baby's scalp with their fingers during an internal vaginal examination, to see whether this produces a rise in the baby's heart rate (a good sign). Though less scientific, this has been shown to be somewhat effective if fetal blood sampling is not available.

If the baby is believed to be distressed, the woman is given oxygen, and if she is hooked up to a Syntocinon drip, it is turned down or off. If the baby does not improve, and the cervix is not fully open, a caesarean is performed.

Fetal distress is usually unavoidable, but there are some things you may want to try to help prevent (or reduce) the chances of it happening. These include:

- **A change of position** since, when lying on your back, blood supply can be reduced to your baby through vena-caval compression. Moving

off your back onto your side, or into a forward-leaning position (if you are able to), may help.
- **Avoiding interventions** including induction, augmentation and epidurals, unless absolutely necessary.
- **Looking after yourself** by eating well, resting, reducing stress and working through any emotional issues before the birth. Remaining relaxed in labour can help keep your adrenaline levels low and possibly reduce the chances of your baby becoming distressed.

ANTERIOR LIP

Most women move smoothly from the first to the second stage of labour. However, occasionally when the cervix is nearly fully dilated the top (or front) of it swells. This is called an anterior lip and it can happen because:
- The cervix is being pinched between the baby's head and the woman's pubic bone.
- The woman has been in one position for a long time, causing uneven pressure on her cervix from the baby's head.
- The baby has been in a posterior position with their head slightly deflexed, causing uneven pressure.

An anterior lip is often accompanied by an early urge to push, before the woman's body is completely ready. Her pushing efforts often sound less forceful or inconsistent and there may be some slightly heavier vaginal bleeding. Pushing with an anterior lip can increase swelling, slow progress and possibly lead to exhaustion and frustration; the baby may even become distressed if it persists.

NOTE: An anterior lip mostly occurs with first babies and is very unusual with subsequent babies.

Caregiver recommendations may include:
- **Resisting the urge to push** – This is easier said than done!
- **Changing positions** – Perhaps try moving onto your hands and knees with your bottom raised and head down. Being in a bath can also help as it removes the gravitational pull on the baby.
- **Having some gas** – This should relax you and possibly reduce the urge to push. An epidural can also do this, but you may want to avoid having one at this late stage.
- **Pushing the cervix back** – The caregiver may try to manually ease the swollen cervix over the baby's head during a contraction, using their fingers during a vaginal examination. This can fix the problem quite rapidly but may be painful if you are not using medical pain relief. Gas can help.

If you have an anterior lip, resisting the urge to push can be difficult of course, taking immense focus to go against the natural urge of your body. However, you can try:
- Blowing out (imagine blowing out a candle), panting, yelling or groaning during the contraction.
- Taking homeopathic remedies. Check your labour kit.
- Pressing on certain acupressure points. The buttock and/or hand point, aiming at letting go (both physically and emotionally) and helping the cervix dilate. These can be pressed during each contraction. (See the acupressure appendix).

SHOULDER PRESENTATION

In very rare cases (0.25% of births) the unborn baby lies with their back or shoulder near the woman's cervix, called a shoulder presentation. This is more common with:
- Women having their second or subsequent baby.
- Preterm babies before 34 weeks.
- Polyhydramnios.
- Placenta previa.
- A second twin (or triplet); usually the first baby is head down.
- A bicornuate uterus.

A shoulder presentation is easily detected by the caregiver feeling your belly at a routine pregnancy visit or during labour. An ultrasound may be performed to rule out placenta previa or a bicornuate uterus. The main concern for babies lying transverse is that if the waters break, the cord could prolapse (see below), which is life-threatening for the baby.

Some caregivers advocate a routine caesarean; others try to turn the baby by manipulating them when feeling the woman's belly. If this is done during early labour, the contractions often push the baby's head down, keeping them in position until the birth. Once this happens, the caregiver may also break the waters to try and remove some of the amniotic fluid in case extra fluid encourages the baby to turn back again. Babies who continue to present shoulder first need to be born by caesarean.

HEAVY BLEEDING

Significant bleeding (soaking a pad or more) during labour is of concern and is referred to as an intrapartum haemorrhage. If this happens, the caregiver recommends:

- Monitoring the baby's heart rate with a CTG machine.
- Monitoring the woman's pulse and blood pressure more closely.
- Starting an intravenous drip (or in severe cases a blood transfusion).
- Lying the woman on her left side to maximise blood flow to her internal organs and the unborn baby. Oxygen is also given.
- Possibly an ultrasound (if there is enough time), to investigate why the bleeding might be happening.

Should the bleeding becomes very heavy, affecting the woman and/or her baby, a caesarean is performed, possibly using a general anaesthetic (if there is no time to insert an epidural or spinal). A general anaesthetic may also be preferred in case the epidural or spinal further lowers the woman's blood pressure. The baby may need to go to the intensive care nursery, depending on their condition at birth.

CORD PROLAPSE

A cord prolapse is a rare complication, in which the umbilical cord falls past the baby, through the woman's open cervix and into her vagina. This can occur if the waters break but the baby is not engaged in the pelvis. The umbilical cord can then become compressed, restricting (or cutting off) blood and oxygen flow to the baby, which is life-threatening. The baby needs to be delivered quickly by caesarean (often under general anaesthetic, unless an epidural is already in place).

In an effort to relieve pressure on the baby's cord, the caregiver normally keeps their fingers inside the woman's vagina, pushing the baby's head (or bottom, if breech) up, off the cord. To help with this, the woman assumes a head down, buttocks up position, either on all fours or by lying on her side with her bottom elevated, using a large pillow under her hip. She also has oxygen given through a mask, and her baby's heart rate is monitored.

If the cord prolapses outside the woman's vagina, it needs to be gently replaced (just inside the vagina) to keep it warm and moist and prevent the blood vessels from going into spasm, which can impede blood flow to the baby more rapidly.

The extent to which the baby is affected by a cord prolapse depends on the degree of cord compression and the length of time the cord is compressed. If the cord is only partially compressed (or intermittently compressed), the baby may be born healthy. If the cord is fully compressed for a few minutes, they will probably need resuscitation at birth and may have problems due to lack of oxygen. If the cord is fully compressed for more than 8 to 10 minutes, then sadly the baby is unlikely to survive.

If your waters break at home and you feel or see the cord protruding out of the vagina, call an ambulance; adopt a knee-to-chest position on all fours, with your bottom higher than your shoulders, and gently push any part of the cord you can see outside the vagina back into the vagina.

CHAPTER 7

Second stage and birthing your baby

The second stage of labour begins when the cervix is fully open (10 cm dilated) and the uterus and vagina become one continuous birth canal. The baby's head moves down and out of the uterus and into the vagina, which is very elastic and stretches to accommodate its passage. Your baby's journey is not a straight line. They negotiate an angle through the pelvis and under the pubic bone to be born, a little like placing your foot into a gum boot.

The second stage consists of four different phases, each with its own characteristics.

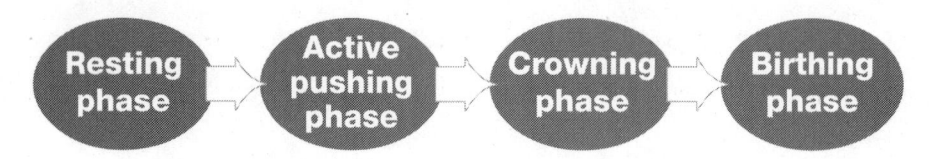

Resting phase → Active pushing phase → Crowning phase → Birthing phase

The second stage requires hard, physical exertion to move your baby through your body.

RESTING PHASE
Moving from first stage into second stage usually brings a lull in the contractions. The cervix is completely open but there is no urge to push yet. The uterus readjusts for a change in the contraction pattern and the baby slowly repositions in readiness to move down the birth canal. The resting phase can last from 5 to 20 minutes or more, with the contractions:
- Fading away completely, or
- Feeling milder, with longer rest periods between them.

While most women are relieved to finally have a break from the intense contractions of transition, it is normal to feel anxious or confused that it has all stopped. Some things to consider are:

- **Don't intervene or panic** – Enjoy the rest, it is normal. Interventions (eg. breaking the waters or natural remedies) are not needed to start the labour again, especially if your baby has been in a posterior position, because the resting phase allows them time to finish rotating round to an anterior position.

  Some caregivers don't recognise the resting phase, or wish to shorten it by asking the woman to push before her body is ready. This can cause problems and is quite ineffective. If you and your baby are well, it is reasonable to allow the resting phase to take its course. Talk to your caregiver during the pregnancy about how they usually manage the second stage. If you prefer to avoid early pushing, ask for more time.
- **Listen to your body** – rest and doze if you need to. Allow time to recover and wait patiently for the active pushing phase to begin.
- **Fetal distress** – If your baby is showing signs of distress you may have to push before you are ready. This can be very stressful, as you try hard to birth your baby while being worried about their wellbeing. In some cases, forceps or a ventouse are used to deliver the baby more rapidly.
- **Epidurals mask the resting phase** – But the caregiver often performs a vaginal examination to confirm the cervix is fully open. You should wait until the epidural wears off before actively pushing, so you push more effectively.
- **Waters breaking** – If the waters have not broken yet, a fluid-filled bag usually oozes down the birth canal, in front of the baby's head. The caregiver normally pierces this bag to release the amniotic fluid.

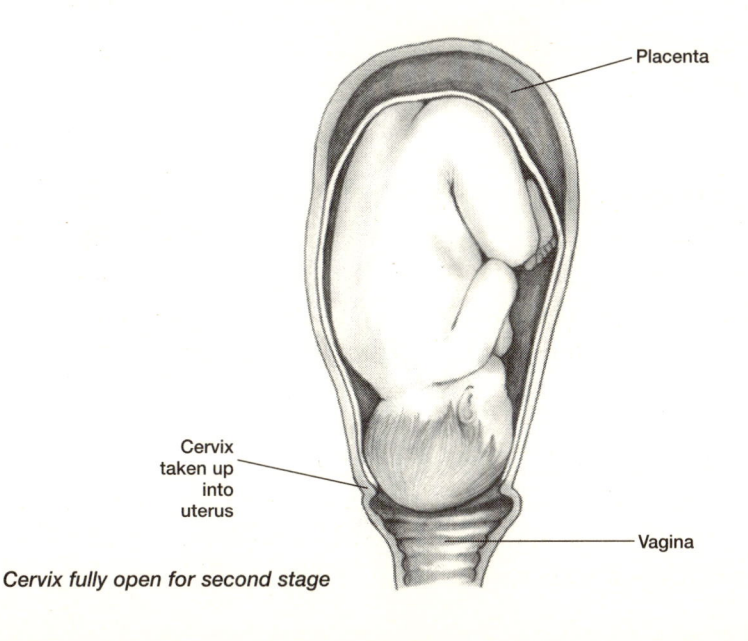

Cervix fully open for second stage

> **Did you know?**
> On rare occasions the sac remains intact until the baby's head is born. They emerge with a fine membrane covering their face, called a caul. Superstition has it that these babies are lucky and will never drown.

Both the woman and her partner/support team can feel tired and anxious, or may enjoy the rest, or be excited about the impending birth!

ACTIVE PUSHING PHASE

The second stage is mostly made up of active pushing. The baby moves lower into the birth canal, applying pressure to the nerve receptors in the woman's pelvic floor muscles, sending messages to her body, triggering a spontaneous urge to push (called Ferguson's reflex).

With each contraction the woman pushes and her baby comes further down the vagina. As the contraction eases, the baby's head moves back up slightly but not quite as far as it was before. This natural process allows the pelvic floor muscles and perineum to stretch gradually. Some women become upset when they feel their baby move back after pushing. Rest assured, this is normal. Your baby comes down further with each contraction and push. However, you only need to push when the contraction is happening – pushing without a contraction will exhaust you.

During the active pushing phase, contractions feel more expulsive and involuntary, and often come less frequently, four to seven minutes apart.

Sensations and progress

The sensations during active pushing tend to change as the baby progresses down the birth canal.

1. Early pushing – As the baby's head presses on the rectum, pressure sensations (mixed with pain) can be felt, similar to wanting to open your bowels.

Some women try to feel their baby's head during the pushing phase to help them keep in touch with how they are progressing. If you were to put your middle finger into your vagina at this point, you would need to insert it all the way in to touch your baby's head.

2. Middle pushing – This can be felt as painful pressure, mixed with a burning sensation at the peak of the stronger contractions. Pressure from the baby's head starts to bulge the woman's perineum and stretch open her anus (distending it out). Caregivers see this as a positive sign that the baby is getting close to being born.

It takes about 1 to 2 hours of active pushing for first babies, and anything from 5 to 30 minutes for subsequent babies, to reach this stage.

If you inserted your index finger into your vagina at this time, you would only need to go in as far as the second joint on your finger to feel your baby's head.

3. End pushing – As the baby stretches the perineum further, burning sensations intensify, until gradually the baby's head can be clearly seen at the vaginal opening with each contraction. The first glimpse often looks like a wrinkled walnut, as the bones of the baby's skull overlap to make their skin look bunched up. Caregivers say the baby's head is now on view.

You might ask for a mirror to see your baby for yourself, or feel your baby's head with your hand at the vaginal opening during each contraction. If you feel your baby's head while the contraction is not there, you would only need to put the tip of your finger inside your vagina.

Things to consider

Pushing instinctively – Many caregivers (and support people) direct women to push in a controlled or strained way, known as the Valsalva manoeuvre. The woman is instructed to take a breath in, hold it and 'push, push – keep pushing', until she can't hold her breath any longer, continuously repeating this for each contraction. Directed pushing is not beneficial and has been shown to:
- Tighten the pelvic floor muscles, impeding the descent of the baby down the birth canal.
- Reducing the amount of oxygen available to the baby, sometimes causing them to become distressed.
- Increase the chances of the woman tearing.[1]

It also exhausts the woman more rapidly and makes her feel as though someone else is taking over. Pushing instinctively may take slightly longer, but your baby will be better oxygenated and you will have more energy.

Occasionally guidance is needed to get into a rhythm, especially if you have an epidural in place and your natural urge is minimal (or absent). However, guidance to help you push does not need to be directed pushing.

Getting off your back – Lying on your back (or in a semi-reclining position) can reduce blood flow and oxygen to your baby, perhaps distressing them. If you can't be upright or forward on your knees, try lying on your side to push. Staying off your tailbone (or coccyx) also increases the size of your pelvis, allowing your baby more room to be born.

NOTE: *It is important you use positions you feel comfortable in. However, your caregiver may have personal preferences to have you on your back and/or in stirrups (called the lithotomy position). You should find out during the pregnancy whether they have a problem with you being in alternative positions. If you and the baby are well, there should be no need to move from your preferred position.*

Letting go – It is normal to instinctively pull back, or withhold the push, due to the pain being experienced (or possibly concerns about the baby or birth). Letting go of this resistance helps your baby come down. You may need your caregiver to talk you through this. A warm, wet compress on the perineum, or getting into the bath, can help facilitate it as well.

Emotions during active pushing

The active pushing phase often brings a change of energy and focus, with many women becoming more aware of their surroundings, talking more and giving clearer directions between contractions. Both the woman and her partner/support person may feel excited, relieved, empowered, overwhelmed, exhausted, fearful or a mixture of all these. Women often have concerns about the pain or tearing. Some people feel embarrassed about the woman opening her bowels slightly, or the noises she is making.

CROWNING PHASE

Soon, about 5 cm of the baby's head can be seen. Now the head advances slightly more with each push, staying where it is after the contraction stops. This continues until the baby's head crowns. Crowning is when the widest part of the baby's head (their crown) emerges and you can see the back of their head to their forehead. Within moments the baby's face and head emerge.

Sensations and progress

The perineum stretches to become paper-thin and an intense burning (or stinging) is felt, lasting for a few seconds. This can trigger panic for some women, causing them to scream, cry or swear. (Common remarks are 'Get it out', 'Get your hands away' or 'Do something!'). Moments later the baby's head is born and the woman experiences enormous relief.

Things to consider

Panting or blowing – Your caregiver may ask you to pant or blow, to help ease the baby's head out and minimise tearing of the perineum. If you are finding it difficult to ignore your body's signals to push, your support people can gently repeat the caregiver's directions, or offer affirmations or words practised during the pregnancy, such as 'Blow', 'Breathe out', 'Our baby is coming.' It may help to try imagining yourself breathing your baby out and rehearsing this during the pregnancy to keep you focused. Remember, all this can be forgotten at the time of birth!

Be realistic – You can only do your best. It is now thought that panting may not make a lot of difference to whether the perineum tears or not (although it is still widely practised).[2]

Controlling the baby's head – As your baby's head crowns, the caregiver usually places their fingers (or cupped hand) over the baby's head, to gently control the speed of their birth. Again, this aims to reduce the chances of the perineum tearing. Some women use their own hand(s), to help them focus on easing their baby out slowly.

NOTE: *A few caregivers have a habit of putting their fingers inside the woman's vagina to help it 'stretch', or pushing her labia back over the baby's head. This is unnecessary and painful and may cause the genitals to swell and bruise. If your caregiver is making you uncomfortable doing this, ask them to stop. You may wish to discuss this with them during the pregnancy, or include this in your birth plan.*

Emotions during the crowning phase

It is normal to feel frightened and worried by the stretching or burning sensations. You may need to dig to the depths of your being to summon the motivation to persevere for this final phase. Some women feel unable to control their pushing, but others feel very aware and focused.

Partners and support people can also be fearful or anxious, worried about the woman or the baby, or overwhelmed by her sheer efforts and the pain she is enduring. Both of you may be excited to see (or feel) the baby's head, overwhelmed with love, happiness and relief that it is nearly over.

BIRTHING PHASE

Your baby's head emerges. If you were to reach down between your thighs, you would feel the back of their head, because they come out facing your bottom. Your baby won't start breathing until their body is born, but oxygen is still supplied through the umbilical cord. Some babies squirm, or make small gurgling sounds at this stage, but others look calm and serene. It is normal for their skin to look blue-purple in colour, until their body is born and they start breathing.

After the baby's head is born, there is a break of four to seven minutes until the next contraction. During this time their shoulders rotate, so that one shoulder lies under their mother's pubic bone, with the other one at a time close to her tailbone. With the next contraction, the shoulders are born, and the rest of the baby's body slips out quite quickly, often with a gush of amniotic fluid. Once the baby's entire body leaves their mother, this is documented as the time of birth.

Things to consider

Checking for the cord – After the baby's head emerges, the caregiver may routinely check if any cord is around the baby's neck (which is normal for 25% of babies). If present, the loop of cord is usually loose and can be eased over the baby's head, or just allowed to slip over their shoulders and trunk as their body is born, or simply unravelled after the birth.

In the rare circumstance that the cord is tight and preventing the rest of the baby from being born easily, the caregiver may need to clamp and cut it. This means the baby needs to be born fairly quickly now, because their oxygen supply is cut off. You may be required to push before the next contraction starts. A few babies need some oxygen and resuscitation soon after birth, but they usually respond by crying soon afterwards.

Baby born in one contraction – A few babies are born, head and body, with the one contraction. This is more common for subsequent babies, or if the baby is relatively small. The baby may appear a little stunned, and your caregiver may need to stimulate them by rubbing their skin or giving them some oxygen. Again, most babies breathe and cry within a minute or so of these things happening.

Compound presentation – This is when the baby's hand and arm lies alongside their head and are born at the same time (perhaps the baby liked sucking their thumb!). This can increase the chances of the woman tearing, so the caregiver may try to hold the baby's hand back, or gently grasp their hand and extend their whole arm out before their body is born.

Not wanting to hold your baby – Despite the perception that all women want to pick up their baby and cuddle them immediately after their birth, the reality is that many women need time and space before doing this. Feeling initially reluctant to hold your baby is very normal, and it is important you are given time. Your partner or support person might hold the baby while you gather your thoughts and be present with your feelings.

The partner 'catching' the baby – Increasingly, many fathers are having a hands-on role in catching their son or daughter, which is an amazing thrill. If everything is progressing normally, and you are not physically supporting the woman, this is possible and you can ask your caregiver to facilitate it.

Emotions at the birth

As **the woman** you may feel:
- Overwhelming relief.
- Shocked, if it has been very quick.
- Exhausted, if it has been long and hard.
- Joy and exhilaration.
- Like you're falling in love!
- A need to adjust to how your dream baby actually looks.
- 'Thank heavens it's over, I never want to do that again!'
- Spaced out, drunk on emotions as though it's all a bit surreal.
- Frightened and helpless if your baby is unwell and being worked on by staff.
- Traumatised by complications and interventions.
- Excited about, or disappointed with, the sex of your baby.
- A special connection with your partner/support person.

As **the partner or support person** you may feel:
- Relief that they are both all right.
- Excited, emotions flooding through your mind, body and soul.
- Shocked or exhausted.
- Angry, frightened or helpless if your baby is unwell and being monitored by staff.
- Traumatised by complications and interventions.
- Like you're falling madly in love!
- Admiration and awe for the mother's achievements.
- Excited, or disappointed, by the sex of the baby.
- A need to adjust to how your dream baby actually looks.
- A special connection with your partner.

Support strategies

Physical and emotional support needs to continue on from the first stage but may require adjusting. Consider the suggestions described in Chapters 5, 6 and 9, as well as the following strategies.

Support strategies for the woman
Noises and breathing
Listen to your body and follow its cues. If you feel you need guidance, ask your caregiver. Some women try to deliberately push with their contractions, others just go with the flow, letting their body do the work. It is normal to bear down, grunt and groan spontaneously, perhaps unaware you are pushing. A few women sing or shout purposefully, if it helps them cope. Try to keep you voice low and take your energies down to your baby.

Positive attitudes
Having confidence in your body's ability to give birth is important – remember, your body was made for this. Some women try to work with their baby to keep them motivated. Others talk to their baby in between contractions, such as 'Come on, baby, I want to see you.' A few don't have time for any of this.

Addressing concerns
Holding concerns about the birth, your baby, or even parenting, may slow the progress of the second stage. Working through these concerns during the pregnancy is ideal, otherwise talking about them at this time might help. Perhaps request that your caregiver gives you space to do this (providing your baby is well).

Support strategies for the partner/support person
Facilitating her privacy
It is normal to feel vulnerable and on show during second stage as everyone's attention suddenly focuses on your genitals. Caregivers may turn on lights (or use torches) and more staff can enter the room. If there are no complications, perhaps ask for the lights to be dimmed (or have filtered light from an adjoining bathroom). As the partner or support person, if you feel she is vulnerable or exposed, cover her with a sheet or help her into a more private position. Gently request that any superfluous staff leave, and consider that she may not want a camera or video on her yet (even if she agreed to it during the pregnancy).

Body comfort
Pushing is hard work and she may appreciate her brow being wiped with a cool cloth, sips of water or having her hair tied back. Alternatively she may not want to be touched at all and will probably let you know!

A warm compress on her perineum and/or anus can help relax her pelvic floor muscles and relieve burning sensations. This can be applied with a flannel or nappy, moistened with warm water (and wrung out), then placed on the area. Your caregiver may take over using the compress closer to the crowning phase. Be aware that some women don't want their genitals touched. So remove it if she requests this.

Sounds and smells

Keep noise and conversation to a minimum, although she may want her favourite music. Also, newborns can sense their parents' smell at birth, especially their mother's. If you have been using aromatherapy, remove it now so the baby is not overwhelmed. (Don't put essential oils in the birth pool.)

Listening and reassuring

Have confidence in her birthing ability. Listen to her complaints, commands and directions. Offer her praise, affirmations and reassurance. Understand that her frustrations may be misdirected at you. (Having a thick skin can help!) If she screams an order at you, it is not because she does not love you but because she is in pain, exhausted and may not have time to ask nicely.

Staying calm

It is normal to feel nervous or anxious, but be aware of your body tension and try to consciously relax. If you have concerns, ask your caregiver for guidance and reassurance.

POSITIONING FOR BIRTH

Most women instinctively assume positions that feel right during the second stage, but if it is taking a while (more than 60 to 90 minutes), then alternatives may be needed so gravity can assist. It can take a great deal of effort to change positions during second stage and your partner, support person and/or caregiver will probably need to help you. You can try:

- **Standing** – Keep your legs a comfortable width apart, and lean forward onto something (or someone). Sometimes the partner/support person can support you from behind, but they may need to lean up against a wall to support themselves.

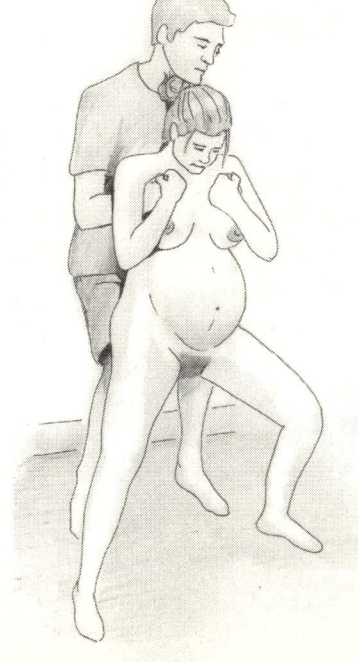

- **Kneeling or on all fours** – This can reduce tearing of the perineum.

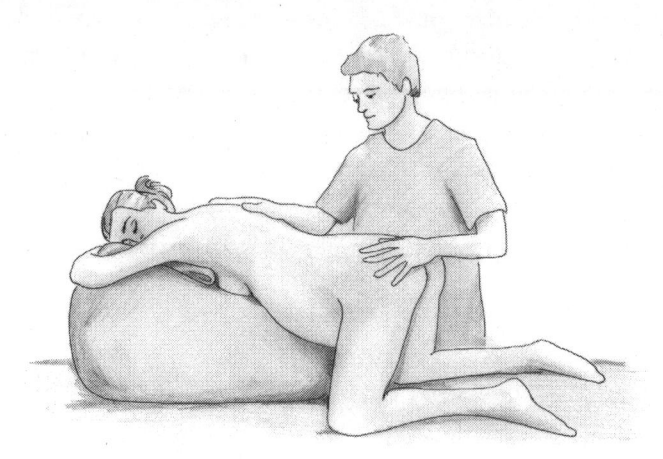

- **Squatting** – This enlarges the pelvis by up to 1 to 2 cm, providing extra room for the baby. Most women don't have the energy or physical ability to squat for the entire second stage, but it may be an option for short periods. You may want to practise squatting during the pregnancy, to strengthen and stretch your legs. You can also try straddling your partner/support person's legs (while that person is sitting), to rest and maintain a type of squatting position while pushing.

- **A birth stool or toilet** – Sitting helps your body let go, because this position feels familiar. Using the toilet can help overcome concerns about opening your bowels or people looking at your genitals.

- **Lying on your side** – This can help you rest between the contractions and is a good position if you are exhausted or have an epidural in place. It can also slow down the baby's progress if the birth is happening too quickly. Your support person or caregiver may help you hold one of your legs up, in a bent position.

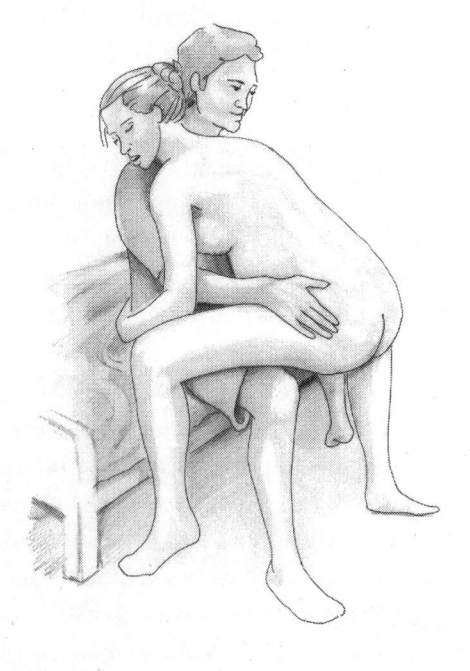

AVOID:
- **Lying on your back** – This is often uncomfortable and can reduce blood flow and oxygen to the baby. However, if your instincts are to lie on your back, trust this and only change position if you are uncomfortable (or your caregiver detects the baby's heart rate is dropping too low). Reclining in the bath is fine, as the water produces weightlessness.
- **Sitting back in a semi-reclining position** – This can reduce the opening of your pelvis, slowing the birth's progress and making it more difficult for the baby's shoulders to be born. It can also place weight from your abdomen and uterus up against your diaphragm (the muscle under the lungs), making it more difficult to breathe.

Expectations for care

Your caregiver stays with you for most of the time now and listens to your baby's heart rate more frequently, every 5 to 10 minutes or so. If a CTG monitor is being used, this is usually maintained until the baby's head crowns. If you have an obstetrician, they will arrive as the baby's head comes in view and normally takes over from the midwife to deliver the baby. The midwife stays to assist the doctor. A paediatrician may be called if there are health concerns for your baby.

As soon as your baby is born (and presuming there are no complications), they are placed on your belly, or in your arms, or between your legs if you are on your hands and knees, and the midwife makes a mental note of the time of birth. Some caregiver's announce the sex of the baby, but you may request that you discover this yourself.

VAGINAL EXAMINATIONS

As you move from the first to second stage your caregiver may want to perform a vaginal examination to see whether the cervix is fully dilated. This is not essential and you may decline it. Experienced caregivers can usually detect this progress by the way you grunt, moan or push, and possibly by noticing a trickle of bright blood from the vagina, and/or the perineum and anus bulging. However, a vaginal examination may be necessary if your caregiver is concerned, or if you have an epidural in place (because the physical signs of second stage are not as obvious). If you have an obstetrician, they will try to organise their commitments to make it to your birth. To do this they may ask the midwife to perform vaginal examinations more frequently so that they have a better idea of your progress (although, again, you can refuse this).

Occasionally the pushing stage arrives faster than anticipated and your announcement of 'I want to push' may be received with some scepticism or even disbelief. If this is the case, trust your instincts (they are usually right) and ask the midwife to check your dilation so that she can be prepared for the birth!

TIME LIMITS

Some caregivers place time limits on the second stage of labour. It is normal for active pushing to last up to 1 to 2 hours for first babies, and 15 to 60 minutes for subsequent babies. If you are given unrealistic time limits (eg. one hour from full dilation for a first baby) before interventions are suggested (forceps, ventouse or an episiotomy), this can make you feel scared and unnecessarily pressured. Caregivers are less likely to intervene with women having subsequent babies, unless there are obvious complications.

If your baby is progressing slowly but surely, and you and your baby are well, there is no need to intervene.

Variations for the second stage

Variations for the second stage can play a part in the length of labour, how the baby is born, and often how a woman ultimately feels about her birth experience afterwards.

TEARING

Sometimes the woman's genitals tear when giving birth. This may be:
- **Grazes of the vagina, perineum or labia** – These are shallow splits in the skin that rarely need stitches but may sting when passing urine. Having regular urinary alkaliniser powders (mixed with water) after the birth can make the urine less acidic and less likely to sting.
- **First degree tears** – These are small tears of the perineum, involving the top layer of skin and some underlying tissue but no muscle tissue. They do not generally require suturing, but some caregivers put in one or two stitches.

- **Second degree tears** – These involve the vaginal skin, underlying tissue and some of the pelvic floor muscles. Second degree tears are almost always stitched to aid healing.
- **Third and fourth degree tears** – These are not common. A third degree tear extends through the pelvic floor muscles and partially through the edge of the anus. A fourth degree tear extends completely through the anus and/or rectum (see Chapter 8).
- **Vaginal wall tears** – These are inside the vagina and are more common with a forceps delivery. They often require stitches, especially if deep, or bleeding heavily.
- **Tears of the cervix** – Also associated with forceps (and/or ventouse) births, these are rare but tend to bleed quite heavily if not stitched.
- **Tears of the labia** – These are relatively common and may be sutured, depending on the nature of the tear. Often this is more for cosmetic appearance and/or the caregiver's and woman's preferences.

In Australia more than 60% of women don't have stitches but no one can predict which women will. Even perineal massage holds no guarantees. As a guide, tearing is *more* likely if:
- It is your first baby.
- You give birth lying on your back, semi-reclining or in stirrups.
- You give birth while standing, squatting or on a birth stool, although leaning forward in these positions can reduce this risk.
- The birth is very fast.
- You have a ventouse or forceps delivery.
- The perineum is swollen (if the pushing is prolonged while squatting or on a birth stool, or if the caregiver manipulates or massages the perineum excessively).
- The baby remains in a posterior position at the time of birth.
- The baby is unusually large (over 4.5 kg or 10 lb), although many large babies are born without the woman tearing, especially if this is not her first baby.

Tearing is *less* likely if:
- It is your second or subsequent vaginal birth.
- You give birth in a kneeling, all fours or side-lying position, or have a water birth in any position.
- You have done perineal massage regularly during the final weeks of pregnancy.
- Your pelvic floor is relaxed. Women who are very concerned about

tearing often do tear, possibly because they tense up their pelvic floor muscles, making them less likely to stretch. Consider trying warm compresses or a water birth. Visualisation, affirmations and homeopathic remedies may reduce fear and aid relaxation during pushing.

Episiotomy

With an episiotomy the caregiver uses surgical scissors to cut the woman's perineum, usually as the baby's head is crowning, with or without local anaesthetic (often the perineum is quite numb at this stage). The cut can range from 3 to 7 cm in length, and is usually equivalent to a second degree tear, requiring stitches.

Episiotomies can be either **midline** (straight down from the vagina towards the anus) or **mediolateral** (going down, but out to one side at a 45° angle). The type used generally depends on the caregiver's preferences. Midline episiotomies cut less muscle and tend to be easier to repair and heal better. However, the chances of it extending through to the anus are increased. Therefore, many caregivers prefer to do a mediolateral episiotomy, even though it damages more muscle tissue.

Whether you 'need' an episiotomy, very much depends on your caregiver's beliefs. Research shows that there are very few valid health reasons for performing an episiotomy. In fact, they can actually do more harm than good. In Australia, the overall episiotomy rate is about 13%, which is much less than other countries, but they still tend to be overused. Episiotomies were adopted long before research into their effectiveness was conducted, and many beliefs about them are now known to be false. As a summary:

- Belief: An episiotomy protects the pelvic floor muscles from tears, especially third and fourth degree tears.
  The research: Episiotomy cuts through the pelvic floor muscles, equivalent to (or worse than) a second degree tear, and increases the chance of extending to a third or fourth degree tear.[3]
- Belief: An episiotomy prevents the pelvic floor from overstretching, therefore helps with urinary and bowel incontinence, prolapse of the vagina or uterus and loss of sexual sensation.
  The research: Evidence does not support this belief. When an episiotomy is performed, the pelvic floor muscles are already at full stretch. Cutting them damages the muscles, which may never have torn, thus increasing incontinence.
- Belief: An episiotomy is needed for a forceps delivery.

The research: Performing a forceps delivery without an episiotomy reduces the chances of deep perineal tears.[4]
- Belief: An episiotomy is needed for a ventouse delivery.
The research: A ventouse birth does not require a routine episiotomy.
- Belief: An episiotomy is easier to repair because it is a clean cut, rather than a ragged tear.
The research: A tear is as straightforward to repair as an episiotomy. Any competent childbirth caregiver should be able to repair both.[5]
- Belief: An episiotomy shortens the second stage of labour.
The research: It may only shorten the second stage by 3 to 5 contractions (15 minutes or so), which could be a valid reason if the baby is distressed. It may also be used if the mother is exhausted.
- Belief: An episiotomy is necessary for a premature baby to prevent bleeding in their brain, mental retardation, and trauma to their skull.
The research: The perineum is soft and flexible and the baby's skull is designed to mould and adapt to birth. There is no evidence to support any of these proposed advantages for premature babies.
- Belief: An episiotomy is needed to help manage shoulder dystocia.
The research: Episiotomy has not been shown to help with shoulder dystocia, as it is the bones of the woman's pelvis holding the baby back, not her perineum.
- Belief: The woman's perineum will not stretch effectively because she is too physically fit (eg. a dancer or someone who rides horses).
The research: Women with strong pelvic floor muscles are more likely to end up with an intact perineum and have fewer problems with urinary incontinence after the birth.
- Belief: Women with fair skin, Asian women, or those having their first baby need an episiotomy.
The research: These perceptions are false and not reasons to perform an episiotomy.
- Belief: The perineum is buttonholing, or starting to tear in the middle, instead of the vaginal edge, and an episiotomy may prevent it from extending to the anus.
The research: The perineum normally tears from the buttonhole upwards, towards the edge of the vagina. Extending downwards towards the anus is more likely with an episiotomy.
- Belief: Injecting the perineum with local anaesthetic is necessary just in case an episiotomy is required.
The research: Injecting local anaesthetic swells the perineal tissues and

increases the chances of the perineum tearing. It also makes the intention of the caregiver to do an episiotomy more likely.
- Belief: The perineum appears white or blanched and looks like it will tear, so an episiotomy is necessary to prevent a large tear.
The research: The perineum often looks blanched or white as it stretches to full capacity, and can remain intact (if given the chance).

It is important to remember that your perineum will only tear to the minimum depth it needs to (if at all). A caregiver usually overestimates what your body needs and may even cause an injury when in fact tearing might never have occurred at all.

How can I avoid an episiotomy?

The best thing you can do to reduce your chances of receiving an episiotomy is to select a caregiver (or birthplace) who is unlikely to perform one. Discuss this during the pregnancy and the circumstances one may be needed (or you would accept one). Ask what their episiotomy rate is. If you cannot come to a compromise, think about changing your care. If you don't know who your caregiver will be, write it in a birth plan or inform them during the labour.

In general, midwives perform less episiotomies than doctors; but midwives working in delivery suites are more likely to perform them than midwives working in birth centres or at homebirths. However, individual practitioners vary. Rates tend to be less in smaller metropolitan and country hospitals than in larger city and private hospitals, and are lowest in birth centres and for homebirths (less than 1%).

FAST BIRTH

Babies born rapidly are said to have a precipitate birth. This usually involves a short labour, with strong, frequent contractions from the start and little rest in between. Fast births are generally not a problem, but may increase the chances of perineal tearing, or result in heavy bleeding afterwards. Some babies are a little stunned at birth, perhaps needing stimulation or oxygen.

Fast births are often seen by others as a piece of good luck. However, women can feel shocked and bewildered by the intensity and pain, and sometimes they feel traumatised. Partners and support people can also feel frightened and helpless witnessing the birth, as the woman appears distressed and often not receptive to preplanned support strategies. Talk about your experiences afterwards (when you feel ready). It is normal to feel negative about it, even though others may say how lucky you were.

Baby distressed
If your baby becomes distressed during the second stage, your caregiver may want to intervene with forceps or a ventouse (or an episiotomy if the baby's head is close to being born). Be aware that it is normal for an unborn baby's heart rate to drop periodically during contractions, but if it remains low, even after the contraction has stopped, this can be a sign of distress, especially if there is meconium present in the amniotic fluid. Depending on the severity of the distress, interventions may need to be performed fairly quickly, with little time for negotiation.

Baby's presentation
In most cases, the crown of the baby's head leads the way – a vertex presentation. However, occasionally the baby's face or brow presents instead. (Breech babies are dealt with in Chapter 4.)

Face presentation
About 0.2% of babies are born face first. This is more common for women having subsequent babies and it is usually not a problem, with over 90% being born normally (the remaining 10% by caesarean, due to the angle of the baby's head).

The baby may have a bruised, sore face and require gentle handling in the early days, with possibly extra help with breastfeeding. A few babies continue to be irritable and unsettled in the weeks following. Some parents consult a cranial osteopath, or take their baby to a specialist chiropractor, to help with spinal alignment. You may want to try baby massage, or your homeopath may suggest a remedy.

Brow presentation
A baby presenting brow first is very rare (0.05%), and also less common for first births. Most require a caesarean, because the diameter of the baby's head is greatly increased in this position. On rare occasions, if the baby is small and the woman has a roomy pelvis with strong contractions, the baby may end up being born vaginally. Brow babies tend to have a slightly misshapen head, which returns to normal within a few days.

Forceps and ventouse
Forceps and ventouse are medical interventions used to vaginally deliver babies more rapidly in the second stage, usually if the baby is distressed or the time taken for the baby to be born is thought to be too long.

Both interventions are usually performed by obstetric specialists or registrars in a delivery suite, although some GPs and midwives undergo training to use them in emergency situations or in remote and rural areas. Women having their first vaginal birth are more likely to have an assisted delivery than with subsequent births (unless the previous birth was a caesarean).

Forceps

Forceps are two separate metal pieces that look similar to a pair of salad servers. When correctly positioned, they aim to provide a protective cage around the baby's head to prevent excessive pressure being applied. Forceps can be used for premature babies and caesareans, as well as vaginal breech births (after the baby's body is born).

Before a forceps delivery can be performed:
- The cervix must be fully dilated (to 10 cm).
- The waters must be broken.
- The baby's head must be engaged.
- The caregiver must perform a vaginal examination to determine the position of the baby's head so the forceps can be applied correctly.
- The woman's bladder must be emptied (usually done with a catheter).
- The woman should have adequate pain relief (an epidural, spinal or pudendal block).

The woman lies on her back, with her legs in stirrups, to stabilise her body and counteract the traction applied by the caregiver to deliver the baby. You may be able to be propped up with a couple of pillows so you can see what is happening and have some eye contact with your caregiver, if this is what you prefer.

The forceps are lubricated with an antiseptic cream and placed in position one at a time, in between contractions. Once in place, with the next contraction the woman pushes as the doctor pulls, until the contraction eases; once the next contraction begins again, the process is repeated. It may take two or three contractions before the baby's head is born. Often an episiotomy is performed as the baby's head crowns (although this is not absolutely necessary). Once the baby's head is delivered, the forceps are removed and the baby's body is born in the usual way.

Unsuccessful forceps and caesarean

A trial of forceps is when forceps are attempted in the operating theatre if the caregiver thinks using forceps might not be successful or could prove difficult, because the baby's head might not come down easily. If this ends up being the case, the forceps are abandoned and a caesarean is performed.

This can be emotional and distressing. Take one step at a time, and try to accept that the wheels are in motion now.

NOTE: *Ideally an episiotomy would not be routinely performed with a trial of forceps, otherwise the woman could end up with an unnecessary episiotomy as well as a caesarean scar. If you are confronted with the prospect of having a trial of forceps, discuss this with your caregiver.*

Ventouse

Ventouse (French for 'suction') is a specially designed metal or rubber cup which is placed on the baby's head to assist their birth (also called a vacuum extraction). The ventouse cup is placed on the crown of the baby's head, avoiding their soft fontanelle, and tubing attached to the cup is connected to suction to create a negative pressure. With the next contraction the woman pushes and the caregiver pulls, until the contraction eases off. It usually takes two or three contractions to deliver the baby's head, after which the pressure is released and the cup removed. The baby's body is delivered in the usual way.

Guidelines for the safe use of a ventouse are:
- The baby's head should start to descend with the first pull and start to emerge after no more than three pulls.
- The cup should not be reapplied more than twice if it has slipped off.
- The cup should not be applied for more than 20 minutes.

Ventouse are used in similar circumstances to forceps. Medical pain relief is not necessarily needed because it merely mimics a normal birth, except it is quicker. For this reason, an episiotomy is also not routine.

Forceps or ventouse?

If you need an assisted delivery, the choice between forceps or ventouse depends on the position of the baby's head, how far they have come down the birth canal and the preferences of the caregiver. Forceps and ventouse both have their pros and cons, and there are no guarantees that either (or both) will be successful. However, in recent years there has been a gradual swing away from using forceps, in favour of ventouse, especially if the baby's head is relatively low in the vagina.

Different caregivers have different points of view about the most appropriate method to be used in different circumstances. However, research suggests overall that ventouse delivery is associated with less injury to the mother and baby.

For some women an assisted delivery is the only way their baby could be born vaginally and a caesarean avoided. Their judicious use can be beneficial,

and in some cases life-saving. However, they can be overused, particularly if the caregiver places unrealistic time limits on the second stage. Some strategies to help achieve a vaginal birth unaided include:
- Using upright positions to push.
- Avoiding an epidural, or allowing time for it to wear off before pushing.
- Avoiding time limits, if you and your baby are well.
- Having continuous, supportive care from a known person throughout the entire labour.
- Using a Syntocinon drip to rectify weak, infrequent or sporadic contractions (if your baby is not distressed).
- Being aware that mild fetal distress diagnosed through continuous CTG monitoring can be inaccurate (unless fetal scalp blood sampling is used). Adopting a sensible wait-and-see approach may help avoid unnecessary interventions.

Consider negotiating these strategies with your caregiver during pregnancy.

Baby after an assisted delivery

The baby may have swelling, bruising and grazing on their scalp, ears or cheeks after an assisted delivery, and be agitated or unsettled. Handle them gently and try to avoid applying pressure to their head. Take care when attaching them to the breast and only hold their head at the base of their neck. You may find warm baths help relax them in the days following the birth. Some women use homeopathic remedies.

SHOULDER DYSTOCIA

If the baby's shoulders have difficulty being born, this is called shoulder dystocia. Most shoulder dystocias are mild to moderate, only briefly delaying the birth of the baby's body. This is often because their shoulders have not rotated yet, or the woman is lying on her back, or in a semi-reclining position, pushing her tailbone inwards and reducing the size of her pelvis. In most cases it is relieved by moving to a hands and knees position, or lying on your side.

Severe shoulder dystocia happens when the baby's shoulders are too large to fit easily through the woman's pelvis, and the baby's top (or anterior) shoulder becomes wedged behind the woman's pubic bone. This is a rare complication, occurring in about 0.2% of vaginal births, but the risk is increased if the baby weighs more than 4.5 kg (10 lb).

Unfortunately there is no way to reliably predict shoulder dystocia. However, some caregivers suggest inducing labour early, or having a caesarean just in case, even though these interventions may be unnecessary.[6] Using

ultrasound or trying to measure the woman's pelvis are both inaccurate and unreliable,[7] as are other supposed risk factors such as:
- Having a previous shoulder dystocia birth – This does not mean the next baby will, and some women go on to birth bigger babies without trouble.
- The woman being overweight – This is not a predictor, unless she has uncontrolled diabetes.
- The mother being over 4.5 kg when she was born – This may mean she is more likely to have larger babies, but cannot predict shoulder dystocia.
- The father's size at birth, or as an adult – This is unrelated to the size of the baby or shoulder dystocia.

How is shoulder dystocia managed?

The most common way to manage shoulder dystocia is to change the woman's position. If she is able to move, getting onto hands and knees, and usually raising one leg (like a kneeling lunge), is highly effective.

If she has an epidural in place and cannot move easily, the caregiver may get her to lie on her side, or bring her knees up to her chest (called the McRobert's manoeuvre) to free her coccyx bone. Sometimes another caregiver will apply firm pressure onto the woman's lower belly (just above the pubic bone) to try and release the baby's shoulder. In the majority of cases these strategies are effective, particularly if enough time is allowed.

Occasionally the caregiver may need to internally manipulate the baby's position by placing their hand inside the woman's vagina and rotating the baby's shoulder to free it and/or pull the shoulder down, or one arm out, to free the opposite shoulder.

Health concerns for the baby

Fortunately most babies with shoulder dystocia are born healthy, although they may require some oxygen at birth and could be irritable or unsettled for a while, especially if their neck and spine have been twisted. You may want to consult with a paediatric chiropractor or osteopath in the weeks afterwards.

If the dystocia was severe and manipulation was required, the baby's arm or clavicle (the bone from their shoulder to lower neck) may fracture, their muscles may be strained and sometimes nerves injured, possibly causing temporary paralysis to one arm (called Erb's palsy). This usually heals within months.[8] If the baby remains wedged for a prolonged period, reducing their oxygen supply, this can be life-threatening, or lead to them having developmental and learning difficulties.

Health concerns for the woman
Depending on the manipulations used, the woman may need to recover from bruising or extensive vaginal tears. There is also an increased chance of a postpartum haemorrhage, and in very rare cases a ruptured uterus.

Shoulder dystocia is a rare, unpredictable emergency. Many caregivers may rush into the room and take over with a sense of urgency. This can be frightening and upsetting, particularly if invasive techniques are used. If shoulder dystocia does occur, try to stay calm and remember that most cases do resolve easily. Ideally, your caregivers should also stay calm and give you clear explanations and directions as much as possible.

GIVING BIRTH TO TWINS
If you are pregnant with twins, your decision to have a vaginal birth will depend on your preferences and the position of the babies, particularly the first twin (the one closest to your cervix). As a guide:
- As long as both babies are head down (40% of twins) they can be born vaginally, unless there are other health complications.
- If the first twin is head down and the second twin is breech (28% of twins), a vaginal birth may be considered, depending on how you and your caregiver feel about vaginal breech births (discussed in Chapter 4). This also applies to when both babies are breech (9% of twin pregnancies).
- When the first twin is head down but the second is lying transverse (7% of twins), it is possible to plan a vaginal birth. This is because often the second twin moves automatically into a head-down position after the first twin is born, or the caregiver manipulates them into position (discussed below).
- If the first twin is breech but the second twin is head down (7% of twins), a caesarean is recommended, because the heads may become interlocked as the first twin moves down the birth canal, inhibiting their birth.
- If the first baby is breech and the second is transverse (4% of twins), usually a caesarean is planned.
- A caesarean is always performed if both babies are transverse (1% of twins).

The labour
The vaginal birth of twins is similar to that for single births. It is no more painful and you don't need to go through the labour twice, although you obviously need

to push out two babies. More than 50% of twin pregnancies progress without complications. If the twins are not born prematurely, labour often starts around 37 to 39 weeks, meaning induction is often unnecessary. The babies' heart rates may be continuously monitored with a twin CTG machine, or the midwives may listen with two Dopplers periodically.

Decisions about pain relief for labour should ideally be your choice. Some caregivers recommend a routine epidural if the second twin is not head down, in case they need to manipulate them after the first twin is born. Discuss this with your caregiver during the pregnancy.

The birth

Once the first twin is born, their cord is clamped and cut. Then there is a resting phase of 15 to 30 minutes or more, before active pushing starts again for the second twin. (Sometimes the second twin is born within a few minutes.)

The ideal time interval between the birth of twins is controversial. Some caregivers prefer to facilitate it as soon as possible (15 minutes or less), while others are happy to wait. If the second twin's heart rate is normal, there should be no need to hurry, with 30 minutes to an hour being acceptable. However, concerns about waiting can include limiting the risks of:
- The second twin's cord prolapsing, requiring an immediate caesarean.
- Early separation of the placentas before the second twin is born (fairly rare).
- The woman's cervix partially closing after the first twin is born, making it more difficult to deliver the second twin rapidly if they become distressed.

To speed up the resting phase the caregiver may:
- Break the waters of the second twin's amniotic sac.
- Start a Syntocinon drip to stimulate more contractions, or commence the drip 10 to 15 minutes after the first twin's birth.

Once contractions resume, the second twin moves down and the woman feels an urge to push again. Most women are surprised at how quick and easy the birth of their second twin is. Afterwards, their cord is clamped and cut, and then both placentas are delivered in the usual way.

Manipulating the second twin

If the second twin is lying transverse after the first twin is born, the caregiver will try and manipulate them into position. Some caregivers use a portable ultrasound machine during the resting phase to visualise the position of the second twin. Manipulations can be:

- **External cephalic version** – In an ECV the caregiver moves the baby by feeling the woman's belly (successful in up to 75% of cases).
- **Internal podalic version** – Here, the caregiver reaches up into the uterus (through a vaginal examination) and gently grasps the baby's feet, before guiding them down the vagina to facilitate a breech birth. This may be attempted if the external version is unsuccessful or too difficult.

If these methods are unsuccessful, a caesarean is performed for the second twin.

People present for the birth

Many parents are a little shocked by the amount of people present at their multiple birth. Because twins are less common, junior staff are interested in the learning experience, meaning you often have extra 'helpers' present. The minimum you can expect is the doctor delivering the babies and perhaps another doctor assisting them; two or three midwives, to assist the doctor and receive the babies; and perhaps two paediatricians, to attend to the babies once they are born, particularly if problems are expected. If you are keen to have as few people as possible, you could have one doctor, one or two midwives and one or two paediatric staff (or the paediatric staff can wait outside the door and be called in if needed). Discuss these options with your caregiver.

Baby born before arrival at the birthplace

About 0.4% of Australian babies are born before their mother gets to her birthplace (or before the caregiver arrives for a homebirth). This is called BBA or born before arrival. Take heart that most women do make it, and if they don't, most births are straightforward.

Women having their first baby normally have plenty of time. Even if you stayed at home until you were ready to push, it is usually another one or two hours before your baby is born. Try not to move before you are ready. Arriving too early can be disheartening and may increase your chances of medical intervention.

Women having a subsequent baby often don't feel really uncomfortable until they are 7 to 8 cm dilated (unless the previous birth was a caesarean with little, or no, dilation, then it is the same as for a first baby). Leaving it until this late stage means the baby can be born within an hour, even if your last labour was very prolonged. Therefore, plan to move to your birthplace once you are sure you are in labour, rather than waiting until you have very strong pains.

What to do

If it looks as though your baby will be born before you leave home, call an ambulance. As the woman, don't drive yourself to the hospital. Try to stay calm. Complications are unlikely.

If you are driving the woman to her birthplace, and the baby is coming, pull over and be with her. Ring for an ambulance to meet you (if you have a mobile phone).

As a guide for partners:

- Stay calm. Her body will know what to do. If you are taking directions over the phone, let the person know what is happening and they will guide you.
- Maintain her privacy (if in the car). Cover her up. Perhaps get someone to hold up a blanket. Ask audiences to go away!
- Once you see the baby's head, they will be born soon. If they have the cord around their neck, lift this over their head once they are born.
- The baby will look quite purple and it often takes 30 seconds to a minute before they breathe and cry (although this will seem like an eternity). Cover them with anything dry (a blanket, shirt, towel or jumper). It is important the baby is kept warm.

Reviving the baby

It is rare for a baby to need anything more than a rub-down and a blanket around them. However, if they don't seem to be responding, you may need to help them breathe. This can be done by:

- Lying them flat on their back, with their head lying straight, **not** tilted back.
- Holding their chin with your fingers (being careful not to lean on their neck).
- Placing your mouth over the baby's **nose** and **mouth** and **puffing** every two seconds – **do not blow**. Use only as much air as you can keep in your cheeks to inflate their lungs with each breath; usually half-a-dozen breaths are enough. On rare occasions, you may need to continue this until help arrives.

NOTE: *Heart compressions on newborns are done with 2 fingers in the middle of their breastbone, to a depth of 2 cm, and a rate of 2 per second. However, it is generally only recommended that people trained in cardiac massage should attempt this. You may consider doing a course during the pregnancy. It is a good skill to have anyway. Be aware that most babies who are not breathing still have a good heart rate.*

The cord, placenta and bleeding

In most cases cutting the cord is unnecessary. The blood vessels soon spasm and it is not a problem if the placenta comes away with the cord still attached. The placenta normally separates 15 to 30 minutes after the birth. Hopefully by then you will be at the hospital (or help has arrived).

The woman pushes to deliver the placenta, with blood coming away (about a cupful). She may need to sit up and squat (or sit on the toilet, if still at home) to help the placenta come. Sometimes she can gently ease it out herself by wrapping the cord around her finger, similar to removing a tampon. However, if it does not come easily, leave the cord alone and wait for help or make your way to the hospital. If the placenta delivers, wrap it in a towel or place it in a plastic bag, and keep it close to the baby, as it is still attached to their belly by the cord.

If the woman is bleeding heavily, wait for an ambulance to come. Sometimes rubbing her lower belly can make the uterus contract, to control the bleeding, especially if the placenta is already out.

Having a baby like this can be frightening, overwhelming and possibly undignified, and the woman may feel forgotten in all the drama, especially if everyone is giving attention to whoever attended the birth. This can downplay her wonderful achievement in birthing her baby. Feelings of shock, embarrassment and disappointment for the birth experience are common, and it may seem surreal, taking a while to accept the experience. Sharing your thoughts and feelings with someone you trust, and your partner being sensitive to your needs, can help.

STILLBORN BABY

A baby dying is one of the most devastating experiences a parent could ever face. The profound pain that follows is all-consuming and often misunderstood by family and friends. Many babies who die are born very prematurely. Others have an abnormality or an inherited disorder. A few die for no apparent reason. Certainly many more babies survive today compared to 20 years ago, due to advances in technology. Yet even with the best of care, just over 1% of babies still die in Australia.

The scope of this book cannot possibly cover the many experiences, procedures and emotions that may accompany the unanticipated tragedy of a baby dying. Even so, if you are reading this during the pregnancy, you may want to put some thought towards the types of choices parents make, in the short time they have to say goodbye to their baby.

These days, the death of a baby is acknowledged, and given the recognition

it deserves. Parents are given every opportunity to spend time with their baby (be this for hours or days afterwards). Saying goodbye in your own way helps enormously with grieving. Some things parents consider are:
- Seeing and holding their baby to help come to terms with their existence and death. Even parents who are told that their baby has a physical deformity find it is not as severe as anything they could have imagined. They invariably acknowledge the beauty of their child. Their perfect toes, their curly hair or their rosebud lips.
- Bathing and dressing their baby, to have intimate contact and to do some nurturing things for them. Many parents feel they have been robbed of their parenting role and this is their chance to take on this role with their child.
- Keepsakes are important and can remind parents and others that they did indeed have a baby. These may be photos, a lock of hair, foot and hand prints, the baby's identification bracelet, hospital record card or the bunny rug they were first wrapped in.
- Naming the baby allows them to be referred to by name and helps others relate to the baby as a person, who was very real. Some people hold a special naming ceremony, or a religious ceremony, as part of their farewells.

Grieving

There is no correct way to grieve. Individuals feel differently at different stages, moving through many emotions, such as numbness, disbelief and shock, as well as feeling disconnected, disorientated, angry, guilty, sad and lonely, despairing and depressed. These come and go in cycles, with no order or predictability, over months and years after the baby's death, at times feeling very intense, overwhelming and frightening. Commonly parents feel that no one else understands, and different expressions of grief between couples can cause relationship strains. Hopefully over time, and with love, support and many people to listen to and be with the pain, parents can move through their grief without it overwhelming their lives. Parents often need the help and support of professionals, or other parents who have had similar experiences. Contacts for organisations are in the resource section.

CHAPTER 8

Third and fourth stages of labour

The third stage

The third stage begins from the moment the baby is born until the delivery of the placenta, cord and membranes (or afterbirth). Over 95% of Australian women have an actively managed third stage in which they are given an injection of Syntocinon to deliver the placenta. The remaining women choose to have a natural third stage, which is generally facilitated in birth centres and homebirth.

The expulsion of the placenta is a complex process that consists of three phases.

1. Resting phase

Natural management: Once the baby is born, the uterus stops contracting for 10 to 20 minutes (ranging from 5 minutes to 1 hour). Most women use this time to rest and recover, enjoying their new baby.

Active management: An oxytocin injection is administered to the woman (usually into her thigh) as the baby's body is born. This makes the uterus contract within two to five minutes, preventing the resting phase from occurring.

2. Separation phase

Natural management: On seeing and holding her baby, the woman experiences a rush of emotions, accompanied by a surge of her own natural oxytocin hormone. This makes her uterus contract and tighten, becoming smaller and firmer (often felt as mild cramping or discomfort). The inner walls of the uterus shrink and the centre of the placenta detaches. It folds down over itself to shear the remaining outer rim and membranes (or the sac the baby was encased in) from the rest of the uterine wall.

Active management: The caregiver waits for signs of placental separation after the birth, which are:
- The uterus contracting (felt by touching the woman's lower belly).
- A trickle of blood from her vagina.
- The umbilical cord slightly lengthening.

The caregiver then holds the cord with one hand, using gentle traction to detach the placenta and membranes from the wall of the uterus. At the same time they put their other hand on the woman's lower belly to support her uterus (called controlled cord traction).

3. Expulsion phase

Natural management: After the placenta separates, the muscles of the uterus contract and retract, making the uterine space even smaller and pushing the afterbirth out through the partially opened cervix and into the woman's vagina. If she is upright, the weight of the placenta makes it come away effortlessly (literally falling out). However, if she is lying down or sitting, she may need to push the soft placenta out (or her caregiver assists with gentle traction on the cord, similar to removing a tampon). Both the separation and expulsion phases take place with one contraction.

Active management: The caregiver continues to draw down on the cord until the placenta becomes visible at the vaginal opening. They then place both hands on the placenta to ease it out, with the membranes following.

The fine membranes can sometimes be caught up if the cervix closes up before they can be delivered (oxytocin injections tend to do this). If this happens, the caregiver gently moves the placenta up and down, or in a twisting motion, to help release them. The woman may be asked to push (or perhaps cough), to help open her cervix slightly to assist this. Sometimes a surgical clamp is placed on the part of the membranes seen outside the vagina and twisted (similar to twirling spaghetti) to ease the membranes out, and avoid leaving any inside the uterus.

Once the entire afterbirth is delivered, the third stage is complete.

NATURAL VS ACTIVE MANAGEMENT

Most caregivers recommend actively managing the third stage to decrease the chances of a postpartum haemorrhage (PPH). Studies assessing the most appropriate way to manage this stage show clear benefits for routine active management, including:
- An overall reduction in blood loss.
- Less chance of experiencing a mild PPH.

- Less chance of a severe PPH.
- Less need for further oxytocic drugs to control heavy bleeding.
- Less likely to require a blood transfusion.
- Less chance of being anaemic after the birth.[1]

Some caregivers prefer to facilitate a natural third stage because of their philosophical beliefs about birth being a natural process and their desire to avoid intervention. Some evidence suggests that the risks of bleeding, and the amount of blood lost, are only slightly increased in a natural third stage.[2] Be aware, however, that up to 20% of women planning a natural third stage still require an oxytocic injection, either because the bleeding is heavier or to help deliver a retained placenta. Some birth centres recommend an oxytocic injection routinely if the labour is more than 24 hours, the second stage is more than 2 hours or the woman has had a previous birth with an excessive blood loss, because these factors increase the chances of a PPH.

NOTE: Depending on your chosen birthplace, you may need to make your preferences known. For example, birth centres may routinely facilitate a natural third stage and delivery suites routinely administer oxytocic injections. Discuss this with your caregiver before the birth or address it in your birth plan.

CLAMPING AND CUTTING THE CORD

At some stage after your baby is born, their cord needs to be cut. The caregiver places a sterile, plastic clamp on the cord, about 1 to 2 cm from the baby's belly button. They then place another metal surgical clamp on the cord, leaving a space between the two clamps, so the partner, woman or caregiver can cut it. The cord is quite rubbery and can be tough to cut.

> **Did you know?**
> The cord contains no nerves, similar to your hair or fingernails. So when it is cut there is no pain experienced by either mother or baby.

If the third stage is managed naturally, the cord is left to pulsate until the placenta has separated. This allows blood to continue to flow from the placenta to the baby for several minutes (albeit at a greatly reduced rate as the baby's lungs take over). With an actively managed third stage, the cord is clamped and cut within a minute after the baby is born, before it stops pulsating.

Reasons why parents choose to delay the cutting of the cord include:
- Wanting a more relaxed atmosphere.
- Allowing the complex interplay of physiological relationships that normally leads to an uncomplicated natural third stage.
- Waiting until the baby's circulation and breathing become stabilised.

- Allowing the baby to receive extra blood, estimated to be about 75 to 125 ml in total.[3]

Whether your baby needs extra blood is controversial. Allowing the cord to pulsate potentially provides up to 30% more blood volume and up to 60% more red blood cells.[4] Natural birth proponents believe this is part of the normal birth process, providing the baby with additional iron stores and preventing anaemia. Medical birth proponents believe it is not essential, possibly increasing the baby's chances of becoming jaundiced.

At this stage, it is not clear whether delaying the cutting of the cord is beneficial or detrimental for healthy, full-term babies born in developed countries. However, benefits have been shown for small, premature babies and babies in developing countries (who have a tendency to be anaemic).

The cord will need to be cut early if you intend to donate the baby's cord blood (see pages 302–303). Other reasons that may necessitate this include:
- Removing a cord that is tightly around the baby's neck at birth.
- The baby being unwell and requiring medical attention.
- The cord being unusually short, making it difficult to hold the baby, or to bring them to the surface after a water birth. This may simply mean changing position, or leaving the baby between your legs for a while (if not in the bath), if you are keen to leave the cord pulsating.

CHECKING THE PLACENTA

Your caregiver will examine the placenta, cord and membranes soon after the birth. This may be done in front of you if you wish to see the placenta, or in another room. The caregiver takes note of:
- The size, shape, thickness and texture of the placenta.
- Whether any sections look as though they were not functioning.
- Whether all the sections are present and it appears complete (in case some has been left in the uterus).
- Whether there are three blood vessels (two arteries and a vein) in the cord.

The placenta is then disposed of (usually incinerated) unless you wish to keep it (see page 303). If the baby is thought to have an inherited disorder, or is unwell or stillborn, the placenta may be sent to the pathology laboratory for examination and testing before being disposed of.

EMOTIONS

As **the woman** you may feel:
- Relief that you have your baby in your arms and you are both okay.

- Overwhelmed at the sheer enormity of what you and your baby have just achieved.
- Joy at touching and meeting your child. Love for them and your partner.
- Shocked or stunned if the labour and birth were quick, and not wanting to be touched.
- Invincible, you can do anything now!
- Wanting to see your other child(ren) and share the new baby.
- Disbelief – *I really did it! Is it really over?*
- Exhausted and wanting to sleep.
- Excited, wanting to tell the world, buzzing, unable to rest or sleep.

As **the partner or support person** you may feel:
- Relief that mother and baby are okay.
- Love for your partner and child.
- Excited, wanting to ring everyone.
- Disbelief – *Am I really a father?*
- An enormous sense of responsibility for your new family.
- Wonderful to be able to share something so amazing with the person you love, glad you were there.
- Total admiration and pride for her and what she has done.
- Concerned if there are problems.
- Exhausted and wanting to sleep.
- A special moment as the new baby is welcomed to the family.

ISSUES AND CONTROVERSIES
Types of oxytocic medications

Different types of oxytocin injections may be used to actively manage the third stage. The most common one is Syntocinon, but Ergometrine or Syntometrine can be used.

Syntocinon is a synthetic form of the natural oxytocin that closely mimics the normal short, rhythmic contractions of the uterus. It is effective, safe and produces few side effects, working within 2 to 3 minutes of being injected into a muscle, lasting 5 to 10 minutes (or within seconds of intravenous injection, but only lasting a couple of minutes).

Ergometrine is an uterotonic drug that increases the tone of the uterine muscles, causing strong, frequent and sometimes sustained contractions of the uterus. It works within 5 to 7 minutes of being injected into a muscle, lasting 2 to 4 hours (or within seconds of intravenous injection and lasting 45 minutes).

Compared to Syntocinon, Ergometrine further reduces the total amount of blood loss but can at times cause severe side effects, such as nausea, vomiting, continual painful or labour-like contractions, a rise in blood pressure, dizziness, ringing in the ears, headache, palpitations and occasionally 'entrapping' or retaining of the placenta (if it has not been delivered yet).

Routine Ergometrine is now used less for actively managing the third stage, but may be used if the woman's bleeding is not adequately controlled after a Syntocinon injection.

Syntometrine is a mix of Syntocinon and Ergometrine which makes the uterus contract sooner than Syntocinon alone, also sustaining more intense contractions for a longer period of time after the birth. However, the side effects of Ergometrine remain. Recent studies show only slight differences in blood loss for women given Syntometrine when compared to just Syntocinon alone.[5] You may wish to ask your caregiver which type they prefer to use.

Rhesus negative blood group

At birth it is normal for a small amount of the baby's blood to cross over into their mother's bloodstream, usually as the placenta separates. For women who are Rhesus negative, this may set up a reaction called isoimmunisation (see Chapter 4). Therefore the caregiver takes a sample of blood from the baby's cord attached to the placenta (after it is clamped and cut), to test and determine the baby's Rhesus factor and blood group. If the baby is Rhesus positive, the woman requires an injection of anti-D immunoglobulin within 72 hours of the birth to prevent antibodies forming. If her baby is Rhesus negative, no injection is required.

Most hospitals also perform an additional blood test on the woman in the hours following the birth to measure how much of the baby's blood (if any) has passed into her bloodstream, so that the correct dose of anti-D immunoglobulin can be given.

A few women choose to decline anti-D. This may be due to religious or personal beliefs about accepting blood products, or because they feel they will not have any more children (although soon after having a baby is not the ideal time to make definite decisions about further children). If you do decline, it is advisable to have a blood test 6 to 12 months after the birth, or prior to conceiving another child, to see whether antibodies have formed.

Cord blood donation

It is possible to donate your baby's cord blood to the Australian Cord Blood Bank, to treat children and adults suffering from leukaemia and some cancers.

However, this is not available in all hospitals or birth centres (check with your caregiver), and is not possible with homebirths.

Most women are able to donate their baby's cord blood, but some circumstances make cord blood unsuitable for donation:

- Women carrying HIV/AIDS or Hepatitis B or C.
- Women who have spent at least six months in the UK between 1 January 1980 and 31 December 1996, in case of mad cow disease.
- Having a fever during labour or the baby being less than 36 weeks gestation.
- The baby having a known inherited abnormality, being distressed during labour or unwell at birth.

If cord blood donation is available at your birthplace, ask your caregiver for a leaflet explaining the procedure, a consent form to sign and a questionnaire to fill in. When you arrive at your birthplace let your caregiver know you intend to donate your baby's cord blood (or include this in your birth plan).

The labour and birth proceed as normal, but the third stage is actively managed to ensure enough blood is collected. The baby is also placed on the woman's belly (or in her arms) for up to a minute before clamping the cord to increase the amount of blood available for donation. Once the cord is clamped and cut, blood is taken from the cord and placenta.

The cord blood is transported to the Australian Cord Blood Bank laboratory within 36 hours, where it is tested, processed and labelled with a nonidentifiable number before being frozen until required by a compatible child or adult needing a transplant. It can be stored for up to 20 years. Personal details of each mother and baby are kept confidential and separate from the cord blood.

There are now private companies who offer to collect your baby's cord blood for a fee in case stem cell research is developed to treat diseases such as heart disease, Parkinson's, Alzheimer's, multiple sclerosis, diabetes or cancer. This is controversial and in reality there is only a very small chance of your baby's blood being useful. As a guide:

- Within your family the only use for the cord blood at this stage is for treating leukaemia, and then only if the child's sibling or perhaps a close family member has leukaemia, as it is not recommended to donate a child's own stem cells back to them because their cells are obviously susceptible to the disease.
- Using it for diseases the baby may contract is unlikely, even assuming the science is perfected, as the blood can only be stored for up to 20 years.

Private donations are different from donating to the Australian Cord Blood Bank (which is free). They cannot be registered to help other children with leukaemia and are only kept for the family paying for it.

Placenta rituals

Rituals involving the placenta or afterbirth have been with us since ancient times. A popular ritual today is to plant the placenta under a special tree for the baby.

NOTE: The placenta needs to be buried at least 40 cm or deeper (or placed in a very large pot, so the rich placenta does not burn the tree's root system). Most local councils place restrictions on burying human body parts, especially in public areas.

A less common ritual is to eat the placenta (either raw or cooked) in the belief that it contains hormones and nutrients that promote a healthy recovery. Placentas are actually high in zinc, which is known to alleviate postnatal depression.

Did you know?
- Aborigines use the cord to make necklaces for the child to wear to ward off disease.
- The Sudanese consider the placenta to be the infant's 'spirit double', and it is buried in a place that represents the parents' hopes for their child (eg. close to a hospital to become a doctor).
- In Yemen the placenta is placed on the family's roof for the birds to eat, in the hope that it will guarantee love between the parents.
- Malaysians see the placenta as the child's older sibling, with the two being reunited at death. The midwife carefully washes it and wraps it in a white cloth to be buried.
- The Chinese consider the placenta a powerful medicine. It is dried and powdered and placed in capsules for the woman to take at various times in her life, including menopause.

If you are planning a ritual, your caregiver places the placenta in strong plastic bags, or an airtight container, for you to take home. It may be placed in the freezer until you are ready to carry out the ritual.

A **lotus birth** involves leaving the cord unclamped and uncut while it dries and separates naturally from the baby's belly button (taking 5 to 10 days). The placenta is usually washed and salted, or smothered in herbs or essential oils a couple of times a day to help with the smell. It is wrapped in a towel and/or kept in a plastic bag, so it can be held comfortably with the baby while they are being fed and cared for. Lotus births are a Buddhist tradition believed to nurture good health and a long life.

The fourth stage

The first hour after the placenta is delivered is the fourth stage. The woman rests, recuperates, eats, drinks and gets to know her new baby. The fourth stage is generally spent where you gave birth, and if all has gone normally, you might use the time to take photos, freshen up, ring relatives and friends, and perhaps have a small celebration. However, for a few parents it is spent dealing with unexpected complications that have developed with the third stage, or with concerns because their baby is unwell. During the first hour after the birth the woman's body stabilises. Her physical recovery will depend on the type of labour and birth she had and if there were complications.

PHYSICAL RECOVERY
Bleeding

The average blood loss at birth is 200 to 400 ml (equivalent to a blood donation), but can range from 50 to 500 ml. When blood is spread over bed sheets, it can look like a lot, but your caregiver is aware of what is normal.

The uterus continues to contract to control the flow of blood where the placenta was attached. These contractions can sometimes be strong after pains (more common with subsequent babies). During the fourth stage it is normal for the bleeding to be heavier than a normal period, often soaking a pad. This will settle in the hours to follow.

Shivery and shaky

It is normal to shiver and shake; a warm blanket, removing wet linen from beneath you, having a warm drink and something to eat can help. Some women take Bach or bush flower remedies such as Rescue Remedy or Emergency Essence.

Removing drips, epidurals and catheters

Most women are keen to shed any attachments they may have, such as:
- **An intravenous drip** – This may be left in until after you pass urine (usually within an hour or two of the birth).
- **A urinary catheter** – If the bleeding is normal, the catheter can be removed soon after the placenta has been delivered.
- **An epidural catheter** – This is taken out soon after the birth, but it may be an hour or two before full sensation returns. Don't attempt to get up unaided.

EMOTIONS
The fourth stage is usually a special, exciting time, full of mixed emotions. You may find it is quiet and reflective, or perhaps intense, as the preceding labour events still hang in the air. You may feel:
- **Alert and euphoric** – Your hormones can make it difficult to sleep (even if the labour was long and exhausting). Many women have a need to share the experience, finding their minds are buzzing while their partner or support person falls asleep!
- **Exhausted and lethargic** – Perhaps you've literally run out of steam, with no energy or inclination to even hold the baby. You may need some space to rest and be nurtured yourself.
- **Empty** – Some women experience a profound sense of unexplainable loss and physical emptiness.
- **Shocked, overwhelmed, out of control and/or anxious** – This is especially the case if complications are now unfolding or the baby is unwell.

SUPPORT STRATEGIES
After completing the amazing task of giving birth, physical and emotional support is still required. Even if you feel you are on an invincible high, don't underestimate the enormous experience your body has just been through and the adjustment it is still making. The new baby can easily (and unintentionally) absorb the attention of your partner or support people and they may need gentle reminding that you still need their support.

Some parents plan for a specific environment soon after the birth (dim lighting, people talking quietly, playing certain music), as well as making breastfeeding the baby a priority. You may request that your caregiver delay weighing and measuring your baby to facilitate this.

Getting comfortable
Most women are aware of several discomforts (or pain), including sore, stinging and swollen genitals, lower backache, haemorrhoids, afterpains, perhaps even a sore throat from making noise during the birth. Ask for help to get comfortable, especially if you want to breastfeed. Get others to place extra pillows where you need them, and lower or lift the head of the bed (if adjustable), or lie on your side to take the pressure off your perineum and bottom. Possibly ask for some painkilling tablets or a heat pack for cramping. Small ice packs can be placed on the genitals or haemorrhoids. Some women take homeopathic remedies (such as Arnica). Consider asking your support person to manage one last massage!

Getting up for a shower
It can be great to wash, change clothes and clean your teeth after the birth. Take care when moving around. Ask your caregiver if it is okay to get up. Have someone physically help you to the toilet or shower when needed.

Hungry and thirsty
It is not unusual to feel ravenous after the birth. If you've used up your supply of favourite foods and treats send your support person out for a takeaway.

As **the partner or support person** you need to:

Remain sensitive to her needs
She still needs your support, so try not to pull back or shut down amidst the excitement of the new baby arriving. Shower her with admiration. If she does not wish to hold her baby yet, hold the baby close by until she is ready.

The caregiver will usually remain present until the woman and baby are stabilised, making her comfortable. However, sometimes they are busy (or preoccupied because the baby is unwell) and may leave you alone for periods of time. In some cases the woman is left physically uncomfortable, or emotionally vulnerable, and it may be up to you to meet her needs. Cover her if she is feeling cold or exposed. Find some extra blankets (ask the midwives) and make her comfortable with pillows. If the sheets are wet, gently place dry towels underneath her and get her a sanitary napkin. Make her a cup of tea or a cold drink and get her something to eat. If she is looking shocked or overwhelmed, stay close and give her a cuddle.

If you are worried about the amount she is bleeding, or the baby's health, ask (or buzz) for help straightaway.

NOTE: *Don't remove her legs from stirrups if she is in these, and stop her if she attempts to do this herself. Two people are needed to do this in the correct manner to avoid nerve and ligament strain.*

Physical help
She will probably feel a bit weak and shaky. Make sure the caregiver gives the okay for her to get up to the shower or toilet. Stay close by in case she feels light-headed or faint. Hold her arm and walk with her. Sit with her while she showers. She may need a plastic chair in the shower if she feels weak. Help her dry her legs and put on her underwear for her so she doesn't have to bend down. Walk with her back to the room.

Support yourself

While the woman is still your priority, it is also important to support yourself. Have something to eat and rest with the baby. If the bed is big enough, you may be able to curl up together for a short nap. When calling relatives and friends, consider how long it will be before they arrive on the doorstep. Perhaps delay contacting them or ask them to wait a while.

EXPECTATIONS FOR CARE

Your caregiver frequently checks the physical wellbeing of you and your baby (Chapter 12 deals with your baby's care). This may include:

- Checking your blood loss every 15 to 30 minutes (or if you feel the bleeding is heavy).
- Feeling the fundus of the uterus to make sure it is hard and contracted.
- Possibly taking your blood pressure and pulse (if concerned).
- Checking your genital tears or grazes, and placing stitches in if necessary.
- Assisting you to feed your baby (if required).
- Helping you to the shower and toilet, or getting support people to do this.

If you have a private obstetrician, they normally leave once the placenta is delivered (or after suturing any genital tears or an episiotomy). If you have a homebirth, the midwife generally stays for at least two hours to make sure you have passed urine, the bleeding is controlled and the baby is well and has fed. The midwife should be on call to return at short notice if needed (or arrange for another midwife, if they are too tired or unavailable).

Are stitches required?

The decision to suture a graze, tear or episiotomy depends on:

- How extensive the injury is.
- Whether the tear is expected to cause problems or pain in the long term if not stitched.
- The preferences of the caregiver.
- Your own preferences. (Genital injuries are discussed in Chapter 7.)

In recent years it has increasingly become the view that caregivers tend to 'overstitch' childbirth injuries, because many heal well on their own. A woman's genitals are made of similar tissue to the human mouth. Both these areas generally bleed heavily and swell immensely but have an amazing capacity to heal. As stitching has only become routine in the last century, it seems reasonable that women should take part in deciding whether stitches are required or not. Discuss this during the pregnancy.

Making the choice – Caregivers will vary in their preferences and flexibility with suturing. They may like to put a stitch or two in, no matter how slight the injury, or be happy to let small tears and grazes heal on their own. Some women prefer stitches, while others wish to avoid them unless absolutely necessary.

You can ask your caregiver for a mirror to see first-hand what the injury involves. Bear in mind, however, that it can be difficult for an untrained eye to tell how severe the injury is when the genitals are swollen and covered in blood. If the tear is small, neat and not too deep, you may ask your caregiver to leave it. However, if the two edges of the tear do not meet up, or it's deep or in an awkward position, you may be more inclined to accept stitches.

The stitching – In most cases the stitching is done soon after the birth, but it may be delayed until you feel more recovered and/or the baby has fed (ie. an hour or so). When being stitched, you need to lie on your back on the bed, with your bottom just over the edge and your legs supported in stirrups (or chairs if at home). A strong light is shone on the area, to help the caregiver see clearly.

If you had an epidural or spinal and it is still effective, this normally provides adequate pain relief. If not, then a local anaesthetic is used. This can sting as it is being administered and you may need to 'breathe through' it or ask for some gas. Some caregivers add sodium bicarbonate to the local anaesthetic to reduce the sting.

It takes a few minutes for the anaesthetic to take full effect. If the stitching is hurting, ask your caregiver to wait, or for more anaesthetic. Try to consciously relax your bottom. This makes the procedure more comfortable for you and easier for your caregiver to insert the stitches. There are many different types of suture materials. All dissolve and do not need to be removed (unless they're causing problems). Stitches can take two weeks or up to three to four months to completely dissolve, depending on the type.

> **Did you know?**
> Many women ask, 'How many stitches?' However, because long, continuous stitches are often used, as well as separate stitches, the number is only a rough estimate. The more stitches you have, the deeper the tear, not necessarily the larger the size, because the injury needs to be repaired in separate layers.

Once the stitches are in place, the caregiver gently checks inside the vagina to make sure the stitching is complete. If the tear (or episiotomy) was deep, they may also place one finger gently inside the anus to make sure the stitches have not accidentally gone through to the rectum (otherwise the stitches will need to be removed). Local anaesthetic provides good pain relief to the area for a couple of hours, after which some ice to the area and/or pain relieving tablets can help.

Variations for third and fourth stages

Variations during these final stages can affect the early postnatal experience and the opportunity to connect intimately with your baby. Many women feel saddened, distressed and upset if this time is filled with worrying complications, and often they need to grieve for this lost time.

DIFFICULTY URINATING
Your caregiver will encourage you to pass urine within an hour or so of having your baby (even though this may be the last thing you feel like doing). Emptying your bladder allows the uterus to keep well contracted to control the bleeding and also lets your caregiver know that everything is in working order. If you had a catheter during labour, or passed urine while pushing your baby, it may take a couple of hours for your bladder to fill again, so drink plenty of water.

It can sometimes sting to pass urine if you have sustained grazes around the labia. If this is the case, try:
- Passing urine in the shower or bath, while sitting in a bowl of warm water, or while pouring a jug of warm water onto the genitals (on the toilet).
- Leaning backwards, if the grazes are near the labia, or leaning forwards if they are towards the base of the vagina.
- Taking urinary alkalinisers every four to six hours to make the urine less acidic.
- Putting ointment on the grazes (pawpaw or calendula). Avoid vaseline or zinc, which don't promote healing of the tissue underneath.

Nerve damage to the bladder
On rare occasions the nerves to the bladder can be injured from pressure during a vaginal, forceps or caesarean birth, or if the bladder becomes overfull when an epidural or spinal is in place. Signs of nerve damage are normally evident during the first two days after the birth, and can include:
- Difficulty passing urine.

- Not being able to sense or feel when you need to go to the toilet.
- Urine dribbling away in small amounts uncontrollably.
- The bladder feeling full, even though you have just been to the toilet.

To help the nerves heal and to stop the bladder from overfilling, a urinary catheter is inserted for a few days. The nerves often return to their full function after this time, so when the catheter is removed you can empty the bladder normally. However, for a few women this can take weeks, possibly requiring a consultation with a physiotherapist or continence advisor. The strategies used to help pass urine during labour in Chapter 6 may help.

FEELING FAINT

Losing the normal amount of blood at birth can lower your blood pressure and make you feel faint, weak and shaky. Sometimes women momentarily pass out, especially if they stand up too soon, have been bleeding heavily or were anaemic during pregnancy. Some women even have difficulty sitting up in bed and need to delay getting up for several hours.

- Allow your body time to stabilise. Delay getting up for at least 45 minutes to an hour, longer if the blood loss was heavy. Lie on your side to breastfeed if you need to. Maybe wait until after a good night's sleep, if the faintness continues.
- Drink at least four large glasses of water, or diluted juice, during the hour after giving birth, and have something to eat.
- Limit (or avoid) champagne or other alcohol, which can lower your blood pressure further.
- Get up slowly, once your caregiver says it is okay. Sit up first, then hang your feet over the side of the bed and stay there for a minute. If that feels fine, then slowly get up. Make sure someone is with you, and sit down again if you feel faint. If getting up from a mat on the floor, or out of the bath, go onto your hands and knees first.
- Always have someone with you or nearby when you're up. Have a plastic chair in the bathroom and don't make the shower too hot. Ventilate the room and take a cool drink with you.
- You may want to try some Bach or bush flower remedies (Rescue Remedy or Emergency Essence). Aromatherapists often recommend rejuvenating oils on a tissue to smell (lemon or tangerine). Avoid lavender, bergamot or ylang ylang, which can further lower your blood pressure.

A vasovagal

In rare circumstances the woman may experience a vasovagal episode. This can initially be mistaken for fainting, but within seconds can resemble something more serious, because she temporarily stops breathing and turns blue. Vasovagals are fairly short-lived, with the woman recovering within 30 seconds to a minute or so, but are quite scary to witness and disorientating for the woman as she regains her awareness.

This dramatic reaction is a normal response to stimulation of the vagus nerve, often because a blood clot is sitting inside the woman's cervix.

HAEMATOMAS

If the vulva, vagina or perineum abnormally swell within a few hours of the birth, blood may be collecting under the skin or stitches (similar to a bruise). This is called a haematoma and can make the area feel full, dragging, throbbing or heavy, often becoming increasingly painful as the hours pass.

A doctor may need to gently lance the area to allow the blood to be released, normally bringing great relief. Sometimes the stitches are removed to allow bleeding blood vessels to be tied off, or have pressure applied to them, before restitching the area. Ice packs to the genitals can be soothing afterwards, especially if you have needed to be re-stitched. Homeopathic Arnica (for bruising) may be helpful.

PRIMARY POSTPARTUM HAEMORRHAGE

A primary postpartum haemorrhage is excessive bleeding within 24 hours of the baby being born (either vaginally or with a caesarean). This can complicate around 6% of births. A PPH is normally caused by the uterus not contracting efficiently after the placenta is delivered, or with severe tears of the vagina or cervix. Factors that can increase the chances of a PPH include:
- An abnormally long or fast labour.
- A full bladder soon after the birth.
- Very large fibroids in the uterus.
- Placenta previa, placental abruption, twins (or more), polyhydramnios or a large baby (more than 4.5 kg or 10 lb).
- Experiencing a PPH with a previous birth.
- Taking some medications in the days just before the birth (for blood pressure or premature labour, a general anaesthetic, aspirin or heparin).

A few women bleed if feeling distressed, perhaps because their baby is unwell, making their body release adrenaline, which suppresses uterine contractions.

Women increase their blood volume by up to 50% during pregnancy, to around 6000 ml. A normal 200 to 500 ml blood loss at birth is about 3 to 10% of the total blood volume. In the days following, large amounts of urine are passed to excrete this excess fluid. Therefore, haemorrhaging during the first 24 hours does not affect women as much as excessive bleeding after this time.

Postpartum haemorrhages are classified into grades of severity:

- **Class 1** – 700 to 1000 ml (11 to 15% of blood volume), accounts for most PPHs and is regarded as mild. The woman shows minimal physical signs, perhaps feeling a little faint and weak.
- **Class 2** – 1100 to 1500 ml (18 to 25% of blood volume), moderate to severe. Physical signs include a low blood pressure, fast pulse, breathlessness and unable to get up without feeling light-headed and/or fainting.
- **Class 3** – 1600 to 2100 ml (26 to 35% of blood volume), uncommon but severe. The woman is quite unwell, with rapid breathing, feeling cold, clammy and sweaty, looking pale and possibly passing out or collapsing, requiring intravenous fluids, oxygen and perhaps a blood transfusion.
- **Class 4** – Over 2400 ml (40% of blood volume), very rare but life-threatening, requiring urgent medical attention and immediate blood transfusion.

When treating a PPH, the main aim is to deliver the placenta as soon as possible (if this hasn't happened already) and stimulate the uterus to contract. The caregiver rubs the woman's lower belly, administers further oxytocic injections and starts an intravenous drip to replace fluids (or in case a blood transfusion is needed). If the woman cannot urinate, a catheter is inserted.

A recently introduced treatment is to administer prostaglandin medications, as an injection or tablet (or suppository into the vagina or anus). This can be an effective emergency measure before the blood loss becomes excessive, but may cause side effects such as nausea, vomiting and diarrhoea (sometimes accompanied by abdominal pain).

NOTE: *Some women choose to decline a blood transfusion unless their haemorrhage is life-threatening, preferring just to rest, eat well and take iron supplements. However, depending on the severity of the blood loss, this may mean being slowly nursed back to health by family and friends for over 6 to 12 weeks.*

Recovery after a PPH usually involves resting, eating well, taking iron supplements and being helped with your mothering and domestic duties for six to eight weeks. It is common to feel weak and to tire easily, perhaps being more prone to feeling depressed. Patience is needed to allow your body time to heal.

A severe PPH can affect breast milk supply, perhaps taking longer for the milk to come in and fully establish. It may be necessary to feed your baby more frequently to increase milk production in the early weeks.

Natural therapies may include regular massages and/or acupuncture. Herbalists may suggest fennel seed and nettle (for milk supply), and possibly lady's mantle, squaw vine and/or raspberry leaf for building energy and uterine muscle tone. Homeopaths may recommend Cocculus, Kali phosphoricum, Nux vomica, Staphysagria or Phosphoric acid for exhaustion. Consult your practitioner.

Retained placenta

Occasionally the placenta does not readily expel from the uterus after the baby is born and is said to be retained. The placenta may:

- Not separate at all, meaning bleeding is minimal and there is time to wait and use alternative measures to encourage it to come, before medically intervening.
- Separate partially, but remain inside the uterus, making bleeding heavy from the area where the placenta has detached. Bleeding continues until the placenta is fully expelled from the uterus, meaning interventions are quickly needed to prevent excessive bleeding.

Sometimes a small section of the placenta is retained after the placenta is delivered. This is usually expelled with a blood clot during the hours (or days) after the birth but may cause an infection, and sometimes heavy bleeding, if it remains in the uterus, requiring antibiotics and perhaps a D&C.

If the bleeding is not heavy (and your caregiver is prepared to wait), you may wish to try some natural therapies to encourage the expulsion of the placenta. These include:

- Nipple stimulation to trigger a release of natural oxytocin hormone (see Chapter 10), or offering the baby the breast to suckle.
- Emptying the bladder, changing position to being more upright, or moving to the toilet.
- A firm massage to the lower back.
- Herbalist remedies, such as blue or black cohosh, or pennyroyal leaf.
- Aromatherapy; perhaps clary sage, geranium or frankincense, diluted in a carrier oil and massaged onto the lower back, or as a warm compress to the lower back and/or abdomen.
- Homeopathic remedies – Arnica, Cimicifuga, Pulsatilla or Secale.
- Acupressure to the foot point, ankle point, or hand point for one

minute, every three to four minutes, until the placenta comes. (See acupressure appendix.)
- Visualising the placenta separating and coming away, and the uterus contracting. (See visualisation appendix.)

If the bleeding is heavy, or natural interventions are unsuccessful, medical interventions will be required, which may include:
- Administering more oxytocic drugs.
- The doctor manually removing the placenta under an epidural or general anaesthetic. Although, if the bleeding is excessive, there may be little time to administer these and gas may be used.
- An umbilical vein injection, which involves injecting a solution of salt water and Syntocinon into the vein of the umbilical cord leading to the placenta (after it has been cut and the baby separated). This can reduce the rate of manual removal of the placenta from 28% to 4%.

Placenta accreta

In very rare circumstances the placenta attaches to the muscles of the uterus instead of the lining and will not separate (called placenta accreta). The doctor may try to cut it away in the operating theatre under anaesthetic, but occasionally a hysterectomy is required. If there is not much placenta attached, it may be left inside the uterus in the hope it is naturally reabsorbed (which has varying degrees of success).

Women who lose their uterus have a great loss to grieve, needing counselling and support to help them come to terms with this devastating outcome.

THIRD AND FOURTH DEGREE TEARS

These injuries involve the woman's perineum tearing down to and partially through the edge of the anus (third degree) or completely through the anus and/or rectum (fourth degree), damaging the anal sphincter, the double ring of muscle that opens and closes to release wind and bowel motions. The incidence of third and fourth degree tear rates is not really known because they are generally underreported, but they range from 0.2% to 4%.[6]

These tears are unpredictable but tend to occur more often if:
- It is a first baby.
- An episiotomy is performed, especially a midline episiotomy.
- Forceps are used, or to a lesser extent a ventouse, or the birth is complicated by shoulder dystocia.

- The baby weighs over 4.5 kg (or 10 lb) or is born in a posterior position or as a compound presentation.
- The birth is unusually fast.

Third and fourth degree tears need to be repaired meticulously by an obstetrician or a senior obstetric registrar, using a local, epidural, spinal or light general anaesthetic in the delivery suite or operating theatre. If the tear extends into the bowel, some obstetricians ask a colorectal surgeon to perform the repair.

Caring for a third or fourth degree tear is similar to caring for other tears. Often antibiotics are prescribed to prevent an infection developing. Avoiding constipation is also important and your caregiver may prescribe laxatives and advise taking painkillers with codeine.

Physical recovery can be a slow and difficult process. The majority of women recover well without long-term problems, although it is widely believed that complications are underreported. For a few women, ongoing health issues can persist for weeks, months or longer, and these may include:
- Anal incontinence, including an inability to control wind, or less commonly faeces. There may be feelings of urgency to get to the toilet before the motion is accidentally passed (more common with fourth degree tears).[7]
- Continued perineal pain, which can be quite debilitating and difficult to cope with. Hopefully this will improve over time as the muscles heal and strengthen. A few women have further corrective surgery, which may or may not be successful.
- Painful sexual intercourse. This may improve over time or the woman may have a further operation, which may or may not be successful.

Your caregiver may order tests to assess how the tear has healed, especially if ongoing problems are being experienced (such as incontinence). These can include an ultrasound of the lower rectum, using a probe inside the anus or measuring rectal pressure with a probe placed into the rectum.

For women planning another baby, opinions vary about the best options for giving birth. Women with a previous fourth degree tear, and increasingly women with a previous third degree tear, are advised to have caesareans for subsequent births, particularly if they have experienced problems with their tears or if it is believed the tear was caused by a complication that may reoccur, such as shoulder dystocia or a large baby.

Taking a just-in-case approach may suit some women but not others. Be aware that up to 95% of women who have had a third degree tear do not sustain further anal sphincter damage at the next birth.[8] So ultimately it is your choice. This may be a difficult, emotional decision and you need to consider factors such as the extent of your injuries, how they have healed and your personal wishes for future births.

The thought of a tear involving the anus is distressing, with the birth and/or repair being potentially traumatic. Fears about how your body will recover and whether you will have long-term problems are normal and can be hard to deal with when mothering your baby, in some cases leading to feelings of depression. A few women even feel angry at their baby for doing this to them, or angry with their caregiver if they were not happy with the way the birth unfolded.

It is important you have support, understanding and help around you. Try to express your feelings honestly with your partner, family or friends. Tell your caregiver, even though you may feel your injuries are private or embarrassing. You may wish to talk with a professional counsellor or phone the Australian Continence Foundation (1800 330066) to speak with an expert continence nurse advisor for confidential and professional advice.

ANAL FISSURES

An anal fissure is a superficial tear, or small ulcer, just inside the anus. Anal fissures can develop in any person at any time of their life, through straining and passing large bowel motions, but a few women have them as a result of their anus stretching during childbirth.

An anal fissure can cause sharp pain when opening the bowels, persisting for several minutes, up to one or two hours afterwards, and possibly bleeding slightly. Most heal within two to four weeks after the birth, but some women find that they continue to be painful and irritating for several months.

Some support strategies include:
- Avoiding constipation.
- After opening the bowels, filling the bath (or a bowl) with warm water and sitting in it for a few minutes. You may wish to add 1 part salt to 10 parts water.
- Trying calendula or pawpaw ointment.
- Applying a paste with slippery elm powder, water, vitamin E oil and comfrey root powder. Check with your herbalist for measures.

Medicated creams may be prescribed to help decrease any inflammation (usually containing small amounts of steroids). If the anal fissure continues for several months, you may be offered an operation to repair it. However, this carries the risk of damaging and weakening the anal sphincter, possibly leading to anal incontinence.[9]

Uterine inversion

An inversion of the uterus is a rare complication, occurring in about 1 in every 100,000 births (or 0.001%). The top of the uterus is pushed (or pulled) down, coming through the woman's cervix and into her vagina, straining the supporting uterine ligaments and causing sudden, sharp pain, as well as a sensation that something is in the vagina. If it is sudden, the woman may collapse from shock. Uterine inversions normally occur when caregivers try to deliver the placenta without a contraction (while it is still attached to the uterus) or while trying to deliver a retained placenta.

The caregiver aims to replace the uterus to its normal position as quickly and gently as possible. A narcotic injection may be administered for pain relief and sometimes a light general anaesthetic is used while the uterus is being replaced. Treatments can also include:

- Intravenous medications to help relax the uterus while it is being replaced.
- Oxygen and intravenous fluids for the woman to reverse the physical shock.
- An oxytocin injection or prostaglandin medication to make the uterus contract strongly and remain in its normal position.

A uterine inversion should not affect a woman's fertility or her ability to carry another baby. However, there is a slightly increased risk of experiencing another uterine inversion with a subsequent vaginal birth.

CHAPTER 9

The pain of labour

The thoughts of a pregnant woman frequently turn towards the impending birth and the pain involved, especially as the baby's due date draws near. When talking with other women, debates about dealing with labour pain often polarise into two camps. One side viewing the pain as pointless and to be avoided at all costs, so 'take any drug you can'; the other camp seeing medical pain relief as having potential side effects, besides 'women have been doing it naturally for years.' However, many women approach their labour somewhere in between these ideas, often taking a wait-and-see approach and being open to accepting pain relief under certain circumstances.

Pain is a complex, private and very personal experience, which can at times feel isolating. However, physical pain sensations are only part of the whole picture. The woman's mind, body and emotions influence her pain, going beyond the physiological process of her labouring and birthing body.

The physiology of pain

We have many inbuilt physical mechanisms that help us deal naturally with pain. Understanding these can ensure you gain the maximum benefits from your chosen pain-relieving options, when the time comes.

Pain is transmitted to the brain by three types of sensory nerves:
- **A-beta fibres** – large nerves that sense heat, cold, light, touch and massage.
- **A-delta fibres** – medium-sized nerves that sense brief, sharp, jabbing or pricking-type pains.
- **C fibres** – small nerves that detect longer-lasting, burning or aching sensations.

All these nerves come into play at various stages of the labour and birth.

When part of the body is stretched, changed, irritated or injured, the tissues release a chemical called bradykinin, which attaches to the receiving ends of nerve fibres, transmitting the message of pain to the spinal cord. Here they meet ascending nerve fibres which relay the pain messages up the spinal cord to the brain, where it is interpreted as a pain sensation. However, we know of two physical mechanisms that can naturally modify this process so the sensations seem less painful.

Endorphin release

Endorphins are opiate-like substances manufactured by the body in the presence of pain. They act as natural analgesics, and it is thought that pregnant women manufacture more endorphins just prior to labour.

When labour reaches a certain pain level, endorphins are released by the spinal cord nerves, preventing some pain messages from reaching the brain and decreasing the woman's sense of discomfort. For many women endorphins also positively alter their memory of the birth by creating an amnesic effect. This has the potential to provide an internal protection against the intensity of labour and giving birth.

The gate control theory

The large nerve fibres that sense touch, heat, cold and pressure carry messages to the spinal cord more rapidly than smaller nerve fibres, which sense sharp, burning or aching pains. This gives large nerve fibres priority, so they can override or shut the gate to pain messages.

This is why we instinctively rub our bodies when we are hurt, and why heat packs and massage can alter the intensity of labour pain. Other triggers for the gate control are changing position, walking, rocking, stomping and pelvic rocking, because large nerve receptors are activated in the moving muscles and joints.

If pain increases to a very high level, the gate can be pushed back open to a degree, making the sensation stronger and methods relying on the gate control less effective. However, the release of endorphins usually compensates at this point.

THE PAIN OF LABOUR AND BIRTH

As labour begins, pain messages are sent along the small nerve fibres to the spinal cord and brain to be interpreted as pain. Stimulation of large nerve fibres, with touch, heat, cold or massage, intercepts some of the pain messages by reaching the spinal cord first. The final pain sensation is modified before reaching the woman's brain to be interpreted, and then expressed, as a physical response to pain.

As labour progresses and intensifies, the woman's conscious pain sensations increase. This triggers a release of endorphins, diminishing the pain messages relayed to her brain, making her perceive it as less intense.

During transition, the labour intensifies to the point that the gate control is overridden, making touch, heat, cold or massage less effective. The woman's body releases more endorphins as she attempts to lessen her perception of pain. Many women become drowsy and sleepy, appearing introverted, less responsive and spaced out, with their eyes glazing over. This is also the part of labour that seems hardest to remember afterwards, because of the amnesic effect of the endorphins.

During the second stage, the larger nerves of the vagina, pelvic floor, anus and perineum start to sense pain from pressure and stretching as the baby moves down the birth canal. Applying warmth to the area with warm compresses (or a bath) helps close the gate again to the intensity of the pain.

The woman's perception of her labour pain

Each woman's labour experience is uniquely her own. For many it is hard but manageable. For others it is all-consuming and overwhelming. A few find it tolerable, or merely uncomfortable, perhaps virtually painless. Rarely, it has been described as orgasmic and pleasurable. All these experiences are possible, but for most women, labour *is* painful.

Each woman responds to labour pain in her own way, but the amount of discomfort she feels can also be influenced by her:
- Fears and concerns.
- Past pain experiences.
- Psychological approach and pain threshold.
- Expectations.
- Partner's or support person's influence.
- Caregiver's expectations.
- Feeling in control.
- Social, cultural and spiritual beliefs.

The labour experience brings vulnerability, stress and varying levels of distress, all expected reactions to the process the body is going through. How a woman interprets her pain affects her choices about managing, or controlling it, and ultimately how she feels about her labour and birth afterwards.

Fears and concerns

Some women approach their labour in a very open and accepting way, confident in their body's ability to give birth and to deal with their pain. Others are not so sure, or are admittedly nervous, scared or even terrified of what may lie ahead. Fear of the unknown and concerns about the what-if?s are fairly normal during pregnancy. However, suppressing your fears may only make them resurface in some way, shape or form during labour, increasing the level of pain felt.

Some cultures believe that fear is the main cause of a labouring woman suffering in childbirth. This theory does have a physiological explanation. A woman's underlying fears can make her body tense, often without realising it. Adrenaline is then released, inhibiting her endorphins, which are needed to help relieve pain. Adrenaline also inhibits contractions, prolonging the labour. Increased pain and a prolonged labour can create anxiety, making her feel she is not coping or progressing, adding to her fears and increasing the pain. This ends up being a vicious cycle of:

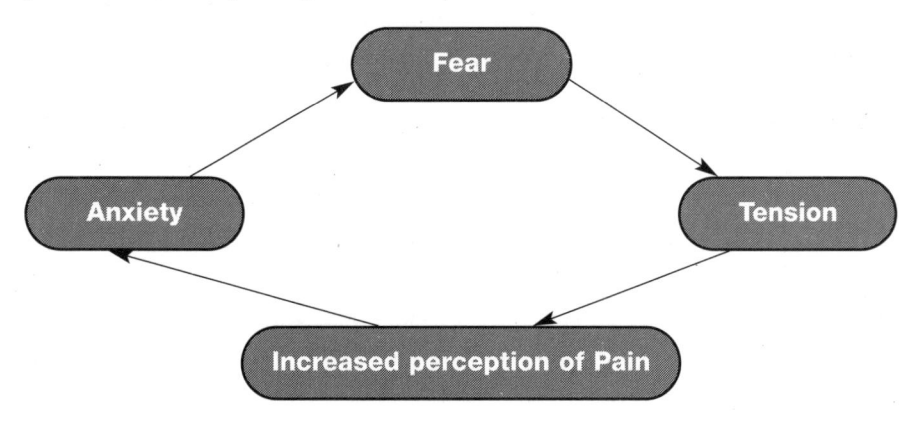

```
         Fear
        ↗    ↘
   Anxiety  Tension
        ↖    ↙
   Increased perception of Pain
```

Feeling fearful, anxious and in unmanageable pain can lead to requesting pain relief sooner and/or becoming exhausted prematurely, as more energy is used to fight the labour, rather than going with it. This type of experience also creates feelings of not being in control and seeing the whole labour process as negative, perhaps leading to feelings of failure, if you expected to cope better.

Often by identifying and openly acknowledging your fears (for example, fear of the perineum tearing), you can devise some coping strategies (such as using a warm compress on the area, or being in the bath when pushing). Sharing your fears can also help your caregiver and partner/support person work with you through this phase of the labour, to help calm and reassure you, and hopefully assist you to tolerate the pain.

Choosing a birthplace and caregiver you feel comfortable with can help allay fears and reduce tension, encouraging endorphin release and helping your labour progress. Other ways to mentally prepare for labour are discussed in support tools, later in this section.

Bear in mind that fear can sometimes be positive. One theory is that during the pushing phase, some fear is expected and normal, as the baby comes down the birth canal, energising the woman to push more vigorously. In this instance, accepting the fear, rather than avoiding it or trying to prevent it, may be necessary.

A factor in labour is the intense sensation. It is beyond the expectations of anyone who has never given birth. It is simply a part of the whole labour – nothing more, nothing to be afraid of, and nothing to waste your time and energy fighting against.

Past pain experiences

Sometimes women use past pain experiences (such as bad period cramps, dealing with an operation or accident) to try and gauge their pain threshold and imagine how they may cope with labour. However, labour is a unique experience, far different from any other pain sensation and many women are taken by surprise when it turns out to be nothing like they anticipated.

If the labour is unexpectedly more painful, this can make you suddenly fearful and anxious, increasing your pain sensations. So it is important to approach your labour with an open mind and not rely too much on past experiences.

If a previous birth was very painful, it is normal to feel apprehensive about a repeat performance. On the other hand, women who have had a positive experience may rely on this body memory to help them through the next time in a relaxed and more accepting way. Bear in mind that each labour is different and it may be better or worse. Remain open to what may come.

Birth stories

Hearing other women's birth stories may create fears (or add to them), perhaps leaving you upset, bewildered, angry or anxious about the impending labour. However, listening to a variety of birth stories, even scary ones, can help you gather ideas so you can explore different support tools that might be useful.

For all the positive birth stories you hear, perhaps ask: 'What worked for you?' or 'What made a difference?' For all the negative stories, perhaps ask: 'How did that make you feel?' or 'What would you do differently next time?'

Things to remember when listening to birth stories are:

- Each woman's experience is unique. While most women describe their labour as painful, this does not necessarily mean it was unpleasant.
- Labours vary immensely. Other women's stories cannot bring you to a full understanding of what your labour pain will be like. You need to remain open and just wait and see.
- If feeling overwhelmed, remind yourself that this was their experience. You are not this woman and your birth will be different. You and your baby will have your own unique story.
- Good birth stories can have a positive and powerful effect, so listen out for them. Some women find they are a great source of relief and motivation when preparing for their own labour and birth.

Psychological approach and pain threshold

Women often rely on their perceived pain threshold to envisage how they will cope with their labour. This can help them feel confident if they believe their threshold is high, or perhaps scared and uncertain if they think it is low. However, it is probably not useful to think of your pain threshold as such, because dealing with labour is more about your psychological approach to the pain, rather than your pain threshold.

The notion of a pain threshold is more complex than just being able to tolerate a certain level of pain. A person's threshold for pain can change dramatically, depending on the circumstances, how they view the pain and how they are feeling emotionally at the time. For example, if a person is feeling motivated to want to deal with the pain, in control of the situation and calm and accepting, because they feel they are working with it and there is a purpose to it, they are better able to tolerate very intense pain sensations. However, if they are feeling despondent, exhausted, threatened, out of control or less willing to accept the pain, this can make even mild pain intolerable. Ways to help you approach your labour pain in a positive frame of mind are discussed in helpful tools.

Expectations

Living up to your own, and other's, expectations can be very hard for a woman to deal with, because there are no guarantees of how an individual labour and birth will unfold.

Unrealistic expectations can place incredible pressure on you to behave in a certain way or accept certain methods of pain relief. Unmet expectations can also make you feel less motivated to want to deal with the pain, lowering your tolerance of it.

Your expectations need to be flexible, so you are not set up for failure (such as not achieving a drug-free birth), possibly leading to disappointment, anger and/or depression in the days, weeks or months after the birth. If you are feeling disappointed with how things are unfolding during the labour (for example, a vaginal examination revealing your cervix is not very dilated), have a cry if you need to, and try to let go of your expectations. Deal with where you are now and the labour you are experiencing, rather than where you would like it to be, and the labour you would prefer. This can help you approach your pain in a more positive way and increase your tolerance. Often if you are given the space to reconsider how your labour is unfolding, you can re-group and become more motivated to continue.

Pain relief

If medical or natural pain relief methods do not relieve your pain as much as expected, this can leave you feeling fearful, agitated, tense and anxious, increasing the pain sensations and making you less tolerant of them. In some cases, the pain relief is adequate, but the side effects are unexpectedly unpleasant. For example, during pregnancy you may plan to rely on the bath, or acupuncture, or a pethidine injection to be the 'one thing' that gets you through your labour. However, if they don't, this can make you feel less able to cope with your pain, as your motivation wanes and you feel unsure about your next plan of action.

Try to be open to various pain relieving methods. Read about how they work and the range of effects they can have, and don't rely on only one. Labour tends to be a rollercoaster of intensity and respite, and your pain relief methods may need to change and adjust as the labour unfolds.

Partner's or support person's influence

Sometimes a woman's partner or support person has attitudes towards labour pain that are very different from her own. This can affect how she labours and how competently they can support her. Be aware that 'support person distress' is not a valid reason to give a woman pain relief. Support people should *never* ask caregivers to 'give her something', because *they* feel uncomfortable. Women can make distressing noises, yet actually feel they are coping, drawing on inner strengths and resources and only using these vocal cries as a form of release. Each woman needs to express her own needs when she is ready.

Caregiver's expectations

Caregivers have their own beliefs about labour pain, and their personal approaches can be affected by what is considered routine in a birthplace, or the attitudes of their peers. Ideally, caregivers should modify their suggestions for pain relief to meet each woman's individual needs, but in reality this is not always the case.

It is common for women to receive messages about their caregiver's expectations during pregnancy visits, such as them indicating it will be very likely the woman will need an epidural. This can undermine her confidence in dealing with the pain, making her feel less motivated to want to deal with it, perhaps because the epidural seems inevitable.

Another common practice during labour is for caregivers to offer a woman gas, pethidine or an epidural, as soon as she starts making birthing noises, even though she may feel she is dealing with her pain. But because the caregiver is the trusted expert, the woman can start to question her coping abilities, perhaps feeling she should accept pain relief because her caregiver 'thinks she needs it'. Caregivers should wait for women to ask for pain relief, rather than offer it before being requested. You may wish to include this in your birth plan.

FEELING IN CONTROL

Feeling in control of the decisions you make about accepting or declining pain relief helps you feel less anxious and more relaxed about what is going on, because you can personally gauge how you are coping with your pain. This also promotes relaxation and endorphin release to decrease pain perception, as well as helping you feel motivated and positive about dealing with your labour.

When entering a hospital, it can be an automatic response to take on the role of a patient requiring treatment, giving over to a caregiver who will now look after you. This is referred to as being a passive patient. Subtle actions like changing into a hospital gown, or being directed to lie on a hospital bed, can contribute to feeling like a guest on the caregiver's territory. A guest is polite, asks permission and does not want to put anyone out by deviating from the expected routine. This environment can also modify a woman's reactions to her pain and how she should manage it, sometimes feeling pressured to 'keep it together' because she feels self-conscious or embarrassed.

Many women ask their caregiver to do 'what's best', but it can be hard for caregivers to get it right, because they don't really know what each woman needs or wants. When considering this situation, ask yourself:

- Will my caregiver always make the right decision for me?
- If the labour does not go according to plan, who is responsible for the decisions that have been made?
- Do I feel comfortable questioning their choices?
- What are the possibilities or consequences of choosing one option over another?

If you avoid ownership and responsibility for your pain relief decisions, you may end up feeling like 'They did this to me', rather than 'We all decided this was the best.' Playing a role in the decision-making process can help you accept the way your labour unfolds, because you feel more in control. However, you need to have an understanding of what is happening and of your pain relief choices, to make these decisions. Finding out all you can during the pregnancy will help with this.

Some women prefer to be a passive patient, because it is often easier to hand over decisions to their caregiver. This is also a choice, but it is important to think carefully about the implications. Try not to confuse this with the argument 'that's what I am paying them for'.

Raising a child involves making thousands of personal decisions on behalf of your baby. Pregnancy, labour and birth are ideal opportunities to start practising this role.

SOCIAL, CULTURAL AND SPIRITUAL BELIEFS

Strong cultural and religious beliefs can play a role in how each woman deals with her labour pain, even dictating acceptable behaviour and choices for pain relief. For example:

- Some Christians believe labour pain is what God intended and encourage women not to accept pain relief but to trust that their experience is part of God's plan.
- The Church of Scientology advocates that women should not make noises during labour, nor accept medical pain relief.
- Women from Middle Eastern and Mediterranean cultures are expected to scream and cry uncontrollably so support people can provide love and sympathy; sometimes their reactions may not equate to the level of pain they are feeling or their need for pain relief.
- Japanese women tend to suppress their emotions and not readily show distress, yet they verbally express how painful their labour is.

Western culture generally views labour pain as something that should be fixed or stopped, often embracing medical pain relief. However, since the 1980s there has been a growing trend to use natural therapies to reduce the need for medication in labour, incorporating more hands-on physical and emotional support instead.

Other factors
The way a labour unfolds, how long it takes, unforeseen complications and physical and emotional exhaustion, can all influence a woman's motivation and pain tolerance.

Exhaustion
Feeling tired is a normal sign of endorphin release during labour. In reality, true exhaustion is not that common, but can come about if the established labour lasts beyond 18 to 24 hours. If the labour continues for longer than anticipated, the woman can feel less motivated to want to deal with her pain, lowering her tolerance of it. This can be made worse if her support people are tiring around her.

If feeling exhausted:
- You may need to call in some fresh support people with enthusiasm and energy to help you get through this final phase of the labour.
- Try something different. Often just a change of position or scenery, such as moving to the bath or shower, can re-energise you to continue.
- Consider asking your caregiver to leave you for a while to try and rest, recover and re-group.
- Sometimes medical pain relief, such as an epidural, may be a judicious choice, depending on the circumstances.

Complications arising
Complications and unexpected interventions can feel threatening, triggering sudden fear that can make a woman tense and anxious, increasing her pain. Sometimes interventions are welcomed because they can indirectly give permission to accept pain relief, because the decision is taken out of the woman's hands.

If it is not an emergency, take one step at a time. Having one intervention does not necessarily mean you have to accept others. For example, it may be decided you need a Syntocinon drip to speed up the contractions, but you may still prefer not to have an epidural (which is often suggested as well). Continue to use natural forms of pain relief (or gas or pethidine), remain active and use pre-planned birth positions. Try to maintain some essential elements of your birth plan to make it a more positive experience.

EXPLORING BELIEFS AND PERCEPTIONS

There is some mental preparation you can do to help with your pain perception, and you may wish to consider using some support tools to assist you during the labour when the time comes. Believe it or not, fears, worries and concerns can be great motivators to find out more about your pain relief options, and devise coping strategies.

By exploring your and your partner/support person's beliefs and perceptions about labour pain, you can start to nurture some positive attitudes to help you deal with any fears or concerns. Some women feel that they need to explore their issues with a professional counsellor (or their caregiver or childbirth educator). You may also consider homeopathic remedies for emotional support.

Try working through the following to identify, or clarify, your approach to labour:

1. Have you ever experienced strong physical pain before? Do you believe labour will be similar?

2. Do you expect labour pain to be:
   Not very painful   Mild   Strong   Very strong   Excruciating?

3. Is labour pain something you have to suffer, or is it something you work with? Or a bit of both?

4. Is labour pain manageable? Do you see it as purposeful?

5. If labour continues for several hours, how do you think you will manage? How do you expect to be supported during long periods of pain?

6. Do you believe your body can get through the labour and birth? Does your partner/support person believe you can cope?

7. Will you feel comfortable being vocal and making loud sounds? How does your partner/support person feel about hearing you in labour?

8. Do you question the need to have to endure pain? What do you think about women who use medical pain relief? And what about women who decline pain relief?

9. Are you worried about the possible side effects of using medical pain relief? Are you worried about coping, if you choose not to use them?

10. How do you think your environment and the support you receive will help you manage labour?

11. Do you think your partner/support person and caregiver will support how you choose to manage your pain, whatever this may be?

12. If this is not your first baby, how do you think your past experience(s) will impact on your choices for managing labour pain with this pregnancy?

Nearly everyone holds some negative beliefs about pain, but these can be changed into positive attitudes if labour is seen as healthy and natural, something to work with rather than feel a victim of. Positive attitudes can help you accept labour as normal. It may be stressful and painful, but it is *normal*. If you can see labour as purposeful, a vehicle that brings your child, then the pain can be perceived as a tool that actively moves your body through the process. You may still feel frightened and challenged at times, yet throughout it all you are aware that it is a positive means to an end.

Setting realistic, achievable goals can also help you work towards an outcome you can feel good about. It may not be your ideal outcome, but if you can look back and say you gave it your best shot, you are more likely to feel positive about the experience. This can leave lasting, and sometimes profound, impressions, ones that are capable of supporting your transition into parenting.

Identifying qualities and strengths

One effective way to support positive attitudes is to identify the strengths and qualities you and your partner (or support person) will bring to the labour. This can be done by reflecting back on how you have dealt with stress or difficult situations in the past, and can be a wonderful way to share your feelings, vulnerabilities and strengths, as well as acknowledging what each person sees in the other.

Write these out on a piece of paper independently, and then share them after the exercise (you will need six pieces of blank paper).

1. What are your fears and concerns? (Eg. performance anxiety for the woman, or not knowing how to help for the partner/support person.)

2. Identify the qualities you normally draw strength from in times of difficulty or when faced with a stressful situation. (Eg. determination, keeping calm, or being a good communicator.)

3. Identify the qualities you believe the other person will bring. (Eg. the woman seeing her partner as strong and protective; or the partner seeing the woman as determined.)

This process of identifying strengths can give you a sense of the positive coping strategies you already have for dealing with labour.

Helpful tools

We have listed some helpful support tools that may be implemented during labour (perhaps in combination with various natural forms of pain relief). Often by practising certain techniques during the pregnancy, they become familiar and relaxing, helping you to work with the pain, especially when feeling fearful or anxious. However, these strategies are not guarantees that you will have a painless labour.

Key words can help you focus when the pain feels overwhelming. They should be short, simple and personal, so they feel familiar. For example: 'Release . . . relax . . . open . . . flow . . . flop . . .' Repeat your chosen key words to yourself on a regular basis during the pregnancy. As you do this, allow your body to relax and release tension, so you can lay down a word-associated memory to be used during labour. Your partner or support person can remind you, or gently repeat your key words (unless, of course, you ask them to stop).

Affirmations aim to reinforce positive attitudes and are also more effective if you use your own wording. Examples are:
- 'My body is working and progressing with each contraction.'
- 'This is not forever. It will end with my baby in my arms.'
- 'I am strong and healthy. Labour is normal.'
- 'Take one contraction at a time, and then let it go.'
- 'I will work with the labour I have and accept the way I labour.'

When you find affirmations that feel right for you, write them down and place them where you can see them daily, to help reinforce them. Again, you can repeat them to yourself during labour, or your partner or support person can say them to you.

NOTE: *For some women, the intensity of labour (especially towards the end) makes it virtually impossible to implement any of these planned support strategies. It may be all they can do to lapse into survival mode, just accepting the experience of pain. If labour is progressing rapidly, knowing it will be over soon may help you cope.*

Medical forms of pain relief

It is hard to know what your labour will bring. To be able to communicate effectively with your caregiver and work towards a positive birth experience together, it is important to be aware of your pain relief options, their effectiveness and any potential side effects for you and your baby.

The timing of accepting pain relief can have a flow-on effect to other interventions as the labour progresses. One method of relief may sustain you for a few hours, but as the pain sensations return or intensify you can be left feeling unprepared to deal with this new level of pain, especially if it is likely to be a while before the baby is born. This can lead you to request stronger pain relief, and so the cycle continues.

That is not to say you cannot accept pain relief early, but it is important to be aware of what your choices may lead to. For example, some women request pain relief as soon as the pain starts to feel a little harder, rather than waiting until it is actually unbearable. This is often because they feel anxious about how they will cope in one or two hours time. Yet by waiting 30 minutes or so, natural endorphins may be released and the pain may become more tolerable.

Take a moment to think about your use of pain relief. If you choose to have something at 2 to 3 cm dilation, what will you have at 5 to 6 cm, or 8 to 9 cm? Also, what are the implications of the prolonged use (or increasing doses) of your chosen method?

GAS

The gas used for labour pain relief is nitrous oxide (Entonox), or laughing gas, similar to that used by dentists. It is colourless and odourless, and usually diluted with oxygen (50:50), hence the nickname 'gas and air'. Higher mixes of nitrous gas may be used (70:30), if a stronger anaesthetic is required for medical interventions.

Nitrous oxide is inhaled and absorbed into the bloodstream from the lungs, moving rapidly to the brain within 10 to 15 seconds. Here, it depresses the brain's normal functioning, changing how you perceive pain. Nitrous is also a sedative and can have an amnesic effect. Once you stop inhaling the gas, it takes one to two minutes to be expelled from your system altogether.

Gas is available in all delivery suites and most birth centres. A homebirth midwife may be able to supply it, or you may have to hire it.

Why gas?
Gas tends to be the first line of action, generally because:
- It is easy to administer, and quickly reversible.
- It has the least amount of side effects for mother and baby.
- When labour is very advanced, it is preferred over a narcotic injection or epidural.
- It can relax the woman to allow her labour to progress.
- It can help avoid early pushing, if the cervix is not fully dilated or with an anterior lip.
- It can be used quickly for unexpected medical interventions if there is not enough time to administer a narcotic or insert an epidural.

Caregivers may discourage the use of gas during the pushing phase if a woman appears not to be pushing effectively, because it can be hard to inhale gas and push at the same time.

NOTE: *A few women assume they will not like the gas because they are worried the mask over their face will make them feel claustrophobic. However, many birthplaces now use mouthpieces that can be placed inside the mouth rather than over the face.*

Gas is generally **not** recommended for women who have:
- Suffered decompression sickness in the past (the bends), or who have had serious lung problems such as a pneumothorax (a hole in the lung causing it to collapse).
- Severe folic acid or vitamin B12 deficiency, because nitrous oxide inactivates these vitamins in the woman's system, possibly causing functional disturbances in the spinal cord and nervous system.[1]

Using the gas
For optimal pain relief you need to time breathing the gas with the contractions. Your caregiver will help you with this. As a guide:
1. Start breathing the gas as soon as a contraction starts.
2. Continue to breathe, deeply and slowly, for the whole contraction. This allows the gas to build up in your system and provide adequate pain relief.
3. Once the contraction passes, stop using the gas.

It often takes two to three contractions to get a good effect, so don't give up after the first contraction.

NOTE: *It is important for the woman to hold the mask or mouthpiece, not her partner or support person. This prevents her overdosing on the gas and passing out. Once you've had enough, the mask or mouthpiece falls away, stopping further gas from being released.*

Effects on the woman

Gas is considered the safest form of medical pain relief for women in labour, but potential side effects can include:

- **Suppression of breathing** – A few women become heavily sedated and unable to be roused, especially if they continue the gas between contractions. If the sedation is heavy enough, it can suppress the woman's breathing and oxygen intake (as well as the baby's). If this happens, the gas is usually taken away for several minutes, or not used between the contractions. The caregiver may also turn the nitrous level down.
- **Nausea and vomiting** – These can be experienced by some women (although this is less likely compared to gases used in the past). Be aware that starting pain relief of any kind often coincides with an increase in the intensity of labour, which is also the time many women feel nauseous and/or vomit. If the gas is effectively relieving the pain, you may wish to persevere for a while to see whether the nausea and vomiting subsides.
- **Hallucinations** – Being 'off with the fairies' can make communicating with others difficult. Some women feel scared or panicky. The caregiver may remove the gas for a while, or increase the levels of oxygen in the mix.
- **Enhancing narcotics** – If nitrous oxide is combined with a pethidine injection, it can make you quite drowsy or spaced out. On the other hand, if pethidine is not very effective, gas could add to the level of pain relief.

Effects on the baby

Nitrous oxide rapidly crosses the placenta to the baby, so the baby's blood concentrations are equal to the mother's while she is using it. However, gas excretes rapidly through the baby's lungs after birth and is out of their system altogether five minutes later. Nitrous oxide does not affect the baby's ability to feed and, at present, it is believed that it does not have any long-term effects on the baby.

> **Did you know?**
>
> It is now recognised that other pregnant women in the labour room exposed to nitrous oxide exhaled by the labouring woman are at a slightly increased risk of miscarriage, preterm birth and having a low birth weight baby.[2] The room should be well ventilated, and pregnant caregivers or support people should minimise their exposure. If the midwife caring for you is pregnant and you start using nitrous oxide, they may ask another midwife to care for you.

Women's experiences with gas

Surveys of women who have used gas have found that 50% regard it as being very effective, 20% found it gave them some pain relief and 30% found it to be ineffective.[3] So it is important to have realistic expectations about what gas can provide. Nitrous oxide does not remove the pain altogether, but many women say it takes the edge off it, or they feel mentally removed from the pain. Others describe it as feeling as though they are floating, disorientated, drunk, stoned, confused, out of it, nauseated or claustrophobic. The beauty of gas is that you can always stop it if you don't like it.

Support strategies

Time the gas, as many women doze in between the contractions, only waking when the pain is strong, rather than when the contraction is just starting. This may be too late for the gas to work effectively. The support person can place their fingertips on the woman's belly, to feel the uterus tensing, usually about 5 to 10 seconds before she feels any pain, then gently nudge her awake so she can start breathing the gas. If you are having difficulty doing this, ask your caregiver to show you.

Some women want to continue using the gas during the pushing phase. This can be achieved by starting to inhale about 30 seconds before the next contraction is due, and then stopping to push with the contraction.

Help wet her mouth and lips, as these can dry out when using the gas for prolonged periods. In between the contractions the support person can:
- Put a wet cloth or sponge in her mouth, letting her breathe in and out through her nose.
- Offer her sips of water or ice chips to suck on.
- Use a fine water spray on her face.
- Use lip balm or lanolin on her lips.

NOTE: *It has been known for partners or support people to use the gas in between the woman's contractions, while the caregiver is out of the room. This is not allowed and not recommended as it makes you a less effective support person, besides proving rather embarrassing if staff catch you at it.*

PETHIDINE

The most common narcotic medication used for pain relief during labour is pethidine. Occasionally other narcotics are prescribed, such as morphine or Fentanyl (Sublimaze). Narcotics act like potent endorphins.

Pethidine is injected into the buttock, leg or arm muscle and absorbed into the bloodstream, before attaching to nerve fibres in the spinal cord. It takes 15 to 30 minutes to be fully effective and is broken down by the liver, before being excreted through the kidneys over the next 3 to 6 hours.

Pethidine is available in delivery suites and most birth centres. Women planning a homebirth need to ask their local doctor to write a script and have this filled in the weeks before the birth.

NOTE: Although uncommon, narcotics may be administered intravenously, using Patient Controlled Analgesia (PCA). This involves the woman periodically pressing a button to give small, measured doses through an electronic dispenser, with an inbuilt mechanism to prevent overdosing.

Why pethidine?

Pethidine tends to be used if the gas starts to become ineffective, or the woman wants to avoid (or delay) an epidural. It affects your mental clarity, making you feel drowsy, possibly inducing short periods of sleep, as well as counteracting muscle spasm.

Pethidine tends to be more effective during the early and active phases of labour, from 3 to 4 cm, up to 7 to 8 cm dilation. If it is administered too early, it may slow, or stop, the contractions (this may be the desired effect if experiencing a prolonged prelabour). Occasionally the relaxing effect of pethidine encourages the cervix to dilate, assisting the labour's progress.

The caregiver usually performs a vaginal examination before administering pethidine and may discourage its use if the cervix is more than 7 to 8 cm dilated and the labour is progressing rapidly. This is because the baby is expected to be born within a couple of hours and is more likely to experience side effects. Pethidine is also less likely to be effective in relieving the more intense pain associated with transition.

Pethidine is generally ***not*** recommended if:
- The baby is premature or suspected of being unwell.
- The woman is allergic to narcotics (say, a rash or swelling soon after having the medication, not vomiting), although allergies are rare.
- Certain antidepressants were taken two weeks before labour. (Check with your caregiver.)

NOTE: Women addicted to narcotics in the past can have pethidine if they wish. However, if you are concerned about triggering an addictive response, let your caregiver know that you don't want narcotics under any circumstances (or write this on your birth plan). It is not necessary to disclose the reasons why.

Effects on the woman
- **Feeling nauseated or vomiting** – About 15 to 30% of women feel nauseated (and occasionally vomit) after having pethidine. Your

caregiver may administer an antinausea medication with the pethidine injection (usually Maxalon), or this may be given as a separate injection later if vomiting does occur.
- **Increased perspiration** – Your partner or support person may need to wipe your face frequently and make sure your clothes and sheets are comfortably dry, as well as encourage you to drink fluids.
- **Drowsiness** – This is normal with pethidine, but a few women become heavily sedated and not easily roused, perhaps remaining affected for a while after the birth. This can make you disinterested in interacting with, or feeding, your baby, just wanting to be left alone to sleep for a while.
- **Suppression of breathing** – Opiates tend to slow the natural breathing rate slightly, but with an injection of pethidine this is mild. However, narcotic PCA increases the chances and severity of this effect. If the breathing becomes severely suppressed, oxygen intake can be low and the caregiver will need to stop the infusion. They may also need to administer an injection of naloxone (Narcan), even though this can take all the pain relief away within minutes.
- **Disorientation** – Pethidine may make you say, or imagine, unusual things, or feel out of control, confused and less able to remember events surrounding the labour and birth. Some women don't mind this, but others find it unpleasant.
- **Dizziness** – Pethidine slightly lowers your blood pressure and may cause dizziness. Women are advised to stay in bed for a few hours after the injection (using a bedpan if needing to go to the toilet, or being assisted to walk to the bathroom). If you request pethidine while in the shower or bath, you will be encouraged to lie down on the bed, or kneel on a mat on the floor.

NOTE: *All potent narcotics have the potential to lead to addiction. However, it is believed that one or two injections during labour will not lead to addiction, or the risk is extremely low.*

Effects on the baby

Narcotics cross the placenta to the baby within 30 minutes after the mother is injected, reaching peak concentrations in the baby's blood after 1 hour, and starting to decline after 2 hours, but lasting 4 to 6 hours, as the mother's body excretes the drug. Narcotics reach the baby within two minutes if given intravenously with PCA. If the baby's heart rate is being continuously monitored with a CTG trace during labour, their heart rate tends to stay around the same speed, rather than fluctuating from 120 to 160 beats per minute. It is not clear whether this is a problem or not, but it does indicate the baby is sedated. It can also be difficult to know whether the baby is distressed. Usually their heart rate is observed more closely.

If the baby is born with pethidine in their system, it takes them up to three days to excrete it, because their liver and kidneys are less mature and their blood levels of the drug are comparatively higher. The following side effects for babies are more likely if they are born within one to two hours after their mother has the injection.

- **Baby's breathing at birth** – Opiates can suppress the baby's desire to breathe at birth. Up to 25% of babies are affected in this way.[3] Babies affected by pethidine usually have a lower Apgar score and may be slow to respond (not breathing themselves), requiring the caregiver to ventilate their lungs with a special face mask and oxygen.

  Occasionally the baby is given an injection of naloxone to reverse this effect, although this only lasts for four hours. Naloxone may need to be repeated if the baby becomes drowsy or stops breathing again after this time. Often the baby is observed in the intensive care nursery for four to six hours after having naloxone, in case their breathing becomes suppressed again.

  NOTE: Naloxone cannot be used on babies whose mothers have been addicted to narcotics during the pregnancy, as it can cause a sudden, severe withdrawal in the baby, possibly making them experience a seizure. Women addicted to narcotics, or taking methadone, may consider not accepting pethidine during labour for this reason.

- **Suck reflex after the birth** – The baby may be sleepy and less able to suck for a few days following the birth, making them disinterested in feeding or causing difficulty latching on the breast. While this rectifies after a few days, it can make a woman feel that breastfeeding is too hard, or not working, and contribute to her giving it up. Try and be patient with your baby and trust that their feeding will improve. Newborns have plenty of fluid and fat reserves to last them for a few days until the pethidine wears off and they are more alert.

- **Connecting with your baby:** Some babies have slightly different behaviour patterns in the days following the birth. They can be less enthusiastic at making eye contact, less reactive to sounds and movement, and less inclined to 'curl up' in the fetal position. The significance of this is unknown. At present, no long-term effects have been proven – although it can be bewildering if your 'extra good' baby suddenly wakes up and becomes a normal demanding newborn as the pethidine leaves their system! A few babies are more irritable, cry more readily when disturbed and can be more difficult to settle to sleep. Again, this should improve after a few days.

Women's experiences
Reported pain relief varies from very good to very little; some women just feel more calm and relaxed. As with gas, pethidine doesn't remove the pain altogether, but it can dull it and make it more tolerable. Some women describe feeling removed from their pain or less anxious about it, and so more able to cope.

Others find the side effects make their labour a negative experience. Descriptions include feeling drugged, dreamy, floating, nauseated, disorientated, confused, dizzy, isolated, sleepy or euphoric.

NOTE: *Increasing the dose of pethidine or giving an additional injection is not generally recommended because this does not make it more effective, but only increases the side effects such as nausea, vomiting and disorientation.*

Support strategies
Help her to move if she needs to change position, or pass urine.

Time her contractions, as described in support strategies for gas. Some women wake suddenly with pain after drifting off to sleep, making them feel tense or out of control.

Communicate with her, in case she feels isolated or is unable to communicate. Perhaps she can hear and is aware of what is happening, but has difficulty speaking. Don't presume she is totally unaware, even if she looks asleep, especially if discussing issues about her care with the caregiver. Try whispering what you wish to communicate to her in her ear. Continue to give her occasional reassurances and encouragement (but still let her rest a bit!). If she becomes agitated with your efforts to keep in touch with her, it may be that she just wants to be left alone.

Help her connect with the baby, if she is still quite affected after the birth. She may be disinclined (or too sleepy) to hold the baby, or worried she may drop them. Try placing the baby on her belly, or close to her. Put up the bedsides and pack pillows around to keep the baby safe. Alternatively, hold the baby nearby and try not to take them out of the room for long periods. Encourage the baby to feed during the first hour, or at least nuzzle at the breast, if the woman is feeling drowsy.

EPIDURAL AND SPINAL ANAESTHESIA
Epidurals and spinals involve medications being injected into the lower back area by an anaesthetist. Both methods are called regional anaesthetics because they prevent pain (and to a degree, touch and temperature sensations) from being felt in a specific region of the body; in this case, from the waist down.

Epidurals and spinals require different insertion techniques and have different side effects. The main differences are as follows:
- **The epidural needle** is inserted only as far as the epidural space, located just outside a layer of tissue called the dura mater which encases the spinal cord and spinal fluid.
- **The spinal needle** is inserted a little further, piercing the dura mater, reaching the spinal fluid (which surrounds the spinal cord and flows around the brain).

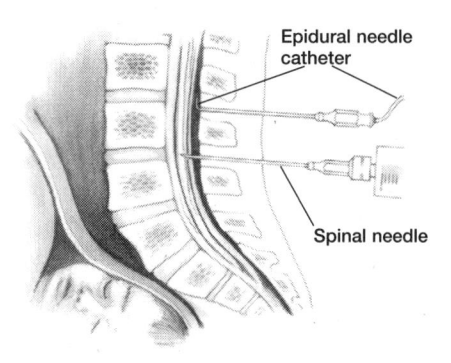

Epidural and spinal needles being inserted

- **An epidural** uses a fine hollow catheter (the width of fishing line), which is fed through the hollow needle into the epidural space before the medications are injected. The needle is removed, leaving the long catheter in place (taped up the length of the woman's back), to enable more medications to be added later if needed.
- **A spinal** involves the medications being injected directly into the spinal fluid, bathing the nerves, before removing the needle altogether. No catheter is left in place, making it a 'once only' procedure.
- **Epidurals** generally take 10 to 30 minutes to relieve the pain (but can start making a difference after 10 minutes) and last 1 to 2 hours, before wearing off (or requiring a top-up).
- **Spinals** take 5 to 10 minutes to relieve the pain and last for 1 to 2 hours, but cannot be topped up.
- **Epidurals** are technically harder to insert than a spinal and therefore are less likely to be successful.
- **Spinals** use lower doses of medications because they are injected directly into the spinal fluid where the nerves are located.

In recent years, there has been an increasing trend to combine an epidural with a spinal, called a CSE. This method aims to take advantage of the rapid effectiveness of a spinal (while the epidural takes full effect), yet have the ongoing use of the epidural catheter for additional pain relief, especially if the labour is long, or further medications are required for a forceps, ventouse or caesarean birth.

Epidurals (or combined epidural–spinals) are more commonly used during labour, and spinals are more likely to be used for caesareans. The type administered often depends on the anaesthetist's preferences, and sometimes the hospital policy. Your preferences (if you have any) may also influence the decision.

Epidurals and spinals can only be administered in delivery suites of larger public and private hospitals. Women choosing birth centres, or homebirth, need to transfer to the delivery suite to have one. They also may be unavailable (or restricted) in some smaller metropolitan and rural hospitals, due to the cost and availability of an anaesthetist's services. Some hospitals limit the use of epidurals to medical interventions such as a forceps or caesarean birth. Check with your caregiver or hospital during the pregnancy.

Medications used

Up until the 1990s, high doses of local anaesthetics were used, such as lidocaine (Xylocaine) or bupivacaine (Marcaine). However, it became apparent that while they were effective for pain relief, they also numbed the woman's sensations so she couldn't feel *anything* and was less likely to have a normal birth. These days, anaesthetists use lighter doses of local anaesthetics, mixed with narcotics (such as fentanyl, sufentanil, morphine or pethidine). This is regarded as the gold standard of epidural anaesthesia because it can provide adequate pain relief but reduce the side effects of the local anaesthetic.

Continuous epidurals

Continuous epidurals are given slowly through a measured infusion pump. Many women prefer them because they take away the rollercoaster effect that is sometimes associated with intermittent top-ups. A few hospitals use Patient Controlled Epidural Anaesthesia (PCEA) so the woman can self-administer to control her own pain.

Walking epidurals

Walking or light epidurals only use narcotic medications. They relieve some labour pain but don't cause muscle weakness, allowing you to move around and feel the baby coming down the birth canal. However, many women find they don't relieve their pain adequately, so anaesthetists tend to mix the narcotic with some local medications (making you less able to move). Narcotic epidurals can take 10 to 30 minutes to take full effect and last for 4 to 24 hours, depending on the type of medication.

Medical considerations

Epidurals and spinals may be recommended for women with high blood pressure, because one of the side effects is to lower the blood pressure. In the past, epidurals were routinely recommended for women having twins, a premature baby, a posterior or breech baby, or for women planning a vaginal birth after a previous caesarean. This was generally in case interventions were needed to help deliver the baby(s). However, there are no benefits for using epidurals routinely in these circumstances.

A few reasons why an epidural or spinal may **not** be recommended include:
- Bleeding tendencies, if a woman has a blood-clotting disorder, or is taking medications to thin the blood (aspirin or heparin), or has abnormally low platelet levels. The concern is that the epidural needle may cause heavy bleeding in the spinal area.
- Heavy vaginal bleeding caused by placenta previa, or a placental abruption, as the epidural may further decrease the blood pressure.
- A blood infection (septicaemia), which is very rare. If the woman has a high fever and a blood infection is suspected, the concern is that this may spread to the spinal cord and brain.

An epidural is your choice and can always be declined. If you are in two minds about having one, consider why it is being recommended, and remember, you have a right not to accept it.

> **Did you know?**
> Generally back injuries, lumbar disc operations, inherited abnormalities of the spine or bone diseases of the spine do not prevent women from being able to have an epidural or spinal anaesthetic. However, these factors can increase the chances of an epidural not being fully effective, or present difficulties for the anaesthetist inserting the needle.

Inserting an epidural or spinal

Epidurals and spinals are usually given after 3 to 4 cm dilation to avoid slowing or stopping the contractions. They are generally not recommended after 9 to 10 cm, because it can be difficult to push your baby out. However, one may be administered for an anterior lip, or a forceps, ventouse or caesarean birth. A vaginal examination is required before the epidural is inserted.

Depending on how busy the anaesthetist is, the anaesthetic may be administered within minutes or be delayed for half an hour or so. An intravenous drip is required for extra fluids, to help counteract any drop in the blood pressure. Try to pass urine beforehand, as this may be difficult once the anaesthetic is working. Some caregivers routinely recommend inserting a catheter into the bladder.

The anaesthetist usually explains the procedure and briefly lists the potential risks. You should also be given an opportunity to ask questions; however, most women are quite distressed with pain at this point, and generally not receptive to long-winded explanations. There are ethical and legal dilemmas of consent under duress when women ask for epidurals (and other pain relief) whilst in labour, because they are not really in a position to give fully informed consent. This is why it is important to read about your options during the pregnancy and know the possible risks.

You will need to curl up in a fetal position, usually on your side on the bed, or sitting up and leaning over a pillow on your lap. This curves your back and helps separate the bones of the spine. Local anaesthetic is injected into the skin (which may sting), then you need to remain as still as possible for one to three contractions while the anaesthetist inserts the needle (it feels like pressure and prodding). Your partner or caregiver may help by gently holding you in position.

Once inserted, the epidural catheter is fed in – you may feel a tingling, or shooting pains down one leg for a second or two – and the medications are administered. Your caregiver checks your blood pressure regularly and the baby's heart rate is usually monitored with a CTG machine for at least 30 minutes.

Effects on the woman

Many women have epidurals and spinals without problems, and they are relatively safe procedures when performed by an experienced anaesthetist. However, they are also capable of producing, or leading to, more side effects and complications than any other pain-relieving methods for labour, and have a greater potential to affect the way your baby will be born. As a guide:

- **Lowering the blood pressure** is normal and expected. However, this can sometimes be severe, possibly reducing blood flow to the baby, and can occur in up to 18% of women having an epidural, and about 10 to 12% of women having a spinal. Spinals, however, tend to lower the blood pressure more suddenly and more severely then epidurals. Intravenous fluids are given to try to counteract this effect. In rare circumstances the baby may need to be delivered by caesarean.
- **Shivers and shakes** are physical reactions to the local medications, even though you don't feel cold. They usually settle after a while.

- **Developing a fever** (above 38°C) has been linked with having an epidural for more than 4 hours (for 25% of women, and up to 50% if it is in for over 8 hours). 'Epidural fever' may not be an issue in itself but can be confused with a possible infection, meaning treatments with antibiotics just in case, and possibly the baby being closely observed and having a septic work-up (a range of tests for infection).
- **Nausea and vomiting** can be periodic, or ongoing, until the epidural wears off. Antinausea medications can be given as an injection, if there is continual vomiting. Acupressure on the wrist point has been shown to help in up to 50% of women (see acupressure appendix).
- **Itchy skin** can be experienced by 40 to 80% of women when narcotics are used in the epidural or spinal. This is usually all over the body, but particularly around the face and neck, lasting for up to 24 hours. The baby is not affected. Itching is not a sign of being allergic to the medication, it is simply a physical reaction to the narcotic being administered in this way.

    Some caregivers prescribe antihistamines, which can make you feel drowsy and sleepy. Small amounts may transfer to the baby in breast milk, but not usually enough to show any effects. Some caregivers prescribe low doses of naloxone, or mix this drug with the epidural narcotic, to try to reduce itching without reducing the pain-relieving effects.
- **Urine retention** may result as the nerves of the bladder are also anaesthetised, blocking the sensation of wanting to pass urine. If the bladder becomes overfull and distended, it is possible to have longer-term problems with emptying the bladder. You may need a urinary catheter to keep the bladder empty during labour. This may be left in place for several hours after the birth, to avoid nerve damage.
- **Backache** caused by an epidural or spinal is controversial, but is reported in up to 30% of women. During the days after the birth, this is expected, but for long-term backache the picture is not clear. Evidence suggests that back pain may be linked with lying in awkward positions for long periods of time, rather than the actual procedure.[4] Support people and caregivers need to pay attention to the woman's position and to move her from side to side every hour or so without twisting her back.
- **Slowing the labour** is a possibility as epidurals and spinals can affect contractions and slow the first and second stages of labour, significantly increasing the need to augment the labour. This is less likely if their administration is delayed until at least 5 cm dilation. They relax the

pelvic floor muscles and reduce the ability of the baby's head to rotate and descend down the birth canal, increasing the chances of needing a forceps or ventouse birth. If you can delay the active pushing until the epidural wears off (or turn down a continuous epidural), this can help you avoid becoming tired or requiring these interventions. However, some women find it hard to push when their pain returns and may need a lighter top-up, or additional narcotic in the epidural, to help them push effectively.

- **Severe headache** may occur. Spinals can sometimes cause small amounts of spinal fluid to leak from the puncture site once the needle is removed. This reduces fluid pressure around the spinal cord and brain, causing a severe headache within 12 to 48 hours for around 2 to 10% of women.[5] Headaches do not happen with epidurals, unless the needle inadvertently reaches the spinal canal (about 1% of the time), effectively becoming a spinal.

    Spinal headaches usually go away on their own within a few days, but may last for a week or more. The headache is generally worse when you sit or stand up, and relieved when lying flat (not ideal for a new mother!). Other symptoms can include nausea, vomiting, dizziness, stiff neck, hearing a 'ringing' sound and not being able to tolerate bright lights.

    Treatments include lying flat, taking mild analgesics, drinking stimulants (tea, coffee or cola), although these may stimulate the baby if breastfeeding. If the headache is prolonged and severe, then a blood patch may be used. The anaesthetist takes blood from a vein in your arm and inserts it into the epidural space to create a blood clot to seal up the hole. However, studies suggest that the possible complications of blood patching (pain, infection, nerve irritability and difficulty inserting epidurals at a later date) may offset the benefits of the procedure.

- **Slow breathing** may be caused by narcotic medications, so reducing oxygen to mother and baby. In these (rare) cases oxygen is administered and an injection of naloxone is given.

- **Numbness and weakness** in the lower limbs (possibly reducing bladder and bowel control) is experienced by around 0.03% of women. These can also be caused by forceps births and using stirrups. Up to 99% of nerve injuries resolve within 3 to 6 months, but some may take longer. Your caregiver may refer you to a neurologist. Some women use acupuncture to stimulate the nerves to heal more rapidly.

- **Local anaesthetic in the vein** can result if pain relief is unintentionally injected into a vein and enters the bloodstream, causing fits. This can be life-threatening. Measures are taken by the anaesthetist to try and prevent this, but on rare occasions it still happens.
- **Infections** are extremely rare (1 in 500,000) but can be serious and life-threatening. Physical signs can include:
  - Severe back pain, usually within 24 hours.
  - Severe headache.
  - Neck stiffness.
  - A fever.
  - Possibly leg weakness or permanent paralysis.

  Treatment involves large doses of intravenous antibiotics. Rarely, the infection turns into an abscess, which may need to be surgically drained.
- **Overstimulating the uterus** is a possibility as spinal anaesthetics used during labour can hyperstimulate the uterus, making it contract too much. This is more likely for women having a subsequent baby, when the contractions are already very strong. Hyperstimulation can stress the baby and may lead to an emergency caesarean (or a ventouse or forceps delivery if the cervix is fully dilated). Spinals are not recommended for labouring women who have had a previous caesarean, as this could put unnecessary strain on their scar.
- **A total spinal** (or high block) occurs when an epidural accidentally becomes a spinal and larger doses of medications are injected into the spinal canal (spinals need less medications to be effective). This is very rare but life-threatening, as excess local medication rapidly travels up the spinal cord, numbing the nerves to the woman's chest and neck, causing:
  - Very low blood pressure, slow pulse, nausea, looking pale (or blue), sweating, dizziness, drowsiness or passing out.
  - Feeling numb or weak in the arms and hands.
  - Having difficulty breathing, being unable to speak, or only whisper.

  Intravenous fluids and drugs are given to help raise the blood pressure and oxygen is administered, but the woman may need to be attached to a ventilator machine to breathe for her until the spinal anaesthetic wears off (after two to six hours). The baby also needs to be delivered as soon as possible, usually by caesarean.
- **Permanent paralysis** is very rare, but can happen for around 1 in 250,000 to 1 in 1,000,000 women if spinal nerves are damaged during the insertion of an epidural or spinal.

Effects on the baby
- **Distress** – This can occur due to a lowering of the woman's blood pressure, possibly leading to a caesarean.
- **A non-reactive CTG trace** (see effects of pethidine on the baby).
- **Sedation** – Depending on the amount and type of narcotic used, and how long the baby was exposed before the birth, they may be lethargic and reluctant to feed in the days following. At present there are no known long-term effects.
- **Baby being unwell** – An epidural-induced fever in the woman may increase the chances of short-term effects for her baby, such as a lower Apgar score, requiring oxygen or resuscitation, being floppy and having less muscle tone, and possibly needing transfer to the nursery for observation.

Women's experiences of epidurals and spinals
Epidurals and spinals are the most effective way to relieve labour pain; they allow you to remain mentally alert, while providing a break from the contractions, especially if the labour is prolonged. They can also help when you are feeling anxious and may reduce (or reverse) stress-related responses in the body, by stopping hyperventilation, lowering adrenaline levels, increasing oxygenation and improving blood flow to the placenta (if the blood pressure does not fall too low).[6] However, epidurals and spinals are not guaranteed to produce the desired effects. Even if administered without technical problems, only 80 to 85% of women are pain free, with 12 to 15% experiencing a patchy block (so, for example, one side of the body still feels pain), and 3 to 5% obtaining no pain relief at all.

Sometimes the pain relief does not meet expectations. A few women feel distressed if they can sense *any* discomfort, and others are disappointed at how little sensation they can feel. In a few cases women feel dissatisfied because the relief is timed poorly, perhaps being given too late.

Support strategies
Lie her on her side to avoid further lowering of her blood pressure through aorto-caval compression. This also encourages the baby's head to rotate to an anterior position. If she needs to lie on her back for a vaginal examination (or other procedures), place a small pillow under her right side to slightly tilt her towards the left (moving the uterus off the vena cava blood vessel).

Change her to the other side periodically. Be aware of her positioning, to ensure her back is not twisted. Support her with pillows, including one or two between her legs. If she has some strength in her legs, suggest she kneel over some pillows or a beanbag.

Remind her to empty her bladder every one to two hours if she doesn't have a catheter in place. Ask the midwife to help with a bedpan.

Keep her cool throughout. If she develops a fever, give her ice to suck; using a cool sponge or fan may also help.

Keep supporting her, although support people should take this time to refresh themselves. Don't withdraw all your support from her – she still needs your help, comfort and encouragement.

Natural therapies and other methods of pain relief

Natural therapies are popular forms of pain relief during labour. However, like medical methods, they may not always produce the desired effects, and it can be hard to know what will actually work for you until you're using the therapies in labour. Try not to rely on a single method, as you could be left feeling disappointed, frustrated or even a failure if it does not meet your expectations.

Acupuncture

Acupuncture can help reduce pain and increase relaxation. One study compared 90 women using acupuncture with 90 women who did not, and found that 58% of the acupuncture group had no medical pain relief, compared to 14% in the non-acupuncture group. Both groups had similar labour lengths and uses of augmentation.[7]

Bear in mind that using acupuncture can make it hard to move around and labour in the shower or bath. However, flat ear-press needles can be taped in place on the earlobe to stimulate points with your fingers as needed. You will need to find an acupuncturist who is familiar with treating pregnant women and who can be on call for you when the labour starts (or becomes established).

Acupressure, shiatsu and reflexology

Acupressure, shiatsu and reflexology work on similar principles to acupuncture but are easier to use because you don't need a qualified acupuncturist to administer them. However, they tend to be less effective when compared to acupuncture. Your partner or support person can learn to find the points. You could even place ink marks on your skin during early labour to make locating them easier.

Reflexology points

Used for labour pain. Pressure is applied to one foot (or both feet) during each contraction and then the pressure is eased as the contraction subsides. The woman may be lying on her side, kneeling, or sitting on a chair or the toilet while this is being done.

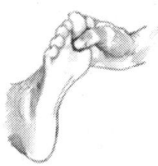

Big toe point – The point lies between the fleshy pads under the big toe and next toe. The partner or support person holds the woman's foot firmly and applies strong pressure with their finger or thumb.

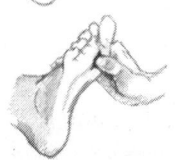

Ball of foot point – The point lies just below the centre of the ball of the foot. Strong pressure is applied by the partner or support person with their finger or thumb.

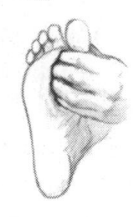

Half moon point – A set of points lie in a half moon shape from where the toes join the foot to the farthest end of the ball of the foot. The partner or support person wraps four fingers around the ball of the foot, applying pressure.

AROMATHERAPY

Essential oils aim to calm and relieve muscular spasms and may be diluted in water as warm compresses, evaporated on a burner or added to carrier oils for massage. Common oils used are:
- Lavender for stimulating circulation, calming, mild analgesia and relieving headaches.
- Nutmeg for calming, assisting with anxiety, stimulating circulation and for mild analgesia.
- Jasmine for relieving muscle spasms, calming, relaxation, optimism and confidence.
- Clary sage for mild analgesia, helping with breathing, calming and a contraction stimulant.
- Black pepper for muscular aches, pains, tired and aching limbs, stimulating circulation and assisting with stamina where there is

frustration. (Usually not burnt as it has a very strong smell, but may be used for backache as a compress.)

Consult with a qualified aromatherapist during the pregnancy and test a small patch on your skin before labour to rule out allergic reactions.

BACH FLOWER AND AUSTRALIAN BUSH FLOWER ESSENCES

These aim to treat emotional states and can be used to balance moods and calm the mind. The Bach flower Rescue Remedy or Australian Emergency Essence may be taken for stress, fear, panic, shock, trauma and labour pains. Consult a practitioner during the pregnancy.

BREATHING AND BIRTHING NOISES

Breathing exercises were first introduced in the 1940s and are the basis of the popular Lamaze method, which uses psychoprophylaxis (or mind prevention). Women are trained to use their breathing and distraction techniques, to disassociate their mind from their bodily pain sensations. The success of breathing techniques is extremely variable between individual women. However, there are two common questions.

Can breathing help relieve labour pain? For some women, yes. Breathing can be effective for part (or perhaps all) of their labour, particularly when combined with other natural methods of pain relief. The idea is to keep the breathing as natural as possible, allowing your mind to focus on the in and out breaths, which shifts your awareness away from the pain. However, other women find controlled breathing unproductive. They focus on trying to breathe the 'right' way, becoming tense and perhaps slowing their labour.

NOTE: *Using patterned breathing too early in labour can tire you prematurely. Leave them until the labour is well established (more than 3 to 5 cm dilated).*

Will I know how to breathe? Your body knows how to breathe without focusing on strict regimens. To help make breathing work for you, try:
- Keeping it simple. Breathe naturally, using your own pace and rhythm.
- Breathing in through your nose (or mouth), and releasing your breath out through a relaxed throat and jaw. Start this at the beginning of the contraction, keeping relaxed for as long as possible until the pain intensifies. Then bring your breathing back to normal as the contraction eases.

- Imagining your breath going deep down into your body to your baby. Relax your neck, shoulders and mouth as you breathe out. Relaxing the mouth helps to relax the vagina, which in turn releases tension in the cervix, allowing it to open.
- Allowing your breathing to match the intensity of the contraction, rather than fighting to contain the breath or pain. Work with it rather than against it. As the labour steps up, often the breathing will follow. Try not to panic. This can restrict your breathing. Have faith in your ability to adjust as the labour progresses.
- Releasing sounds if this helps. Sigh or moan, feel it vibrating down your throat. (You can practise in the shower during the pregnancy.) If you need to scream or swear, this is fine. Just try to keep your throat as open as possible.
- Avoiding fast, rapid breathing (hyperventilating). This can tire you and cause light-headedness and tingling lips and hands (due to too much oxygen). Your support person or caregiver should remind you to slow down and breathe normally between contractions. You may need to breathe through cupped hands over your nose and mouth (or in and out of a paper bag) for a minute or two to lower your body's oxygen level.
- Pounding your fists or stomping your feet to the rhythm of the in and out breath. Match this to the intensity of the contractions.
- Singing or talking as a distraction during each contraction. We know of one professional singer who recited her melodic scales, and another who counted 'One thousand, two thousand, three thousand . . .' until the contractions was over. A few women like their support person to talk to them, or tell them stories, as a means of distraction.

A breathing exercise

When you have some quiet time, sit comfortably and close your eyes. Become aware of your breathing. Focus on the in and out breath for around three to four minutes, then just concentrate on your out breath. You can make sounds if you wish, such as 'aah'. As your breath releases, mentally associate this with letting go or releasing. This is what your body and mind need to do for labour. As you continue to consciously release with your out breath, your body should begin to feel more relaxed. This can be practised three to four times a week, or whenever it suits you, particularly during the final weeks of pregnancy, so it becomes automatic when labour is in progress.

HERBS

Herbs may provide support when you are feeling tired, exhausted or anxious during labour, helping you to cope better with the pain. They may be infused as a tea or administered as a tincture in a concentrated liquid form. Some common herbs used include ginger root, raspberry leaf and skullcap. Consult with a qualified herbalist during the pregnancy.

HOMEOPATHY

Homeopathic remedies may help with emotional and physical reactions to the pain, especially if they are inhibiting the progress of labour. Common remedies include Aconite, Caulophyllum, Chamomilla, Coffea, Kali carb, Pulsatilla and Sepia. Consult with a qualified homeopath and have a labour kit made up during the pregnancy. Some women use tissue or cell salts to help with muscle pain and cramping.

HYPNOSIS

Hypnosis can help with relaxation and an acceptance of the labour pain. It introduces word association, for example 'Labour pain is purposeful', to view labour pain as positive (called hypnobirthing). Using hypnosis in this way does not mean you are asleep or unconscious, nor do you lose control over your mind or feelings. You will need to see a professional hypnotherapist, who is experienced in working with pregnant women, for a number of sessions before the birth.

MASSAGE

Massage stimulates skin nerve fibres to lessen the perception of labour pain and is also relaxing. The massage can range from light, fingertip touching to moderate stroking, to deep kneading pressure, possibly incorporating acupressure, shiatsu or reflexology. Many women like quite firm pressure to their lower back at the sacrum, or either side of the upper buttocks, applied with the heel of their support person's hand (or knuckles), or a hand-held massage device. Try different styles of massage during the pregnancy.

Some women want continual physical contact during labour, while others don't want to be touched at all (and this can change at various times). Partners and support people need to follow the woman's lead.

Movement

Movement is an underestimated method of pain relief. Changing position, walking, stomping and pelvic rocking activate nerve receptors in the joints to help diminish pain. Movement also helps the baby into a favourable position to take pressure off areas such as the lower back.

Most women instinctively move during labour and tend to use more upright positions if not instructed to get on a bed. You may wish to try:
- Pelvic rocking, where you rotate your hips in a circular fashion, or to and fro in an all-fours position. It may feel good to match the rocking to the intensity of the contraction.
- Walking between contractions. However, don't make yourself walk if you feel exhausted, or if it doesn't feel right for you.
- Stomping your feet. As the contraction begins, lean on something and move from side to side, using a light stomping action, adjusting to the intensity of each contraction.
- Squeezing a soft ball to the pace of each contraction. Some women tap their fingers or drum their hands, using an open hand to slap, beat or hit a soft surface such as a bed, beanbag or mat.

Music

Music can act as a distraction, or have a calming, relaxing or motivating influence on you. It can also help with rhythmic breathing and massage strokes, or blocking out other sounds. Some women use music to aid their visualisations or assist with hypnosis. Music can also facilitate the relaxation and positive attitudes of staff, partners and support people.

Transcutaneous Electrical Nerve Stimulation (TENS)

TENS is a noninvasive method of pain relief, but not widely utilised in Australia. The TENS machine consists of a small battery-driven pulse generator, connected to one or two pairs of electrode pads, which are adhered to the woman's middle and lower back over specific skin nerve-endings. When turned on, the pads stimulate these areas with rhythmic, electric pulses, causing buzzing or tingling on the skin.

The woman can adjust the hand control unit to make the pulses low frequency and intermittent, or high frequency and continuous. Low frequencies tend to help stimulate endorphin release, while higher frequencies aim to override the sensations of pain using the gate control theory.[8]

TENS is more likely to be effective during early labour and if the stimulation is turned to a point where it is nearly uncomfortable or painful. TENS machines are portable and usually need to be hired, as most hospitals don't supply them. Ask your caregiver.

Visual focus
While many women close their eyes during a contraction, a few like to open them and focus on something. This might be a clock, a circular drawing with a central point, or their partner/support person's eyes.

Visualisation
Visualisations can be practised during the pregnancy. They incorporate positive attitudes to labour pain by imagining a dress rehearsal for the birth, so when labour starts for real, they are used to help release fearful emotions. The visualisation may also include seeing the unborn baby as resilient and the contractions as stimulating or massaging them in readiness for the outside world. To create your own visualisation, see the visualisation appendix.

Water
Warm water can help soothe, calm and relax the body and help you cope with the pain, especially during the pushing phase. Midwives often refer to baths as natural epidurals. Showers can help release tension and soothe tired muscles. Some women like the protectiveness of a confined shower space or bath and feel more comfortable about releasing birthing sounds.

Water injections
Water injections involve the caregiver injecting small amounts of sterile water into four strategic locations under the surface of the skin in the lower back area, corresponding to the borders of the sacrum. Injections may also be used in the groin area. These aim to override pain sensations using the gate control theory.

Water injections need to be administered by a caregiver experienced in the technique. They can initially sting when being injected, but then they reduce pain, lasting for an hour or two. Water injections are not widely used in Australia. Ask your caregiver.[9]

CHAPTER 10

Inducing or augmenting the labour

Induction

Inducing labour involves artificially stimulating the uterus to contract, rather than waiting for labour to begin spontaneously. If an induction is 'successful', the labour continues until the cervix is fully dilated and the baby is born.

How labour starts largely remains a mystery. It is thought that either the baby or the placenta releases chemical messages to tell the woman's body it is time, or that amniotic fluid levels naturally decline, making the uterine space smaller.[1] We do know that the woman's cervix releases prostaglandins during late pregnancy, which ripen the cervix and can stimulate contractions. This also happens when the waters break. Perhaps it is a combination of many things.

Induction may be suggested when a caregiver believes there are risks involved in waiting for labour to start spontaneously. In some cases this is well before the baby's due date, even though the baby will be premature. Medical reasons to induce labour include:
- A health condition or pregnancy complication for the woman (eg. high blood pressure or cholestasis).
- The baby is thought to be unwell or abnormally small.
- Wanting to prevent a possible infection after the waters break, if labour does not start.
- The pregnancy being one to two weeks overdue.
- The baby dying during pregnancy.

Some caregivers induce labour for a suspected large baby. However, methods used to estimate an unborn baby's weight are very inaccurate, with most well-meaning predictions of a large baby resulting in the birth of a normal-sized baby.

Labour can be induced electively, even though the pregnancy is progressing normally and the woman and baby are well. The caregiver may suggest this when going away on holidays, or the baby is due around a holiday season. Or the woman may request it if she is tired, has aggravating pregnancy discomforts or prefers to schedule the baby's birthday to fit in with family commitments or work leave. Whatever the case, it is important to be aware of the procedures involved so you can weigh up the advantages and disadvantages of inducing a normal pregnancy.

Going 'overdue'

The most common reason to induce labour is the pregnancy going overdue. However, due dates are difficult to estimate because each woman is different. Even siblings can be born at different gestations. So don't rely on past performances (or what your mother or sister did). Some women do have all their babies around the same time (for example, 41 weeks). This may be coincidence, or perhaps a predetermined 'clock' set by their body and baby.

In the 1800s a Dr Naegele developed a system to estimate the baby's due date. He declared that a pregnancy lasted 10 lunar months, or 40 weeks (280 days), equal to approximately 9 calendar months. However, we now know a lunar month is 29.53 solar days, so 10 lunar months is 295 days not 280. This corresponds with a study showing the average length of a normal pregnancy to be 40 weeks plus 8 days for first-time mothers, and 40 weeks plus 3 days for women having subsequent babies.[2] Naegele's rule continues to be used, although it is clearly questionable.

When women labour spontaneously, about:
- 5% of babies are born on their due date.
- 88 to 91% are born between 37 and 41 weeks.
- 6 to 8 % are born prematurely (before 37 weeks).
- 1 to 3 % are born after 41 weeks, with a very small percentage born after 42 weeks.

Choosing when to induce

Even if you are fairly sure when your baby is due, choosing the best time to induce labour is not clear cut. Many caregivers suggest 10 days after the due date (taking into account weekends and public holidays, when routine inductions are not performed), but others recommend 7 days, and a few are happy to wait 12 to 14 days.

The advantages of waiting are:
- It allows more time for labour to start spontaneously.
- The induction is more likely to succeed if left until at least 41 weeks, therefore less likely to end in a caesarean because of a failed induction.

The disadvantages are that babies born after 41 to 42 weeks:
- Are at increased risk of becoming distressed during labour.
- Are at increased risk of dying before or during labour (10% chance compared to 1% for babies born before 41 weeks).

This is because the placenta has a limited life span and its function is impaired after this time. Statistically, about 500 routine inductions performed after 41 weeks can prevent 1 baby from dying.

Inducing labour when overdue can be a difficult decision, especially if you are unsure of your dates or wanting to avoid unnecessary interventions. Feeling pressured by caregivers, family or friends to wait longer, or be induced earlier, can also be distressing, making you feel unsure about what is best. Bear in mind that your own feelings are also important. Some women have an innate sense of knowing that their baby is well and, in the absence of health complications, are comfortable waiting longer. Others feel they do not want to go beyond 7 to 10 overdue days and prefer to be induced earlier.

Playing a role in choosing the date can help you feel more in control of the situation and perhaps more positive about the induction (if it is needed). Take one day at a time and assess it as you go. Often your feelings change from day to day. Consider using some natural therapies (if appropriate), and if induction does become inevitable, try to be accepting of it.

Tests when the pregnancy is overdue

When delaying an induction beyond 7 to 10 days past the due date, most caregivers recommend tests to assess the baby's wellbeing. These are only a guide and cannot definitively tell how an unborn baby is coping. However, if they indicate that the baby might be at risk, then labour is induced sooner rather than later.

Testing can vary between caregivers and hospitals, but may include:
- CTG monitoring of the baby's heart rate for 20 to 30 minutes, every second or third day from 7 to 10 days past the due date (until labour starts or is induced).
- An ultrasound measuring amniotic fluid volume around the baby.

Having less fluid is of concern, although amniotic fluid naturally decreases after 37 weeks and can be lower if you are dehydrated. So drink plenty of water for 24 hours before the test.
- A Doppler ultrasound measuring blood flow through the baby's umbilical cord.

A combination of the above tests can be done, called a biophysical profile. Some caregivers also suggest recording the baby's daily movements on a kick chart.

READINESS FOR LABOUR

To increase the chances of an induction being successful (and avoiding a caesarean), a woman's body needs to be ready for labour. The key physical sign of being ready is the 'ripeness' or 'favourability' of her cervix.

As labour nears, the cervix softens, thins and moves forward in the vagina, often opening slightly. If the cervix is long, thick, closed and posterior (towards the back of the vagina), it is said to be 'unripe' or 'unfavourable', and is less likely to respond to induction methods.

About 50% of women being induced have an unripe cervix. Therefore caregivers often use interventions aimed at ripening the cervix as part of an induction. The cervix is assessed with an internal vaginal examination. The caregiver uses five physical signs to determine the favourability of the cervix, these being:
1. Dilation of the cervix.
2. Consistency of the cervix (firm, medium or soft).
3. Position of the cervix (posterior, central or anterior).
4. Effacement or thinning of the cervix (0 to 100%).
5. How far engaged the baby's head is.

Each physical sign is given a score, known as a Bishop's score.

NOTE: *Be aware that the interpretation of these physical signs (and therefore the score given) can vary slightly from caregiver to caregiver.*

Induction methods

Induction methods can involve medications (pharmacological) or mechanical procedures such as breaking the waters. Often a combination is used to optimise the labour's progress and help the induction be successful. The method(s) chosen will depend on:

- The favourability of the cervix.
- Whether the waters have already broken. This makes the woman's body more sensitive to medications (requiring a lesser dose or avoiding them altogether).
- Whether this is a first or subsequent baby. Women who have had a previous baby (vaginally or by caesarean) are more sensitive to most induction methods, generally needing less medications and/or fewer interventions.
- If you have had a previous caesarean birth. Pharmacological methods are often avoided to reduce the rare risk of the uterus rupturing.
- The caregiver's, hospital's and woman's preferences.

When planning an induction, ask your caregiver exactly what is intended and how the procedure(s) will be carried out. Ask them to talk you through all the steps before you agree to being admitted to hospital, so you know what is involved. If you read about an induction method you think you might prefer (but your caregiver has not offered to you), perhaps suggest this as an option.

PHARMACOLOGICAL METHODS

Pharmacological induction methods tend to use either prostaglandin medications or intravenous Syntocinon.

Prostaglandins

Synthetic prostaglandins are usually prescribed as a vaginal (or rectal) gel, or as a pessary with a string attached (like a small tampon). They can also be given as an oral tablet or administered intravenously.

Prostaglandins mainly aim to make the cervix more favourable and the woman's body more susceptible to other induction methods, particularly if the pregnancy is less than 41 weeks. However, prostaglandins will induce labour for up to 50% of women – although this is more likely if the baby is more than 1 week overdue and/or is a subsequent baby.

Prostaglandins are administered during a vaginal examination, normally in the antenatal ward of the hospital. (They are stored in the fridge, so may feel cold when inserted.) The baby's heart rate is continuously monitored with a CTG machine for 20 minutes beforehand and 40 minutes afterwards. If the baby's heart rate remains normal, the machine is removed, so you can get up and walk around.

Prostaglandins normally cause lower abdominal cramping and/or backache as they start to take effect. You can use heat packs or have a shower to help with this. Once labour becomes established or the waters break, the pessary is removed. If a gel is used, often two doses are needed, six to eight hours apart to induce labour. Usually the waters are routinely broken once the cervix starts to dilate, to help stimulate stronger contractions.

Each woman's response to prostaglandins is unpredictable. Some women progress to established labour within 4 to 12 hours, others have two doses and their waters broken, yet their cervix does not dilate (with or without painful contractions). If labour does not establish within 12 hours or so, a Syntocinon drip is then recommended.

The main concern with prostaglandins is the possibility of overstimulating the uterus, making it contract too much (1 to 7% chance). Hyperstimulation is more likely if:

- The cervix is favourable.
- The waters are broken.
- It is a second or subsequent baby.

If hyperstimulation occurs oxygen can be reduced for the baby, so the caregiver may try to suppress the contractions with medications, with varying degrees of success. Sometimes an emergency caesarean is required. Very rarely, the uterus may rupture, although this risk is more likely for women who have had a previous caesarean.

Advantages of prostaglandins:
- There is an increased chance of a successful induction, especially if the cervix is unripe.
- Prostaglandins are associated with a more positive experience, because it feels more natural.
- Once the initial monitoring is completed, you are free to move around, have an active birth and use the shower and bath.
- If the labour is induced, it is often shorter.
- Compared to a Syntocinon drip, prostaglandins are associated with less need for pain relief and less chance of requiring a forceps delivery or caesarean.
- Women planning to have their baby in a birth centre or at home often prefer prostaglandins because they have the option of returning to their chosen birthplace after it is administered.

Disadvantages of prostaglandins:
- They cannot be used if the cervix is too favourable or possibly if the waters have broken, because of the risk of hyperstimulation.
- Prostaglandin gels cannot easily be removed (although pessaries with a string can). Once it's in, it's in. So if hyperstimulation occurs, the

caregiver may perform a vaginal examination to try and scrape what remains of the medication out with their fingers.
- Labour may feel more intense than if it had started spontaneously.
- The medications may cause nausea, vomiting and/or diarrhoea in some women. On rare occasions a local allergic reaction can occur, causing burning and itching inside the vagina.
- From an emotional perspective, waiting for labour to start can be stressful. More so if it does not work and a Syntocinon drip is still required.

Syntocinon

Syntocinon is a synthetic form of natural oxytocin hormone. It is usually given intravenously in the delivery suite (not in a birth centre, nor for a homebirth).

Syntocinon needs to be administered precisely, in a slow, controlled manner with an electric infusion pump. It is started on the lowest dose, then built up gradually every 15 to 30 minutes until the contractions are strong and regular. Once labour is established, the Syntocinon is maintained at the same dose until after the baby is born.

The maximum dose required depends on each woman's individual response. In most cases, the drip needs to run for several hours before labour establishes, although a few women do respond relatively quickly (within an hour or so). Factors that make Syntocinon more likely to stimulate strong contractions are:
- The waters being broken. The longer they have been broken, the more responsive the body tends to be.
- The cervix being favourable, or having prostaglandins before the Syntocinon.
- Already having mild or moderate prelabour contractions.
- Being more than one week past the baby's due date.
- Having a second or subsequent baby.

To optimise its effectiveness, the caregiver often breaks the waters at some stage (if this has not already happened). If the maximum dose is reached and maintained for a couple of hours but labour does not establish (despite the waters being broken), the induction is deemed unsuccessful and the baby is delivered by caesarean.

Advantages of Syntocinon:
- Syntocinon is an alternative if the cervix is too favourable for prostaglandins, or if the waters have broken. It is the next step if prostaglandins were not successful.

- It generally shortens labour (although it can take a while for the contractions to become strong).
- It is less likely to hyperstimulate the uterus and can be turned down (or off) if this happens.

Disadvantages of Syntocinon:
- It is less likely than prostaglandins to succeed at inducing labour if the cervix is unfavourable and/or the pregnancy is less than 41 weeks.
- The baby's heart rate is usually continuously monitored with a CTG machine while the doses are being increased, but most caregivers prefer the monitor to stay on for the entire labour. This restricts your mobility and rules out access to the bath or a shower.
- When compared to prostaglandins, women are more likely to request pain relief sooner.
- Labour may feel more intense than if it had started spontaneously.
- It can be disappointing if you were planning an active birth and/or wanting to have the baby in a birth centre or at home.
- Prolonged use over several hours can have an antidiuretic effect, making the kidneys produce less urine, which can occasionally lead to abnormal fluid retention and overload (called water intoxication). In rare cases this can accumulate in the woman's lungs, becoming life-threatening.
- Prolonged use can also increase the baby's chances of becoming jaundiced after the birth, possibly needing phototherapy.

MECHANICAL METHODS

Mechanical induction methods work by ripening, or dilating, the cervix and/or stimulating the uterus to contract, by increasing the body's natural secretion of prostaglandins or oxytocin. They can be used on their own, or in combination with each other and/or with pharmacological methods.

Breaking the waters

The caregiver may artificially rupture the membranes (called an ARM or amniotomy). This is done through a vaginal examination by using a specially designed implement called an amnihook to create a small tear in the membranes (or bag of waters). Releasing some amniotic fluid can stimulate a natural release of prostaglandins, as well as lowering the baby's head to place more pressure on the cervix.

NOTE: *An amniotomy in itself is not painful because there are no nerves in the membranes. But if the cervix is unfavourable, the vaginal examination required to access the membranes can be uncomfortable (or even painful), because the membranes are difficult to reach (sometimes impossible). Also, if the membranes are very smooth, or particularly tough, more than one attempt may be required.*

Breaking the waters can successfully induce labour for up to 88% of women if the cervix is already favourable. This is more likely if it is a subsequent baby or the pregnancy is more than one week overdue, and/or it is combined with other induction methods.

Soon after the ARM, most women feel a trickle, or gush, of warm fluid coming away. This continues to dribble every time you move, the baby moves or the uterus contracts (you will need to wear a pad). The water can be clear, pinkish or perhaps bloodstained, which is normal. If it is stained with meconium, the baby's heart rate needs to be continuously monitored with a CTG machine. (Bear in mind that the meconium would have been present before the waters were broken and did not happen as a direct result of having the ARM.)

Ideally the baby's head should be engaged when having an ARM, to avoid the rare complication of the umbilical cord prolapsing. If the baby's head is high, the caregiver may try a controlled ARM – meaning they leave their fingers on the baby's head for a minute or so after making a small hole in the membrane, to let the fluid slowly dribble and the baby's head to slowly ease down onto the cervix.

It is normal to experience mild contractions, or cramping, for a few hours after an ARM, but it may take several hours for labour to establish. It is important that you are given adequate time (at least 6 to 24 hours; 2 to 4 hours is not reasonable). In some cases, labour does not start and a Syntocinon drip is required.

NOTE: *While it is possible for an ARM to induce labour for a first-time mother, it is not the preferred method because it could take 24 to 48 hours to work. Even then, a few women will still need Syntocinon to induce labour.*

Advantages of an ARM:

- It can be performed in any birthplace, by a midwife or doctor.
- If combined with other induction methods, it increases the chances of the induction being successful.
- It is close to being natural.
- The contractions intensify slowly, as they would for a normal labour, so there is less chance of you requiring pain relief.
- You can move freely and use the shower and bath (although the bath should be avoided until the contractions are strong, in case the induction takes a while).
- Women who have had a previous caesarean can use it, if the cervix is favourable.

Disadvantages of an ARM:
- It is less effective (or not always possible) when the cervix is unfavourable or the baby's head is not engaged.
- It can increase the risk of infection if labour does not start within 12 to 24 hours.
- It is not recommended for women having an active herpes outbreak or carrying HIV/AIDS, as it increases the chances of the baby becoming infected with these viruses.
- It may slightly increase the chances of the baby becoming distressed during labour because the cushion of fluid minimises pressure on the baby's cord during labour. However, up to 19% of women spontaneously break their waters and most healthy babies are not bothered by this.
- If the membrane is lying very close to the baby's head, the caregiver may slightly scratch the baby's scalp with the amnihook when performing the ARM.

Sweeping the membranes

Sweeping (or stripping) the membranes is often called a strip and stretch. This old induction method involves the caregiver performing a vaginal examination, then placing one finger through the opening of the cervix and moving their finger in a circular motion, which separates the membranes from the lower segment of the uterus. If the cervix is tightly closed, they may try massaging it instead.

Sweeping the membranes aims to trigger the release of natural prostaglandins to ripen the cervix. Some caregivers routinely do this at weekly pregnancy visits from 37 to 38 weeks. It can cause period-like cramping (or irregular contractions) for several hours and often a small amount of vaginal bleeding for a day or so after the procedure (which may persist as a brownish discharge of old blood for several days).

Advantages of sweeping the membranes:
- It is an easy procedure performed by a midwife or doctor.
- It may ripen the cervix and reduce the chances of going overdue.
- Sweeping the membranes may induce labour, although this is unpredictable and can take several hours (or days).
- It may increase the chances of other induction methods succeeding.[3]

Disadvantages of sweeping the membranes:
- It can be uncomfortable or painful.
- It only has a small chance of successfully inducing labour (12–15%).

- Some women find the procedure personally invasive and distressing.
- It holds a small risk of accidentally breaking the waters, which can lead to time pressures to start established labour and possibly needing a Syntocinon drip (or a caesarean if the Syntocinon is not successful – this is more likely if the pregnancy is less than 40 weeks). Therefore, some caregivers prefer to delay sweeping the membranes until 40 to 41 weeks.

NOTE: *Sweeping the membranes is not a routine part of pregnancy care and most caregivers don't use it unless requested or the pregnancy is going overdue. Be aware that some caregivers do not prewarn women that they are about to sweep their membranes. So if a vaginal examination is suggested towards the end of pregnancy, ask your caregiver if they intend to do this.*

Foley's catheter

Foley's catheters have been used for several years to induce labour but have recently gone out of vogue, with the increased popularity of pharmacological methods. A Foley's catheter is normally used to empty the bladder of urine. However, instead of placing it in the bladder, the soft rubber tip is placed inside the cervix during a vaginal examination. The caregiver then gently inflates a small balloon in the end of the catheter with water to expand inside the cervix and apply even pressure. The aim is to ripen and dilate the cervix and/or stimulate the release of prostaglandins to induce labour.

Pressure on the cervix often causes cramping and possibly irregular contractions. You may need a heat pack or a shower to help with these discomforts. You can walk around with the catheter in place, but the end of the tube hangs outside the vagina. Some caregivers place gentle tension on the catheter by taping the end of the tube to your inner thigh.

Once the cervix dilates to 2 to 4 cm, the catheter usually falls out. At this point the caregiver often breaks the waters to help establish labour. A Foley's catheter should work within 6 to 12 hours or so. If the catheter is unsuccessful, then prostaglandins or a Syntocinon drip may be recommended.

NOTE: *An Atad double-balloon catheter may be used. This has two balloons, one that inflates just inside the uterus (but outside the bag of waters) to keep it in place, and a second which inflates inside the cervix.*

Advantages of a Foley's catheter:
- It can be inserted by a midwife or doctor.
- There are no side effects, making it a good option for women who have had a previous caesarean.

Disadvantages of a Foley's catheter:
- If the cervix is unfavourable, it may be difficult (or impossible) to insert.
- It can take a while (or several attempts) to insert correctly.
- It may fall out too early if it is not in an optimal position or too much tension is applied.
- Occasionally the waters can be unintentionally broken, which can introduce time pressures if labour does not start within 12 to 24 hours.

Laminaria tents
A Laminaria tent works on similar principles to a Foley's catheter. It is a thin, rounded stick of sterile seaweed (or a synthetic hydrophilic material called Lamicel), which the caregiver gently places inside the cervix with the assistance of a speculum. As the tent absorbs moisture, it gradually swells to stretch and dilate the cervix, hopefully inducing labour.

RISKS AND PROBLEMS WITH MEDICAL INDUCTIONS
When Syntocinon was developed in the 1960s, caregivers (and women) were so enthused by its potential to control labour that by the 1970s up to 60 to 90% of pregnancies were induced, despite little research having been done. Eventually it was realised that routine inductions could be harmful, with only a few mothers and babies who really needed it for medical reasons actually benefiting. Even with this knowledge, many women are still induced unnecessarily. The WHO recommends induction rates of 10 to 15%, but in Australia, induction rates tend to be around 26%, ranging from 3 to 35%, depending on the caregiver or birthplace.[4]

Did you know?
An Australian study of 171,157 women showed vast differences in induction rates, depending on the woman's chosen place of birth and caregiver, despite all the women having similar rates of complications. For women:
- With their own doctor, in a private hospital, having their first baby, the rate was 25.7%; for women having their subsequent baby, it was 22.9%.
- With their own doctor, in a public hospital, having their first baby, the rate was 21.1%; for women having their subsequent baby, it was 18.9%.
- Who were Medicare only, in a public hospital, having their first baby, the rate was 15.7%; for women having their subsequent baby, it was 12.9%.[5]

Many people believe inductions are virtually risk free. However, once the natural process of labour is disturbed, there are increased risks and problems that can manifest. Apart from the direct side effects of each method, there are also many indirect flow-on effects, referred to as the cascade of intervention. This is essentially a chain of events that carry on from the initial procedure, and may be an accepted part of induction for some women and caregivers, or a motivating reason to try and avoid induction for others.

The cascade is complex and interrelated, but may unfold in the following ways:

- Prostaglandins or mechanical methods may not work, leading to a Syntocinon drip, and the baby's heart rate being continuously monitored. This restricts your mobility (often to the bed), increasing your perception of pain and ruling out the use of showers and baths for pain relief. As a result there is an increased chance of you requiring pain-relieving medications.
- Pharmacological methods tend to accelerate labour pains over a short period. The early phases of the first stage are often skipped, moving straight into strong, established labour. This does not allow your body time to release natural endorphins, making some women panic because they feel unprepared, so they request pain relief sooner.
- The early use of pain relief can lead to the need for additional pain relief as the labour intensifies; for example, gas, then pethidine then an epidural, or simply an early epidural. The labour's progress can be slowed, possibly requiring more Syntocinon to keep the contractions strong. This increases the chances of hyperstimulation, which may distress the baby. Slow progress and/or a distressed baby may lead to a caesarean, or a forceps or ventouse delivery.
- Inductions often have unreasonable time limits. It is not unknown for an induction to be started at 8 am, then for the caregiver to walk in at 6 pm and say to the woman, 'You've had enough time', before performing a caesarean (or forceps or ventouse if the cervix is fully dilated). Time pressures also come into play once the waters are broken.
- Time pressures make it difficult to relax. If the woman is anxious and concerned, her body releases adrenaline, which suppresses contractions, increasing her need for more Syntocinon. If the labour is prolonged, time pressures become a real threat, with the induction viewed as being 'unsuccessful', leading to a caesarean.

NOTE: *If there are medical reasons for inducing labour, then the risks of the induction usually far outweigh the risks involved with continuing the pregnancy. Also, bear in mind that while the cascade effect is possible, it is not inevitable. Many women are induced without additional interventions or complications.*

Natural methods

Natural therapies can be used to ripen the cervix, finetune the body for labour and perhaps induce contractions. Natural methods don't provide a quick result, often taking hours or days, depending on the situation. As with medical induction methods, the body is more likely to respond after the baby's due date, during prelabour or once the waters have broken. Also, bear in mind that if a therapy does not produce results, trying it again in a few days time may stimulate a better response because by now the body is primed.

Some sceptics view natural therapy inductions as a coincidence, saying labour was going to start anyway. This is hard to prove or disprove.

NOTE: Women with medical conditions may not be able to use natural therapies because of their effects or because they take too long to work. Check with your caregiver and/or practitioner.

Acupressure

Acupressure points can prepare the body for labour and/or stimulate contractions. They include the ankle, hand, buttock or foot points (see the acupressure appendix). A TENS machine may also be used to enhance the stimulation of these points.

Acupuncture

A qualified acupuncturist can target points with needles (moxibustion) to finetune and balance the body by raising or lowering energy levels. This aims to create the best possible environment for labour to start. If appropriate, points may also be used to stimulate contractions. When being induced, you often need two treatments, a day or so apart. The first tunes the body and the second stimulates contractions.

Aromatherapy

You may want to try an aromatherapy massage, or burning clary sage or rose (only after 38 weeks of pregnancy). Other oils are jasmine, lavender, chamomile, mandarin and geranium. Consult your aromatherapist.

Bowel stimulation

When labour starts, the smooth muscles of the bowel work hand in hand with the smooth muscles of the uterus, which is why diarrhoea is often experienced during prelabour, and why things like hot curries and drinking prune juice may be recommended.

The most common bowel stimulant to induce labour is castor oil, although individual responses are unpredictable. Some women find it successfully induces labour within 12 to 24 hours, but others just experience cramping and/or nausea. Castor oil tends to be a last resort when facing induction. Midwives often recommend 1 to 2 tablespoons (10 to 20 ml) mixed with a glass of juice (as it tastes awful), repeating this an hour later. Check with your caregiver. Consider taking it in the morning so you are not up all night on the toilet!

Herbs
Herbalists may recommend black or blue cohosh to stimulate contractions. In recent years raspberry leaf tea (or tablets) has become popular to take during late pregnancy to reduce the chances of going overdue. Consult your herbalist.

Homeopathy
Caulophyllum is a common homeopathic remedy used to stimulate contractions, especially if the waters have broken. It tends to be more effective when combined with acupuncture or acupressure. You may have this made up as part of a labour kit. See your homeopath.

Massage
Massage can relax the mind and body and may be combined with shiatsu or reflexology points for balance or to stimulate contractions.

Nipple stimulation
When the nipples are stimulated close to the time of labour, it triggers a release of natural oxytocin to make the uterus contract. Some women do nipple stimulation each day during the last few weeks of their pregnancy to help ripen the cervix and reduce the chances of going overdue.

NOTE: Nipple stimulation is only recommended for women experiencing a normal pregnancy, as it is not clear whether it is safe for the baby if there are medical health conditions complicating the pregnancy.[6]

Nipple stimulation aims to mimic the timing of contractions. This is how it's done:
- Take one nipple between the thumb and forefinger, and roll it gently between them, or gently pull the nipple down and out, from the areola, until it becomes erect. Your partner can also lick or gently suck the nipple. Some caregivers suggest using a breast pump for a few pumps.
- Once the nipple is erect, continue stimulating for about one minute, then leave it for two to four minutes.

- Next, go to the other nipple and repeat the same procedure, waiting two to four minutes afterwards before returning to the first nipple, and so on. You can do this for 30 minutes to an hour or so, repeating it in a few hours time or the next day.

Relaxation

Feeling pressured to perform can be stressful, with your body releasing adrenaline that can suppress, or stop, contractions. On the other hand, low levels of adrenaline can delay labour until things are in place, such as finishing the renovations, moving house, finalising a project, when Christmas Day passes, your other children are asleep or your mother arrives (or leaves!).

Sometimes letting go mentally, or organising things that may be holding you back, can help. Try a massage, a dinner out, possibly a small glass of wine or using a relaxation visualisation (see visualisation appendix).

Sex and orgasm

Orgasm stimulates the release of natural oxytocin, causing the uterus to contract and possibly starting labour (if it is near the baby's due date). The man's semen also ripens the woman's cervix because it contains prostaglandins. If intercourse is not desirable (or feasible, or not recommended because the waters are broken), then orgasm through masturbation may be an alternative.

Visualisation

Visualisation may prime your body, or help labour to start. (See the visualisation appendix to help you create your own.)

COPING STRATEGIES

If an induction is planned, or becomes inevitable, you may wish to consider some strategies to help make it a more positive experience. Obtain all the facts as to why your caregiver feels an induction is necessary. If you are unsure, or uncomfortable about being induced (or the methods being offered), ask about other options. If you feel you need a second opinion, follow your instincts.

Depending on the method(s) chosen, you may want to negotiate some aspects of your care to help avoid the cascade of intervention.
- If there are no complications, consider delaying the induction until 7 to 10 days past the due date. This maximises your chances of the induction being successful, or avoiding it altogether if labour starts

spontaneously beforehand. The lead-on risks of induction are greatly reduced if the pregnancy is at least one week overdue.
- If prostaglandins or Syntocinon don't work, and the waters are not broken (and there are no complications), consider repeating it in a day or two. Often the second attempt is more successful.
- Once the required dose of Syntocinon is reached, request that the baby's heart rate be intermittently monitored every 30 minutes or only continuously monitored for 20 to 30 minutes, every hour or two (if the baby's heart rate is normal and/or the amniotic fluid is not meconium-stained). Alternatively, your support person may be able to hold the CTG monitor in place on your belly to allow you more freedom of movement.
- If not continuously monitored, you should be able to use the shower or bath with Syntocinon. Most electric infusion pumps run on batteries. Perhaps request an extension of the intravenous tubing to allow more freedom and ask that the drip be put in the hand you don't favour (for example, the left hand if you are right-handed).
- If you wish to avoid or delay medicated pain relief, try holding out for 30 to 45 minutes after the strong contractions start. This allows your body time to release natural endorphins, helping you cope better. Often women who try this find they feel more relaxed and in control because they are on top of the pain rather than being engulfed by it.
- **Don't** feel pressured into having your baby during business hours. If you need help at 2 am, that is when you need it. It is your right to have medical care when it is necessary, not when it is convenient. If you are well and the baby is well, time is on your side.

EMOTIONAL CONSIDERATIONS
Depending on how you view induction, you may experience a range of emotional reactions:
- Disappointment in your body and yourself.
- Fear that you are handing over control.
- More in control if the induction is your choice.
- Relief that the pregnancy is ending and you can meet your baby.
- Upset if you are not able to give birth where you planned (in the case of a birth centre or homebirth).
- Worried that the induction will be more painful.
- Unhappy with having to be monitored and restricted in your movement.

- Grief in letting go of how you would have liked the labour to be.
- Feelings of becoming a number in the medical system.
- Concerned (or invaded) by all the procedures.
- Worried about whether you and your baby will be all right, particularly if the induction is happening because of health complications.

Emotions can cloud your whole labour and birth experience. Being able to work with them is usually easier than dealing with them weeks down the track when you are consumed by your new mothering role. If the situation doesn't require immediate induction, ask for some time to be with your feelings. Try to identify what is surfacing for you and allow the emotions to be felt. Cry if you need to. Don't let others hurry you out of your feelings with comments like 'You'll be all right.' Yes, you probably will be all right, but your emotions should not be negated.

Some strategies that other women have found helpful are:
- Letting go of the labour they would have liked and trying to go with the flow.
- Talking with their partner or family, letting them know their feelings. Ask them how they feel about the induction.
- Writing down feelings, fears and disappointments.
- Being aware of all their choices and becoming involved in the decisions-making process.

Pregnancy, labour and birth involve working with the unknown. They bring you into the moment and demand you work with what is happening at the time. If you are flexible and realistic, it is easier to deal with the unexpected. This is not to say that you shouldn't question or negotiate what is being offered, but if all else fails, work with the situation you are in to help retain some essence of what you originally planned.

Augmentation

The word 'augment' means to increase or enlarge. When labour is augmented, interventions are used to intensify the contractions because they have become weak (hypotonic), irregular, too far apart and/or not lasting long enough, or have stopped altogether. Labour contractions need to be strong and efficient to dilate the cervix and allow the baby to be born.

Your caregiver may suggest augmentation if they feel the labour is not progressing, or is progressing too slowly. Adequate progress should take into account:

- The pattern, length and intensity of the contractions, usually 2 to 4 minutes apart and lasting 50 seconds or more.
- How quickly the cervix thins and dilates (at least 0.5 cm an hour during the first stage for first babies, quicker for subsequent babies).
- The baby's head flexing and descending lower into the pelvis (and/or sitting more snugly on the cervix).
- Two hours of active pushing for first babies and one hour for subsequent babies.

A slow, steady labour can be normal. If mother and baby are well, then augmentation may not be necessary. There is a tendency to overuse augmentation in Australia, and rates can range from 18 to 35%, depending on the caregiver and the birthplace.

Medical reasons for labour slowing include:
- Being dehydrated and/or ketotic (often accompanied by the woman feeling exhausted).
- Having a narcotic injection or epidural before 4 cm dilation, or using the bath too early.
- The baby's head being deflexed and not sitting snugly on the cervix.
- The baby being in a posterior position and taking a while to rotate towards the front.
- The labour being truly obstructed because the baby's head remains deflexed, or is in a face or brow position.
- The contractions not being coordinated, despite seeming strong, intense and close together. This is called incoordinate uterine action and occurs when the uterine muscles don't contract in partnership, making the uterus tense and tender to touch even after the contraction passes. This is uncommon but can happen if the baby's head is deflexed, and may possibly lead to the baby becoming distressed. It is unlikely to happen again with a subsequent baby.

Other factors that may be at play when labour slows can include:
- A natural lull in the contractions, or a temporary pattern change.
- Feeling fearful or anxious with external threats (eg. interventions being suggested, complications unfolding or too many people in the room), or internal concerns (eg. worry about the pain ahead, losing control, the baby's wellbeing, parenting abilities or the baby's sex).

If there appears to be no apparent medical reason, you may choose to wait, rest and recuperate for a while, or to look at natural therapies to help intensify the contractions. On the other hand, if you are feeling tired, frustrated and despondent, you may readily accept (or request) augmentation. Bear in mind that many caregivers don't recognise these natural influences, or are simply impatient or not comfortable with waiting.

Medical methods
Medical augmentation methods are similar to medical induction methods, with some slight variations.

Breaking the waters
An ARM is often the first option to augment labour, unless the waters have already broken. Amniotic fluid can trickle away from a hole in the sac behind the baby's head (called a hind-water leak), leaving a bag of forewaters in front of the baby's head that can still be broken to augment labour.

An ARM done when the cervix is 3 to 9 cm dilated can rapidly intensify the contractions. If it is done after 9 cm, it tends to make the baby's head come further down the birth canal, increasing the urge to push (usually the desired effect).

Some caregivers like to routinely break the waters at some stage during labour, regardless of whether it is progressing slowly or not. This may be out of habit to facilitate a faster labour, or to see whether the amniotic fluid is meconium-stained (or to internally monitor the baby's heart rate with a CTG). Research shows both benefits and risks for a routine ARM before 5 cm. It may shorten the labour by up to 60 to 120 minutes and reduce the likelihood of needing a Syntocinon drip, but it can also increase the chances of the baby becoming distressed (due to compression of the umbilical cord) and is associated with a higher chance of requiring a caesarean.[7]

Intravenous Syntocinon
A Syntocinon drip can:
- Stimulate contractions after the waters have broken.
- Establish the labour after a prolonged prelabour.
- Intensify contractions that have slowed, weakened or stopped, due to dehydration or pain relief.
- Strengthen contractions to help the baby's head to flex and move down the birth canal.
- Hasten the labour's progress.
- Regulate incoordinate contractions.

Intravenous Syntocinon can take up to two to three hours to establish labour, then another two to four hours before changes in the cervix are noticeable. Waiting an hour or two is not reasonable.

Syntocinon can be the catalyst for achieving a vaginal birth, but it is the final card. If labour still does not progress, then a caesarean is needed. Up to 30% of labours augmented with Syntocinon also involve the baby being distressed, which may lead to a forceps, ventouse or caesarean delivery.

Rehydration
Giving extra fluids intravenously can help with dehydration and ketosis, and may be all that is needed to help the contractions return. If this does not work within two to four hours, then intravenous Syntocinon may be suggested.

Pain relief
While pain relief can slow labour, it can sometimes help it to progress, especially if a woman is feeling apprehensive about moving from one phase of labour to the next (typically around 3 cm, 7 cm, near full dilation or when pushing). Pain relief may facilitate relaxation to let go and enable labour to progress, but it will not really help if you are less than 3 to 4 cm dilated. Instead you could try:
- A bath.
- The gas, especially during the transitional phase.
- A narcotic injection, although its effects can be difficult to predict and may end up slowing or stopping the labour.
- An epidural, although again, it may slow labour and Syntocinon may be required.

NATURAL THERAPIES
You may want to try some natural therapies to augment labour before embarking on medical interventions. However, this may involve negotiating some time to see whether they work. Most methods are similar to those used to induce labour, but there are a few variations for some.

Homeopathy
Some homeopathic remedies address the woman's psychological state, such as anxiety or fear if the cervix is not dilating, or painful but ineffective contractions. Homeopathic labour kits often come with a range of remedies and directions that describe different emotional states so these can be treated.

Massage, acupressure and reflexology
Massage and the use of acupressure, shiatsu and reflexology can stimulate contractions, but also help the woman relax and let go.

Orgasm

Setting up an environment to achieve an orgasm in hospital may be tricky, although it is not unheard of for a woman (alone or with her partner) to go into the bathroom for a bit of privacy to attempt it!

SUPPORT STRATEGIES

Many support strategies described in Chapters 5, 6, 7 and 9 can help you avoid augmentation. These include:
- Using gravity and mobility (eg. standing, sitting, kneeling or all fours, walking or pelvic rocking) and forward leaning positions to assist the uterus to contract efficiently and help the baby rotate towards the front.
- Staying well nourished and hydrated. Sports (or electrolyte) drinks can help if the labour is turning out to be a marathon event.
- Working with your fears before the birth, perhaps using relaxation techniques or visualisations.

Effective communication and negotiation skills may be needed if augmentation is being suggested. As with all professions, caregivers will have different approaches and varying communication skills, and how they present the pros and cons of an intervention will often depend on their personal style and opinion. In reality, not everyone is able to provide information in a nonbiased manner, but if you are unaware of alternative approaches, then you will need to trust their judgment. To help you negotiate for reasonable alternatives to augmentation, you should try the following:
- Choose your caregivers and birthplaces carefully.
- Learn about interventions even though you don't want to face the possibility of needing them.
- Consider doing a birth plan.
- Negotiate tactfully, especially if you wish to divert from what is being suggested. Do this in a non-threatening way. Confrontation often does not work, unless it is a last resort. Professionals commonly react with irrational responses like 'Do you want to risk your life or your baby's life?' There is very little comeback for this.
- Be aware that no matter how experienced your caregiver, *no one* can accurately predict 100% of the time the outcomes of various interventions. They can only give you a general idea of the range of possible outcomes. Sometimes it can be hard to know whether your choices are the right ones. You can only take it one step at a time.
- Don't feel pressured. A few hours are comparatively short in the scope

of your whole pregnancy and birth experience. Sometimes waiting (if there are no complications) can mean the difference between a normal birth and a caesarean.
- Be aware that you have the right to:
  1. Fair and clear information.
  2. A second opinion if you feel you need it.
  3. Make decisions about your care, including the right to decline interventions or ask for an alternative, if available.

CHAPTER 11

Caesarean birth

A caesarean birth involves delivering the baby and the placenta through a surgical incision in the woman's lower belly and uterus. A caesarean performed before labour begins is elective (or planned); and if performed during labour, it is an emergency (or unplanned) caesarean, even though the situation may not be a true medical emergency.

Before the twentieth century, caesareans were a last resort to save a baby if the woman had just died. By the early 1900s 1% of births were caesareans. Improvements in surgical and anaesthetic techniques made caesareans safer and more acceptable, and by 1970 the rate was 5%, which has since escalated sharply to 20 to 30% in the new millennium.

> **Did you know?**
> Caesareans originated in Roman times when Julius Caesar decreed that a woman dying in childbirth should have her baby delivered by cutting her belly open, to increase the low population at the time.

Caesareans are performed when health concerns for a mother and/or baby indicate that labouring and/or giving birth vaginally hold more risks than the possible risks of the operation, or the birth needs to happen fairly quickly. Medical reasons include:
- Placenta previa or placental abruption.
- Fetal distress.
- Cord prolapse.
- The woman or baby being unwell.
- The baby being in an unusual position (eg. deflexed head, breech, transverse, brow or face presentations).
- The first stage of labour not progressing.
- Unsuccessful induction or augmentation.
- Twins or more (see Chapter 7).
- Very premature babies not in a head-down position, or who require immediate delivery.
- Some types of previous uterine surgery.

- A fourth degree tear with a previous vaginal birth.
- HIV or hepatitis C with high viral loads or an active outbreak of genital herpes when the waters break, or labour commences.
- A large baby (more than 4.5 kg or 10 lb).

NOTE: *Most babies 'fit' unless they are in an unusual position, but the baby may be unusually large if the woman has uncontrolled diabetes or the baby has an abnormality. However, research indicates that estimations are frequently incorrect, with many unnecessary caesareans performed on normal-sized babies.*[1]

Intervening to perform a caesarean for non-medical reasons is when the risks of the caesarean do not outweigh the possible risks of having the baby vaginally. These include:

- Having had a previous caesarean. These account for 40% of caesareans, but are not discouraged because women are having smaller families and the risks of repeating the operation multiple times is less of an issue.
- Unreasonable time limits during first stage of labour.
- Routine CTG monitoring, with 'false positive' interpretations (where it is thought that the baby has a problem but is in fact well).
- 'Precious baby', a term used for babies conceived with fertility treatments or if the woman is having her first baby after the age of 40.
- Woman's choice, to avoid labour and/or a vaginal birth, to schedule the birth or simply because she views caesareans as 'better'. These reasons need to be weighed up against the possible risks involved.
- Caregiver's preference, just in case complications arise or possibly to avoid litigation (although, one woman has successfully sued for having an unnecessary caesarean).

If a caesarean is suggested and you are not sure whether the reasons are valid, discuss your options with your caregiver or seek a second opinion.

What a caesarean operation involves

The care, procedures and interventions involved with a caesarean are unique. The following is a guide to what you can expect before, during and soon after the operation.

BEFORE THE OPERATION

Several routine procedures are carried out pre-operatively. When the caesarean is planned, these often take place hours beforehand. If the caesarean is unplanned, they are done just prior to the operation. In the rare circumstance that it is a true medical emergency, procedures are done within minutes, perhaps simultaneously, by multiple caregivers.

Signing a consent form
This is a legal document stating that the reasons for the operation have been explained to you and that you give your consent. The woman usually signs this, but if she is unwell, her partner or support person may do this on her behalf.

Talking with the anaesthetist
The anaesthetist administers and supervises the anaesthetic. They listen to your heart and lungs with a stethoscope and order blood tests in case a blood transfusion is required. Questions are asked about your health and the pregnancy, to anticipate any possible problems and help choose the most appropriate anaesthetic. Allergies to medications, iodine (the antiseptic used) or sticking plaster dressings are important. Metal allergies are also relevant in case the surgeon prefers to use small, metal staples instead of stitches. If you are unwell, or too distressed with labour pain, your partner or support person may be asked to answer on your behalf.

Removing jewellery, make-up and underwear
Jewellery gets in the way when inserting drips and applying monitoring equipment, although a wedding band may be taped over. Lipstick, nail polish and foundation are removed, so the anaesthetist can observe the colour of your skin, lips and nail beds (a guide to whether you have adequate oxygen). In an emergency, the polish from one fingernail may be removed, or the anaesthetist may rely on an oximeter to measure oxygen levels.

You wear a hospital gown and need to remove your underpants and bra.

Being shaved
Shaving or closely clipping pubic hair helps prevent infections.

Other preparations
An intravenous drip is placed in your arm to administer fluids and medications. Many hospitals routinely give a small drink of sodium citrate. This is a bitter-tasting fluid that helps neutralise stomach acids, aiming to prevent aspiration (see Chapter 6). A urine catheter is routinely inserted to keep the bladder empty and out of the way during the operation.

When wheeled into the operating theatre, you are moved onto a high, narrow bed and a triangular sponge is placed under your right side to tilt your body towards the left and prevent aorto-caval compression. You have an oxygen mask, heart monitor wires on your chest, a blood pressure cuff on your arm and perhaps an oximeter strapped to your finger.

Your belly is washed with a brown iodine antiseptic solution and is covered with green sterile drapes. One drape is used as an upright screen like a small curtain, in front of your chest to prevent you from witnessing the operation. (You may ask for this to be lowered when the baby is born.)

Your partner/support person's role

Generally, only one extra person is permitted into the operating room, and only if the woman is awake (having an epidural or spinal anaesthetic). Some hospitals request that you read and sign a conditions of entry form. You need to change into special theatre clothes. Once everything is set up, and the operation is close to commencing, you are shown into the operating theatre and directed to sit on a low stool next to the woman's head and shoulders, shielded from seeing the operation with a cloth screen.

ANAESTHETIC USED

The type of anaesthetic used is ultimately the decision of the anaesthetist. However, if you have no health complications, you may be able to play a role in this choice and discuss your preferences before the operation.

Epidurals and spinals

The majority of caesarean births involve an epidural or spinal anaesthetic or a combination of the two (CSE). These are fully explained in Chapter 9. Epidurals and spinals are preferred to a general anaesthetic because:
- They tend to be safer for mothers and babies.
- You don't miss your baby's birth and can participate to a degree. Some women find this a scary thought, but most are surprised at how positive the experience is.
- You can hold and feed your baby sooner after the birth and not feel drowsy.
- Your partner or support person can be present and involved in the birth.
- The baby is more likely to be alert, have a better Apgar score, not need resuscitation and be keener to feed soon after the birth.

The choice of an epidural, spinal or CSE will generally depend on:
- Whether an epidural is already in place, just needing to be topped up.

- Whether the caesarean needs to be performed quickly; if it does, it usually means a general anaesthetic or perhaps a spinal.
- Whether epidural pain relief is preferred after the operation.
- The preferences of the anaesthetist, the woman and the surgeon.

If you are having an epidural or spinal, it is inserted in the delivery suite or an anaesthetic room attached to the operating theatre. Once it is effective (tested by the anaesthetist touching your skin with a piece of ice or the tip of a pointed object), you are wheeled into the operating theatre.

General anaesthetic

A general anaesthetic involves intravenous medications and/or breathing gas to make you unconscious (or asleep) for the operation. Up until the late 1970s most caesareans were done using a general anaesthetic. However, with the introduction of epidurals and spinals (which have less health risks), they are now only used for around 5% of caesareans.

Reasons for a general anaesthetic include the following:
- A rapid anaesthetic is required because it is a medical emergency.
- The epidural is not working effectively (12 to 15% chance).
- A previous back injury, lumbar disc operation or inherited abnormality of the spine can make the insertion of an epidural or spinal needle difficult. The anaesthetist will usually try to insert the needle first. It may be worthwhile having a consultation with the anaesthetist during the pregnancy, or taking past X-rays, scans or doctor's letters with you to the labour.
- You have health conditions that lower the blood pressure (heavy bleeding during late pregnancy) or predispose you to bleeding (liver disorders or low platelet levels), because an epidural or spinal may risk bleeding in the spinal area.
- You strongly prefer a general anaesthetic. Be aware that it is possible to have an epidural or spinal and then be given a general anaesthetic during the operation if you begin to feel distressed about being awake.

General anaesthetic used for caesareans tends to be light to moderate, aiming to give good anaesthesia but also to minimise the side effects. The following are a few things to be aware of:
- Your partner (or support person) cannot be with you because you are unconscious and unable to communicate. Some operating theatres have a viewing window that allows them to see the baby being born (but not view the operation).
- The anaesthetic passes rapidly to the baby via the placenta. Your baby

is more likely to have a low Apgar score and require resuscitation by the paediatrician soon after birth.
- You may be drowsy, groggy, nauseated and possibly vomit when you wake up from the anaesthetic. This makes it difficult to interact with your baby for a while (ranging from a short period to several hours). A few women take a number of days to feel right again. Injectable medications may be prescribed to stop the nausea or vomiting.
- Depending on the hospital, you may not see your baby until you transfer from the recovery room to the postnatal ward, a couple of hours after the birth. Consider requesting that your partner wait in the recovery room with the baby, so you can see them both when you wake up from the anaesthetic. Perhaps include this in your birth plan.

THE OPERATION

The operation commences once all preparations are carried out, the anaesthetic is working effectively and your partner or support person are seated beside you (if this is possible). Some doctors talk you through, step by step, or you may prefer them not to do this. A few women choose to listen to music with a portable player, or wear earplugs or talk with their partner to take their mind off what is happening.

Depending on the hospital, there could be many people in the operating room, including some or all of the following:
- The woman (hopefully!) and her partner or support person.
- The anaesthetist.
- The surgeon (your private obstetrician or the hospital's obstetrician or senior obstetric registrar).
- An assistant for the surgeon, usually a resident or registrar training in obstetrics.
- An assistant for the anaesthetist, usually a resident or registrar training in anaesthesia.
- A 'scrub' nurse, who sets up the surgical equipment and passes instruments to the surgeon.
- A 'scouting' assistant (nurse's aide), who fetches anything that is needed, answers or makes phone calls as required, and checks on the woman and her partner to see how they are coping.
- An anaesthetic nurse, who attaches monitors and assists the anaesthetist.
- A midwife, who receives the baby from the surgeon soon after the birth.
- A paediatrician (or paediatric resident or registrar), who attends to the baby soon after birth, especially if complications arise.

- Possibly a midwifery or medical student, present for observational purposes.
- If it is a multiple birth, an extra midwife and paediatrician are present for each additional baby.

Sensations for the woman

When having an epidural or spinal anaesthetic, you are awake and hear noises, and possibly feel sensations but should not experience pain. Many women describe feeling warm, heavy and a dead weight from the waist down. A few feel the incision like someone drawing on their skin, but no pain. You may feel movement and unusual rummaging sensations in your belly as the baby is being delivered.

Most sensations are momentary, usually passing within a few seconds. Staying awake to see your baby may help you to tolerate them. Rarely, a woman feels she is not dealing with them very well or is sensing some pain. In this situation the anaesthetist can administer a general anaesthetic very quickly (or place more medications down the epidural catheter, although this takes several minutes to be effective). It is important to know that this is possible so you feel some control over the situation.

Types of caesarean incisions

There are three types of incisions that can be used to perform a caesarean:
1. A low, transverse (horizontal) incision in the lower segment of the uterus (LSCS). This is preferred because the lower segment, when compared to the upper segment:
   - Is thinner, less muscular and has less blood supply, minimising blood loss.
   - Heals better, with less scar tissue.
   - Has a minimal chance of rupturing with a subsequent labour.
   - Is positioned away from the woman's intestines, reducing the chances of scar tissue forming.
2. A vertical incision (classical or CS). This goes up the middle of the uterus, involving the upper segment, but only tends to be used if:
   - It is a true medical emergency, because it is quicker to deliver the baby this way.
   - The baby is in a transverse position; a vertical incision helps the surgeon reach the baby higher in the uterus.
   - This is a multiple pregnancy, to reach all the babies.
   - The baby is very premature (less than 28 weeks), because the lower segment only forms during the last 12 weeks of pregnancy.

3. A low vertical incision. This is in the lower segment of the uterus but can be extended to a vertical incision if necessary; it may be preferred if the surgeon is unsure whether a classical incision will be required. Low vertical incisions have the same advantages as low horizontal incisions (unless extended into the upper segment).

The actual operation

The following information aims to explain the procedures involved with a LSCS (the most common type) in order to help you prepare for a caesarean if one is required. If you feel tense or apprehensive, we suggest you stop or skip sections and return to it at another time, when you feel ready to read it.

A 15 to 20 cm incision is made horizontally, through the skin, across the top of the bikini line. Then the two long abdominal muscles that naturally meet in the middle of the belly (lying vertically from the pubic bone to the breastbone) are gently pulled to each side, exposing the bladder and front of the uterus. The bladder is moved down, out of the way, exposing the lower segment of the uterus. A 10 to 12 cm incision is made horizontally, across the lower segment of the uterus (similar to the incision on the skin). When this happens, amniotic fluid from around the baby gushes out. A small suction tube is used to collect the fluid. You will probably hear loud, liquid sucking sounds, similar to a bath tub emptying.

NOTE: *The procedure is the same for the caesarean birth of multiple babies.*

If the baby is full term, and in a head-down position and engaged, their head is usually lower than the incision, so only their shoulder is seen. (If the baby is breech, their lower back is seen.) The surgeon uses their hands to bring the baby's head (or bottom) up and out of the pelvis and through the incision. Sometimes small lift-out forceps are used on the baby's head. Delivering the baby can require some pressure and movement, which you may sense if awake.

Once the baby's head is born, the caregiver may suction amniotic fluid from their nose and mouth (more sucking noises), especially if it is meconium-stained, before the rest of their body is pulled up and out of the uterus to be born. Once the baby's entire body leaves the uterus, this is documented as the time of birth. It takes around 5 minutes from the first incision to the birth of the baby (or 10 to 15 minutes for multiple babies).

If the baby is well, the surgeon may lift them above the cloth screen for you to see, before clamping and cutting their umbilical cord and passing them to the midwife. The baby is taken to a resuscitation table, where they are labelled, dried and wrapped warmly before being passed to you. Some hospitals wrap the baby's body in gladwrap, or a soft sheet of silver wrapping (a space blanket), to retain their body heat. If your baby is well, and not too small or premature, you may ask to have some skin-to-skin contact, with the blanket on top of them and you.

In most cases the partner or support person leaves with the baby after 10 minutes or so, accompanying them to the postnatal ward for weighing, measuring, bathing and administering of vitamin K. You may ask that these procedures be delayed so your baby can stay and perhaps breastfeed (or until you can join them on the ward). If you have a general anaesthetic, the baby is taken out of the operating theatre (after being checked, wrapped and labelled) to spend time with your waiting partner or support person.

Babies who are unwell need to have their cord cut and clamped immediately and be taken directly to the resuscitation table for the paediatric doctor to attend them. This is usually located to one side of the operating room, making it feel as though your baby is miles away. As the partner or support person you can usually be with the baby. Just ask staff to escort you so you don't trip over equipment or contaminate sterile drapes.

Once the baby is stabilised, the midwife wraps them warmly and passes them to you to hold. However, if the baby remains unwell, they need to go directly to the intensive care nursery in an incubator. Your partner or support person can go with them.

The surgeon delivers the placenta by gently pulling on the cord (cord traction) through the incision the baby was born out of, or by using their hand to gently sweep the placenta from the wall of the uterus (manual removal). Research indicates that cord traction decreases the amount of blood lost and is less likely to cause a uterine infection.[2] You may wish to check which technique the surgeon uses. At the same time, the anaesthetist administers intravenous Syntocinon to help the uterus contract and control the bleeding (as for a vaginal birth).

The placenta is checked by the midwife and placed in a plastic bag. If you wish to see the placenta, donate cord blood or keep your placenta for a ritual, let the midwife know or include this in your birth plan.

The surgeon closes the incisions in layers. The uterus is repaired in two layers, and then the abdominal muscles and fat layers, all with dissolving stitches. The skin is closed either with separate stiches, or one long continuous stitch threaded underneath the skin (either dissolving or a type that needs to be removed). A few doctors use small metal staples to hold the skin together. Stitching takes up to 30 minutes or more. Occasionally a small plastic tube is left in the wound to drain away excess blood, which is collected in a small container attached to the end.

The recovery room

Once the stitching is completed, you are lifted off the operating table onto a trolley bed and wheeled into the recovery room adjacent to the operating theatre. Here you are closely monitored for an hour or so. The midwife takes your blood pressure and pulse, checks the caesarean wound, feels your uterus, and monitors the vaginal bleeding. If you had a general anaesthetic, they make sure you rouse from this normally. If you start requiring pain relief, they may administer a narcotic injection or an epidural top-up.

Once you are physically stable, you are wheeled to the postnatal ward for the remainder of your hospital stay. If your baby has been taken to the intensive care nursery, you can usually go there first to spend time with them. Most hospitals have Polaroid cameras, so you can take a photo of your baby with you to the postnatal ward, or your partner or support person may take photos with your own camera.

NOTE: *Some people want to take photos or video footage in the operating theatre. This will depend on the hospital and the operating surgeon.*

Early care and physical recovery

Your physical recovery will depend on your health at the time of the operation, whether you had a long and difficult labour beforehand, how smoothly the operation went, and whether there were any complications.

First 24 to 48 hours

The first 24 hours involve resting, sleeping and recuperating. An intravenous drip provides fluids, routine antibiotics and possibly pain-relieving medications, and a urinary catheter keeps your bladder empty. These attachments make moving, and holding your baby, restrictive. To help keep pressure off your tender belly, breastfeed lying on your side or sitting up, with your baby on a pillow. Many women find the football hold ideal. Ask for help from staff and your family to lift, change and handle your baby. Your partner may be able to stay overnight if you are not sharing the room with another woman.

The drip is removed after 48 hours or so. The wound drain (if you have one) is removed once the blood loss is minimal (1 to 2 days), and the urinary catheter is removed once you are moving around (12 to 24 hours).

Pain relief
The first couple of days can be quite difficult, even if all is going well. You will need strong pain-relieving medications for 24 to 48 hours (epidural top-ups through an intravenous drip or narcotic injections). These can make you feel sleepy or drowsy. Some women also use natural therapies, including heat packs, acupressure, TENS machine or homeopathic remedies.

Diet and wind pain
You can have fluids (juices, jelly, ice cream, water, etc) for 12 hours to 24 hours, and solid food when you feel you can tolerate it. Restricting fluids and food until passing wind is no longer routine. However, it is normal to experience wind or gas pains during the early days, regardless of your diet. These often come in waves and can be quite painful. Peppermint water or peppermint tea can help.

Moving around
You will be encouraged to get out of bed and move around as soon as possible. Ideally, within 24 to 48 hours. This promotes healing, reduces wind pain and prevents the rare complication of a thrombosis (or DVT). Ask for pain-relieving medications at least half an hour before getting up. Take it slowly and have someone with you, in case you feel weak or wobbly.

While it can seem like an impossible task to get out of bed so soon after a major operation, most women are quite surprised at how well they move and how much better they feel, both mentally and physically, after showering. Aim to get out of bed once or twice a day for short periods in the early days, while continuing to rest and recover in between.

The stitches
The caesarean wound is covered with a surgical dressing for two to four days. This is usually waterproof, so you can shower. When the dressing is removed, getting it wet is not a problem. Consider wearing highcut underpants that cover the bikini line, so your stitches aren't irritated. When walking or going to the toilet, pad your incision with a folded nappy, towel or cushion, to gently support the area.

NEXT ONE TO TWO WEEKS
The next one or two weeks are still recovery time, but most women comment on how each day feels like a major improvement. The normal hospital stay after a caesarean is five to seven days. A few women choose

to go home earlier if all is well, having a midwife visit them at home for several days.

Many women tend to be more active once going home. However, this can quickly deplete your physical reserves, making you weak, tired and the stitches more painful, possibly with heavier vaginal bleeding. For a few women, overdoing it leads to infections, because their body's resistance is lowered. It is important to rest and take care of yourself at this vulnerable time. Try not to do too much too soon. It may still be difficult to lift and care for your new baby, so get your partner, family and friends to help (especially if you have other children to care for).

Pain relief

After the first couple of days you will rely on strong pain-relieving drugs and/or suppositories. These will be needed fairly regularly for a week or so, before taking milder analgesics. Gentle postnatal exercises can be started five to seven days after the birth to assist your body's recovery (if you are feeling up to this).

The stitches

Nondissolving stitches (or staples) need to be removed after five to seven days. This is normally done by the staff before you go home, or by the midwife doing home visits if you leave hospital earlier.

It is normal for the scar to have a watery ooze, look reddened and feel tender in the first few days. Some incisions initially look crooked or uneven, but this usually improves over time. A few women notice numb areas around their stitches. Normal sensations return over the following months. Things to be concerned about are:
- The skin 5 to 10 cm around the scar becoming red, inflamed and painful (indicating an infection).
- Pus or offensive-smelling fluid oozing from the wound.
- A fever (above 38°C) and/or the vaginal bleeding increasing dramatically or smelling offensive.
- Lower abdominal pain worsening over time rather than improving.

Let your caregiver (or the hospital) know if you are concerned.

Support strategies

Try exposing your scar to fresh air occasionally, to discourage infection. Stand or sit tall to help air circulate around the stitches (this also supports your lower back), or place a clean handtowel in the crease to separate the skin. Perhaps expose it to a little sunlight each day (but be careful not to sunburn).

Pat the scar with a clean towel after bathing or showering. Avoid talcs or creams until the scar is well healed. After 10 to 14 days, you may wish to rub vitamin E, calendula cream or pawpaw ointment in to help with healing. Acupuncture has also been known to help.

Two to eight weeks

You will probably feel you can do more, but are unlikely to feel a hundred per cent. Bear in mind that a caesarean is a major operation, taking up to six weeks to recover from fully. Taking short walks may be manageable, but the weekly shop can be too much. Try to make arrangements with family, friends, neighbours or other parents to help with siblings, household chores and any unavoidable running around.

Driving

Car insurance companies often don't cover the driver in an accident if they have had a major operation in the previous six weeks (even though this is not against the law). If you are feeling well after a few weeks, your doctor may write you a letter stating you are fit to drive. Contact your insurance company about your policy. Alternatively, catch taxis, take public transport or arrange for others to drive you.

Physical changes

The vaginal bleeding is similar to bleeding after a normal birth, but perhaps a little lighter. The scar may be a dark, deep purple colour, which fades to pink and then white over several months (possibly shrinking a little in size). The pubic hair grows back, concealing the scar, which can feel itchy. Most women have a medical check-up six to eight weeks after the birth to make sure everything is healing.

Resuming sex

Some women feel like resuming sex after three to six weeks, which is fine from a physical perspective, but many women do not yet feel ready emotionally. A few women experience some pain with deep sexual penetration. This should improve over time, but if it doesn't, let your caregiver know. Be conscious of contraception if you don't wish to conceive again. Most caregivers consider that conceiving a subsequent baby at least three months after a caesarean is reasonable, if you want another baby soon.

Two months and beyond

Some women recover remarkably quickly. Others take several months to feel back to normal. Caring for a new baby requires a lot of energy. So try to take it easy and deal with each day as it comes. After two to three months your physical recovery should be just about complete, although you may notice a lack of energy on some days, especially if you are overdoing things.

Risks and problems associated with caesareans

Vaginal births and caesareans both carry risks. However, overall, vaginal births are much safer for women, and caesarean births are marginally safer for babies. At present, the caesarean rate in Australia is around 24%, even though the WHO recommends 10 to 15%. Caesarean rates, like induction rates, vary greatly between caregivers, hospitals, states and countries.

> **Did you know?**
> An Australian study of 171,157 women (mentioned previously) showed vast differences in caesarean rates, depending on the woman's chosen place of birth and caregiver, despite them all having similar rates of complications.[3] For women:
> - With their own doctor, in a private hospital, having their first baby – 4.1% elective caesareans + 12.3% emergency caesareans = 16.4%; for women having a subsequent baby – 14.5% elective caesareans + 3.5% emergency caesareans = 18.0%.
> - With their own doctor, in a public hospital, having their first baby – 2.9% elective caesareans + 10.9% for emergency caesareans = 13.8%; for women having their subsequent baby – 10.2% elective caesareans + 3.3% emergency caesareans = 13.5%
> - Who were Medicare only, having their first baby – 1.5% elective caesareans + 8.5% emergency caesareans = 10.0%; for women having a subsequent baby – 6.5% elective caesareans + 2.9% emergency caesareans = 9.4%.

Possible variations for the woman

Reported complications for caesareans vary from 5 to 28%, compared with 1.6 to 3% for vaginal births, and range from fairly minor to quite severe.

Infections

Caesareans are 5 to 20 times more likely to lead to an infection, when compared to vaginal births. This can involve the wound, blood (septicaemia), urine or the lining of the uterus (endometritis). Intravenous antibiotics are routinely given during and soon after the operation to try to prevent an infection developing, lowering the chances by 50 to 75%. However, an infection is still possible for up to 9% of planned caesareans, and up to 27% of unplanned caesareans.

If an infection does develop, you will need a longer course of antibiotics and possibly a longer stay in hospital (10 to 12 days), or to be readmitted to hospital with the baby for treatment. Be aware that up to 19% of women develop post-operative fever, which may not be linked to an infection. However, your caregiver will probably prescribe antibiotics just in case.

Make sure you rest and have physical and emotional support and help with the baby. Eat healthy foods and include garlic, fish and foods rich in zinc and vitamin C to help boost your immune system. Some women use herbal or homeopathic remedies.

Blood loss

Blood loss for caesareans ranges from 500 to 1000 ml (compared to 250 to 400 ml for a vaginal birth). This can mean you are more likely to be anaemic, tired and lethargic in the following weeks. Although not common, a blood transfusion may be required. Consider taking iron supplements for four to six weeks. Eat iron-rich foods and rest as much as possible.

Adhesions and damage to internal organs

A caesarean involves handling the internal organs, which causes scar tissue or adhesions to form. Small adhesions don't generally cause problems, but may make the next caesarean more difficult to perform. The more caesareans you have, the worse the adhesions can become, possibly leading to long-term pain and difficulties with the functioning of these organs. Most caregivers recommend no more than four caesareans. Adhesions have also been linked to reduced fertility for 10% of women and future ectopic pregnancies when conceiving a subsequent child.[4]

On rare occasions, internal organs (bowel, bladder or uterine arteries) can be unintentionally cut, or damaged, during the operation. This is more likely if it is a medical emergency and the operation is being done in a hurry. However, it can also occur when trying to divide adhesions from a previous caesarean. If organs are damaged, they are repaired during the operation. However, bleeding may be excessive, or an infection may develop, and in some cases the functioning of the organs can be affected on a long-term basis.

Blood clots in the vein
A deep vein thrombosis (DVT) is more likely to develop after a caesarean because you tend to be less mobile. Moving around and getting up as soon as possible reduces this risk (see Chapter 13).

Placenta previa and placenta accreta
Caesareans increase the risk of placenta previa with a subsequent pregnancy. If placenta previa does occur, it is more likely to be complicated by a rare condition called placenta accreta (explained in Chapter 8).

Complications of the anaesthetic
Complications may occur with a caesarean as a direct consequence of the anaesthetic used rather than the surgical procedure itself. Side effects for epidurals and spinals are described in Chapter 9, and general anaesthetics are covered previously in this chapter.

Woman dying
In the very rare circumstances that a woman could die in relation to childbirth, the risk is about four to six times higher with a caesarean than a vaginal birth. Around 30 women die each year in Australia from around 250,000 births (0.012%).

POSSIBLE VARIATIONS FOR THE BABY
Breathing difficulties
Planned, elective caesareans make babies prone to transient tachypnoea of the newborn (TTN or wet lung). This is where the baby has healthy, mature lungs, but excessive amniotic fluid remains in them, making their breathing faster. It used to be thought that TTN was caused by the fluid not being squeezed out of a baby's lungs (because they were not born vaginally). However, it is now believed that labour stimulates low levels of adrenaline in the baby, making their lungs absorb most of the excess fluid before birth. TTN is unlikely to occur if the caesarean is conducted during labour. Some women request that their caesarean be performed after labour starts (if possible), rather than scheduling it routinely. Treatments for TTN usually involve close observation and oxygen therapy for about 24 to 48 hours in the intensive care nursery.

Prematurity
Elective caesareans performed prior to 41 weeks have an increased chance of delivering a premature baby, mainly because the due date has been miscalculated. This is less likely these days with the use of early ultrasounds, but you may wish to wait until labour starts before having your caesarean, or delay it until one week past the due date if there are no urgent medical complications.

Physical injury and cuts
Occasionally the baby is physically injured, either through the surgeon's efforts during the delivery or as a result of being accidentally cut, especially if it is a medical emergency. The chance is about 1.9% for babies lying head down, and 6% for babies in alternative positions, such as breech.

Effects of the anaesthetic
Babies are more likely to be affected if the woman has a general anaesthetic (discussed earlier in this chapter), but epidurals and spinals can also have side effects (see Chapter 9).

Emotional reactions

Some women feel very positive about their caesarean experience. Others accept the caesarean but feel disappointed. A few feel devastated or traumatised. If the caesarean was unplanned, there is little time to adjust, creating issues that may take a while to resolve.

EMOTIONS FOR THE WOMAN
Nervous about the operation
The unknown can be scary. For a lot of women, having a baby is their first contact with a hospital and having an operation, which can feel overwhelming. It may help to talk with others who have had a caesarean, although be aware that their experience will be different to yours. Perhaps ask your hospital for a tour of the operating theatre beforehand (although not many hospitals do this).

Feeling comfortable
You may prefer to have a caesarean, especially if you are not keen on experiencing labour or a vaginal birth. Caesareans are done so frequently these

days, this attitude is becoming increasingly accepted by society. Caesareans may also be appreciated as another success story of modern technology, helping women achieve motherhood (similar to fertility treatments). Some women appreciate that they have not had to recover from a long labour with an elective caesarean, or feel they know no different if they have never had a vaginal birth.

Feeling different from other women

A few women consider themselves different from, or envious of, women who have had a vaginal birth, perhaps feeling they need to justify their caesarean. A few feel it is unfair, or that their body has let them down. Occasionally this can be expressed as feeling less of a mother, or that their child is deprived in some way. Responses from well-meaning others, such as 'At least you have a healthy baby', may be true but can undermine your feelings, which are valid and normal.

Feeling shocked

Many women don't expect to have a caesarean and may feel the birth was taken out of their control. Anger, disappointment or feeling traumatised can be part of this, especially if you feel you weren't given a chance to have a vaginal birth, or aren't sure exactly why the caesarean was needed. A few women even feel obliged to be grateful to their caregivers, yet find this difficult to reconcile if they are feeling angry.

Knowing this was the only way

If the labour was long and difficult, many women feel they did everything possible but ultimately the caesarean was needed, bringing relief and positive feelings, possibly mixed with sadness and disappointment. The caesarean may also be welcomed if you think the baby may be unwell – at last you can see and hold them and stop worrying.

Unable to witness the birth

If a general anaesthetic is required, missing out on those early hours of contact with your baby can impact on your feelings about the birth. If you have no recollection of your baby being born, it can be hard to believe the baby is really yours. A few women express jealousy or even anger that their partner or support person spent more time with their baby or saw their baby first.

Let others know you need time to accept what has happened. If you feel it will help, ask your partner to retell the birth story to help fill in the gaps of lost time.

Hearing 'Told you so!'
If you were planning a natural birth, thoughtless comments such as, 'I told you so' (in relation to not achieving a normal birth) can be undermining and hurtful, perhaps reinforcing feelings of failure. Be selective about who you have around you and create a safe, emotional cocoon, only allowing those in who will validate and nurture your emotional needs. Don't take on others' perceptions of your birth 'not being good enough'.

Frustrated with the pain and debilitation of recovering
Struggling with recovering from a major operation, combined with the demands of a new baby, can be extremely difficult. This is compounded with the common social expectation that a caesarean is nothing serious, or that the recovery is similar to recovering from a vaginal birth. Try not to be superwoman. Ask for support and understanding.

Intact genitals
While most are reluctant to admit this openly, a few women take comfort that their genitals are 'undisturbed' after a caesarean. Critics of this approach often quip with the saying 'Too posh to push'.

Upset that your body is scarred
Some women find their caesarean scar upsetting and distressing, and need an enormous amount of adjustment to accept their new body image. This can affect their self-esteem and how attractive they feel, which are normal feelings. Perhaps ask your partner to look at the scar and share your feelings with them to help you come to terms with it.

Feeling the birth is just one day in a lifelong relationship
Having a baby is the ultimate goal, and how this is achieved can pale into insignificance once parenting starts. Some women don't put much emphasis on their birth and merely see it as a means to an end. If people start fussing about the caesarean, they simply don't agree that it was anything to dwell on. They have produced their child and are now parenting, and that is all that matters.

EMOTIONS FOR THE PARTNER/SUPPORT PERSON
Nervous about being present
Most people have reservations about witnessing an operation. However, being present at a caesarean does not entail seeing anything of great note, except a

lot of equipment. A few people find the noises or smells disturbing, perhaps due to a previous negative hospital experience. Be aware that it is extremely rare to faint, but you do have the option of leaving at any time. Discuss these issues with the woman as part of your birth preparations. Most people are very pleased they took part (and most women appreciate their presence).

Happy because you feel it is the best option

Some partners prefer their baby to be born by caesarean. Perhaps this is how they were born, or it may seem more convenient and predictable (or a relief because they no longer need to support her during labour). It may also be welcomed if the woman and/or baby are unwell, or the labour has been long and difficult.

Privileged to bond with your baby

Caesarean routines often mean that the partner or support person is alone with the baby for an hour or so before the woman leaves the recovery room. This can be a special time to get to know your child and to realise you are a parent, and it is often a significant part of the birth experience.

Feeling helpless

Unplanned caesareans can bring mixed feelings of frustration, disappointment and possibly anger, or a sense that it is out of your control. You may feel disappointed that your baby will be born this way, or upset if you were playing a vital role in her labour support. This may be compounded by not being allowed into the operating room (if she has a general anaesthetic) and can bring up issues of not protecting her and your baby from intervention. A few partners express fears that their partner or baby will die.

Try to stay calm. Be close with her for as long as possible, holding her hand and telling her you love her. Talk about your feelings after the birth. Listen to her as well – she may be feeling the same. Be sensitive to each other's needs, so neither of you feel guilty or blamed. Debrief the birth with her caregivers if you need to.

Vaginal birth after caesarean

Many women choose to explore the option of a vaginal birth after previously having a caesarean (VBAC, pronounced *vee-back*). Research indicates that VBACs are safe and involve similar risks to any healthy woman having a baby.[5]

HEALTH FACTORS RELATING TO VBAC
Most women can plan a VBAC unless there is a medical reason to repeat the caesarean.

Conceiving the next baby
There are no strict guidelines as to when you can conceive your next baby. The caesarean scar heals completely by two to six weeks, and most caregivers consider at least three months afterwards is a reasonable time if there were no complications, such as a wound infection, which may prolong the healing process. However, women who conceive earlier than this can still plan a VBAC.

'Once a caesarean, always a caesarean'
This term was coined by an American obstetrician in 1916, when caesarean rates were 1% and vertical (classical) incisions were used, making attempting a VBAC more risky. The use of low transverse incisions over the last 30 years, has made planning a VBAC a safe and achievable option.

If the previous caesarean was a vertical incision (which is not common), then a VBAC is generally not advisable, because the risk of uterine rupture is about 10%, when compared to less than 1% with a lower segment scar. NOTE: *Some women have scars up the middle of their belly but have had a low horizontal incision on their uterus. You may need to obtain a copy of your medical records, or a letter from your previous caregiver, to confirm the type of incision that was made.*

More than one previous caesarean
Having more than one previous caesarean should not in itself be a reason to exclude you from planning a VBAC. In studies where women laboured after 2 previous caesareans, 60 to 70% gave birth vaginally, without increased risk.

Previous uterine surgery
Surgery involving cutting through the full muscle thickness of the uterus can affect the safety of a VBAC, in the same way that a previous classical caesarean can. This kind of surgery might include removing a large fibroid or a uterine septum. However, sometimes these operations just involve scraping the wall of the uterus. You may need to obtain a copy of your medical records to find out what was involved.

Large baby
Women who have had a caesarean for a large baby have up to a 70% chance of a vaginal birth with a subsequent pregnancy. The first caesarean may have

been done because the baby's head was deflexed, or the caregiver misjudged the size of the baby (which is common), or the woman was not given enough time to progress in her previous labour. Even women who had difficult first births (ie. forceps or ventouse deliveries) are unlikely to encounter the same difficulties with a subsequent birth.

Medical conditions

Caesareans are often performed because of a complication during the pregnancy or labour, such as high blood pressure, a breech baby or fetal distress. If this reason no longer exists for a subsequent baby, then planning a VBAC is reasonable. Other issues can include:

- **The previous labour not progressing** – This may have been a result of not being given adequate time to dilate last time, or an induction or augmentation failing. Be aware that subsequent labours are much quicker up to the point to which your body progressed last time. However, from this point onwards the progress is usually similar to having a first baby (for example, one to two hours of pushing). If labour does not start spontaneously, consider waiting until you are at least 10 days past the due date before using mechanical methods of induction. Pharmacological induction methods are generally not recommended as they significantly increase the chances of a uterine rupture.[6]
- **Twins** – There is increasing research evidence that supports the safety of having twins vaginally after a previous caesarean.[7]

ARGUMENTS FOR AND AGAINST VBAC

In the past, planning a VBAC was controversial because some practitioners argued it was unsafe. These days it ultimately comes down to your personal choice once you have considered the risks and benefits. On the whole, parents should be encouraged to have a VBAC, but their choice to have a repeat caesarean should be respected. For every three women planning a VBAC, at least two will achieve a vaginal birth if they have a supportive birthplace and caregiver.[8]

Advantages of a VBAC

The main advantage of a vaginal birth is to reduce the risk of caesarean complications. Other benefits include:

- Decreased pain, increased mobility and faster recovery. This allows you to return to normal activities more quickly, making parenting a little easier, especially if you have other small children to care for.

- Experiencing a vaginal birth. This can be very important for some women and is often linked with their body image and belief that a vaginal birth is a physical task their body was created for. A few women feel incomplete, unfulfilled or traumatised by their previous caesarean. Planning a VBAC plays a vital role in their healing process, even if this leads to another caesarean, because they feel like an active participant in the process.
- Bonding and feeding. A vaginal birth increases the likelihood of spending the early time after the birth with your new baby and partner, breastfeeding early and bonding.
- Lower cost. While this is unlikely to affect your decision, it may be of interest to know that a caesarean birth costs the health system more than twice as much as a vaginal birth.[9]

Disadvantages of a VBAC

The main health complication people focus on when planning a VBAC is the small possibility that the previous caesarean scar may break down and the uterus will rupture. This is more likely to happen during labour, although it is possible (but rare) for it to happen during the last few weeks of pregnancy.

A uterine rupture occurs when the scar separates and perhaps tears further. It happens for less than 1% of women planning a VBAC. Women who are induced, or augmented, with medications are more at risk, while women who have already had one successful VBAC are less at risk.

NOTE: *While quite rare, it is possible for the uterus to rupture in women who do not have a caesarean scar. This is often associated with hyperstimulation of uterine contractions with medications, especially for women having a subsequent baby.*

If the uterus does rupture, it can be life-threatening for 25 to 30% of unborn babies. Some babies survive without problems if a caesarean is performed rapidly (within 15 to 20 minutes), but a few surviving babies are left with developmental delays and brain damage. In very rare circumstances it is life-threatening for the woman.

Physical signs of rupture can include:
- The baby being distressed (80% of cases).
- Excessive vaginal bleeding.
- The woman appearing pale and sweaty, with low blood pressure and a fast pulse.
- The uterus not contracting, sometimes associated with constant abdominal pain.

NOTE: *Scar tenderness is not a reliable sign but was used frequently in the past. In reality, women normally feel pain in this area during labour because their cervix is dilating.*

Once a ruptured uterus is diagnosed, an emergency caesarean is performed using a general anaesthetic. In rare cases, a blood transfusion and/or hysterectomy are required.

ACHIEVING THE OPTIMAL OUTCOMES
Where to have the baby

Choosing a supportive birthplace is important. Generally, birthplaces with low caesarean rates tend to have higher VBAC rates (birth centres and smaller public hospitals, for example). A few women choose a homebirth if their hospital is not supportive.

The ideal birthplace is a contentious issue. Some caregivers argue that the chances of a major medical emergency for a woman planning a VBAC are similar to the chances for any healthy labouring woman, making the birthplace her choice. Others recommend a hospital with 24-hour emergency facilities and a doctor and anaesthetist *on site* (rather than just on call), so a caesarean can be performed within 15 to 20 minutes if a rupture occurs.

NOTE: *It is arguable that all maternity hospitals should have 24-hour medical cover on site, but this is not the case for some private hospitals and smaller public or rural hospitals. Ask your caregiver about the emergency arrangements at your birthplace.*

Supportive caregivers

If you have supportive caregivers, your chances of achieving a vaginal birth are 60 to 85%, depending on the circumstances. However, planning a VBAC in Australia may not be as easy as it is in other countries,[10] because:

- It is difficult to find a sympathetic caregiver who is willing to support a planned VBAC. In many cases non-medical reasons are given to repeat the caesarean or discourage the VBAC, or a caesarean is performed after the slightest variation in the labour pattern.
- For women who do find a supportive caregiver, achieving a vaginal birth is often impeded by medical interventions, such as continuous CTG monitoring or unrealistic time limits.
- Medical terms and attitudes tend to dramatise the risks and are loaded with negative terminology, including, 'trial of scar', 'trial of labour', 'unsuccessful' or 'failed' VBAC, undermining women's confidence in their ability to give birth vaginally.

Finding a caregiver in tune with your needs is important and you may have to do some research to optimise your chances of achieving a vaginal birth. If you feel your caregiver is not being supportive, consider obtaining a second opinion. Caregivers who believe in the safety and appropriateness of

VBAC should support your decision but know when to intervene, and have the ability to inspire and care for you with confidence, experience and expertise. Local VBAC support groups, midwives and childbirth educators can be instrumental in helping you find an appropriate caregiver.

You may consider employing an extra support person with some birthing expertise to help you achieve your goals and make the experience positive. This may be a childbirth educator, midwife or professional doula (see Chapter 5).

Expectations for care and support strategies

Depending on your birthplace and caregiver, the labour care can vary. You may want to negotiate some aspects of it and include your preferences in your birth plan.

Early arrival at hospital – You may be asked to come to your birthplace as soon as labour starts, so your baby's heart rate can be continuously monitored with a CTG machine. A few women find this reassuring, but others feel it is unnecessary and inhibiting, possibly increasing their chances of another caesarean. Coming in early may also place pressure on you to perform, making it difficult for the labour to establish and creating time pressures. The more normally you are treated, the more likely you will have a vaginal birth.

Support strategies: Consider negotiating to come in when the labour is becoming more established. If it makes you feel more comfortable, you could come for an earlier check then go back home for a while.

IV cannula or drip – Your caregiver may suggest a routine intravenous cannula or drip, in case fluids or a general anaesthetic need to be administered. A blood test is also taken, in case a blood transfusion is required (which is not common).

Support strategies: You may choose to decline this. Alternatively, ask for the cannula to be placed in your left arm if you are right-handed (or visa versa) and do not have the drip attached, so you can move freely and use the shower and bath.

Induction and augmentation – As a general rule, medications to induce or augment labour contractions should be avoided as they increase the risk of uterine rupture; mechanical methods are acceptable. However, some caregivers believe that for a few women a vaginal birth is only possible if small amounts of intravenous Syntocinon are used.

Slow progress: There is no evidence to support an increased risk of a uterine rupture if the labour is prolonged. If you and the baby are well, and you are happy to continue, time is on your side.

Continuous monitoring – Some caregivers insist on continually monitoring the baby's heart rate for the entire labour. Others criticise this because it has a tendency to increase caesarean rates if it incorrectly diagnoses fetal distress. A few women say it makes them feel like a disaster waiting to happen, although other women find it reassuring.

Support strategies: You may prefer intermittent monitoring and only accept continuous monitoring if a problem is suspected. Be aware that your anxiety levels can sometimes play a role in the baby becoming distressed, and this should be a factor when considering whether to accept (or decline) continuous monitoring.

Pain-relieving medications – Pain relief should be a matter of your choice. The advantages and disadvantages of each method are covered in Chapter 9.

Support strategies: If you can do without narcotics or an epidural, wonderful! But if you decide you really need them, try holding out until you are at least 4 to 5 cm dilated to reduce the chances of them slowing your labour's progress.

Manual exploration of the uterus – In the past, caregivers routinely 'explored' the woman's uterus after a VBAC, to check whether the scar was intact. This is rarely done these days, but a few caregivers may still perform the procedure. A manual exploration involves the caregiver feeling inside the uterus soon after the birth, through a vaginal examination. It can be quite uncomfortable (if you don't have an effective epidural), and increases infection and bleeding rates. By rights, this should not be part of your VBAC care.

A repeat caesarean – For every woman planning a VBAC, there is the constant thought that a repeat caesarean may be necessary. Be realistic and plan for this by putting strategies in place to make it a positive experience and help you regain control of the situation.

Try to be honest about how you feel. Some women go along with the idea of a VBAC because their caregiver or family feel it is best. However, if you are not consciously committed, then it rarely succeeds because it is difficult to relax and allow the labour to progress. Some research shows that quite a few women will request a repeat caesarean within five hours of their labour starting, with caregivers being more likely to concede to this request when a VBAC is planned.

Emotions when planning a VBAC
Emotions for the woman

Planning a VBAC brings up unique emotional issues. Sometimes these are enough to impede a vaginal birth. It can be worthwhile exploring how you feel before the birth so you can work through your emotions before they confront you in labour.

Fear in all its forms, is a common reaction and can include:
- **Fear of disappointment** – Even with the best possible preparations, a caesarean may still eventuate. However, sometimes the subsequent labour reinforces the need for another caesarean. Not planning a VBAC means that you will never know whether a vaginal birth was possible. Surround yourself with people who are willing to support you, no matter what the outcome.
- **Fear of losing control** – Planning a VBAC can be an exercise in trying to regain control.
- **Fear of the unknown** – Trying something new is always hard. Take one step at a time. Even women having a second vaginal birth have fears as there is no knowing what the labour will bring.
- **Fear of the pain** – Particularly if you have never experienced labour, or your last labour was long and difficult. Balancing this fear with not wanting to jeopardise your chances of a vaginal birth can be difficult. Read all you can on pain-relieving options (see Chapter 9).
- **Fear of complications** – Concerns about the scar splitting are especially common. This can be dwelt on frequently during the pregnancy and often surface during labour. Talk with your partner or a friend and share your feelings. Try to make the decision that is right for you and avoid others who are not supportive. Some women use homeopathic remedies to help, or visualisations or hypnosis to create positive thoughts (for example, 'My uterus is strong and resilient').

Feeling alone – It can sometimes feel as though you are on a lone crusade when planning a VBAC. Prepare yourself for negative comments, and contact local support groups to meet women who are planning or have achieved a VBAC.

When labour starts – You may feel excited, as well as anxious, that your moment of truth has arrived. Try to stay calm, keep your breathing slow and take each contraction as it comes. Remember the purpose of all your preparations.

Experiencing deja vu in a subsequent labour can bring up past unpleasant experiences or feelings. Talk about this and try to separate this labour from your previous one. They are different, and you don't want to set yourself up for a similar ending. It is normal to feel anxious and pessimistic until you reach the stage of labour you got to last time. This can be an emotional and physical hurdle, but once it passes, you will usually feel more relaxed and optimistic.

Remember conceiving, growing and parenting a child are amazing tasks. Be proud of your body in being able to produce your children, and nurture yourself whatever the outcome.

Emotions for the partner/support person

As the partner or support person you may feel very in tune with her VBAC plans, or perhaps at odds with what she is trying to achieve. You may want to support her but can't identify with the importance of a vaginal birth, or feel she is obsessed. Alternatively, you may feel it is important for her to give birth vaginally (or for your baby to be born this way), but feel she is not committed to a VBAC. These are all issues you need to discuss and work through before the birth.

If you are united and committed, then you are more likely to achieve your goals. Prepare positively for the birth, but remain flexible and open. Go over any issues that are concerning you. It is better to do this beforehand rather than during the labour or when parenting. The woman needs to feel supported, but she also needs to commit to planning a VBAC, as ultimately it is her body that will be giving birth. It is important that she feels supported, no matter what eventuates.

CHAPTER 12

Your baby soon after birth

The first moments after birth are monumental for your baby. On leaving the womb, their body undergoes amazing adjustments to adapt to the outside world to be an independent person.

At birth your baby's first gasp of air causes pressure changes in their heart and lungs, diverting blood flow away from their umbilical cord (and placenta) to their lungs to absorb oxygen. This incredible changeover takes seconds, creating a new circulatory system that lasts for a lifetime.

Your baby takes their first breath because they:
- Sense less oxygen as their umbilical cord collapses.
- Feel cooler and are stimulated through touch, light and noise.

Breathing starts within 60 seconds, but the baby's lungs are not fully functional for an hour or so.

Body temperature regulation

Newborns can't shiver and move around to keep warm. Their main source of heat is brown adipose tissue body fat (BAT), similar to that found in hibernating animals. BAT requires extra oxygen and glucose to metabolise, so if a newborn becomes cold, their blood sugar levels drop rapidly and they become disinterested in feeding as they try to compensate.

Your baby is born into room temperature (21 to 25°C) having left your uterus which is at a temperature of around 37.5°C, if not kept warm; their temperature can quickly drop to 33 to 34°C. Amniotic fluid on their skin, cool drafts and contact with cool surfaces can accelerate this heat loss. To minimise this, babies need skin-to-skin contact and/or a prewarmed blanket placed around them. Some birthplaces also place a bonnet on their head.

NOTE: *If your baby needs medical attention, the examination table is heated, and the caregiver dries and covers the baby as much as possible while attending to them.*

The role of the birthing environment

A baby's reactions to labour and birth are a mystery. Some parents want to welcome their child into calm, peaceful surroundings as they move from their warm, dark, watery environment into a world of bright lights, cool air and loud sounds. A few caregivers, however, believe this stimulation is necessary to trigger the baby's breathing.

In the 1970s, French obstetrician Frederick Leboyer put forward his beliefs about the benefits of setting up a gentle birth environment to minimise the shock of being born.[1] Many parents (and some birthplaces) have adopted these concepts to varying degrees, such as:
- Dimming lights or darkening the room.
- Being quiet, talking only in whispers.
- Immersing the baby in a warm bath when they are first separated from their mother, to bring them 'back to the womb'.

Water birth is also believed to slow this transition by delaying gravity and allowing the baby to breathe moist air soon after birth. It is true that babies born into water don't tend to cry as vigorously and have a very relaxed muscle tone. However, being born into a gentle environment is not something that has been proven to be beneficial, nor have other environments been shown to be detrimental. Care must be taken not to interpret the Leboyer method, or other similar approaches, as a way of making your baby 'better' or 'worse', and you should not feel guilty if your ideal environment does not eventuate. Some birthplaces are not designed (or inclined) to accommodate requests for a gentle birth environment. However, if it is important to you, discuss it with your caregiver and/or include it in your birth plan.

> **Did you know?**
> - The Mansi women in Siberia hang their most beautiful kerchief in the birthing hut, to please the mythological woman who sends children.
> - In Zaire the Mbuti woman gives birth wherever she is at the time.
> - In Madagascar, the Tanala woman stuffs every opening in the house with rags or newspaper, to shut out evil spirits.

Routine procedures and possible interventions

THE APGAR SCORE

The Apgar score uses five physical signs to allocate a possible score of 0, 1 or 2 when the baby is one and five minutes old (but may be repeated at 7 and 10 minutes if they are unwell). Apgar scores aim to standardise how caregivers evaluate a baby's physical wellbeing at birth. Yet despite its popular use, opinions vary about its validity and importance. The five minute Apgar score is regarded as more significant than the one minute Apgar score and more reflective of the baby's overall health.

SIGNS	0	1 point	2 points
Colour	Blue, pale	Body pink, limbs blue	Completely pink
Breathing	Absent	Slow, irregular breaths – less than 40 per min	Strong cry – 40 breaths per minute or more
Heartbeat	Absent	Less than 100 per minute	Over 100 per minute
Muscle tone	Limp, flaccid	Limbs have some movement	Actively moving
Response to touch	Absent	Some response	Active Response

The Apgar score is done visually, so you are often not aware it is taking place. Some caregivers gently place their hand on the baby's chest, or umbilical cord, to check the baby's heart rate, but this is presumed to be over 100 if the baby is vigorous and crying. Generally a score of 8, 9 or 10 at 1 minute, and 9 or 10 at 5 minutes, reflects a well and healthy baby, the only difference being the individual way the caregiver scores. A score of 5 to 7 indicates the baby is mildly unwell, 3 to 4 is moderately unwell and 0 to 2 is very unwell (scored at 1 or 5 minutes).

A low Apgar score (usually at one minute) can be due to:
- A fast birth or a ventouse or forceps delivery.
- The cord wrapped tightly around the baby's neck, momentarily restricting blood flow.
- Distress during labour (low heart rate and/or meconium-stained amniotic fluid).
- The mother having a narcotic or general anaesthetic.
- The baby being very premature or having a genetic disorder or physical abnormality.
- No apparent reason.

NOTE: *Many caregivers tend to allocate the one minute score well before the first minute is reached, possibly due to the excitement of the birth or out of habit. This can result in a lower score, even though the baby is well. While this can concern parents, remember that the five minute score is more important and a better indicator of your baby's health. Some hospitals have stop clocks in delivery rooms to guide caregivers.*

ROUTINE INTERVENTIONS AT BIRTH

A few babies require medical interventions at birth to help them adjust to independent life. Some caregivers and birthplaces only intervene if necessary, but others perform procedures routinely, even if the baby appears well.

Stimulating your baby

The caregiver often tries to stimulate the baby to breathe. Methods can include:
- Rubbing their body with a warm towel.
- Tickling their toes or rubbing their feet.
- Gently blowing on their face.
- Talking to them and/or asking you to talk to your baby.
- Gently suctioning their nostrils.
- Briefly ventilating their lungs (helping them to breathe).

> **Did you know?**
> In the 1950s, babies were stimulated to breathe by holding them upside down and giving their bottom a smack!

Suctioning the baby's nose and mouth

The baby's nose and mouth may be suctioned with a flexible, plastic catheter attached to a source of low suction. The tip of the catheter is gently placed just inside the baby's nostrils and/or mouth to clear their airways and help them to breathe. However, this intervention is now questioned because most healthy babies clear their own airways and the 1 to 2 ml of fluid in their nose and mouth is minimal compared to the 75 to 100 ml of amniotic fluid that normally remains in their lungs for up to 24 hours after birth.[2]

Other things the caregiver may do include:
- Using a piece of cloth to wipe excess mucus, blood or amniotic fluid draining from the baby's nose or mouth.
- Placing the baby on their stomach across their mother's belly or sitting them up and forward.

Circumstances that do require suctioning are generally limited to:
- The amniotic fluid being heavily meconium-stained.
- Clearing thick mucus from the back of the baby's throat.

Suctioning the baby's stomach

Routine suction of the mucus from the baby's stomach (gastric suctioning) is no longer recommended because in 3 to 4% of cases it stimulates the baby's pharynx, causing their airways to spasm and possibly triggering an abnormally low heart rate or bradycardia. It can also disrupt their interest in feeding and possibly remove 'good' bacteria from their stomach which are needed to digest milk.

Oxygen and ventilation

If your baby does not breathe within a minute or so, the caregiver places a small facemask over their nose and mouth, and compresses the attached bag to deliver a controlled mix of air and oxygen, artificially inflating their lungs.

The baby's cord is cut so they can be taken to a resuscitation table for this procedure (but it may be done close to you if the equipment is portable). Most babies start breathing after a few ventilations, but occasionally the caregiver needs to continue if the baby is not responding. A specialist paediatric doctor is called to attend if there are concerns and/or the baby needs transfer to the intensive care nursery for further treatments or observation.

IDENTIFICATION AND OBSERVATIONS

Soon after a hospital birth the baby is labelled with two identification bracelets, on their wrist(s) and/or ankle(s) with their mother's name, their date of birth and sex, and sometimes their time of birth and medical record number. Twins are generally identified as 'twin 1' and 'twin 2'.

NOTE: *When admitted to hospital the woman is registered under the name on her Medicare card. Her baby is always identified as 'Baby of . . .' (eg. B/O Jane Smith). This is standard procedure and the only way hospitals can identify a link between mother and baby. If you intend to give your baby a different surname, this is done when you apply for their birth certificate.*

The caregiver regularly observes the baby by listening, watching and touching them. Many newborns are snuffly or gurgly for an hour or two, but this should not interfere with their feeding. Your baby's skin should be pinkish (if fair). Darker babies are noted to have red lips. Your caregiver may use the back of their hand on your baby's forehead to feel their warmth, or check their temperature with a thermometer. They may also use a stethoscope to listen to your baby's heart rate and breathing.

WEIGHING, MEASURING AND BATHING

Weighing and measuring your baby is usually done within 30 to 60 minutes after the birth, depending on the birthplace and how busy your caregiver is. It can be left until later if you want to feed your baby first. Your baby is also given a quick head-to-toe check (five fingers and five toes) before being dressed and wrapped (and sometimes bathed).

These procedures normally happen in the birth room, but some birthplaces take the baby to another room. If so, your partner or support person can go with them or you can ask that this be delayed until you are able to go with your baby. (Don't forget the camera!) Babies, who are unwell are swiftly weighed on arrival in the intensive care nursery in case medications or intravenous fluids are required, as dosages are calculated by their weight.

Weight: Your baby is weighed with no clothes on electronic scales and the weight is recorded in grams or kilograms. The average weight of a term baby is 3.3 kg (7 lb 4½ oz), but can range from 2.8 to 4.5 kg (6 lb 3 oz to 9 lb 15 oz).

Head circumference: The average head circumference of a newborn is 35 cm, ranging from 33 to 37 cm. This is measured again before going home, as the size often 'grows' a centimetre or more because their previously moulded head (from the birth) becomes more rounded in shape.

Length: A baby's average length is 50 cm (20 inches), ranging from 46 to 56 cm (18 to 22 inches). The caregiver may trail a measuring tape down your baby's back and leg, or place them on a special measuring board. Don't be too concerned if your baby 'shrinks' or 'grows' dramatically after a week, as this can slightly fluctuate depending on the caregiver's measuring methods.

Bathing

Many parents now wait a day or more before bathing their baby, to allow any rich vernix cream to soak into their baby's skin and prevent them from becoming too cold soon after birth. Premature and unwell babies transferred to the intensive care nursery are not bathed until they are well enough (nor are well babies with a temperature below 36°C).

There is no medical reason to bath your baby straightaway and you can ask that this be delayed if you wish. Most babies are born fairly unsoiled, but if you think your baby needs a clean up before visitors arrive, then you (or your caregiver) can wipe their face and scalp and/or their bottom with a warm cloth (known as a top and tail).

Some hospitals routinely use antiseptic solutions to cleanse the baby's skin, stating reasons such as infection control. This practice is questionable and skin specialists believe that excessively bathing newborns with soapy, perfumed or medicated preparations irritates their skin, making it dry and more prone to rashes and skin infections.[3] The 'friendly' bacteria, which protect the baby's skin from other hostile or foreign bacteria, are removed. Using plain water (possibly with sorbelene cream) is best for your baby's skin.

Vitamin K

Vitamin K is necessary to create normal blood clotting and prevent excessive bleeding. Small amounts are obtained from foods, but it is mostly produced by normal bacteria in the bowel and stored in the liver. Babies are born with naturally low levels of vitamin K, but the vast majority build this up by six weeks as their gut bacteria multiplies. In very rare cases this does not happen and the baby's vitamin K levels become lower than they were at birth, creating an unsafe deficiency. This is called vitamin K deficiency bleeding (VKDB), previously known as haemorrhagic disease of the newborn (HDN). As a way of preventing VKDB in a few babies, all parents are encouraged to give their baby some form of vitamin K soon after birth as a precaution.

VKDB is classified into three types, depending on when the bleeding starts.
- **Early VKDB** occurs within 24 hours after birth and is rare, but it can be experienced by 6 to 12% of babies whose mothers took certain prescribed medications during the last few weeks of their pregnancy (aspirin, heparin, anti-epileptics, barbiturates or tuberculosis drugs, to name a few). Daily vitamin K supplements in the last two to four weeks of pregnancy are generally advised for these women, as well as giving the baby vitamin K at birth.
- **Classical VKDB** occurs two to seven days after birth and is more common if the baby's feeding is delayed, or infrequent, in the first few days of life (0.44% of well babies and 1.5% of unwell babies).
- **Late VKDB** occurs from eight days to six months of age (commonly 4 to 12 weeks) and is usually associated with fully breastfed babies who do not absorb, produce or store adequate vitamin K. Bottle-fed babies are less at risk but can still experience late VKDB. The incidence is 0.005% to 0.02%; however, 50% of these babies have had vitamin K injections but are found to have a liver disorder or bowel absorption problem.

The physical signs of VKDB may include:
- Excessive bleeding of some sort (in bowel motions or from their nose or mouth).
- Unexplained bruising.
- Excessive bleeding after an injection.

VKDB is very rare, but 30 to 50% of babies who develop it experience serious bleeding in the brain, making them drowsy and/or less responsive. This can lead to a range of problems from mild to severe brain damage and, in a few cases (0.001 to 0.003%), dying.

Vitamin K injections have been routinely given to newborns since the 1970s. In 1992 a UK study indicated that they may be linked to an increased risk of childhood leukaemia.[4] This prompted caregivers to recommend oral vitamin K for a while. Since then studies have failed to replicate these findings. In 2000 the Australian National Health and Medical Research Council stated that vitamin K injections were *not* believed to be linked with childhood cancer, recommending that all babies be given vitamin K to prevent VKDB.[5]

Vitamin K is usually given as one injection soon after birth, but it can be given as three oral doses at the parent's request. Both methods are generally effective in preventing VKDB. Oral vitamin K is given:
- The day of birth.
- Between four to seven days after birth.
- At about one month of age.

If your baby vomits within one hour of having oral vitamin K, the dose needs to be repeated. When choosing oral vitamin K, it is very important that you remember to give all three doses.

Declining vitamin K

A few parents decline vitamin K for their baby, perhaps because they wish to avoid interventions, or they feel their newborn is healthy and it is unnatural to interfere unless absolutely necessary. Common questions asked include:
- **What if I eat vitamin K-rich foods during pregnancy?** Dietary sources of vitamin K play a very minor role in how we obtain it, passing from mother to baby at 3% of what is eaten, and do not protect against VKDB. Vitamin K produced by a woman's gut bacteria cannot be transmitted to her baby.
- **What if I take vitamin K supplements during pregnancy?** Supplements (usually 10 mg per day for the last three to four weeks of pregnancy) can help prevent early VKDB but does not protect against classical and late VKDB.

- **What if I take vitamin K supplements while breastfeeding?**
Breast milk contains 1 to 2 micrograms per litre of vitamin K (formula contains 30 micrograms per litre). There us no research to demonstrate how effective this is for preventing VKDB. If planning to supplement, taking 5 mg every day until the baby is at least 12 weeks old (fully breastfeeding and no solids) may help with late VKDB, but does not protect against classical VKDB.
- **What if my baby appears physically well after a normal birth?**
The way your baby is born, and their general appearance at birth, does not predict whether they will get VKDB.

Parents who conscientiously object to their baby receiving vitamin K may find they encounter negative comments, criticism and pressure from caregivers. If you have made this decision, then prepare yourself for these types of responses. You may wish to be flexible in your decision if your baby is unwell or not feeding frequently. If you do notice signs of VKDB, it is important to seek medical attention immediately.

Hepatitis B vaccination

Hepatitis B is a virus that infects the liver. About 50% of infected adults show no signs of illness and are unaware they carry the virus unless they have a blood test, with 1 to 12 % of infected adults continuing to carry the virus for years, being able to pass it on to others. They are also at increased risk of having long-term liver disease (25%) and possibly liver cancer (15 to 25%) later in life, usually by middle age.

Babies infected with hep B usually show no signs of illness, but 50 to 90% of them become long-term carriers of the virus and can infect others, as well as being at risk of liver disease and liver cancer later in life.[6] If not vaccinated soon after birth, babies born to women with hepatitis B have a 40% chance of becoming infected with the virus either through a vaginal or caesarean birth, or through breastfeeding. Vaccinated babies can be breast-fed and their mothers are encouraged to do so.

Most Australian babies are at very low risk of contracting hep B if their mother, or others they live with, don't carry the virus. Transmission from child to child (such as in a day-care setting) is unlikely but possible through contact with open sores and wounds of an infected child.

Since May 2000, hep B vaccinations have been routinely offered to all newborn babies as part of the National Australian Immunisation Schedule. This aims to protect babies at risk of becoming infected, and to ensure protection when they become teenagers and are at higher risk through sexual activity and experimentation with injecting drugs, amateur piercing or tattooing (common ways of becoming infected). Be aware, though, that having a hep B vaccination does not guarantee immunity or protection against the virus.

NOTE: *'Vaccination' refers to the injection of a substance that aims to set up an immune response in the body. Some people are vaccinated but still don't develop immunity. The word 'immunisation' describes the body's successful response to being vaccinated.*

Hepatitis B vaccinations are given:
- Within seven days of birth.
- At 2, 4, 6 and 12 months of age.

Hepatitis B vaccines are generally regarded as safe, but they occasionally have side effects, such as:
- Temporary soreness at the injection site (5 to 15%) and/or infection of the injection site (less than 1%).
- A mild fever within 24 hours (0.6 to 3.7%).
- Some adults report nausea, dizziness, tiredness, aching muscles and joints within 24 hours.

Very rare side effects include high fever or an allergic reaction. Some parents use homeopathic remedies for their child to reduce or prevent side effects.

Declining hep B vaccination

Children who are not fully immunised are ineligible for childcare assistance payments and other government family benefits. If you wish to decline the hep B vaccination for your baby (or delay it until they are older), complete a conscientious objection form from the Health Insurance Commission, which needs to be signed by a doctor to be validated.

WELL BABIES NEEDING FURTHER OBSERVATIONS

Hospitals often require well, healthy babies with certain risk factors to have further observations for 24 to 48 hours after birth in case they become unwell. Women planning to go home early may be advised to stay until these observations are completed. If your baby is born at home, your caregiver may return at more regular intervals, or tell you what to look for so you can notify them.

In the past, routine observations were performed in the intensive care nursery. However, these days most hospitals try to keep the baby and their mother together where possible.

Common reasons for a well baby to have more frequent observations include:

- **Meconium-stained liquor** during labour, in case the baby has inhaled a small amount into their lungs and develops breathing difficulties. Their temperature, heart rate and breathing are checked every four hours, or each time the baby wakes for a feed.
- **Group B streptococcus** (found with tests during pregnancy), in case the baby develops breathing difficulties and pneumonia. Their temperature, heart rate, breathing, general appearance and feeding patterns are monitored.
- **Increased breathing rate** (more than 70 or 80 breaths per minute, normally 40 to 60), which is often due to transient tachypnoea of the newborn. If your baby looks relaxed and can feed without pulling off the breast (or teat) to breathe, then they are usually well, but caregivers may be concerned in case it is the early stages of an infection. Their temperature, heart rate and breathing are monitored. They may also have a septic work-up and intravenous antibiotics, just in case.
- **Low temperature** (below 36°C). The baby is often taken to the intensive care nursery to warm up in a humidicrib, and may have heel-prick blood tests for sugar levels and an intravenous drip for fluids, if they are reluctant to feed.
- **Having naloxone** at birth, to reverse the effects of a narcotic injection received by their mother for pain relief. Naloxone wears off after four hours and the baby may become drowsy again and possibly stop breathing. They are observed in the intensive care nursery for four to six hours.
- **Underweight babies** (less than 2.8 kg or 6 lb 3 oz) can have low temperatures and blood glucose levels, requiring temperature checks and heel-prick blood tests for sugar levels, and are encouraged to feed every three to four hours.
- **Overweight babies** (more than 4.5 kg or 10 lb) may be at risk of undetected diabetes during their mother's pregnancy. They are also given frequent blood sugar heel-prick tests and are encouraged to feed every three to four hours.

Early parenting

BONDING WITH YOUR BABY

The concept of bonding between parents and newborns is seen as a desired, positive psychological adjustment, in which the mother (and the father too) openly shows that she wants to be with and care for her baby. The media often portrays this as falling in love and something that occurs within minutes, as if parents are suddenly struck by a thunderbolt of emotions at birth. While this may be the case for some parents, many others find bonding is a gradual process over days, weeks or even months. So don't be surprised or feel guilty if you don't 'fall in love' immediately. These feelings will come, and you are not a bad parent because they are not instantaneous.

It is normal for women to feel overwhelmed and exhausted when the baby is born and to be self-focused for a few days while they recover. It may also take a while for fathers to bond as the reality sinks in. Feelings can range from positive and loving, to intense or unexpected, or apprehensive and scared. Being nervous about holding or handling your little baby can also delay the opportunity to connect immediately.

> **Did you know?**
> Our skin secretes special chemicals called pheromones. Newborns have a heightened awareness of their parents' smell, so they can distinguish them from others.

THE FIRST FEED

Newborns are quite alert for an hour or so after birth before drifting into a long sleep for two to eight hours. So feeding them is a priority (if it's possible). Babies take 5 to 50 minutes to become interested in feeding, indicated by them opening their mouth and trying to latch onto something (called the rooting reflex). It is a myth that all babies go to the breast as soon as they are born.

The first breastfeed

From our experience, babies who breastfeed within an hour or so of birth are more likely to feed without problems for subsequent feeds. However, if your baby is sleepy or disinterested in feeding this early, this is not a huge problem. Your baby's 'first milk' is colostrum. This clear, yellowish fluid is high in protein, minerals, vitamins and anti-infective agents (antibodies). Colostrum is all your baby needs until your milk comes in on day two to five after the birth. Mother and baby can usually work out the first breastfeed in their own time, if left to their own devices. Some caregivers try to physically place the baby on the breast, but this may be before the woman and her baby are mentally, emotionally and/or physically ready, which can feel invasive and upsetting. It is important you are given space and time even if your baby does not feed until a few hours after the birth.

Doing anything for the first time can make you feel hesitant, nervous, anxious or reluctant. Just be aware that breastfeeding is a learnt skill for both of you and your baby, and it takes time to 'come naturally' (even with subsequent babies). Ask for help if you prefer, but consider having a go yourself first. It is surprising how many babies eventually latch themselves, if left near the nipple to search it out. Ask your caregiver to check the way your baby is latched, to make sure they are on correctly. If you feel everyone is watching you, politely ask them to leave so you don't feel pressured to get it right.

The following suggestions can help make the first breastfeed a positive experience. You may want to practise with a doll during the pregnancy and/or attend some breastfeeding information sessions at your hospital.

- **Mother comfortable** – Sitting up is the easiest position. Place pillows behind and around you to get comfortable and support your back. If you have had a caesarean, lie on your side. You may need your caregiver to help you manoeuvre.
- **Baby comfortable** – Support your baby with your hands, or lay them on a pillow in front of you. You may wish to wrap them, or perhaps have skin-to-skin contact.
- **Hands where?** – Hold your breast with the corresponding hand on that same side (left breast = left hand). Make sure your fingers are well back off the areola, as this is where the baby needs to latch. Place your other hand around the base of your baby's neck and upper back (not on their head). This supports and guides them without pushing them onto the breast.
- **Chest to chest** – Your baby's chest should be towards your chest, so they are facing the breast (not lying on their back and turning their head sideways). If they are unwrapped, place their lower arm around your waist.
- **Nose to nipple and chin up!** – Have your baby's nose in line with your nipple. This encourages them to tilt their head back slightly, and avoids their mouth being too far past the nipple.
- **Latching** – Gently brush your baby's top lip with your nipple to stimulate them to open their mouth. Guide your baby, aiming the

nipple towards the roof of their mouth, with their tongue sitting well down under the nipple, to 'milk' the breast. Remember, always bring the baby to the breast not the breast to the baby, otherwise you will end up in an awkward, hunched-over position for the whole feed, or risk the baby slipping off the nipple as you move to get comfortable. Be aware that it is normal for babies to be fussy initially, latching on and off and perhaps crying. If they don't latch first time, this is normal and not reflective of your ability to feed them. Be patient – they are learning too! After a week or so it will be more natural and you won't have to think about it.

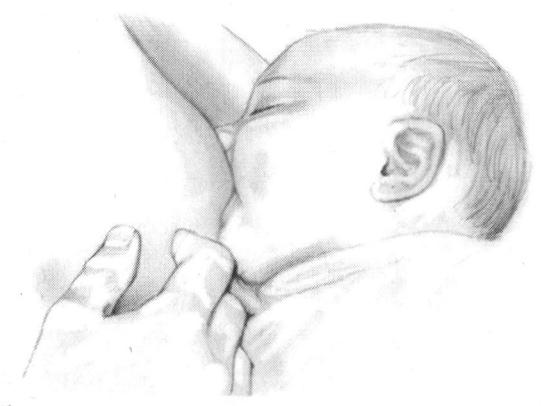

Baby latched correctly

- **Hold them close, chin to breast** – Once latched, don't be afraid to push your baby's chin into the breast. If you let them fall back, they can pull or drag the nipple, possibly causing damage. A baby's nostrils naturally flare out to breathe, but if you are concerned, you can use your finger to depress the breast a little near their nose.
- **How does it feel?** – As the baby latches, there is a moment of slight discomfort as they draw the nipple into the back of their throat. Once the nipple is completely in, the sensation should be strong or dragging, but not painful. If it continues to be painful, place your little finger inside the corner of their mouth to break the seal and get them off. Then relatch. This is better than enduring a painful feed and damaging the nipples.
- **How does it look?** – If your baby is latched correctly, most of your areola cannot be seen and their lips are wide, in a K shape, bottom lip rolled out (not pursed as though kissing the breast). Their jaw, around the base of their ear and earlobe, usually moves as they feed. You shouldn't hear sucking sounds (otherwise they are not creating a seal

and are latched incorrectly). Ask your caregiver to check, if you are unsure.
- **How long?** – Allow your baby to feed for as long as they like (5 to 20 minutes or longer). If they are latched correctly, the nipple will not be damaged. It is not necessary to give them both breasts, but you can offer them the other side if you wish. For their second breastfeed, offer them the breast you did not start on. Breastfed babies don't usually need to burp and many women don't worry about trying to burp their baby at all, despite others' suggestions that this is necessary.

The first bottle-feed

If you choose to bottle-feed from birth, the hospital may provide formula and equipment, or you may be asked to bring your own. Don't worry if the brand of formula they use is not the one you have chosen. They usually have a different formula each month and changing brands is not an issue for your baby.

Soon after the birth, ask the staff to organise a bottle so it is ready when your baby is interested. You can express colostrum into it if you want your baby to receive some of this first milk. When you and your baby are ready, offer them the bottle. Try to avoid letting staff feed them. This is a time for you to connect with your baby and get to know them (and practise feeding). If you don't feel up to it, ask your partner or support person to feed them. When feeding:
- Make sure you are sitting comfortably with pillows for support. Your baby may be wrapped or you may have skin-to-skin contact, perhaps resting on a pillow on your lap.
- The bottle of formula is placed in a jug of warm water, so check the temperature by shaking some milk onto the inside of your wrist. It should feel lukewarm not hot. Giving it at room temperature is okay.
- Avoid screwing the lid of the bottle on too tightly; some air needs to get into the bottle as the baby sucks, so the formula can flow easily.
- Hold your baby close to your chest and gently brush their top lip with the teat so they open their mouth.
- Place the teat into your baby's open mouth, on top of their tongue. Make sure the bottle is held slightly upwards, at an angle, to fill the teat with formula, so air is not being sucked in as the baby drinks.
- Most newborns use regular flow teats. If your baby gags because the formula is flowing too fast, slide the teat out of their mouth and sit them up and forward so they can catch their breath.
- Once the milk is finished, or your baby stops sucking, gently sit them

up and forward to burp them. Support their head by holding your hand under their chin (without being tight around their neck). Or just place them upright, over your shoulder. Not all babies need to burp, but if they do, this will happen within five minutes or so. Newborns drink up to 30 ml of formula milk for their first feed. If they don't drink it all, don't worry. Discard what is left and use a new bottle for the next feed.

Early parenting skills
The first hour

The first hour is typically spent in the room where you gave birth (or in Recovery after a caesarean). If all has gone well, the role of early parenting consists of holding and talking to your new baby. If you have never held a baby before, you may feel nervous. Try to remember that babies are pretty durable, even though they look small and delicate. However, supporting their neck muscles is important during the early weeks.

If your baby is being passed to you from another person, cradle both your arms with your hands facing upwards, overlapping at waist level. Let the baby's neck rest in the crook of one of your bent elbows. If picking up your baby from the bed or cot:

- Guide one hand under their neck and support it with the palm of your hand. Use your fingers to support their head, with the top of their back resting on your wrist.
- Slide your other hand under their bottom, either between their legs or under the side of their bottom, so it rests in the palm of your hand.
- Once you feel both hands are in place, lean towards your baby as you lift them up, holding them near your chest for extra support. Once you are holding them, move the hand under their head along their back until their head rests in the crook of your arm, then move the other hand under their bottom, up the baby's back, stabilising them with your chest. Cradle your baby with their head slightly higher than their bottom.

The first couple of times you pick up your baby can feel awkward. Within a week or so it becomes more natural. Try to:

- Hold your baby gently but firmly, to reassure them and provide the security they were used to when snugly held inside the uterus.
- Talk softly to your baby as you pick them up, or wrap them firmly in a blanket to prevent the startle reflex (where they throw their arms out and often cry).

- When laying your baby down, make sure their head is fully supported with your hand or arm, to avoid their head flopping backwards.

  Did you know?
  People instinctively hold babies on the left side, near their heart, regardless of whether they are right- or left-handed. This has been documented in children as young as three or four years, when cradling dolls.

The following 23 hours

Parenting over the next day consists of feeding and changing your baby, as well as cuddling and gazing at them. Once your baby has been fed, weighed, checked and dressed, they often fall into a well-deserved sleep, so you too can rest. When your baby wakes again, they may just look around, or cry and be fidgety or interested in feeding again (and perhaps need changing). They then fall back to sleep . . . and so the parenting continues!

Your baby's first bowel motion is passed within 24 hours (if not passed during labour). This sticky, dark green substance is called meconium and is quite difficult to clean off your baby's bottom. They should also pass urine once during the first 24 hours, but this might not happen for a while, if they urinate at birth. If you need help to change your baby's nappy, ask your caregiver for guidance.

INTRODUCING THE BABY TO THEIR SIBLINGS

Children attending the birth are introduced to their brother or sister straight away. Allow them to approach the new baby in their own time and reassure them you are all right and that it is normal for the baby to cry. More commonly, though, older children meet their new sibling when visiting after the birth. To make this a positive experience, consider:
- Having someone else hold the baby, or place them in their cot, when your older child first sees you again. This means there is nothing between you and your child, and you can have a big hug before the new baby is introduced. Care and assistance may be needed if you have had a caesarean.
- Sitting the older child on your lap and then placing the baby on their lap, so they can hold their new brother or sister and still be close to you.
- Buying a gift for your child from the new baby, and/or one for the new baby from the older child. Encourage friends to bring small treats or presents for the older child so they don't feel left out.

- Having a birthday cake and candle to sing 'Happy Birthday' to the baby.
- Taking your child to the intensive care nursery if the baby is unwell. Prepare them for what they will see and include them as much as possible.

Your newborn baby's physical appearance and behaviours

A NEWBORN'S APPEARANCE

Parents are often unprepared for the sight of their new creation, especially as most newborns look very different from the perfect TV cherub! Many babies change dramatically during the first week as the crumples smooth out and any swellings go down. Not knowing what to expect can make you feel unsure about whether your baby is normal.

Head

At birth, your baby's head looks large compared to the rest of their body. They may be bald, or have hair, which is generally replaced with new hair of a different colour and consistency before their first birthday. Babies born vaginally usually have out-of-shape heads (called moulding). Their head becomes more rounded within 24 to 72 hours. They may also have some swelling on the top, known as a caput, caused by pressure on their mother's cervix during labour. This gradually disappears within 12 to 24 hours. Babies born by caesarean usually have no caput or moulding, unless their mother was labouring before the caesarean. Babies born with forceps or a ventouse may have pressure marks, and sometimes bruising. If an internal CTG monitor was attached or fetal blood sampling was performed, there will be small marks from these on their scalp. This may also occur when the waters are broken by the amnihook before the birth.

A baby's fontanelle is covered with a strong membrane that protects their brain. You may see this pulsating in time with their heartbeat, or bulge when the baby cries. It can also look sunken at times, but this is not a sign of dehydration, as long as the baby is alert when awake, feeding and having wet nappies. Their fontanelle can close anytime from 4 to 18 months old.

Face

A newborn's forehead often looks large and slopes back, and their face may be puffy and swollen. A few babies have facial contusions, which is a faint bruising all over their face. This is caused by the baby descending rapidly down the birth canal and breaking small blood vessels on the way, but generally disappears after a week or so.

Nose and sneezing

Your baby's nose can look flattened and enlarged with flared nostrils. It is commonly covered with small, white spots called milia, caused by temporary blockages of their sebaceous glands. These normally disappear by four to six weeks and should never be squeezed.

Sneezing is common and helps the baby clear their nasal passages of mucus, dust and sometimes milk, and does not mean they are getting a cold. Babies may also cough when bringing up mucus from the back of their throat and mouth.

Eyes

Most newborns have steel blue or dark grey eyes. Their true colour usually becomes obvious within 2 to 12 months, but it may take longer. The whites of their eyes often look slightly bluish and a few babies have red patches on them, due to small, broken blood vessels caused by pressure from the birth. This disappears in about two weeks. Your baby's eyelids may be swollen and have patches of red or purple on the skin. Often one eye looks bigger than the other.

Newborns squint frequently and have immature eye muscle control, making it difficult for them to focus, or follow a moving object, until six weeks of age. This is why young babies often look cross-eyed. Your baby won't necessarily produce tears during the early weeks, but their eyes have a natural protective film, which prevents dust and fluff from irritating them.

Ears

Your baby's ears can look flattened, folded or creased and misshapen after being compressed in the uterus. This corrects over the following days. Their ears may also be slightly bruised if forceps were used. Be careful not to bump them if this is the case. Your baby's hearing is very acute, so take care not to talk too loudly, or shout at your other children, when their head is near your face. Babies normally startle to loud noises, letting you know they can hear. However, they won't respond if they are distracted, tired, have just fed, or the noise is continually repeated.

Mouth

Your baby's lips look red, but the skin around their mouth can often look whitish-blue, as their fine skin shows the veins underneath. (This is not a sign of wind!) Some newborns have tiny white cysts along the roof of their mouth or gums, called Epstein's pearls. These disappear over the following weeks. Their bottom lip may quiver at times, which is a normal reflex, and not a response to being cold. They may also get hiccups, but are not generally worried by them. These settle on their own.

Body

A newborn's body can be long and thin, or display a plump pot belly. A few babies still have a fine covering of downy hair on their backs and upper arms, which disappears by four to six weeks. They may have some thick, greasy, white vernix cream, if born before 40 weeks.

Your baby may be blood-streaked at birth and may have traces of greenish-black meconium on their skin. Enlarged nipples and swollen breasts are common for both boys and girls, and they can sometimes excrete a little milky fluid, nicknamed 'witches' milk, due to the mother's hormones produced during pregnancy.

Arms, legs, hands and feet

Your baby's hands and feet can often look bluish-purple in colour and feel cool, which is normal as they naturally divert more blood to their head and chest. Their legs can be bow-shaped, but will straighten as they grow older. A newborn's feet normally curve inwards, due to their position in the womb, and generally straighten by the time they are ready to walk. Newborns have long, soft, flexible fingernails, which can cause marks on their face from accidental scratching. If your baby is overdue, their hands and feet could be wrinkled, with dry, peeling skin.

Skin

Depending on your baby's ethnicity, their skin can look pink, pale, ruddy-red or brownish in colour. Black babies don't generally look dark until a few weeks of age, when the melanin pigment in their skin develops, although their genitals and nipples are usually dark. A newborn's immature blood circulation often causes their skin to look mottled, with red-purple blotches, particularly if premature. On the odd occasion, their upper body can look pale, while their lower half looks redder, which is normal. Gently moving your baby around, or massaging them, can help stimulate their blood flow.

Umbilical cord

A small, plastic clamp remains on your baby's umbilical cord stump for two to three days. Once their cord dries, the clamp is removed by the midwife. The stump of the cord slowly shrivels and darkens, becoming smelly and often bleeding a little, before finally separating 7 to 10 days after the birth. No special care is required and you don't need to apply anything, like methylated spirits or alcohol, to the cord, as these chemicals can be absorbed into the baby's system.

> **Did you know?**
> The way the cord is cut or clamped does not make their belly button an 'inny' or 'outy'. This is something your baby is born with.

Genitals

The genitals of both boys and girls usually appear large. A baby boy's scrotum often looks swollen due to a normal accumulation of fluid surrounding his testes. This is gradually absorbed within three months. Up to 98% of boys have descended testes at birth, or descend before their first birthday. Baby girls can have a thick mucus or bloodstained vaginal discharge for a few days, due to lowering hormones from their mother. Girls can also have small skin tags around their genitals, which usually disappear as they grow older.

EARLY PHYSICAL VARIATIONS
Cephalhaematoma

A cephalhaematoma is a swelling on the top of a baby's head, at one or both sides. It becomes noticeable 12 to 24 hours after the birth and is caused by blood slowly accumulating between the baby's skin and the bones of their skull (not inside their brain), due to friction during the birth (from their mother's pelvis, forceps or a ventouse). Cephalhaematomas don't cause health problems and go away after several weeks. A few take 9 to 12 months to totally reabsorb.

Sucking blisters on the wrist

A blister, or broken, bruised skin, on one or both hands or wrists is a sucking blister, which is not harmful, but your baby may continue to suck there. Your caregiver may cover it for a few days if the skin is broken (or bleeding), to avoid infection.

Stork marks
Small, pink or red patches on the baby's eyelids, forehead, nose, top lip, the bridge of their nose and/or the nape of their neck are called stork marks, and are tiny blood vessels visible beneath the baby's fine skin. They are harmless and generally fade within 12 months or so.

Strawberry marks
Strawberry marks (haemangiomas) are caused by an overgrowth of tiny blood vessels underneath the baby's skin. They usually start as tiny red dots but slowly become larger over one to nine months until they are bright red (or purplish), soft, raised, spongy swellings; then within two years they shrink and disappear. Removing them with laser, X-rays, freezing or injecting chemicals is no longer recommended.

Spider marks
Spider naevi are collections of small broken blood vessels (or capillaries) that look like a cobweb underneath the baby's fine skin. They are similar to stork marks, with most disappearing within one to two years.

A Mongolian spot
A Mongolian spot is a patch of blue skin discolouration across the baby's lower back and bottom (and occasionally their tummy), which can look like a bruise. It is caused by an accumulation of pigment under the skin and is mainly seen in darker-skinned babies, being present at birth, or appearing over the days or weeks following, and naturally fading before the child is three.

Birthmarks
Permanent birthmarks stay with a baby for life. We don't really know why they develop, but they are not connected with anything the woman has done during her pregnancy. If it is quite prominent, it can take a while to come to terms with your baby's birthmark, with some parents grieving the loss of their perfect baby and/or feeling concerned about how it may affect their child's life.

Traditional birthmarks (pigmented naevi) appear in a variety of shapes and sizes but don't cause any health problems. They can be:
- Flat and pale (coffee-coloured), enlarging as the baby grows older but not becoming darker.
- Dark and slightly raised, sometimes with hairs growing out of them, often called moles.

Occasionally, the birthmark doesn't become apparent until the baby is a couple of months old.

Port wine stains are caused by dilated capillaries in the skin, appearing bright red to purple in colour. They tend to appear on the baby's face and neck, but can be anywhere on their body. Some parents consult a paediatric dermatologist about using laser treatments to remove them when their child is older.

Normal newborn behaviour

Newborns behave in different ways, as adults do. How your baby reacts during their first day of life will depend on their personality, as well as how their birth unfolded. Your baby may:

- Initially cry at birth, and then be alert and interested in their surroundings.
- Cry lustily on and off until wrapped or held closely by their parent, or once they have fed.
- Be irritable and unsettled, especially if forceps or a ventouse delivered them; possibly not comforted with anything you do. Sometimes wrapping and holding them close can help.
- Remain quiet, looking around in a dreamy way.
- Be sleepy or drowsy and possibly not interested in feeding. This may be their personality, or they may be exhausted or affected by a residue of narcotic medications.
- Be fussy and unsettled, wanting frequently to feed.

Did you know?
Newborns can display mimicking behaviour soon after birth. If the person holding the baby is in a quiet environment and pokes their tongue out, the baby often pokes out their tongue back!

A newborn's physical reflexes

Newborns have many natural reflexes that help them develop inside the uterus and survive after birth. These are automatic physical responses that caregivers use to assess how their nervous system is developing. Premature babies have immature, or absent, reflexes, which develop as they grow. Many newborn reflexes disappear within a baby's first year. A few stay for life.

Rooting reflex

Your baby's rooting reflex is triggered when their cheek is touched. This makes their head turn in that direction, often opening their mouth wide (whether they are hungry or not). Babies display the rooting reflex frequently when awake and it remains strong until three to four months of age.

Sucking and swallowing

Sucking and swallowing reflexes are mature in babies born after 36 weeks. Your baby coordinates these reflexes simultaneously to drink milk in a sucking-swallowing-breathing sequence. A newborn's desire to suck is very strong and not always related to hunger, called non-nutritive sucking. This is an inbuilt mechanism to provide comfort, being present for a year or so. The swallowing reflex remains for life. Babies are also born with a hand-to-mouth response, known as the Babkin reflex. If your baby becomes upset or tired, they may resort to this to try and comfort themselves.

Gag reflex

Your baby has a protective gag reflex. Their throat closes over and their tongue pushes excess milk or mucus out of the back of their mouth, to prevent it being breathed in. When babies start solid foods, they tend to gag a lot until they become accustomed to eating. The gag reflex is important for survival and is closely associated with the swallow, cough and sneeze reflexes.

It is not uncommon for newborns to gag on excess mucus in the first few days after birth, making them momentarily look distressed and turn blue. This is understandably distressing to witness. You can sit your baby upright, or place them over your shoulder, to help them swallow or spit out the mucus, although their gag reflex usually deals with it without your help.

Startle reflex

The startle or Moro reflex occurs in response to a sudden movement or loud noise. The baby flings out their arms, fans their fingers and extends their legs, and then quickly pulls their arms back in towards their body in an embrace position. This often causes them to tremor and cry. Caregivers use the startle reflex to test a baby's central nervous system development and muscle tone soon after birth.

The startle reflex can cause a sleeping baby to suddenly wake and perhaps make it difficult to resettle them to sleep. This is why formal settling techniques recommend firmly wrapping newborns to help minimise this response. It usually disappears by the time they are 8 to 10 weeks old.

Crawling reflex

When newborns are placed on their stomach, they usually draw up their legs under their belly and then kick their legs out, shuffling in a crawling motion. If you apply firm pressure to the soles of their feet this triggers a response for them to push forward, creating the crawling reflex, which is only present for four weeks and is not part of formal crawling.

> **Did you know?**
> In recent years, more babies are skipping the crawling milestone, just going straight from sitting to walking. Paediatricians are not concerned by this, but think it is an interesting result that has evolved since babies have been placed on their backs to sleep to help prevent SIDS.

Grasp reflex

Your baby will make a grasping action whenever something is placed in their hand. This reflex is very strong, even in premature babies, and remains present for three to four months.

Walking and Babinski reflexes

If your baby is held upright, supported under their armpits, with their feet touching a flat surface, this simulates a stepping action, which is present until eight weeks. Caregivers also test the Babinski reflex, by gently stroking the sole of the baby's foot from heel to toe. In response, they turn up their toes and move their foot inwards.

Tonic neck reflex

A tonic neck or fencing reflex is stimulated by turning your baby's head to one side while they are lying on their back. They respond by straightening their arm and leg on the side they are facing, and bending their arm and leg on the opposite side. This is to help protect them from rolling over.

Traction reflex

Caregivers test babies for a traction reflex or head lag in the early days after birth. Your baby is held by both wrists and then lifted forward into a sitting position. Their head should first lag back, then straighten and fall forward.

Galant reflex

The Galant reflex is tested to assess a newborn's spinal nerve development. Your baby is held under their stomach (facing down) while the caregiver gently strokes one side of their back. They should arch their body and pull their pelvis towards the side being stroked. This is thought to be a swimming reflex left over from our amphibian ancestors, and is present for about nine months.

What to expect from your caregiver

Once all the activity surrounding the birth subsides, mother and baby experience an immense transition, being left alone to be with each other, rest and recuperate. Staff normally move you to the postnatal ward within one to three hours. Some birth centres allow you to stay longer, perhaps overnight. Your partner or support person may be able to stay overnight in the postnatal ward if you are not sharing your room with another new mother.

If you and your baby are well, you may choose to go home early, within 4 to 48 hours. The midwife visits you the next day, and is on call if you have any concerns.

If you have had a homebirth, your caregiver will probably leave two to three hours after the birth and be on call to return if needed (or organise another midwife if they are too tired or too busy to come at short notice). They should revisit within 12 to 24 hours after the birth for a routine postnatal check.

NEWBORN EXAMINATIONS

Your baby has several head-to-toe physical examinations at different times, for various reasons. These can be:

- **An initial general check** – This is a brief, overall examination soon after the birth, to make sure your baby is generally healthy and normal. This is usually done when they are being measured and weighed.
- **Daily physical checks** – These are done by the postnatal midwives, aiming to detect any problems with feeding patterns, bowel motions, passing urine, cord stump separating, skin rashes, infections or jaundice.
- **A formal examination** – Usually performed by a paediatrician or local GP, this involves a thorough examination, including the baby's reflexes, hips, abdomen and eyes, and listening for a heart murmur.
- **Growth and development checks** – These are done at regular intervals at the baby health clinic or local doctor's surgery. This involves weighing, measuring and checking the baby's physical and mental development and expected milestones.

Usually your baby needs to be undressed to be examined. Many don't like this and often cry. Also, some parts of the examination may be a little uncomfortable for them. Once it is finished, your baby can be dressed and cuddled. It is probably comforting to give them a feed as well. The examinations described below can be categorised as: general check (G), daily check (D), formal examination (FE), and/or growth and development (G&D).

Head – This involves: measuring their head circumference (G, FE, G&D); checking the fontanelle for size and tension (G, FE, G&D); looking at their head shape, caput/moulding, if a cephalhaematoma is forming, scratches from a scalp electrode or fetal blood sampling site healing (if used during labour) (D); and testing their head lag reflex (FE, G&D).

Eyes – Are their eyes looking normal (G, FE, G&D), and are there any signs of infection, inflammation or pus-like discharge or swelling of the eyelids (FE, D)? An eye test also involves: examining the back of the baby's eyeballs (retina) with a light and checking the eye lenses for clouding (cataracts) (FE); and, from six weeks, seeing if the baby tracks (follows moving objects) with their eyes (G&D).

Ears – These check their ears are normally formed and positioned with normal openings (G, FE), perhaps with a formal hearing assessment (FE, G&D).

Nose – This is to see whether they can breathe while their mouth is closed and while feeding (G, FE).

Lips and mouth – Here, the doctor checks the colour of their lips and the roof of their mouth (for cleft palate), and tests their sucking reflex (G, FE).

Neck – This involves: checking their neck for cysts, lumps, or webbing of the skin (G); and feeling their thyroid gland to see if it is a normal size, and testing their tonic neck reflex (FE).

Arms and hands – This involves: checking both arms are equal in length and that both move, and that there are five fingers on each hand and normal palm creases (G, FE); testing their grasp and startle reflexes (FE); and checking for infection of their fingernail beds (D).

Chest – This involves: checking they have two nipples (G); counting their breaths per minute using a stethoscope, and listening to their lungs and heart sounds (G&D); and screening for a heart murmur (FE).

Skin – These examinations check for marks or birthmarks, if their skin is dry or peeling and if vernix is present (G, FE); and look at the colour of their skin for jaundice and whether they have rashes or spots (D).

Abdomen – This involves: checking their tummy is soft, looking for hernias, making sure the cord is clamped adequately and that there are three blood vessels in the cord (G); making sure the cord is separating normally, with no infection of the bellybutton (D); and gently feeling the baby's kidneys, liver and spleen to make sure they are normal in size (FE).

Genitals
- **For boys**, this involves: checking their penis and scrotum size and shape, if both testes have descended into the scrotum and can be felt (G, FE, G&D); whether there is fluid swelling in the scrotum (hydrocele), and that the opening of the penis (where urine is passed) is correctly situated at the tip of the penis (G, FE); and making sure the urine passes in a good strong stream rather than dribbling (D, FE).
- **For girls**, this involves: checking that their labia and clitoris look normal and that a vaginal opening can be seen when the labia are parted (G, FE).
- **For both sexes**, tests make sure they have passed urine within 24 hours and, once the breast milk is in (after two to four days, sooner for formula), that they are having at least six wet nappies a day (D).

Bottom – This is to check that they have an anal opening (G) and there is adequate space between their anus and scrotum, or vagina (FE); and to make sure they pass their first bowel motion within 24 hours of birth, and that it changes to a yellow colour once the breast milk comes in (or after a couple of days of formula) (D).

Groin and hips – These involve: checking their groin for a pulse, done with the baby's legs in a frog position, and feeling for hernias (FE); and checking their hip joints for stability and any clicks (more common with breech babies, most resolve without treatments as the child grows older) (FE, G&D). The manoeuvre involves the caregiver bending the baby's leg, with their foot on their thigh, then placing two fingers on their hips and moving each leg in a circular outward motion. This can be temporarily uncomfortable for the baby.

Legs and feet – These examinations: check their legs are the same length, with five toes on each foot, and that they can move both legs (G, FE); test the walking reflex (FE); and look for any infection of the toenail beds (D).

Routine screening blood test

Australian babies are routinely screened for rare metabolic disorders which involve a deficiency of a specific enzyme necessary for metabolism. This is called a newborn screening test (NBST) and is done three to five days after the birth, so treatments can be started (if necessary) before the baby shows signs of illness. The four main disorders tested for are:

1. **Cystic fibrosis**, which causes the intestines and lungs to produce thick mucus, affect 1 in 2500 babies.
2. **Galactosaemia**, which causes an accumulation of galactose (a sugar present in breast milk and most formulas), requiring soy-based formula and a lactose-free diet for life, affecting 1 in 40,000 babies.
3. **Congenital hypothyroidism**, where the baby has a small, absent or poorly functioning thyroid gland, possibly leading to physical and mental delays if not treated, affecting 1 in 3500 babies.
4. **Phenylketonuria** (PKU), where the baby lacks the liver enzyme phenylalanine hydroxylase, possibly leading to permanent brain damage if not treated early, affecting 1 in 10,000 babies.

Some laboratories routinely test for up to 30 other rare disorders. Your caregiver should provide written information and give you an opportunity to ask questions before you consent (verbally or in writing). A few parents decline this test for their baby.

The test involves pricking the baby's heel and taking a few drops of blood. It helps if their foot is warmed in some way just before the test, to help with blood flow. Your baby should ideally be awake, and you can feed them just beforehand or afterwards to settle them. It is advisable not to breastfeed them while having the test performed as this can relate the breastfeeding to being a painful experience. However, you can hold your baby if you prefer. Many parents don't want to watch, and ask that their baby be taken to another room.

The drops of blood are soaked into a paper card with 3 or 4 circles about 1 cm in diameter printed on it. All the circles must be filled in for testing. Your baby's heel may be a little bruised for a few days.

The test may need to be repeated if the first one was inconclusive or was done before the baby was 48 hours old. Your caregiver or hospital will contact you if this is the case, or if the initial test indicates that your baby may have a metabolic disorder.

The laboratory can store your baby's blood samples for up to 20 years or longer for:
- Quality control.
- Further testing, to provide additional medical information (with your consent).

- Research, after identifying information has been removed.

Laboratories have strict guidelines regarding confidentiality and how the blood samples can be used for future testing. Ideally parents should be given the choice as to whether they consent to these records being kept and be given some assurances that the sample is destroyed if this is their preference.

Variations for the baby

UNWELL BABY

Premature and/or unwell babies need to be cared for in an intensive care nursery, which can be a foreign and daunting environment. It can be hard to take everything in, especially when dealing with your baby being vulnerable and sick, so try to give yourself time to digest what is happening and don't be surprised if you need to ask the same questions repeatedly. Staff generally work closely with parents and involve them in their baby's care as much as possible. If you know in advance that your baby(s) may need intensive care, arrange to have a tour during the pregnancy.

Thankfully most babies only require intensive care for short periods of time (hours or days). However, a few need to stay for several weeks, or even months, meaning the woman goes home long before her baby does. Early parenting is then spent visiting, watching and waiting for the baby to recover, as well as expressing breast milk, if breastfeeding.

Support strategies

Having your baby in the nursery can be physically and emotionally exhausting, with feelings of sadness and emptiness every time you go back to the postnatal ward, or back home without your baby. Some support strategies can include:

- Staying close to your baby – They know your voice, touch and smell, and can thrive on your love. Interact with them when they are awake, by talking and singing to them; stroke them and cuddle them when possible. These actions can help you form strong attachments and help you get to know their mannerisms and expressions, giving you concrete memories to take with you when you are separated.
- Communicating with staff – Share your concerns; ask them for suggestions and to explain the procedures being performed.
- Getting involved with your baby's care – Even if you feel this is limited, early contact helps alleviate nerves and fears. Be guided by staff.

- Journaling your feelings and thoughts during times of separation – This can be especially useful if you are feeling overwhelmed. It may turn into a special book that you give your child when they are older.
- Taking time out for yourself to eat, drink and rest – If home, have dinner out occasionally, get a massage, see a movie or catch up with a friend.
- Seeking help with your other children so that you can concentrate on your sick baby – Of course, you should include your baby's siblings as much as possible, but it can be hard to meet all your children's needs.
- Accepting offers of help from family and friends – This could be cooking meals, cleaning the house, minding other children, driving you to the hospital or being someone to talk with. Even if you are fiercely independent, the exhausting schedule can take its toll.
- Sharing your feelings – Be open about your fears, pain and vulnerability with someone you trust.
- Focusing ahead on when your baby can come home – Plan a welcome-home party and invite all your family and friends!

JAUNDICE

Jaundice is a yellowing of the baby's skin and eyes, due to the build-up of bilirubin in their system. Bilirubin is produced by the normal breakdown of extra red blood cells during the first week after birth. The baby no longer needs these extra cells because they have stopped sharing oxygen with their mother.

About 30 to 50% of babies temporarily accumulate varying levels of bilirubin in their blood because their liver cannot excrete it fast enough, making the baby jaundiced. Most babies are only slightly yellow, with no health problems. But a few babies accumulate excessively high levels of bilirubin, and if this is not treated, it may lead to a degree of brain damage called kernicterus.

Physical signs of jaundice

The whites of the baby's eyes and their face start to yellow and as bilirubin accumulates, this colouring deepens, moving down their body (over a day or two) to their chest, belly and sometimes upper arms and legs. If the levels become very high, the jaundice spreads to their hands and feet. When bilirubin levels start to lower, the yellow discolouration disappears in reverse; that is, the baby's chest, neck, head and eyes are the last areas to lose their yellow appearance. Very severe jaundice can make the baby drowsy, lethargic and reluctant or disinterested in feeding. However, most babies have treatment commenced before they reach this stage.

There are three types of jaundice:
- **Physiological jaundice**, the most common, does not require treatment because the bilirubin levels remain low. It first appears 24 to 48 hours after the birth, peaking by three to six days, then subsiding after a week or so. The baby is well and appears unperturbed by their yellow appearance. However, very small and premature babies may not process their bilirubin quickly enough and may need phototherapy. Physiological jaundice is not preventable, but early and frequent feeding can decrease the severity of it.
  NOTE: *Supplementing breastfeeding with water, glucose solutions or formula does not prevent jaundice or make it disappear any quicker, and is not recommended.*
- **Breast milk jaundice** is mild but persists for 6 to 12 weeks after the birth. The baby appears slightly yellow but is well, with no treatments required, because the bilirubin levels remain low. The exact cause is not clear, although up to 30% of breastfed babies have it to some degree. It is harmless and should ***not*** be a reason to stop breastfeeding for any period of time.
- **Nonphysiological jaundice** is uncommon and caused by the baby being ill or having a health disorder. It usually appears within 24 hours of birth and can become quite severe, requiring treatments.

Detecting jaundice

The baby is visually observed, or a special jaundice meter is used. This device is placed on their forehead, emitting a brief beam of light onto their skin, measuring the degree of yellowness. If your caregiver believes the bilirubin levels are becoming high, the baby has a blood test (usually by pricking their heel) to accurately measure the level. Levels exceeding 250 imol/L generally require phototherapy. Premature babies are treated at lower levels (150 to 200 imol/L, depending on their gestation).

Phototherapy

Phototherapy exposes the baby's skin to a bright blue light. This turns the bilirubin into a water-soluble substance that can be excreted by the baby's kidneys. Phototherapy can be administered in postnatal wards or the intensive care nursery (depending on the hospital's policy). In recent years, special bili-suits, imbedded with optical fibres, have been used at home after early discharge.

Traditional phototherapy involves the baby being naked (except for maybe a nappy) in a warmed incubator, so their skin is exposed to maximum light. Little soft shields cover their eyes and their temperature is checked regularly. This may be needed almost continuously for several days, with short breaks taken only for feeding and changing. Bilirubin blood tests are performed daily to guide the caregiver as to when the phototherapy can be stopped.

Some babies develop skin rashes and it is common for them to have frequent, loose, green bowel motions. The baby is encouraged to feed regularly (every three to four hours), to help improve their jaundice.

Exchange transfusion

Very rarely the bilirubin levels become extremely high, despite phototherapy. In these cases an exchange blood transfusion is recommended. This involves giving the baby fresh blood and taking away their bilirubin blood to dilute the levels in their system. The transfusion is carried out in the intensive care nursery so the baby's heart rate, breathing, temperature and blood pressure can be continuously monitored during the procedure.

The blood is matched with a blood sample from the mother, as well as the baby's blood type. It may be possible to use blood from a relative of the baby if they have compatible blood types and enough time is available. Check with your caregiver.

The warmed blood is exchanged in slow steps, 5 to 20 ml at a time, every three to five minutes, until the blood volume is completely replaced twice (about 500 to 600 ml, depending on their birth weight). The baby is then closely monitored for several hours afterwards.

FAQs

SHOULD MY SON BE CIRCUMCISED?

You may be thinking of having your son circumcised. At this stage, there is no strong medical evidence to support the routine circumcision of baby boys. Circumcision rates in Australia are presently about 10% and the procedure is usually performed when the baby is 6 to 12 months old (earlier for some religions), with a local or general anaesthetic. Parents who choose to have their son circumcised do so for religious, cultural or personal reasons, including:
- Wanting their son to look like their father (although by the time the baby is a teenager most of his peers will not be circumcised).
- The belief that the circumcised penis looks nicer or cleaner and is

easier to look after. (Others see the uncircumcised penis as more natural and very easy to care for.)
- Possible health benefits and/or to prevent circumcision in later life for medical reasons.

The health benefits of routine circumcision are very small, and at this stage research indicates they do not outweigh the risks of routinely being circumcised.[7] The main issues are:
1. Preventing phimosis (not being able to pull the foreskin back) – This happens for 0.9% of uncircumcised boys by puberty. It is treated with steroid creams, but if unsuccessful, a circumcision may be recommended.
2. Reducing urine infections (occurring in 1% of boys) – These are treated with antibiotics. Circumcision may reduce the changes to 0.02%.[8]
3. Reducing inflammation of the head of the penis (balanitis), happening for 6% of uncircumcised boys and 3% of circumcised boys – This is treated with frequent nappy changes and bathing the penis in warm water. If it becomes severe, a steroid cream and/or a course of antibiotics may be prescribed.
4. Preventing cancer of the penis (rare: 0.00001%).
5. Reducing sexually transmitted infections (eg. HIV/AIDS) – Statistically, passing these infections on can be slightly reduced. However, only wearing a condom can provide full protection.

The main reasons parents choose **not** to circumcise include:
- It is not natural or necessary.
- It is genital mutilation, violating the baby's human rights. The child can choose to be circumcised as an adult.
- 1 to 5% of circumcisions lead to health complications, depending on the experience and skill of the surgeon and the type of anaesthetic used (eg. excessive bleeding, infection, damage to the penis or sepsis, which can be life-threatening).
- It is painful with no anaesthesia, or painful for days afterwards.
- An uncircumcised penis naturally lubricates during sexual foreplay to assist sexual penetration, and the foreskin keeps the area highly sensitive.

Care of the foreskin
Your son's foreskin is naturally adhered to the head of his penis from birth and cannot be pulled back. It does not require special care or cleaning.

Simply bathe your son normally and wash over the outside of his penis when his nappy is dirty. *Never* forcefully pull back his foreskin as this will hurt him and possibly cause bleeding and scarring. By the time he is three to five years old (sometimes older or younger), his foreskin will naturally separate, allowing him to pull it back. You can then start teaching him to gently pull back his foreskin and rinse the head of his penis in plain water (avoid soaps) in the bath or shower.

AT WHAT AGE CAN A NEWBORN TRAVEL BY PLANE?

There is no medical reason why a healthy newborn cannot fly, and domestic flights usually have no restrictions. However, some international airlines have policies that prevent babies less than 28 days old (ie. the neonatal period) from being passengers. Check with your airline.

If going overseas, your baby needs a passport (with a photo) and the application form requires a signature from both parents (if known). You may also need to look into vaccinations for your baby, depending on your intended destination. During the flight, the most important thing is to equalise the pressure in your baby's eardrums when taking off and landing. This is done by encouraging them to suckle (either by breastfeeding them or using a dummy, bottle or your finger). The airline may supply a cradle, or you may prefer to use your own portable bed. Ask for a seat near an exit door or in front of the movie screen, so you have space to put the bed on the floor. You will need to hold your baby during take-off and landing, or through turbulence. Remember to take plenty of nappies, changes of clothes, baby wipes, etc, although the airline may provide a baby kit with a few of these essentials. Good luck with nappy changing in the plane's toilet – not an easy task!

CHAPTER 13

The woman's recovery after birth

Physical recovery

From birth to six weeks is called the puerperium (*pew-pear-e-um*), during this time amazing physical changes and hormonal adjustments are taking place within the woman's body. (See Chapter 11 for recovery after a caesarean.)

Afterpains
The uterus contracts sporadically to control the bleeding, which can sometimes be strong and painful. These afterpains are experienced several times a day, for two days or more, usually when breastfeeding. Heat packs and deep breathing can help. Your caregiver may suggest an analgesic.

Uterus
The uterine muscles shrink and the uterus reduces from 1000 to 500 g within the first 7 days, and is 60 to 80 g by 6 weeks. Your caregiver feels the height of your uterus for the first few days to make sure it is shrinking well. It takes 10 to 14 days to shrink below the pubic bone, where it can no longer be felt.

Abdominal muscles
The abdominal muscles are initially weak and stretched, making the belly still look enlarged, soft and flabby, with the soft intestines behind it. As they regain tone and strength, the belly slowly decreases in size (this takes two to six weeks). The separated abdominal muscles take several weeks to knit back together. Gentle postnatal exercises help with this. Remember, it took nine months for your body to change and grow, and it takes time to heal and recover. Try not to place pressure on yourself to regain your

prepregnant body too quickly. Be realistic and ignore insensitive comments from others.

Stretch marks
Stretch marks usually reduce in size, fade and look more silvery, or pearly-white in colour. A few women notice they looked wrinkled when they lose weight, which can improve over time but never disappears altogether.

Linea nigra
This line up the middle of the belly initially looks much darker as the belly shrinks in size after giving birth, but it eventually fades by three to four months.

Bleeding
Bleeding after birth is called lochia and comes from the raw lining of the uterus, where the placenta was attached. It is initially quite heavy (changing sanitary pads every one to two hours, with small gushes when you get up) and sometimes small blood clots are passed (less than a golf ball size). As a guide:
- After one to two days, the bleeding settles to be more like a normal period.
- From 3 to 11 days, to 3 to 6 weeks, it is mainly pink or brown in colour, with bouts of bright bleeding on and off as the uterus shrinks and the placental site heals. Bright-coloured bleeding can also be triggered when you start doing more.

Eventually the vaginal discharge looks white or yellowish-brown, mixed with mucus. Women who breastfeed tend to lose less blood because breastfeeding stimulates uterine contractions.

While the bleeding continues, don't swim in public pools or the beach as this exposes your body to foreign bacteria. You can have a bath in your home. Some homeopaths recommend Arnica to help with bleeding. Herbalists may prescribe shepherd's purse, yarrow, raspberry leaf, nettle tea or cayenne powder. Check with your practitioner.

Vagina and bottom
The genitals can be very sore, swollen and bruised for a week or so, particularly when walking, but even sitting can be uncomfortable or painful. Try to:
- Walk slowly and avoid sudden movements.
- Begin pelvic floor exercises.
- Avoid doing too much, which can lead to heavy, aching, dragging and throbbing sensations.
- Use the softest toilet paper you can buy.
- Feed your baby lying on your side, or perhaps sit on a rubber ring.

NOTE: *Don't sit on rubber rings for hours on end. They inhibit blood flow and possibly increase swelling.*

Stitches

Stitches to the genitals take two weeks or so to heal and a couple of months to completely dissolve. They don't need extra care. Simply shower or bathe daily, then gently pat the area dry with a soft towel. Some women have regular sitz baths. You can add salt to the water if you like, but this has not been shown to have any benefits (nor do antiseptics or lavender oil).

Ice packs help with swelling and pain on the first day and perhaps mild analgesics.[1] Local anaesthetics may be prescribed (spray, gel, cream or foam), but avoid preparations with steroids as these inhibit wound healing and do more harm than good. Hair dryers, heat lamps and sun exposure are not recommended. These only dry out the skin and inhibit healing. Natural therapies include witch hazel on the sanitary napkin to cool and soothe, or a comfrey infusion sitz bath. See your practitioner.

NOTE: *If your stitches feel as though they are pulling, let your caregiver or local doctor know. One or two of them may be cut to release the tension. Stitches to the labia often need removing as they become itchy and irritating after a week or so.*

Urinating

Urinating large volumes in the early days is normal as the body eliminates excess fluids accumulated during pregnancy. Injured genitals can sting as urine passes over them. Your caregiver may provide powdered alkalinisers, which are mixed with water, to make the urine less likely to sting.

Bowel motions

The bowel naturally rests after labour, and most women don't need to open them for a few days (this is not constipation). Weakened pelvic floor muscles can make it difficult to have sufficient muscle tone to defecate when the time comes. To support these muscles, place a clean pad (or folded toilet paper) on the perineum, keeping your hand there while you open your bowels, providing counter-pressure. Pelvic floor exercises eventually strengthen these muscles and increase blood supply to the genitals to help with healing.

Sweating

It is normal to perspire excessively, especially as your milk comes in. A slightly raised temperature is normal during the early recovery period. However, a fever above 38°C may indicate an infection.

NUTRITION AND GOOD HEALTH

It is important to look after yourself physically, so you can cope emotionally and care for your baby. To maintain your strength and energy levels, try to have regular nutritious meals with plenty of fresh fruits and vegetables, calcium and proteins, and adequate carbohydrates. Drink at least eight glasses of water a day. If your diet is balanced, you shouldn't need vitamin supplements, although some women take zinc to help recovery. If you experienced excessive blood loss, your caregiver may recommend iron supplements for 6 to 12 weeks.

Breastfeeding often makes you feel ravenous, but there is no need to eat for two. If breastfeeding multiples, you may need to eat a little extra to what you are used to. Just make sure it is nutritious. There is no food or drink that increases breast milk supply. There is a myth that stout (beer) does this; which is not true, and drinking alcohol can be harmful for your breastfeeding baby. Generally you don't need to avoid particular foods when breastfeeding, but try not to overeat a specific food that may not agree with your baby.

It is important not to diet while breastfeeding, but even if you are bottle feeding, don't diet for at least six weeks until you recover and have adjusted to the demands of early parenting. Women who breastfeed do tend to lose weight more rapidly than women who bottle feed, because breast milk is high in calories and draws on your fat stores.

EXERCISE

Recovering after childbirth involves strengthening weakened muscles with gentle toning and stretching exercises. These can also help you release tension and give you time out from the demands of caring for a newborn. Rigorous exercise to lose weight or get fit is not appropriate until at least six weeks after the birth. Swimming and aqua aerobics should be delayed until you stop bleeding. Remember to start (or resume) your exercise program slowly, and be aware that demanding fitness regimes can decrease your breast milk supply.

Postnatal exercises focus on stability training to strengthen the abdomen and minimise pelvic discomfort and lower back pain. Even simple posture awareness, like walking and sitting tall, helps with this. Upper back exercises can also help when holding and caring for a new baby. Most women can start postnatal exercises within days and many hospitals run physiotherapy classes (or you may prefer postnatal yoga). If you are recovering from a caesarean or are unwell, you may need to delay exercise for a while. Check with your caregiver. Increasingly, postnatal exercise classes offer childcare facilities or teach exercises that include the baby in the class.

Abdominal exercises

To strengthen abdominal muscles, you need to compress or tense them. Stomach compressions are done by standing or sitting straight, or lying on a supportive comfortable surface, with your knees bent (slightly touching) and both feet flat on the floor (your lower back maintaining a natural curve). Pull your tummy in, imagine you are drawing your navel in towards your backbone, while relaxing the rest of your body. Hold for about five seconds, while slowly breathing in and out. Don't hold your breath. Then relax. Try doing five repetitions, relaxing your abdominal muscles in between. You can slowly increase your stomach strength by extending the length of time you hold each compression.

Side reaches and abdominal rotations

To strengthen your oblique abdominal muscles, down each side of your body, lie on your back on the floor with your knees bent and arms beside your body. Take a breath in, then breathe out, performing a stomach compression and tilting your pelvis towards your belly (by flattening the small of your lower back on the floor). As you breathe out, reach down with one hand towards your heel or foot on the same side. Only stretch to where it feels comfortable (you will need to lift your head a little). Breathe in and slowly return to your resting position. Repeat this on the opposite side. Try two to four repetitions in two to three lots, alternating sides and relaxing in between.

Pelvic tilts

You can do pelvic tilts while leaning your back against a wall, feet slightly apart and knees slightly bent, or lying on your back on the floor with knees bent and feet on the floor. Perform a stomach compression and slowly breathe in and out, then lift your hips off the floor (or away from the wall) towards your belly. Your shoulders should stay on the floor or wall. Pull up your pelvic floor muscles, and squeeze your buttocks, holding for about five seconds, then relax. Try six to eight repetitions.

Middle and upper back stretches

Upper back stretches can be done while on a bench or the edge of a chair, so your back is not leaning on anything. Keep your breathing and body relaxed, your back straight and rest your hands on your legs, close to your knees.

1. Compress your stomach muscles and do a pelvic tilt in a sitting position, keeping your hands on your knees. Hold this stretch, taking a few breaths, and then relax. Repeat four to six times.

2. To increase the stretch, slump your shoulders slightly towards your knees. Slide your hands forwards over (or under) your knees, while compressing your stomach muscles and doing a pelvic tilt. Hold this for a few breaths and then relax. Repeat four to six times.
3. Try sitting with your knees slightly apart and reach with both hands to hold one knee. Pull yourself gently away from this knee, while compressing your stomach muscles and doing a pelvic tilt. Hold for a few breaths before relaxing. Repeat this on the other knee. Repeat about four times on each side.

To quickly give your arms and shoulders a stretch after holding your baby, sit or stand comfortably with your knees slightly apart. Join your hands (interlocking the fingers with palms facing out) and straighten your arms out in front of you, in line with your shoulders. Look down to gently stretch your neck. Perform a stomach compression and pelvic tilt to increase the stretch. Hold for a few breaths before relaxing. Repeat if you want to.

Angry cat exercise

Kneel on all fours on the floor. Breathe normally. On your out breath, arch your back by rounding your spine upwards (with your head down), compressing your stomach muscles and doing a pelvic tilt. Try to keep breathing at a comfortable pace. Hold this for a few seconds then relax, but bring your back into straight alignment (don't let it sag). Repeat four to six times.

Feeding your baby

BREASTFEEDING

The early days of breastfeeding are a dynamic settling-in period. It is a vulnerable, demanding time as you learn, practise and experiment with feeding. Be patient with yourself (and your baby). This transitional period *does* eventually change, and breastfeeding becomes second nature.

First two days

The breasts remain soft, similar to the way they were during pregnancy. Some babies are sleepy and don't feed frequently, but others are fussy and unsettled until the mature milk replaces the rich colostrum. During this time:
- Rest and recuperate as much as possible. Feed your baby whenever they seem interested.

- 'Emptying' the breasts and feeding from both sides are not issues yet. It is just a case of stimulating both breasts through regular feeding, while learning the art of latching your baby onto the breast.
- Try to latch your baby without assistance as much as possible. If it feels painful, take them off the nipple by placing your finger in their mouth and pushing their gum down. You may need to do this several times each feed in the early days. If you are continuing to struggle, ask the midwife for assistance.
- If your baby is impatient, frustrated or upset, try cuddling them or gently placing your little finger in their mouth to suck for a minute until they calm down, before latching them.

Days two to five

Colostrum changes to transitional milk, which looks more watery, around two to three days (up to five days) after the birth. The breasts start to fill, feeling firmer, and the baby may be more interested in feeding (or more relaxed if previously unsettled). Their meconium bowel motions become brownish in colour.

You need to become conscious of draining both breasts now. If feeding from one breast at each feed, then alternate (left breast for one feed, right breast for the next). If feeding from both breasts at one feed, use the second breast as a top-up and start with this breast for the next feed, to ensure both are fully drained. Babies always empty the first breast best.

If your baby is feeding every hour or so, just keep moving from one breast to the other. Some babies seem to prefer one breast, but the more you feed from one breast, the more milk it produces and the less milk the other breast produces. This may encourage your baby to refuse the non-preferred breast, making it difficult to balance feeds. If you think this is happening, try feeding from the other side more frequently, offering this breast first. Usually within a day or so the supply equalises. It is possible to feed exclusively from one breast; however, you need to tolerate being lopsided in breast size.

> **Did you know?**
> Breasts can have different flow speeds. For example, one breast may take the baby 5 minutes to drain, while the other takes 20 minutes.

During this transition period:
- Be patient if the feeding now feels uncomfortable. This improves in a few days.
- Persevere with latching your baby on correctly to avoid damaging the nipples. However, your nipples may still be sensitive, tender and sore for a few days as they adjust.

- Take your baby off the breast if they fall asleep, in case they slip off the nipple and munch on the end. Take care when feeding at night and dozing while your baby feeds.

While there are no time limits on breastfeeding, babies will empty the breast within 5 to 40 minutes.

Milk coming in

By three to five days the mature milk comes in. The breasts enlarge, feeling heavy, firm, full and warm and possibly looking flushed. This is temporary and mainly due to increased blood and lymph supply, making it difficult to judge whether the breasts are drained after feeding. A few women leak milk between feeds, or one breast leaks while they are feeding from the other. You can place a cloth under the leaking breast or wear breast pads inside your bra.

It is crucial to feed your baby on demand now; this keeps the milk flowing and avoids painful breast engorgement. Most babies are quite unsettled, wanting to feed every one to three hours, and sleep less. A few babies cough, splutter or gag if the milk comes too quickly, which is normal. They usually deal with this and continue to feed, but if your baby pulls off the breast, sit them up until they seem okay, then relatch them to finish the feed.

Mature milk looks watery and white at the beginning of the feed (called fore milk). This is your baby's thirst quencher. It then becomes richer, looking whiter or yellowish (called hind-milk) and is high in fat and calories, helping your baby to settle for longer periods between feeds. Babies often drink more than they need at this time, vomiting excess milk while their stomach adjusts to the larger volumes. They also poo frequently and their motions now look yellow, curdy and watery.

While your milk is coming in, remember:
- This often coincides with the teary third-day blues, so try to limit (or ban) visitors for 24 to 48 hours.
- Your nipples can feel very tender as your baby attaches, but this should ease within a few seconds and tends to improve after a couple of days. To soften the areola, and to help your baby fully grasp the nipple (and feel more comfortable when they do), try gently massaging it, or hand express a few drops of milk before latching.
- You can start to wear maternity bras for support or comfort. A few women prefer to leave their bra off and sleep on a towel to catch leaking milk.

Let-down reflex

The let-down reflex is a natural response to your baby's suckling. Oxytocin is released from the brain, causing muscle fibres in the breasts to contract, forcefully pushing milk down and out of the nipples for a minute or so. A let-down usually happens one to two minutes after the baby starts feeding (or you start expressing) and can happen unpredictably at other times when looking at (or thinking about) your baby, hearing a baby cry, or your nipples rub up against something.

Not all women feel their let-down, but some describe it as a tingling, sharp, warm or contraction-like sensation in their breasts (usually apparent after a week or two). The best way to tell whether you are having a let-down is by observing your baby feeding. As the milk flows more rapidly, their sucking pattern changes from being short and frequent to long, deep gulping actions. Milk may also leak from your other breast. It is possible to have multiple let-downs, two to three times during a feed.

The let-down reflex is an important component of ongoing, successful breastfeeding. If it doesn't occur, the baby feeds for longer and/or more frequently, and the milk supply gradually reduces over time. A let-down can be inhibited if you are not feeling relaxed, are stressed or embarrassed, or finding feeding difficult or painful. Sometimes deep breathing, conscious shoulder relaxation and/or listening to a visualisation can help you let go after latching. Another technique is as follows:

- Sit in a quiet place to feed (or express) and make sure you have privacy.
- Then gently massage one bare breast for a minute or so, and use your fingertips to lightly stroke from the top of the breast, down to your nipple, slowly and repeatedly.
- You may already have your baby on the breast, or choose to allow them on once you are more relaxed or the milk starts flowing. You can also do this to the opposite breast while feeding.

Day five to two weeks

The mature milk supply establishes and the breasts soften and return to their pregnancy size. It is now easier to tell when they are full or empty, and latching is often more effortless and the nipples are generally comfortable (unless damaged by the baby not attaching properly).

The baby becomes more settled, feeding less frequently (two to five hours or more) and they usually become more efficient at emptying the breast, making feeds comparatively shorter. Their poos are a bright yellow mustard colour, with watery curds. It is normal for breastfed babies to poo 10 times a day, or once every 10 days, and anything in between!

Beyond two to four weeks

Most women settle into a comfortable pattern of enjoyable feeding. Some find their breasts change even more at 6 to 12 weeks, feeling softer or smaller without that full feeling. You might not leak milk frequently, unless experiencing a let-down. These are normal physical signs and *not* indications you are losing your milk.

To tell whether your baby is getting enough milk, they should:
- Have at least 6 wet nappies over a 24-hour period.
- Look bright-eyed and active when awake, not lethargic and disinterested in feeding.
- Have a consistent increase in their weight gain from 10 to 14 days after birth (babies normally lose up to 10% of their weight during the first week, before regaining it).

Breastfeeding twins or more

Breastfeeding twins and triplets is recommended and certainly possible – your breast milk supply always equals your babies' needs, you simply produce more milk. However, you need plenty of emotional and practical support to look after yourself, so you can breastfeed more than one baby.

Twins (or triplets) are individuals and drink different amounts at different speeds and at different times. However, many women try to coax their multiples into similar feeding and sleeping patterns so they become synchronised. The simplest way to breastfeed twins is offer each baby one breast per feeding time (simultaneously, or at separate times), but they should swap breasts at alternate feeds to:
- Vary their visual stimulation.
- Avoid making your breasts lopsided, if one twin is smaller and needs less milk.
- Prevent the babies from getting used to their side, and refusing to feed from the other, in case you develop blocked milk ducts (and need two babies to fully drain one side), or one baby weans earlier than the other.

Feeding simultaneously can save time. You can use the football hold supported by pillows, or lay the babies crossed over in front of you. Otherwise feed them separately, or feed one baby half a feed, then feed the second baby half their feed, then go back to the first baby to finish off the feed, and so on. In the end it is just a case of working out what is convenient and most enjoyable for you all.

When breastfeeding triplets there is the numerical dilemma of three babies and only two breasts! This is usually accommodated by rotating the babies to allow each one an equal time at the breast (depending on who is crying the loudest). You may want to keep a written record of when and how long each baby feeds, and from which breast they fed. But if they all appear happy, this is probably not necessary.

Physical changes when breastfeeding

Breastfeeding hormones bring about many unique physical changes, which generally disappear once you stop feeding:

- **Delay in menstrual periods** – Many women don't experience periods until their baby is fully weaned off the breast. Others start menstruating once their baby starts solid foods or they supplement with formula milk. A few women experience light periods of pink or light red bleeding every now and then (this can also be a side effect of the minipill, or progesterone injections for contraception). Occasionally periods return as normal each month, even though the woman is fully breastfeeding.
- **Decrease in vaginal lubrication** – Most breastfeeding women need to use some form of water-based lubricant when they have sex. This generally returns to normal once you stop feeding.
- **Hair loss** – Alopecia is usually mild but can occasionally be substantial, the hair coming away in clumps and causing small patches of temporary baldness. This sheds the 'extra' hair grown during pregnancy and new hair grows back once the breastfeeding stops. A few women use natural therapies (creams or oils, such as jojoba) or homeopathic remedies.
- **Allergies and sensitivities** – Some women become allergic, or more sensitive, to certain substances or foods while breastfeeding. On the other hand, allergy specialists notice certain women with allergies experience a remission or improvement during their pregnancy and while breastfeeding.
- **Breastfeeding haze** – The regular release of oxytocin and endorphins from the brain during breastfeeding helps you naturally relax and slow your pace. Many women look back at this time and realise how dreamy and hazy they felt.

Emotional considerations

The breastfeeding experience may be as wonderful as you imagined, or not match your expectations at all, especially if it becomes an ongoing struggle. You may feel ambivalent about how intense and demanding it is, or privileged to have an exclusive bond with your baby. Some women feel tied to their baby, with no escape because it is such an effort to express milk in order to have time away from their baby. Others feel proud of their ability to breastfeed and are gratified to see their baby thriving thanks to their efforts alone. It is important to acknowledge how you feel and be supported by those around you.

BOTTLE FEEDING

When formula feeding from birth, you still initially produce breast milk, triggered by hormonal changes. Once your body realises there is neither the demand nor the stimulation, milk production slowly decreases and finally stops, being reabsorbed into the body.

The breasts feel soft to touch for a few days, then become engorged three to five days after the birth, feeling uncomfortable, hot, hard, lumpy and sore. This usually lasts for 2 to 5 days before improving and feeling normal by 10 to 14 days (sometimes longer). Some doctors prescribe drugs to suppress milk supply, but these can lead to unwanted side effects and rebound lactation, where the milk comes back in once the medication is stopped.[2] In most circumstances women are advised to suppress their milk naturally. Strategies to help with breast pain include:

- Wearing a well-fitting bra and breast pads day and night.
- Using cold (or frozen) compresses for 10 minutes every half hour (when awake).
- Avoiding hot water on the breasts while showering.
- Not expressing milk, although hand expressing a few drops for comfort is okay. Do this as little as possible.

Your caregiver may recommend a mild analgesic (such as paracetamol). Homeopaths may suggest Lac caninum or Pulsatilla. Herbalists may prescribe parsley and sage. Aromatherapists may suggest a few drops of clary sage oil, mixed with a carrier oil (such as almond), and massaging this into the breasts. Do a small skin test first to make sure you are not allergic.

Did you know?

In the past, caregivers recommended cooled, white cabbage leaves on the breasts. However, recent research indicates their effects are similar to those of cool packs.[3]

How much formula milk?

Newborn babies generally feed 5 to 8 times in 24 hours. In the first few days they drink about 35 ml per feed. This is worked out as 60 ml per kilogram of body weight every 24 hours. For a 3.5 kg baby:

3.5×60 ml $= 210$ ml, divided by 6 feeds $= 35$ ml per feed

After:
- 2 to 3 days this increases to 50 ml per feed (90 ml/kg in 24 hours).
- 4 to 5 days it is 70 ml per feed (120 ml per kg).
- 7 to 9 days it is 90 ml per feed (150 ml per kg).

Babies usually stay on 90 ml per kilogram over 24 hours until 3 to 4 months. So as their weight increases, so too does their milk requirements.

NOTE: *These amounts are only a guide. Bottle fed babies (like breastfed babies) drink variable amounts each feed, so only give your baby what they need and don't be concerned if they don't finish every bottle.* **Never** *keep leftover milk for the next feed.* **Always** *give a fresh bottle and discard after one hour.*

Your baby and bottle feeding

Bottle fed babies should be fed on demand and will wake frequently for nourishment because their stomachs only tolerate small, regular feeds. By the time they are 8 to 12 weeks old, they tend to move into a more adult-friendly sleep pattern. Some babies drink their bottle quickly (5 to 15 minutes), others take up to 30 to 40 minutes, perhaps occasionally pulling off the teat to rest. If the milk flow is too fast, they may want to suck more afterwards to feel content. If it is too slow, they may tire before finishing the feed, possibly waking again soon.

It is very important to cuddle your baby close, have eye contact and talk with them while feeding. This helps them grow and develop, as well as being emotionally rewarding for you. You may want to feed your baby against your naked skin at times, to have skin-to-skin contact.

NOTE: *Never feed your baby with the bottle 'propped up' on a pillow unsupervised. They can gag or choke on milk, and it increases their chances of developing ear infections. It also deprives your baby of physical interaction with you.*

The bowel motions of bottle fed babies are similar in consistency to plasticine or playdough, ranging from khaki green to yellow or brown in colour. Many babies initially become constipated until their body adjusts to formula. Constipation has more to do with the consistency of the bowel motion (than with how often they go). If it is dry and hard, or comes away in small pebbles, they are probably constipated. If your baby becomes distressed with this, you may need to see your local doctor.

Preparing formula

If your baby has formula from birth, hospital staff should show you how to prepare it. If starting formula after going home, preparing it can seem quite daunting. However, once you get into a routine, it should be quick and easy.

Tinned formula comes in a powdered form. Check the use-by date on the bottom. Once opened, it needs to be used within one month. Some parents make each bottle as they need it. Others make six to eight bottles at a time. Premade formula needs to be refrigerated until used, and lasts 24 hours, then needs to be discarded if the baby does not drink it within this time.

Formula needs to be prepared in a hygienic way. Sterilise all your equipment, bottles and teats, clean the benchtops and put food away.

1. Wash your hands. Boil the amount of water you need and put it aside to cool until lukewarm. (If unsure about the quality of the water, boil for 10 minutes.)
2. Put presterilised bottles on the clean bench and fill each one with the required amount of lukewarm boiled water. You may prefer to fill a large sterilised plastic measuring jug to make a batch and then pour it into the bottles.
3. Follow the directions on the formula tin and use the special scoop provided. Scoop up the powder and gently tap it on the inside of the tin to take out any air pockets. Then run a sterilised blunt knife over the top rim of the scoop to level off the measure.
4. Place each scoop in the lukewarm water. Avoid distractions when counting the scoops. Perhaps write the number on a piece of paper in case you are interrupted and lose count. It is usually better to make up a little more milk rather than to try to measure half-scoops. The powder will not mix properly if the water is too hot or cold. Always put the lukewarm water in first and the powder in second.
5. Shake the bottles or use a sterile fork or whisk in the jug to dissolve all the powder and mix it in well.

NOTE: *It is important that the correct measure of powder is added to the correct amount of water. If you don't understand the instructions, check with another person, your early childhood nurse or pharmacist.*

- Never pack the formula into the scoop.
- Never add extra scoops to make it richer. This constipates and dehydrates the baby, making them sick.
- Never dilute or water down, the formula. This makes the baby sick and vomit and not put on weight.

Store premade bottles (or the jug) in the main part of the fridge (not the fridge door) and use within 24 hours. Jugs need a lid, or to be covered with plastic wrap or foil, and the mixed formula needs stirring before being poured into each bottle, as it can settle to the bottom. You can use a sterilised, plastic funnel to help with pouring. The jug needs to be resterilised before making up the next batch. If out and about you can:

- Take a thermos of lukewarm boiled water and a separate sterile container with pre-measured formula powder, mixing bottles when needed.
- Take premade bottles of formula that are already refrigerated (cold) and transport them in an insulated cooler (keeping for up to six hours). If going to someone else's house, place the bottle in their fridge when you get there.

Heating bottles

Formula milk only needs to be lukewarm and is best heated by placing the bottle in a jug or saucepan of warm to hot water (not boiling). After several minutes shake the bottle to mix the heated milk through. **Always** test the temperature by dripping some milk on the inside of your arm before giving it to your baby.

If you buy a special bottle warmer, follow the manufacturer's instructions and don't leave bottles in them for prolonged periods (30 minutes or more). If you can't heat your bottle, just give it as is. Most babies are not concerned by the temperature, especially in the summer months.

NOTE: *Microwaving formula makes it less nutritional and heats it unevenly, possibly burning the baby's mouth if you do not shake it and test it on your arm first. If you do use a microwave occasionally, take the lid off the bottle before heating.*

Bottle feeding twins or more

When bottle feeding multiples, the following tips may make the process easier:
- Make a large batch of formula and prepare all your bottles at once. Some women carefully scoop the required amount into a jug, and then use a permanent marker to show how much. Of course, this needs to be adjusted as the babies grow and they need more formula.
- If one baby has a slow teat and the other a fast teat, cut a small piece off the rim of one to easily tell them apart.
- If both babies are awake and crying, feed the one who is screaming the loudest first, or sit both in bouncer chairs in front of you, holding a bottle in each hand. Take care not to strain your back. Interact with them to give them mental stimulation.

Try to hold your babies as much as possible when feeding. You might like to try sitting cross-legged on the floor, with you back supported against a lounge or wall, and placing each baby with their head resting on the inside of your bent knees, with pillows around.

Emotional considerations

Choosing to bottle feed can be an easy, clear-cut decision, or it may come about because breastfeeding didn't work out, for whatever reason. It can be

very disappointing to stop breastfeeding before you feel ready, often impacting on your self-esteem and fragile beginnings as a new mother. Emotional reactions can be:
- A great sense of failure or inadequacy as a woman, or that you are not a good mother.
- Sadness, shame and guilt, especially if others question why you have 'chosen' to formula feed.
- Feeling you are not able to bond as well with your baby (although there are many other ways to establish an intimate relationship).
- Relief. Breastfeeding was a struggle and now an end is in sight.

Give yourself time to grieve. Perhaps share your feelings with someone you trust. Dealing with the opinions and comments of others can also be hard, and some women feel alienated, unaccepted and unsupported.

NOTE: *Once the change is made to bottle feeding, it is very difficult to re-establish breastfeeding. Some women feel regret for not giving breastfeeding more of a chance, or perhaps for not sourcing professionals to help them resolve their problems.*

STERILISING FEEDING/EXPRESSING EQUIPMENT

Bottles, teats, breast pumps and formula preparation equipment need to be sterilised. Before sterilising, everything needs to be cleaned to remove any milk.
- Soon after feeding, discard unused milk and rinse the bottle, teat and cap in cold water. Do the same with breast milk pumps or formula preparation equipment.
- Scrub everything with warm to hot soapy water, using a bottle brush to clean inside bottles and teats (or turning teats inside out) and squirting water through the teat holes.
- Rinse thoroughly in cold water so they are ready for sterilising.

Sterilised equipment can be used straight away, or placed in a clean, covered plastic container and stored in the fridge for up to 24 hours. Some parents just cap the bottles and store separately. After 24 hours, unused equipment needs resterilising.

Boiling

You need a large saucepan with a lid, which should be kept exclusively for sterilising. If you do cook in it, make sure it is cleaned thoroughly. Check that jugs, funnels and stirring implements can be boiled (baby feeding and expressing equipment is designed to tolerate boiling). Take care when boiling water around children.

1. Place all your equipment (except teats or dummies) into a saucepan of clean, cold water. Fill the bottles with water and submerge them sideways. The water should be deep enough to cover the equipment.
2. Bring the water to the boil with the lid on and continue boiling for another seven minutes. Add teats and dummies and boil everything for another two to three minutes.
3. After a total of 10 minutes boiling, remove the saucepan from the heat and allow everything to cool with the lid on (or saucepan covered).
4. When the water has cooled, wash your hands and remove the equipment.

Cold sterilisation

Cold or chemical sterilisation uses antibacterial solutions (or tablets) added to water. You can also buy special plastic soaking containers, with lids and grids to keep everything submerged, or you can make up something similar yourself. Parents of multiples often use a large bucket with a lid (used only for this), rather than multiple small containers.

The sterilising solution is replaced every 24 hours and the container is cleaned with warm soapy water and rinsed before making a fresh solution. Metal utensils cannot be cold sterilised because they corrode. A plastic knife and fork for formula preparation is recommended.

1. Wash your hands. Follow the manufacturer's instructions for making up the solution.
2. Place the cleaned, rinsed equipment into the solution. Fill bottles to remove large air bubbles (don't worry about tiny ones) and squeeze the solution through teat holes.
3. Keep the sterilising container out of direct sunlight and allow the equipment to soak, undisturbed, for at least one hour.
4. Wash your hands before removing any equipment. Shake the solution off but *don't* rinse, otherwise it needs to be sterilised again.

NOTE: *If you remove or add any equipment, everything in the container is no longer sterile and you need to wait another hour without disturbing the solution.*

Steam sterilisers

Steam sterilisers are quite expensive, but quick and easy, taking 10 minutes or so. Electric sterilisers are generally automatic, switching themselves off when the process is completed. Microwave sterilisers heat water to sterilise. Always follow the manufacturer's instructions.

Emotional changes and support strategies

New mothers experience a range of emotions that stem from hormonal changes, as well as the sheer physical, emotional and spiritual experience of giving birth. This is mixed with feelings about mothering and influenced by how much practical and emotional support is forthcoming. Fathers also experience a range of emotions as they integrate the birth, support the woman and start their parenting.

From days one to three, you may be feeling:
- Surreal, cocooned in your own world, with everything in slow motion.
- Euphoric, floating on an amazing high and unable to sleep.
- Numb and exhausted. Aware of the baby but feeling removed.
- The labour scenario is playing over in your mind. Needing to retell your story.
- In awe of your beautiful creation.
- Disbelieving: *Is this baby really mine?*
- Pride in yourself, or invincible for getting through the labour.
- Shocked and traumatised if the experience was negative.
- Lonely when your partner leaves (or when leaving your partner and baby behind).
- Missing your other child(ren). Worried how they are coping.
- Relieved that you and your baby are well, or scared and anxious if either of you are unwell.
- Confused and unsure about mothering and feeding. Upset if your baby is not behaving the way you expected.

From days three to five, you may be feeling:
- More aware of what is going on in the outside world.
- Suddenly exhausted, overwhelmed and teary.
- Tender, vulnerable, irritable and sensitive. Upset if feeding is not going smoothly or your baby is unsettled.
- The significance of parenting is exciting and/or daunting.
- That visitors are more of a hindrance than a help. Just wanting to go home.

From days five to seven, you may be feeling:
- Relief. Happy to be home.
- Frightened, anxious or lost without the reassurance of staff on call.

- Unsure: *Am I doing this right?* Worried when your baby is unsettled or cries for long periods.
- Confident and happy to be doing things your way now.
- Tired and exhausted, still recovering.
- Overwhelmed with taking on the domestic role again.
- Worried about your other child(ren). Guilty, if you don't have enough time for them.

From days seven to fourteen, you may be feeling:
- Comfortable as you become more in tune with your baby's needs.
- Wanting to brave the outside world.
- Still very tired and exhausted. Just wanting to sleep.
- Out of your depth. Continually thinking, *Am I a good mother (or father)?*
- Sad, disappointed and/or isolated if there is little support, especially if your partner returns to work; as the partner, feeling you don't want to return to work, or happy to walk out the door!

The blues

The blues are experienced by up to 80% of women, usually around 3 to 5 days after the birth, lasting for a day or two, and generally coinciding with the milk coming in and tiredness catching up. The blues may manifest as:
- Feeling sensitive, irritable, shaky and teary. Finding it hard to understand or describe why you are feeling this way.
- Tears flowing, yet actually feeling okay.
- Feeling like nothing is going right, advice is conflicting and/or support is not forthcoming.

Some women quietly move through their emotions. Others have outpourings of emotion, or sudden mood swings. A few don't notice the blues at all. It is important for family and friends to be understanding and supportive so you don't lose your confidence. Partners can also feel upset and helpless if they don't know how to respond. Generally, just being there, giving her a cuddle and realising it is normal is all that is needed. It may also be a good idea to restrict visitors and to concentrate on your baby and resting and eating well until you are back on track.

SUPPORT DURING THE EARLY WEEKS

Emotional and physical support needs continue for several weeks as you heal and adjust to mothering. Some people create a babymoon (like a honeymoon) by taking time out to celebrate and rest for one to two weeks. This is often a special time of discovery, intimacy, sharing and relationship building with this new person, as well as delaying going back to normal.

Woman's self-support

Your body is still recuperating and producing breast milk (if you are breastfeeding). Care is needed when moving around, and energy levels may be low until the baby is in a more predictable feeding and sleeping pattern (six to eight weeks). So take it easy.

Slowly increase your physical activity. Avoid attempting too much too soon. Even if you think you have bounced back quickly, don't underestimate the enormous experience your body has been through. Efforts to do it all may only end up physically draining you or manifesting as heavier bleeding, pain, heavy sensations in the perineum and anus, and possibly developing mastitis. Plan to spend the first couple of weeks mostly at home.

Realistic expectations: If this is your first baby, your thoughts and expectations may be influenced by what you have experienced in your own family, or based on fantasy images portrayed by the media. This is where the woman raises a family, runs a successful business, has a spotless house and looks effortlessly gorgeous all the time! However, this is far from the reality of changing dirty nappies and sorting through how differently both you and your partner are parenting.

Try not to place pressure on yourself to be the perfect mother by getting it right all the time. Negotiating the early weeks means learning many new things at once, which can be both exciting and nerve-racking. However, it takes time for you and your baby to learn about each other. The more you do, the more comfortable and confident you will become. Bear in mind that newborn babies are pretty durable and it takes a lot for them to notice anything is amiss, and don't forget to acknowledge the fantastic job you are doing.

Rest and recovery: Many mothers cry from exhaustion at various times in the early weeks, feeling helpless and frustrated because the responsibility always stops with them. Limit domestic duties to a bare minimum. Sleep when your baby sleeps and get others to take your baby out occasionally so you can fall into a deep sleep (albeit possibly a short one) because you don't feel on call. Turn the phone off and leave a 'Do not disturb' note on the front door. Avoid open house and ask visitors to ring first. Get help with your other children, especially for pick-ups and drop-offs at childcare or school.

Communication is important. Some women find it easy to ask for help, or it may be forthcoming without them requesting it. However, if you find it difficult to ask people to help you out, you may be left doing everything because you unintentionally give out the vibe 'I am doing fine'. Be aware of how you respond to offers of help. Most family and friends want to help but feel unsure of what you need or want, so let them know. Many women grieve the loss of their belly and all the attention that went with this. It may even feel as though you are invisible and the baby is now the most important person. To help with your emotional needs, try:

- Sharing your feelings, even if they seem wrong or unmotherly, overwhelming or frightening. It is important to let others know.
- Journaling your present experiences.
- Accepting that your lifestyle changes are a temporary but necessary part of having a baby.
- Doing something for yourself every day – a positive thought, a long shower, a massage or just time out.
- Creating some space to sit with your feelings and allowing them to surface; crying may be enough to release them.

Strategies for partner, family and friends

New mothers continue to need emotional and physical support. Partners also need to balance their own needs, so discuss how you can both enjoy this time as well as recover, care for the baby and run the household. If possible, try to have time off work when she comes home, or work half-days. Encourage family and friends to pitch in and lighten the load.

Her physical needs will depend on how the birth unfolded, how the feeding is going and how demanding the baby is. Practical support can include:

- Lifting and carrying heavy objects so she doesn't strain her back.
- Being conscious that entertaining visitors can be draining, perhaps making it necessary to restrict (or stop them) or make space for her to go into the bedroom to sleep or breastfeed.
- If family and friends offer help, take it. Perhaps allocate jobs around the house or the care of your other children.
- Make sure she eats nutritiously. If you are returning to work, have plenty of quick, easy snacks in the house and don't expect dinner on the table when you get home.

Many women worry about taking on the domestic role again, on top of having a new baby. While you may not expect her to do anything, she can put pressure on herself to 'return to duties' as soon as she is home. Remind her to slow down or stop.

Her emotional needs can fluctuate; she may feel confident at times, unsure at others. You might also experience this as you become involved in your baby's care. Providing meaningful support can often be challenging, especially if your partner can't explain why she is feeling the way she is. Holding her when she cries can help her feel you are connecting with her. Talking about how you are both feeling keeps communication open. Reassure her that she is doing well and the baby is fine (as is usually the case). Be patient with each other as you learn the ropes.

If your partner is breastfeeding, positive emotional support is essential, even if the feeding is proving difficult. From a practical perspective, working as a team, in caring for the baby and keeping the household running, supports her breastfeeding. Other strategies include:
- Making time and space for her to share her feelings. Listen, and try not to feel you always have to fix the problem.
- Nurturing her to help her feel good about herself.

Relationship survival tips and other support strategies are covered in Chapter 14.

Expectations for care

If the birth has been in a hospital, most women go home with their baby around three to five days after a vaginal delivery, and up to six to seven days after a caesarean. If either you or the baby are unwell or develop complications, this may be extended. The midwives and mothercraft nurses provide guidance about caring for your baby and assistance with feeding. Some women rely on hospital staff frequently. Others prefer to do their own thing.

If you have opted for early discharge (going home within 4 to 24 hours after the birth), the midwife visits you at home daily or every other day, for an hour or so, depending on your needs and the service offered in your local area. Visits continue for 5 to 7 days after a vaginal birth and up to 6 to 10 days after a caesarean. Mother and baby are checked, your questions are answered, and help is given with feeding and baby care. The midwife should let you know what to expect in the following 24 hours and be on call by phone for urgent advice. If there are health concerns for you or your baby, they organise for you to go to back to the hospital.

If the birth has been at home the midwife generally visits daily for 7 to 10 days or more or every other day, depending on the service they provide and how you and your baby are doing, carrying out similar care as for early discharge. They are available by phone (or to visit if necessary) in between, and up until the six to eight week postnatal check.

If you are not immune to rubella, you will probably be offered a routine vaccination just before being discharged from hospital (or during a home visit). This aims to provide immunity for any future pregnancies, as well as reducing the incidence of rubella in the community.

Home alone

The reality of life with your new baby may only sink in when driving home or stepping through the front door. It can also take your baby a while to adjust as they settle into their new surroundings. So be prepared for them to be a little out of sorts for a day or so.

It can be hard to leave the constant support of professionals and you will need to start sourcing various community services, depending on what is available locally. These can include your GP, early childhood or baby health centre, mothers' or parents' groups, postnatal exercise or yoga classes, 24-hour telephone counselling services and volunteer support groups, especially for breastfeeding, postnatal depression and caring for multiple babies or babies with special needs. You may also be able to access live-in parenting services. Your caregiver should provide contact details for these before you go home, otherwise see our support resources at the end of this book.

YOUR SIX TO EIGHT WEEK POSTNATAL CHECK

A routine postnatal check is offered around six to eight weeks after the birth to check your physical recovery and how you are coping emotionally. This visit is not compulsory but many women find it beneficial. If you experienced health conditions during the pregnancy (for example, diabetes or high blood pressure), a postnatal check is advisable to make sure the condition has stabilised. This may also involve making another appointment with a specialist.

Many professionals can perform a postnatal check, including private obstetricians, midwives, maternity hospital clinics, some birth centres, your local doctor, family planning or women's health services. Your choice will depend on who cared for you during the pregnancy, what is convenient and your own preferences.

Postnatal checks take 30 to 45 minutes, depending on your needs and what you want to discuss. Many women take their new baby, but it may be handy to take someone else to mind them while you have your physical examination. Write a list of any questions you have. Things that may be discussed include:
- The details of your labour, birth and recovery.
- Your general physical and emotional health – are you getting enough support?

- Diet and exercise.
- Your bleeding since the birth, and whether you are opening your bowels and passing urine normally.
- How you are feeding your baby and any difficulties you may be experiencing
- If in a relationship, whether you have resumed sexual intercourse yet and what you are doing for contraception.

The physical examination often entails checking your:
- Blood pressure.
- Breasts and nipples, whether breastfeeding or not.
- Abdominal muscles, for separation and tone; the caesarean scar (if appropriate).
- Genitals for the healing of tears or an episiotomy; using a speculum to look at the cervix, and possibly do a pap test if required. An internal vaginal examination may be performed to check the size of the uterus and make sure there is no tenderness. The caregiver may also check your pelvic floor tone by asking you to 'squeeze' their fingers by tightening your pelvic floor muscles.

NOTE: If you are still feeling sore and sensitive you may ask your caregiver not to perform a vaginal examination.

Sometimes a haemoglobin blood test is done if you lost a lot of blood at the birth. A rubella titre may also be done if you were vaccinated after the birth, to see if you were successfully immunised.

UNEXPECTED OUTCOMES/UNMET EXPECTATIONS

When care during the pregnancy, labour, birth or postnatal period brings unexpected outcomes and/or unmet expectations, some women question the quality of care they received, or wonder whether things could have been done differently. If you are feeling this way, you may consider providing feedback, or even filing a complaint, in an effort to resolve your feelings or contribute towards the type of care other women will receive.

Constructive feedback contributes to the improvement of poor services and helps caregivers reflect on their practice. If an organisation receives repeated complaints, this can prompt them to change their policies, or look at counselling or disciplinary action for the person involved. If you feel you want to act on this, you may consider:
- Discussing the issue directly with the person involved, or writing a letter.

- Letting the head of the department know.
- Asking to speak with the patient advocate or liaison officer of the hospital.
- Writing a letter to the hospital's chief medical officer or director of nursing. They are obliged to investigate complaints and reply in writing about any changes or resolutions.
- Write a letter to the Health Care Complaints Commission in your State or Territory.
- Instigate legal action if you feel you may be due compensation of some nature. Be aware that this is a lengthy, expensive and emotional process. It is important to obtain honest legal advice and assess the personal and financial implications of pursuing this.

Regardless of what you choose, or whether you choose to do nothing at all, it may be important for your emotional wellbeing to share your feelings with someone you trust, or seek out the services of a qualified counsellor to help you work through your issues.

Variations for the woman

BREASTFEEDING VARIATIONS

Sore nipples

Sore nipples are usually caused by the baby not being positioned or attached properly on the breast. Visible injury can be noticed on the nipple, ranging from a blister, bruise, graze or a crack that bleeds. The nipple often looks flattened, or has a whitish crease across the end of it, as soon as the baby stops feeding, and the damage continues to worsen until the baby attaches correctly.

Incorrect attachment often leads to a spiralling cycle of feeding problems because the baby cannot milk the breast efficiently, meaning they feed for longer and/or more frequently, increasing nipple damage and possibly leading to engorgement, blocked milk ducts or mastitis. Once the attachment is corrected, the nipple starts to heal and everything else begins to fall into place. Strategies to help can include:

- **Changing the way your baby is positioned** – Try lying down to feed or using the football hold as a temporary solution to keep the feeding going, until your baby learns to latch properly.
- **Expressing breast milk for 24 to 48 hours from the affected**

breast(s) – Give this milk to the baby in a bottle but take care with breast pumps as overzealous pumping can increase nipple damage. When introducing your baby back to the breast, start with feeding occasionally, or every second feed, or having shorter feeds then expressing the rest.
- **Using a nipple shield** – Some caregivers believe that these should never be used, but others think they have a place, if supervised adequately. While not a first-line option, it may mean the difference between giving up and continuing to breastfeed.

  Nipple shields reduce stimulation of the nipple and can gradually reduce milk supply if used for prolonged periods. They may also make it difficult to encourage correct attachment or for the baby to return to the breast. However, ways to avoid problems can be to:
  - Only use a shield on the affected breast if all other options have failed, and then with professional supervision.
  - Try to use the shield for a few days until the nipple starts to heal. Don't rely on it for weeks.
  - When you are ready, start feeding with the shield and then finish the feed with the baby directly on the breast, or try feeding without the shield for some feeds, perhaps when the baby is happy and content.

Irritated skin – Sometimes the nipples look reddened or pink, dry, flaky or shiny. They may also feel itchy and/or have a burning sensation. To relieve skin irritations, it is important to:
- Avoid soaps, creams, oils and ointments (unless prescribed by your doctor).
- Gently pat the nipples dry with a soft towel after showering or bathing.
- Change breast pads frequently, and don't use plastic-backed pads.
- Wear a well-fitting bra to stop friction, and perhaps have some bra-free time.

Thrush in the nipples – This can be transferred from vaginal thrush, or develop after taking antibiotics. In some cases the baby develops thrush and passes it to their mother. Physical signs include:
- Sharp, deep, needle-like pain or a burning sensation while feeding.
- No visible damage to the nipples, but the skin may look dark pink or orange, dry and flaky.
- Pain continuing throughout the feed, which may worsen when the feed finishes.

Treatment involves an antifungal gel placed on the nipples (and inside the baby's mouth) after each feed, and regular bra-free time. If your baby has a dummy, make sure this is boiled for five minutes every day, and replace it with a new dummy after the treatment starts working. Some women use natural therapies, such as plain yoghurt on the nipples after a feed or a mixture of 1 cup of water with 1 teaspoon of baking soda, boiling for 20 minutes and applying the cooled mixture to the nipples.

Milk blisters – These occur if skin grows over a nipple opening and breast milk collects behind it. The milk thickens, causing considerable pain. It may burst as the baby feeds, or you may need to *gently* squeeze the blister with clean hands or a damp cloth. Be careful not to bruise the nipple. If this does not work (or it is too painful), see your doctor or early childhood nurse to have the blister opened.

Engorged breasts

Milk engorgement normally occurs to some degree when the milk comes in during the early days. However, it can become a very painful problem if the baby is not fed on demand, or is sleepy and disinterested and not feeding regularly. Engorgement can also happen when your baby is older if you:
- Limit feeding times or stretch out the time between feeds.
- Give the baby water or formula supplements.
- Miss breastfeeds without expressing to replace them.
- Do not latch the baby on correctly.
- Wean rapidly, or intentionally suppress your milk supply to bottle feed.

Breast engorgement causes the breasts to swell, feel hot, hard, tender and painful. The best way to fix it is to allow your baby to feed freely and correct any attachment problems. You may also want to try:
- Using warm compresses just before feeding (a clean hand towel or nappy dampened with warm water), and cold or frozen compresses in between feeds.
- Massaging the breasts and areola just before a feed and perhaps gently hand expressing a few drops of milk to soften the nipple.
- Wearing a well-fitting maternity bra between feeds and taking it off completely to feed, encouraging milk flow.
- Just feeding from one breast each feed, or expressing more milk after the feed if you feel the breast is still uncomfortable.

Some women use acupuncture or homeopathic remedies such as Belladonna or Bryonia (be aware you need to stop taking Arnica while using these), or parsley, sage or phytolacca (see your herbalist).

Blocked milk ducts

A tender red lump on the breast may indicate a blocked milk duct, which can be due to:
- Damaged nipples and milk engorgement.
- Bruising or injury to the breast, a tight bra, compression from a baby sling or seat belt, or sleeping for prolonged periods on your tummy. Even strapless dresses or clothing pulled up under the armpits while breastfeeding can result in a blocked duct.
- Using your fingertips to keep the breast away from your baby's nose, or holding the breast tightly while feeding.

Treatments include:
- Making sure the affected breast is fully emptied regularly. Feed from this breast first for the next couple of feeds and perhaps express more milk after the feed if you feel the breast is still full.
- Positioning the baby's chin in the direction of the lump as much as possible. For example, if the lump is near your armpit, try the football hold. Some women lay their baby on a rug on the floor and feed kneeling over them to drain all areas of the breast.
- If using your fingertips to clear the breast from the baby's nose, try moving them regularly or changing the baby's position during the feed.

Strategies for engorgement can also be used, as well as gently but firmly massaging the lump towards the nipple during and after feeds (use some vegetable oil to minimise skin friction). The lump should clear within 12 to 24 hours.

Mastitis

Mastitis occurs for 10 to 20% of women at some time during their breastfeeding. Physical signs include:
- A section of the breast becoming swollen, reddened, throbbing and painful, with the skin feeling hot and tender.
- Flu-like symptoms, feeling weak, lethargic, aching all over, headache, a fever, chills and sweats.

Mastitis can develop following sore nipples, a blocked milk duct or engorged breasts, injury to the breast or if the baby suddenly weans or sleeps through the night. It can also occur when returning to work and milk is not expressed regularly, and can coincide with being tired, stressed, ill or run-down.

Mastitis may be one of the following:
- **Noninfective**, usually resolving with strategies used for blocked milk ducts and engorgement.

- **Infective**, caused by bacteria entering the breast, usually through a damaged nipple, which needs antibiotics. It is important you wash your hands before handling your breasts, especially after nappy changes.

Noninfective mastitis should improve within 36 to 48 hours, but can progress to infective mastitis despite all attempts to rest and drain the breast adequately, requiring antibiotics. It is very important to continue feeding your baby and/or expressing milk frequently, so that the mastitis does not turn into a breast abscess. If you were weaning your baby, delay this until you are well again. Breastfeeding with infective mastitis (or while taking antibiotics) does not harm your baby, but can be extremely painful, even to the point where some women consider giving up their breastfeeding. However, if you have support and persevere, these painful sensations while feeding will pass after a day or two.

To help recover from mastitis use the treatments for engorgement and blocked milk ducts along with:

- Taking your baby to bed and feed, feed, feed (if possible). If your baby is not feeding frequently, express your milk every three to four hours.
- Trying deep breathing through the pain when feeding. You may need to take a mild analgesic (such as paracetamol) to help with pain and fever.
- Seeing your baby health clinic or GP for support and advice if you feel very unwell or the mastitis does not seem to be resolving. If considering natural therapies (see 'Engorged breasts', page 466), these need to be commenced as soon as you realise you have mastitis.
- Letting your partner or family know you need lots of help to get though this. Arrange for others to look after your other children and prepare meals.
- Eating nutritious foods and drink plenty of water.
- Continuing resting and looking after yourself when you start feeling better to help prevent mastitis from recurring.

Breast abscess

Although relatively rare, if mastitis is not treated effectively or soon enough, it can develop into a breast abscess, in which pus collects inside the breast tissue. Physical signs are similar to mastitis, but swelling over the reddened area fluctuates and has pitting oedema – when you push your finger into it, a small impression, or pit, stays for a few seconds after you have taken your finger away.

Treatments include antibiotics (sometimes intravenously in hospital) and/or an operation to drain the abscess. You can take your baby with you to hospital and continue to feed after the operation if it is not too painful, otherwise gently hand express for a couple of days until the incision is more healed. This keeps the breast empty and reduces pressure from where the abscess was removed.

NOTE: *Breast milk may leak from the incision, which can persist for a few weeks. However, breast milk contains anti-infective and healing agents that help prevent further infections. You can place a clean gauze dressing over the incision and change this regularly until it heals completely.*

INFECTIONS

An infection directly related to the birth takes 24 to 48 hours to develop physical symptoms. When an infection is suspected, the caregiver does tests to try to identify the source. These can include a urine sample, vaginal swab test or a swab of abdominal stitches (if you had a caesarean). Results take 24 to 48 hours, but antibiotics are often commenced before the results are known.

Of the uterus

An infection of the lining of the uterus is called endometritis and it happens for 1 to 3% of women after a vaginal birth, and 10 to 30% after a caesarean. It can happen within two to three days of the birth (most common) or up to six weeks afterwards (if a small section of placenta was left inside the uterus). Physical signs include:
- A fever and rapid pulse.
- Lower abdominal pain and a tender uterus.
- Offensive smelling vaginal blood loss and possibly heavier bleeding.
- Headache, sweating and shivering.

The main health concerns are that the infection will spread to the fallopian tubes, affecting future fertility, or will result in a blood infection (sepsis), which can be life-threatening. Antibiotics are prescribed (intravenously in hospital if the infection is severe). It is important to rest, eat well and have help with caring for your baby while recovering.

Of stitches to the genitals

An infection of the genital stitches is not common, but if it does develop, physical signs are noticeable within a week of the birth, with the stitches feeling more painful, hot or full with pressure, reddened and/or oozing pus, but not causing a fever. Treatments involve removing the stitches and washing the area with antiseptic, or placing a gauze dressing soaked in antiseptic on the genitals and changing this daily, allowing the genitals to heal without stitches. Sometimes antibiotics are prescribed.

Of the bladder and/or kidneys
About 12% of women develop bladder infections (cystitis), which sometimes develops into a kidney infection. Cystitis is more likely if a catheter was used during labour, or with a caesarean. Physical signs include:
- Pain or burning when passing urine.
- Needing to pass small amounts of urine frequently.
- A slightly raised temperature (37.5 to 38°C).

If the infection spreads to the kidneys, you may notice:
- Pain in the middle of the back and sides.
- A fever above 38°C and a rapid pulse.
- Sweating and shivering, nausea and vomiting.
- The urine smells offensive and/or is bloodstained.

Treatments include antibiotics (intravenously if the infection is severe), drinking three litres of water a day, and taking mild analgesics for pain and fever and urinary alkalinisers to reduce the stinging sensations. Natural therapies include unsweetened cranberry juice or tablets, parsley, barley water, dandelion tea and possibly uva ursi. Consult your herbalist.

THRUSH AND GARDNERELLA
In the weeks after the birth, a combination of a lowered resistance, continual vaginal bleeding, wearing plastic-backed sanitary pads and being tired and stressed with caring for a new baby makes many women prone to developing thrush or Gardnerella. These infections may require medical treatments if they become severe (see Chapter 2).

HEAVY BLEEDING
A secondary postpartum haemorrhage is abnormally heavy bleeding after 24 hours and up until 6 weeks after the birth (affecting 1% of women). It generally involves cramping, sudden gushes of blood and/or passing blood clots larger than a golf ball and is often caused by an infection of the uterus and/or a small part of the placenta being retained. You should return to the hospital immediately; if the bleeding is very heavy and unrelenting, call an ambulance. Depending on the cause, treatments include antibiotics, a D&C, an intravenous drip and, in rare cases, a blood transfusion.

Thrombosis
The risk for developing a thrombosis continues for up to six weeks after the birth and can be potentially life-threatening if the clot dislodges (called an embolus), as it is carried through the bloodstream to the smaller blood vessels in the lungs or brain.

Superficial inflammation
Thrombophlebitis is when surface veins in the legs become inflamed but don't develop a blood clot. This is more common for women with varicose veins. The skin becomes hot, red and inflamed, with the tissue underneath feeling hard. Treatments involve supporting the area with a firm bandage and keeping the feet raised when resting. Some women use witch hazel compresses to help with the discomfort. An ultrasound of the leg may be done to make sure a blood clot is not forming.

DVT
If a deep vein thrombosis develops, the leg may be swollen and painful. The pain worsens if the toes are pushed back towards the shin. Some women have a slight temperature, but not everyone experiences physical signs. If a DVT is suspected, an ultrasound is done to detect blood clots. Treatment involves bed rest and having medications to thin the blood, possibly spending several weeks in hospital until the clot dissolves. Your baby can stay with your during this time.

Embolus
A small blood clot can lodge in the lungs (pulmonary embolus), causing severe breathlessness, chest pain and coughing-up of blood. If the blockage is severe, the woman may collapse. You need to seek immediate medical attention.

Postnatal depression
Postnatal depression affects about 15% of women at some time during the year following the birth of their child, with 40 to 70% of women noticing signs before their baby is 3 months old. Unpleasant and distressing feelings can persist for several weeks, with most women feeling better within three to six months, but the feelings can last up to a year or longer. Postnatal depression should not be confused with other psychological reactions such as:
- The third day blues.
- Puerperal psychosis.
- Grief after the death of a baby.

- Reactions from the labour and birth bringing up traumatic memories from past sexual abuse.
- The normal anxiety felt by new mothers.
- Post-traumatic stress disorder after experiencing a particularly difficult or traumatic birth (see page 475).

The causes of postnatal depression still remain unclear, but it is probably the result of many factors, physical, psychological and social. It affects women from all walks of life and all cultural backgrounds. Possible risk factors can include:
- Experiencing depression in the past.
- Having relationship difficulties and/or lack of practical and emotional support.
- Dealing with many stresses (eg. financial difficulties, moving house, the death of a close relative).
- Having unrealistic expectations about mothering.
- Having a negative birth experience.
- The baby being demanding and/or frequently unsettled.
- Being a person who tends to have a negative outlook on life or someone who is used to having a lot of control and order in her life.
- The pregnancy being unplanned, or the baby being adopted, or conceived with fertility treatments.
- Having a partner who is depressed.

Women, who experience postnatal depression are at increased risk of experiencing depression again later in life. However, this is not a given.

Signs of postnatal depression

Postnatal depression can be mild and intermittent, or involve severely distressing feelings and thoughts that never seem to go away (or progressively worsen). Some signs that may be noticed are listed below:

Feeling:
- Very low or flat; constantly feeling sad, guilty or ashamed.
- Low self-esteem, lack of confidence, feeling worthless, inadequate or a failure as a mother.
- Exhausted, empty or tearful.
- Out of control; a sense of helplessness or hopelessness.
- Numb.
- Anxious or panicky.
- Fearful for the baby (or of the baby); fear of being alone or going out.
- Angry and resentful towards yourself and/or your baby.
- Fear of being rejected or unwanted.

Physical signs:
- Low energy, lethargy, wanting to sleep all the time.
- Insomnia, unable to sleep, even if tired.
- Frequent nightmares.
- Lack of concentration; poor memory.
- Inability to think clearly or to make decisions.
- Lack of interest or pleasure in usual activities.
- No interest in relating to others or having sex.
- Loss of appetite, or comfort eating.

Behaviour:
- Not motivated to do anything.
- Withdrawing from social contact.
- Obsessive behaviour; wanting to pace, walk or clean all the time.
- Not looking after personal hygiene.
- Inability to cope with the daily routine.

Thoughts:
- Wanting to run away.
- Not wanting to be a mother; wishing to be someone else or that the child was older.
- Frightened about harming yourself and/or your baby.
- That the baby would be better off without you; ideas about suicide.
- Worried about your partner leaving, or harm coming to your partner or your baby.

These signs for short periods of time can be normal. However, if you notice a combination of more than four signs for at least two weeks or more, you are probably depressed and need to seek help.

Because depressive feelings can seem scary or wrong, many women are reluctant to tell others. However, these feelings are a normal part of a psychological illness and not reflective of you as a person. Sharing what you are going through with someone you trust can help deal with the depression and be the first step in getting the help you need to recover. Many women are relieved when they have an explanation for how they are feeling, and partners often cope better after the diagnosis and are more able to provide support.

Support strategies

The woman's relationships with her partner, other children and extended family and friends may suffer as a result of postnatal depression. It can also be difficult to support, or even be with, someone who is very depressed. Healing takes time, and patience is needed. Support strategies for the woman and her partner are similar to those for antenatal depression (discussed in Chapter 3).

Many partners feel forgotten or left out when the woman they love is depressed. There is some evidence that men also suffer from depression more frequently after the birth of their baby compared to other times in their lives. If you think you need help, acknowledge this and seek support.

Professional help

Despite how disabling postnatal depression can be, women do go on to lead happy and productive lives if given the right amount of time to recover, appropriate coping strategies, practical and emotional support, professional help and in some cases medication. Maternity caregivers should be aware of local support networks. However, some women feel they are not receiving the help they need. If this is so, seek out alternative services. It may help to ask local support groups who they recommend. Also, try to be realistic about your expectations. If you are expecting a quick fix, or that the professional should solve all your problems immediately, changing caregivers may not help. It is important you feel you are making some progress and that you can comfortably work with your caregiver towards eventual recovery.

Treatment for postnatal depression depends on what is available locally and the degree of depression you are experiencing, as well as your individual needs and preferences. They may include:

- **Individual counselling** – This is usually useful for mild depression, incorporating day-to-day self-help strategies. Partners may also benefit from counselling.
- **Individual psychotherapy** – This may be required for moderate to severe postnatal depression (if a clinical psychologist or psychiatrist is available), and aims to identify thoughts and behaviour patterns to try to come to an understanding of the feelings associated with depression.
- **Couple counselling** – Couple counselling aims to provide information and support to assist parents to adjust to their new roles and deal with changes in their relationship.
- **Support groups** – These groups aim to help women feel they are not alone, encouraging them to share their feelings more freely in confidence and normalising the depression.

Anti-depressants

Anti-depressants may be appropriate with moderate to severe depression, especially if the sufferer is experiencing prolonged insomnia, tiredness, weight loss, difficulty achieving tasks, or having suicidal thoughts. They are used in conjunction with counselling, psychotherapy and/or support groups. It may take one to three weeks for medications to be effective and they normally need to be continued for several weeks (or months). Finding the right medication and the correct dosage can take time, as each person is different. If breastfeeding, discuss whether you should continue to feed your baby. Antidepressants do pass into breast milk, but the effects on babies are not clear. Some medications also reduce breast milk supply by inhibiting a let-down reflex. If you continue to breastfeed while taking antidepressants, the baby may need to be regularly seen by a paediatrician to monitor their progress.

NOTE: *It is important that medications are taken exactly as prescribed.* **Never** *self-prescribe by increasing or decreasing daily doses on good or bad days. This can worsen the depression and may be dangerous to your health.*

Natural therapies

Natural therapies may be appropriate for mild to moderate depression and/or in combination with other approaches or treatments. Always tell your doctor and natural therapist what you are taking, to ensure treatments do not interact with each other. Therapies thought to help can include:
- Eating fish high in omega oils (tuna and salmon).
- Zinc supplements.
- St John's wort (*Hypericum perforatum*).
- Bergamot, neroli or ylang ylang essential oils.
- Homeopathic remedies specific to your individual physical signs.

POST-TRAUMATIC STRESS DISORDER

Up to 1 to 5% of women experience post-traumatic stress disorder (PTSD), particularly after a difficult birth or an emergency caesarean. This may not surface until months after the birth, or can be mistaken for postnatal depression. Women with PTSD often describe:
- Feeling frequently anxious.
- Having flashbacks, intrusive thoughts and nightmares.
- Feeling detached from others and their baby, avoiding sexual relationships.
- Having reduced self-confidence or struggling with feelings of failure.
- Experiencing problems with breastfeeding, parenting or their relationship.
- Feeling fearful of childbirth, even though another baby is wanted.[4]

If you think you may be experiencing PTSD, communicate this to your partner, caregiver or a trusted friend. You may need professional counselling to help resolve your feelings.

POSTNATAL PSYCHOSIS

Postnatal psychosis is a rare mental illness experienced by 0.2% of new mothers. It generally comes on quite rapidly, usually between three days and six weeks after the birth. Women who have experienced manic depression (bipolar mood disorder) or schizophrenia in the past are at increased risk. Physical signs include:
- Insomnia.
- Not eating or drinking much, often leading to dehydration.
- Confusion, hallucinations (imagining or believing unusual things), feeling frightened, delusions (eg. believing the baby is Jesus), and not realising what time it is, where they are, who they are, or who others are.
- Severe mood swings and erratic behaviour.

Postnatal psychosis requires immediate treatment. The woman may be at increased risk of inflicting injury on herself (possibly attempting suicide) and/or hurting her baby. Treatments include admission to a psychiatric hospital (with the baby, so they are not separated) and initially being sedated to help her rest, eat and drink, and starting appropriate medications before supportive counselling and therapies are commenced. The continuation of breastfeeding depends on the types of medications prescribed. Most women make a full recovery; however, treatments (in hospital and then eventually at home) may continue for several months. She is also at increased risk of experiencing psychosis again, after a subsequent pregnancy.

CHAPTER 14

Transition to parenting

The birth of a parent

With the birth of a baby comes the birth of a parent or the extension of an existing parenting role. Every baby and parent is uniquely different, each bringing their own personality, idiosyncrasies and histories into the dynamics of a family. You will create your personal parenting style as you go. So trust your instincts and bear in mind that whatever you do, and however you do it, your baby will love you, because no one else can care for them just the way mum or dad do!

Becoming a parent is a life-changing event and it lasts forever. It is a difficult job being on call 24 hours a day, 7 days a week, with no rostered time off, no holidays, no pay or sick leave and little status. However, try not to lose sight of how enjoyable, rewarding, hilarious, fun and exciting parenting can be and the many joys your child will bring you.

Early parenting can seem daunting or exciting. It may feel as though your world has been turned upside down, or it can unfold naturally and smoothly. You may even feel so enthralled by your baby that any difficult demands are taken in your stride. Emotions come and go, ranging from wonder, self-doubt, love, guilt, joy, disappointment, amazement to worry, protectiveness, stress, surprise and a sense of immense responsibility, to name but a few. Amid these amazing challenges, somehow you find your way. If you can learn how to accept the changes rather than question them, the transition will be smoother.

REALISTIC PARENTING EXPECTATIONS

Most people want to be good parents, but common attitudes and myths can mean we measure ourselves against others to an unreasonable degree, which can lead to disappointment, guilt and self-blame if your parenting doesn't unfold as expected. Unfortunately, other parents rarely share *exactly* how difficult it is. For some reason everyone puts forward the impression that they are coping beautifully, which makes everyone else wonder why they aren't.

Mother's expectations

Women can feel intimidated and overwhelmed by their new responsibilities, yet remain unaware of how normal their mothering experience is. Myths that perpetuate unrealistic expectations can include the following:

- Myth: Mothers are always happy and motherhood is the ultimate fulfilment for all women.
  Reality: Most women experience unhappy and/or difficult phases, and/or don't see motherhood as their absolute life goal or achievement, even though they love their children very much.
- Myth: Mothers immediately love their baby and instinctively know how to care for them and comfort them.
  Reality: It can take days, weeks or even months to fall in love with your baby. Mothering is usually learnt and takes a lifetime to master.
- Myth: Mothers are on holiday from paid work. All they do is stay at home and care for the baby, with plenty of free time to socialise, cook and do housework.
  Reality: Caring for a newborn baby and doing basic household tasks is a 24-hour-a-day job, with little sleep or time out. Socialising with other mothers is one of the few things that stops you going insane, as well as giving you emotional support.
- Myth: Mothers cause difficult behaviour in their babies.
  Reality: Each baby's behaviour is individual to their personality and not generally a reflection of the parenting they are receiving.
- Myth: Mothers have to be constantly available, always putting their baby's needs first, and they should just get on with it if they are experiencing difficulties.
  Reality: Mothers are human, and parenting is difficult. Women need to nurture themselves and acknowledge when it is hard, so they can take time out to replenish their reserves. This helps them continue to be the wonderful mothers they are.

Try to avoid getting caught up in a competitive cycle with other mothers – this can undermine your confidence in your own ability to mother your baby.

Father's expectations

The reality of fathering is often mixed with feelings of being unsure about what their role should be and how to do things. Common myths that perpetuate unrealistic expectations can include the following:

- Myth: Fathers won't bond with their baby unless they are at the birth.
  Reality: Being at the birth may enhance rapid bonding, but many men find their involvement in the baby's care is the best way to feel close to their child.
- Myth: Fathers should be strong family providers and protectors.
  Reality: Men are human too, and need love, support and understanding, as well as space to be vulnerable and cry. Even if circumstances mean the role of breadwinner naturally becomes his responsibility, it may not be because he wants it this way.
- Myth: Fathers are not capable of giving proper emotional care to nurture, settle and soothe their baby.
  Reality: Parenting is a learnt skill for mothers and fathers. However, women usually get more practice. Being involved will see you become a skilled and loving father to whom your baby responds positively.
- Myth: Caring for babies and household duties is women's work. A father shouldn't have to come home and change dirty nappies.
  Reality: Many women feel their day never ends and look forward to their partner coming home to share the load, otherwise they quickly become overwhelmed and exhausted, in some cases leading to postnatal depression. Domestic duties are the responsibility of both men and women, and you need to participate in running the household.
- Myth: Having a baby will not change a man's interest in his work, sex life or recreational activities.
  Reality: Many men are surprised by how focused they become on their new baby and family. Being a father brings many life changes, with an increased tenderness towards your partner, bringing positive feelings and enhancing your life and relationships.

RELATIONSHIP SURVIVAL TIPS

The first 6 to 12 weeks can be all consuming and very stressful. Coping with constant tiredness, mood swings, a partner's return to work, mismatched expectations and differing approaches to parenting can place incredible demands on even the most stable of relationships as personal needs are pushed into the background. Both parents need time to learn and adjust, and it is important you are sensitive to each other's needs. How you communicate can determine whether you help or hinder each other. If you are constantly correcting or criticising your partner, this can make them feel inadequate or hurt, and inclined to withdraw their help, which does not help you. Respecting each other as competent carers fosters confidence in both of you, encouraging you to persevere with improving your parenting skills.

Communication needs to be clear and ongoing. Caring for your baby is a priority, but it is important not to lose sight of each other and your relationship, which is more than being the other parent to your child. Try to remember, your relationship was there before the children, your relationship created your children, and your relationship is all you will have once your children leave you. It is important to nurture your relationship and not to always put your children first.

Support strategies
- Learn together. Be prepared to live in chaos and unpredictability for a while. It is just a phase, and it will pass as your baby grows older.
- At least once a week, set aside time to talk about how you are both feeling. If this is too hard, even a brief encounter is better than nothing.
- Work as a team and treat each other as competent equals. Don't criticise the other parent if a nappy is not put on correctly, or something is not done the way you would do it. Encourage each other's participation and acknowledge you are both learning.
- Compliment each other. You are both doing a marvellous job.
- Try to be understanding. This is a tremendous adjustment in your lives; even if you are feeling tired and irritable, try not to react angrily.
- Reassess how household chores are divided, and try to come to an agreement about sharing responsibilities. Modify your expectations of how much housework should be done (or how much you expect your partner to do), at least for the first few months.
- Try not to make other major changes unless absolutely necessary (eg. moving house or changing jobs). This creates needless stress and conflict. You have enough to deal with.
- Seek professional help and support to deal with difficult issues.
- Talk about intimacy and sex; acknowledge the reality of what you need and help each other know when the time is right for sexual contact.
- Try to organise some regular 'couple time'.
- If one parent is working, contact each other at least once a day and include a message of love such as 'I'm glad I'm with you', rather than 'Can you pick up some nappies?' or 'I'll be home late from work.'

- Many women feel they need to hand over the baby as soon as their partner walks through the door. This may be okay sometimes, but he may need to adjust from being at work. Talk about how you can achieve a balance.
- Surprise each other with flowers or a card for no special reason. Light some candles with dinner or give your partner an unexpected neck massage.

When caring for your baby

Newborns have unsociable feeding, sleeping and crying behaviours which can impact on how you feel about yourself, your relationship and your parenting. When lack of sleep accumulates, previous coping mechanisms fall away, making dealing with your baby's needs more difficult, and keeping it together, near impossible. Therefore, ongoing support strategies are important.

- Value yourself as a mother or father. Remind yourself you are performing one of the most important jobs anyone can do.
- Try to maintain a sense of humour and focus on what is positive and working, rather than always thinking about what is going wrong.
- If you are a single parent, set up a support network of family and friends, and make caring for yourself, your baby and sleep priorities over housework. When you feel ready, organise a babysitter to have a break, or swap babysitting favours with other mothers.
- Access 24-hour phone helplines and other community support services when necessary.
- Maintain the 'call before you visit' protocol. If someone does visit, ask them to mind your baby while you shower or eat. If your partner works, use the weekends to have a break.
- As the partner, ask what you can do to help and try to look for what needs to be done rather than waiting to be asked (or told). Try not to avoid the parenting role by taking on more work, sporting or social commitments.
- If you have other children, organise for them to be cared for occasionally.
- Go for a walk when you can, or simply be outdoors to lift your spirits after being inside all day.
- Let go of the bad phases and wake each day afresh.
- Take opportunities to share how you are feeling with someone you trust and don't be afraid to ask for support when you need it or to accept offers of help when they come.

- Join a parents' group and/or a postnatal exercise or yoga class, to share your experiences and alleviate the isolation that often comes with early parenting.
- When feeling up to it, organise social activities (outside your home or where others entertain), to nurture relationships with people you care about.
- If you are finding it difficult to cope, cut back on commitments until you feel you can manage them again.
- Use visualisation and relaxation techniques to wind down and relax. Try to have a little time out each day.
- Be kind to yourself and don't expect to always get things right.

Advice — take it or leave it?

Being a new parent makes you a target for advice — and usually lots of it! This may be helpful or confusing, fact or fiction, 'tried and true', common sense or a perennial myth that has filtered down through generations. Essentially babies haven't changed, but modern research and health treatments have, making some things we survived as babies no longer acceptable or safe. As new approaches evolve, so do our methods of parenting. Dealing with advice, whether it comes from your GP or grandmother, can be difficult, and it's often hard to know whether to take it on board or reject it.

Professional advice

Expert advice can be invaluable, and a caregiver's patience and helpful tips may be timely and appreciated. However, sometimes well-intentioned professionals give conflicting advice that is based more on their personal preferences and beliefs than up-to-date research. This may not worry some parents, but others find it undermines their confidence as they try to find their way.

It is hard to determine what information you should rely on from professionals, and many parents feel confused, annoyed, helpless or concerned as they struggle with the merry-go-round of advice. If you are being given conflicting advice, you could:

- Ask for clarification and the benefits of what the caregiver is suggesting. Consider whether you agree and perhaps experiment with the approach.
- If you are being corrected, tell your caregiver you were told something different by another practitioner and ask them why their way is better. Perhaps check with others to confirm it.
- Ask only to be assisted when you request it.

- Seek out one supportive caregiver and use their advice if it seems to work for you and your baby. Consider visiting an alternative caregiver (eg. local doctor, early childhood nurse or pharmacist) for a second opinion.
- Perhaps sit with the information for a while before deciding whether any changes really need to be made.
- If you are feeling overwhelmed with conflicting advice, be aware that you are with your baby 24 hours a day and you know them best and what works well for both of you.
- Use services for what they were designed for. For example, a local doctor may be good if your baby is ill, but may not have expertise in breastfeeding, sleep and settle techniques, and colic. Your early childhood nurse or local support group may be better.

On a positive note, a diverse range of advice can give you a wide range of strategies to choose from. Take what you need and discard what you don't find helpful. See it as reassuring because there is no absolute right way to be a parent.

Health professionals as parents

Many health professionals don't feel comfortable asking their peers for basic advice and/or their peers may not offer it readily because they think you already know. Try to approach your new parenting role first and foremost as a parent. It can be extremely difficult to be objective when it is your own baby, but asking for information and help (no matter how simple) is part of your new role. Perhaps seek out caregivers who are willing to treat you as a mother or father and are not intimidated by your professional knowledge.

Advice from family and friends

Opinions and advice from family and friends may be easier to disregard than professional advice, but harder to deal with diplomatically (or escape from!). People often think their advice is useful because it worked for them, but this is based on their personal experiences (or what was common practice when they were parents). What works for others may not necessarily work for you and your baby. If it doesn't feel right, this does not mean you are parenting incorrectly. It is simply a matter of the suggestions not being suitable. With this kind of advice:

- Be flexible. A piece of advice may work for a while and then not be helpful. Continue down the suggestion list.
- Consider all advice as suggestions only. Use trial and error to find what works and privately discard what doesn't.
- Take the view that 'out of a mountain of advice can come a few pearls of wisdom'.

- Trust your instincts, they are often right! Sometimes the suggestion is good but just needs modifying to suit your preferences or circumstances.
- If it is all too much, consider asking family and friends to limit their advice.

Advice from your parents

Advice will no doubt come from your parents (and in-laws), which can sometimes be useful. However, it may be that you are so caught up in family tensions that you refuse to accept it. Your relationship with your parents can influence how you approach your own parenting. You may strive to be as good as they were, relying on their guidance with love and gratitude, or determined to do it all differently, feeling (rightly or wrongly) scrutinised or judged. Changing long-standing family dynamics can be difficult and tactful negotiations tricky, with confrontation resulting in the withdrawal of much-needed support at a time when you need it most.

Understand that new grandparents also need to adjust to the fact that their child is now a parent. Trust to what you feel is right and pave your own way. Like your own parents you will make mistakes and live and learn, but you will no doubt get there in the end.

Advice from your partner

Advice between partners can become an issue if one partner feels more able to give advice about how to do things correctly, or is less accepting of taking advice. For example, a father who already has children from a previous relationship can make his new partner feel sensitive about being compared (perhaps unintentionally) to a previous partner. Take care when making suggestions, and remember that everyone does things differently, but it does not mean they are wrong. Keep communication open and let your partner know if you feel their advice is undermining your confidence.

SIBLING RIVALRY

Sibling rivalry is as old as time itself and there is nothing you can do to prevent it. The reactions of older children vary widely and generally depend on the child's personality, age and how parents react to their behaviour. A sibling (especially a young one) may:
- Be unsettled and misbehave before the birth as they struggle to understand what life will be like when the baby is born, but settle down once the baby arrives.

- Be loving and affectionate when visiting their new brother or sister, but react differently when they realise the baby is permanent, asking, 'When are you going to send the baby back?'
- Gravitate towards their father, or another person close to them.
- Exhibit attention-seeking behaviour, usually when you are attending to the baby. This is normal and improves with time.
- Want to wear nappies, get into the baby's cot and be 'like a baby'. This is usually temporary.
- Regress – for example, start wetting the bed again. Be patient.
- Be angry or teary. Avoid telling them they should not feel this way, even if they say hurtful things like 'I hate the baby!' Mirroring back these feelings can help. For example, 'I can see you feel angry with the baby. Maybe you wish you could have Mummy all to yourself.' Try to respect and understand their feelings rather than deny them. This is a big life change that brings with it many conflicting emotions.
- Noticeably grow up all of a sudden.

Support strategies

A change in your older child's behaviour is normal and expected. However, the following strategies may help them accept the new baby.

- Avoid big changes around the time of the birth, such as toilet training or moving into a big bed.
- Involve your child in caring for the baby.
- Encourage time between your child and partner before the birth, so this can be carried through after the baby arrives.
- If your older child sleeps with you, consider a mattress or bed beside yours, so they can remain close by.
- Bring out a favourite toy, activity or food when you are about to feed the baby.
- Put aside some special time with them when the baby is asleep, to help them feel secure and loved.
- Try to overlook some of their disruptive behaviour; if they are being extremely naughty, reinforce discipline in the normal way.
- Don't ask your older child to share with the baby just yet. Even if they never play with a certain toy, it is theirs. It can feel threatening if they think the baby gets everything as well as their mother. There is plenty of time to teach sharing.
- Don't leave a young sibling alone with the new baby. Toddlers like to poke eyes, put pillows on faces and may attempt to pick up the baby or force-feed them (all of which is quite normal).

- Obtain help with caring for the older child, but try not to have them taken away constantly. This can make them feel unwanted and unloved.

Sex, sexuality and contraception

RESUMING YOUR SEXUAL RELATIONSHIP

Pregnancy and giving birth is a life-changing event and the way partners relate to each other sexually can change considerably. A woman's physical and emotional readiness to resume sex varies greatly between individuals, but it is thought to be physically safe to have intercourse any time after the bleeding stops, usually around three to six weeks after the birth. A few couples engage in sex within a week or two (while the woman is still bleeding). At present there is no research to support or reject an increased risk for an infection of the woman's uterus, unless the man has a sexually transmitted infection.

Pelvic floor

Your pelvic floor muscles are naturally weaker after carrying your baby and can be further weakened with a vaginal birth. It is normal for the vagina to feel loose for several weeks, making intercourse sensations different for both partners. Daily pelvic floor exercises increases their strength and tone over time. Information on how to do pelvic floor exercises is in Chapter 4.

Breasts

A woman's breasts look and feel different after having a baby, whether she breastfeeds or not. If you are breastfeeding, they are enlarged, the nipples may be more sensitive (or less so) and touching them (or your orgasm) can trigger a let-down reflex, making milk trickle (or spurt) for a few seconds. Some women find their breasts very sexy. Others don't like the changes or feel the multiple demands of breastfeeding on their breasts very claustrophobic.

Some men see the breasts as very sexy or more functional (no longer exclusively 'theirs'), or are put off by the presence of milk. It is important to discuss how you both feel, so you can work out ways to adapt your sexual style to the changes a baby brings.

Vaginal dryness

Low levels of oestrogen when breastfeeding cause vaginal dryness, making penetration uncomfortable. Using a water-based vaginal lubricant (such as K-Y gel) helps with this; these are available at supermarkets and pharmacies.

Stitches to the genitals
It takes about two to three weeks for genital injuries to heal, but possibly up to two to four months for sex to feel completely comfortable again. This varies depending on the severity of the injury and the type of stitches used, as well as how everything has healed. Bear in mind that even women without stitches can initially feel raw and tender because their vaginal walls were grazed, which takes several weeks to heal.

Approaching intercourse
Expecting pain rather than pleasure naturally makes a woman tense her vaginal muscles just before penetration, possibly causing (or increasing) discomfort. Consider:
- Looking at your genitals in a mirror to see how they are healing. Be prepared for them to look a bit different, uneven, or to have small skin tags. This is common, and usually returns to normal after three to six months. Some women need time to adjust to their body and may be more concerned about this than their partner.
- Feeling for tender areas inside your vaginal area, and placing light pressure on spots you think may be sore. If this feels painful, then intercourse will probably feel the same. Repeat this every so often to see how the sensations are improving.
- Experimenting with different sexual positions. Being on top of the man (either sitting or lying) tends to give you more control over how quickly penetration occurs. Depending on where the stitches were, vaginal entry from the rear (the man being behind the woman) may put less pressure on the perineum. Have a water-based lubricant readily available for that unpredictable first time.
- Talking about how you are feeling, and communicating what is happening for you during lovemaking. Understanding and respect can make the encounter more relaxing and less stressful for both of you.

Ongoing pain
If sex continues to be painful, you should seek medical advice. Your caregiver may prescribe a cream, and sometimes daily perineal massage helps. You may also be advised to see a physiotherapist specialising in women's health. Occasionally surgery is recommended to cut and restitch the area. This can make a great improvement or little difference, or perhaps more or different pain. However, being told, 'It will be better when you have the next baby' or 'It's all in your mind' are not valid responses. You should try to discuss any possible treatments with a sympathetic caregiver.

SEXUALITY AND INTIMACY

A new baby is now part of your postnatal relationship (as if you hadn't noticed!) and finding the time or space to engage in uninterrupted sex becomes a challenge. This is exacerbated by being tired and often stressed. The fact that you have shared your baby's birth may create renewed intimacy and a special rediscovery of each other, or it can make the expression of your sexuality more difficult.

A few women feel traumatised and not comfortable with being touched for a while. This needs to be respected. It is important to be honest and communicate what is going on for each of you and how this is affecting your relationship. If problems continue, then counselling (individually or as a couple) may be needed. To help nurture your sexual relationship try:

- Being inventive about where you have sex. (Sometimes you have to take your opportunity where you can!)
- Softening the environment. Light candles or make love in the dark, if this makes you feel more comfortable with your changed body image.
- Explaining why you are wanting or not wanting sex. Look at what you can do to replace the sexual act yet maintain intimacy; for example, massage, touching, cuddling and caressing.

Making each other feel loved and nurtured outside the sexual act is important for your libido. Many women need the rest of their relationship to feel close and supportive to make them feel inclined to want to make love. Believe it or not, helping with housework and the baby can make many woman more inclined to want to have sex!

Emotions

As the woman, you may be feeling:

- Insecure and unattractive; worried about how your partner sees you physically and sexually.
- Empowered and sensual.
- So tired and exhausted that the choice between another hour's sleep and having sex means you'll gladly take the sleep!
- You want to avoid physical contact, because it may lead to sex you are not ready for yet.
- Overwhelmed by the demands of your baby. You cannot give anymore of yourself to anyone.
- So absorbed by your new baby that your relationship with your partner takes a back seat.
- Surprised by the increased genital sensation you have after giving birth.
- Upset or embarrassed if sex feels different.

- In love again, as you both rediscover each other in your own time.
- Worried that you may conceive again, if you haven't started contraception.

As the partner, you may be feeling:
- Unsure about when and how to start.
- That you want to make love but are aware she needs time and space.
- The need to reassure her about how she looks, and that you still find her attractive.
- Concerned that you may hurt her, especially the first time.
- Stressed, tired and exhausted from juggling all your commitments.
- Jealous of her intimate relationship with your new baby.
- Isolated, rejected or guilty for even thinking about touching her when she does not seem interested.
- Very close to your partner after sharing the birth of your baby.

CONTRACEPTION

It is possible to conceive another baby as soon as four to six weeks after giving birth. However, women who fully breastfeed may not ovulate, or have regular periods, for up to four to six months or longer. Even so, breastfeeding as the sole form of contraception is only reliable for 30% of women, but can be up to 97% effective if you are fully breastfeeding day and night, with the baby having no extra foods, fluids or a dummy. Generally, it is not advisable to rely on breastfeeding for contraception.

Women who bottle feed from birth usually have a period within 6 to 10 weeks, or 2 to 6 weeks after fully weaning from the breast to the bottle in the early months. When considering whether you might be fertile again, it is important to remember that you will release an egg **before** you get your first period, so contraception is needed from four to six weeks after having the baby. Discuss your options with your partner and caregiver.

Male condom

A male condom is a fine rubber sheath placed over the penis when erect, just prior to intercourse. It prevents semen being released into the woman's vagina. A new condom is needed each time you have sex and spermicide can also be used if you wish. Condoms can be up to 97% effective if they are put on and taken off correctly and a water-based lubricant is used each time. Before putting on the condom, pinch the end of it with your fingers so a space is left for semen to be released into. After sex, hold the base of the condom before removing the penis from the woman's vagina, so it does not slip off inside her. Wrap the condom in a tissue or toilet paper after use and place it in the bin (not the toilet).

NOTE: *Never use oils or Vaseline as lubricants; these can damage the rubber. Store your condoms in a cool place and use before their expiry date.*

Side effects: None, unless you are allergic to latex rubber or the water-based lubricant being used (or spermicide, if using this).

Breastfeeding: Male condoms can be used when a woman is breastfeeding, but not with spermicide.

Advantages:
- Relatively cheap and easy to buy at chemists and supermarkets.
- Very effective in protecting against sexually transmitted infections, including hepatitis B and HIV/AIDS.
- Can be stopped at any time to conceive another baby.

Disadvantages:
- You need to have one handy.
- They may reduce the spontaneity of sex. Some men find they lose their erection while trying to put one on.
- They can sometimes break during sex, or come off, if not put on and removed correctly and lubricant is not used.

Female condom

The female condom is a thin, soft, polyurethane pouch, designed for women of all ages. It is placed inside the vagina, with a flexible ring at each end to keep it in place. Female condoms are up to 95% effective if used correctly. They come pre-packaged with a generous amount of silicone-based lubricant, but extra lubricant can be used if you wish. Some women also use spermicide. A new condom needs to be used each time you have sex. Wrap it in a tissue or toilet paper after use and place in the bin (not the toilet).

NOTE: *A female condom cannot be used at the same time as a male condom, as they can make the female condom move and/or the male condom come off.*

Side effects: None.

Breastfeeding: Female condoms can be used when breastfeeding, but not with spermicide.

Advantages:
- They are available at pharmacies and family planning clinics or by mail order – no need to see a doctor.
- They can be used if allergic to latex rubber or water-based lubricants.
- Up to 70% of women and their partners like using them. The

polyurethane conducts heat and is like a second skin, making sex feel more sensitive and natural for the woman. The man is not constricted with a tightly fitting male condom.
- It does not need to interrupt sexual spontaneity if put in beforehand.
- They can be used during the woman's menstrual period.
- They are highly effective in protecting against sexually transmitted infections, including hepatitis B and HIV/AIDS.
- You can stop using them at any time to conceive another baby.

Disadvantages:
- The woman or man may not like using them. You should try it at least three times before deciding.
- They may take some practice to insert correctly.
- The man's penis may need to be guided into it, so the condom doesn't bunch up, or his penis doesn't slip down the side of it.
- They may make noise during intercourse. Using extra lubricant can help.

For more information, visit www.femalecondom.org.

Diaphragm or cap

A diaphragm is a thin, rubber dome with a firm, flexible rim that a woman places inside her vagina to cover her cervix. A cap is a smaller dome-shaped device that fits more snugly over the cervix. Both aim to prevent semen entering the uterus to fertilise an egg. The diaphragm or cap must be left in place for at least six hours after intercourse, until all the sperm in the vagina die. Diaphragms are generally around 94% effective and caps around 89% – if used every time and inserted correctly. Spermicide can also be used, but this does not seem to make them more effective.

Check your diaphragm or cap regularly for holes by holding it up to the light, and make sure it does not feel tacky, as this means the rubber is perishing. Wash it after removing it with warm water and a mild soap; rinse and dry carefully, and store in its container away from heat. Some women use a little cornflour to keep it dry. *Never* use perfumed talc.

Side effects: None, unless you are allergic to rubber.

Breastfeeding: Diaphragms and caps can be used when breastfeeding, but not with spermicide.

Advantages:
- They are washable and reusable, usually lasting up to two years.
- Can be worn continuously, and just removed once every 24 hours for washing, before being replaced. Make sure it is more than six hours since last having sex.

- Can be worn while menstruating, but should only be left in for 12 hours at a time.
- Doesn't interrupt sexual spontaneity if already in.
- May be used with the man wearing a condom as well, if you want extra protection.
- Can be stopped at any time to conceive another baby.

Disadvantages:
- Need to be fitted for correct size by a health professional experienced in doing this.
- May need to be refitted after having a baby, or gaining or losing more than 5 kg in weight.
- May not last for two years if worn continuously.
- May take some practice for the woman to insert correctly.

The minipill

The minipill contains small amounts of progesterone hormone and is taken by the woman every day. It makes the mucus in her cervix very thick, so sperm cannot enter the uterus to fertilise an egg. If an egg is fertilised, the minipill also thins the lining of the uterus and slows the passage of the egg down the fallopian tube so it is less likely to implant and survive. For some women it stops ovulation.

The minipill is about 96% effective, but more than 99% effective if you are fully breastfeeding and each pill is taken within three hours of the usual time every day. It may not work if you have diarrhoea and/or vomiting, or if taking certain medications (such as antibiotics). You need to use alternative contraception (such as condoms) while taking the medications, and for seven days after stopping, while continuing to take the minipill. Check with your doctor or family planning service.

Side effects: Possibly irregular menstrual periods or no periods at all, or light spotting between periods. If the minipill fails to prevent a pregnancy, it is more likely to be ectopic. Let your caregiver know straight away if you think you might be pregnant. Occasionally, the minipill can cause an ovarian cyst, with low abdominal pain, similar to an ectopic pregnancy – again, see your doctor. A few women notice a slight weight gain, nausea, headaches and/or a loss of libido.

Breastfeeding: The minipill can be taken while breastfeeding, but is not started until three to six weeks after giving birth. A very small amount of progesterone can pass through breast milk, but at this stage it is not thought to affect the baby.

Advantages:
- It can be used instead of the normal pill while breastfeeding. You may choose to swap to the normal pill once you stop breastfeeding, or continue using the minipill if you prefer.
- It is safer than the normal pill if you smoke, have high blood pressure or a family history of blood clotting abnormalities, strokes or heart attacks.
- It can be stopped at any time to conceive another baby, with fertility returning within two to four weeks.

Disadvantages:
- It needs to be prescribed by a doctor.
- It is not recommended if you have had a previous ectopic pregnancy.
- You need to be *very* strict about taking it on time. If you are more than three hours late, take the minipill when you remember and then take the next one at the usual time. Use alternative contraception (such as condoms) for 48 hours.

Progesterone injections

Progesterone hormone can be given as an injection to the woman, called DMPA. It lasts for 12 to 14 weeks before another injection is given to continue the contraception. DMPA works by stopping ovulation, as well as thickening the mucus in the cervix to prevent sperm from entering, and thinning the lining of the uterus to discourage implantation. It is about 99.8% effective.

Side effects: Possibly irregular menstrual periods or no periods, or light spotting between periods. Periods may last longer when they do come, but are not heavier. The longer you continue DMPA, the more likely you will not have periods. Some women experience significant weight gain, headaches, loss of libido and/or depression.

Breastfeeding: You can use DMPA while breastfeeding, but it is not started until three to six weeks after giving birth. Some progesterone can pass to the baby through breast milk, but long-term studies of children up to teenage years have not shown any effects on their growth, intelligence or development.

Advantages:
- No need to remember to take a pill every day.
- It is more effective than the minipill.
- Decreases the risk of breast cancer.

Disadvantages:
- It needs to be prescribed and administered by a health professional.
- If you don't like the side effects you need to wait three months for the injection to wear off.
- It can delay the return of fertility (and normal periods) for as long as 10 to 18 months after the last injection wears off. DMPA is not recommended if you wish to have another baby within 12 to 18 months.
- May not be recommended if you have previously suffered from depression.

The pill

The pill contains a combination of oestrogen and progesterone hormones. It is taken daily by the woman for 21 days, usually followed by a break (or taking sugar pills) for 7 days. The break triggers a withdrawal bleed, or pretend period. The pill works by stopping ovulation and is more than 96 to 99% effective if taken correctly. It may not work if you have diarrhoea and/or vomiting or if taking certain medications (such as antibiotics). You need to use alternative contraception (such as condoms) while taking the medications, and for seven days after stopping, while continuing to take the pill. Check with your doctor or family planning service.

Side effects: Each woman reacts differently to different types of pills but side effects may include nausea, sore breasts, spotting in between periods, feeling bloated, weight gain, feeling irritable or depressed, and/or a loss of libido. Many side effects can subside after three months of use. Otherwise the type of pill may need to be changed.

The pill can cause patchy, brown discolouration on the face (chloasma), which may take months to fade after stopping. Wear a hat and use factor 30+ sunscreen. Rare, but severe, side effects are generally caused by an increase in blood clotting (eg. chest pain, thrombosis, blurred vision, severe headache). If this happens, seek medical attention immediately.

Breastfeeding: Not recommended until the baby is fully weaned.

Advantages:
- Regular, lighter periods.
- Possibly less pre-menstrual tension and/or less acne (if you experience these).
- You can take the pill continuously, without the seven day break, if you don't want a menstrual period.
- Health benefits include reducing the chances of cysts on the ovary, anaemia, ovarian cancer and cancer of the endometrium.

Disadvantages:
- It needs to be prescribed by a doctor, having blood pressure checks every 12 months.
- It may take a bit of trial and error, taking different types of pills for three months at a time, until you find the right one.
- You need to remember to take it. If you are more than 12 hours late, take the pill when you remember and then take the next one at the usual time. Use alternative contraception (such as condoms) for seven days.
- Your fertility usually returns within one to four months after stopping the pill.
- It may not be recommended if you smoke, have previously suffered from migraines, high blood pressure, liver or kidney problems or severe depression. You should stop the pill four to six weeks before a major operation.

Implanon

Implanon is a small, thin, plastic rod, about the size of a matchstick (40 mm long and 2 mm wide), containing progesterone hormone. It is inserted underneath the woman's skin, usually on the inside of her upper arm, using local anaesthetic. Implanon works in a similar way to progesterone injections, by stopping ovulation, thinning the lining of the uterus and thickening the mucus in the cervix. It lasts for three years, unless removed before this time and is more than 99% effective. About 0.1% of implants are inserted incorrectly, making them ineffective.

Side effects: Possibly irregular, light spotting, or frequent bleeding. A few women experience acne, headaches, weight gain, breast tenderness, dizziness, depression and/or loss of libido. There may be some bruising around the insertion site for a week or so afterwards.

Breastfeeding: At this stage, Implanon is not officially licensed for use during breastfeeding in Australia, but it is thought not to have effects on the baby, similar to progesterone injections.

Advantages:
- Set and forget; no pills or repeated injections.
- After removal, fertility usually returns to normal within three to four weeks.

Disadvantages:
- It needs to be inserted and removed by a doctor trained to do this. (Many GPs can insert them.)
- The effectiveness may wear off after two years for women who are overweight for their height.

Emergency pills

Emergency pills contain high doses of progesterone hormone. They work by delaying ovulation, if this has not occurred yet in the menstrual cycle. If an egg has been fertilised, the pills can prevent it from implanting in the lining of the uterus. Emergency pills used to be called morning after pills, but they can be taken much later than the next morning. The first of two doses must be taken within 120 hours (5 days) of unprotected sex; the second dose is taken 12 hours later. However, the sooner you take them the more effective they are – 98.4 to 99.9% effective within 24 hours; 97 to 99.7% effective within 25 to 48 hours; 93.9 to 99.1% effective within 49 to 72 hours; and 87.5% effective after 72 hours.

Side effects: You may have some vaginal bleeding for a few days afterwards, otherwise nothing really noticeable. Most women have a normal period at the expected time (if not fully breastfeeding and naturally missing periods).

Breastfeeding: May be used. Some progesterone can pass to the baby through breast milk. At this stage it is thought that this does not affect the baby. Some women choose to express and discard their breast milk for 24 hours and give their baby stored breast milk or formula instead.

Advantages:
- They can be used with unplanned unprotected sex, or with mishaps such as a broken condom or taking out a diaphragm too early.
- They can be used more than once in the same menstrual cycle if necessary. Although this should be avoided, if possible.
- They are now available over-the-counter at pharmacies in Australia.

Disadvantages: Unlike male and female condoms, and the pill, emergency pills are not ideal as a main form of contraception. They are strictly for emergencies only.

Intrauterine device (IUD)

An IUD is small, flexible plastic device with a fine nylon string attached. It is placed inside the uterus by a doctor using local anaesthetic, with the string left protruding just outside the cervix (but still within the vagina).

The two most common types are:
- Copper IUD – This has fine copper wire wrapped around the stem to stop sperm surviving in the womb. It also affects the lining of the uterus, preventing the egg from implanting, and is 95 to 98% effective.
- Progestogen IUD – This contains progesterone hormone, which thins the lining of the uterus to prevent a fertilised egg implanting, thickens

mucus in the cervix to prevent sperm from entering, and may stop ovulation for up to 30% of women. It is more than 99% effective.

Side effects: A copper IUD can sometimes make menstrual periods heavier and more painful. A progestogen IUD may cause irregular spotting and lighter periods for the first six months, becoming less frequent or no periods after this time. Progestogen IUDs may also cause vaginal dryness, flushes, headaches, nausea, acne or mood changes in a few women.

Both types have a small risk of causing an infection of the uterus within a week or so after insertion. Occasionally the IUD can fall out within a few weeks of insertion. You can feel the string with your finger to check it is still in place. Rarely, the IUD can pass into, or through, the wall of the uterus during insertion.

If a pregnancy does occur with an IUD, there is a higher chance it will be ectopic. If the pregnancy is in the uterus (confirmed with an ultrasound), the IUD should be removed as soon as possible and there is a 30% chance of miscarriage.

Breastfeeding: Both types of IUDs can be used while breastfeeding. A very small amount of progesterone can pass to the baby through breast milk with progestogen IUDs. At this stage it is thought that this does not affect the baby (similar to the minipill).

Advantages:
- They are set and forget, and can be left in place for five years or more, or removed before this time if you want to conceive another baby.
- After removal, fertility usually returns by the next menstrual cycle.

Disadvantages:
- They need to be inserted and removed by a doctor experienced in doing this.
- They cannot be used if you have large fibroids or an unusual-shaped uterus.
- Not recommended if you have different sexual partners, due to an increased risk of sexually transmitted infections causing a uterine infection.
- Not generally recommended if you want to have another baby within 12 to 18 months.

Natural family planning

Natural family planning (NFP) involves the woman observing physical signs daily (eg. vaginal mucus, temperature, position of her cervix) and perhaps using a commercial ovulation predictor kit, to determine her fertile phase each month (see Chapter 1) and avoid sexual intercourse when it is 'unsafe'. Sometimes condoms or a diaphragm are used during unsafe times to prevent pregnancy. This method is thought to be about 94% effective, depending on how well the woman interprets her physical signs and how disciplined a couple are at abstaining from sex. Some couples use other forms of sexual expression during unsafe times instead of intercourse.

Side effects: None.

Breastfeeding: Natural family planning can be used while breastfeeding. However, ovulation may not occur for several months. Vaginal mucus changes and the absence of periods while breastfeeding makes it difficult to tell when it is unsafe to have sex. Generally, changes in the cervix (becoming soft, open and high in the few days just before ovulation) are the most reliable predictors.

Advantages: Using natural family planning as a method of contraception does not require medications or devices that could affect a woman's health or her fertility.

Disadvantages:
- Couples need to be committed and disciplined, and should attend a natural family planning course to help them understand the physical signs and how to interpret them accurately.
- If using ovulation predictor kits, this can be expensive and they are not always reliable.
- The woman cannot have sex when her libido is usually at its highest.

Male sterilisation – vasectomy

Vasectomy is a simple operation involving cutting and tying the two vas deferens tubes inside the scrotum at the top of each testicle. This prevents sperm getting into a man's semen. Local anaesthetic is used but sometimes sedation or a general anaesthetic is recommended. After a vasectomy the man still ejaculates and has normal sexual function. It takes about 16 ejaculations to clear the remaining sperm, with new, unused sperm being reabsorbed back into his body. Alternative contraception (such as condoms) needs to be used for two months, until a specimen of semen is tested to make sure no sperm are present. About 1 in every 500 to 1000 vasectomies fail because the tubes aren't fully closed or they grow back together; or very rarely the man has three vas deferens and one is missed.

NOTE: *A man does not need his partner's permission to have a vasectomy.*

Side effects: Some swelling, pain and bruising of the groin and/or testicles for a few days. Occasionally, bleeding or an infection can develop after the operation. Very rarely, pain in the groin area continues for several months. This usually improves over time, or may require another operation to try to rectify it.

Breastfeeding: Not applicable.

Advantages:
- It is a permanent form of contraception.
- It allays concerns about conceiving an unwanted pregnancy.

Disadvantages:
- It requires an operation and possibly a few days off work, if your job entails strenuous physical activity. Normal activity is fine.
- It is not easily reversed. Even if the tubes can be put back together successfully, the sperm may no longer be capable of fertilising a woman's egg. You need to be *very* sure that you do not want any more children. Take into consideration if an existing child dies, or if your current relationship ends.
- It often involves a period of grief for the loss of your fertility, which is normal, even though you do not want any more children.

Female sterilisation – tubal occlusion

Tubal occlusion involves an operation to close off the woman's fallopian tubes so that sperm cannot reach her eggs at ovulation. Unused eggs are reabsorbed into her body. It does not affect a woman's sexuality, her menstrual cycle or menopause. The tubes are either cut and tied, burnt with electrolysis or closed off with clips or rings through a laparoscopy or abdominal incision, using a general anaesthetic. You may need to stay overnight in hospital. About 2 to 9 per 1000 operations fail (soon after the operation or years later). If a pregnancy does occur, it is more likely to be ectopic.

Essure is a new method of occlusion, which uses two small soft, flexible, titanium wires. They are inserted into the fallopian tubes via the vagina with a local anaesthetic, taking about 30 minutes. It then takes three months for tissue to grow over them to totally block off the tubes (confirmed by a pelvic X-ray); other contraception needs to be continued until the tubes are completely blocked. Essure has a less than 1% failure rate.

Side effects: With a laparoscopy, abdominal and shoulder tip pain are common for a couple of days. You may react to the general anaesthetic with nausea and feeling lethargic for a few days. Occasionally bleeding or an infection can occur after the operation. With Essure, there may be some light bleeding and mild cramping for a day or so, but you should be able to return to normal activities the next day.

NOTE: *A woman does not need her partner's permission to have a tubal occlusion.*

Breastfeeding: You can have a tubal occlusion while breastfeeding, but you may wish to wait until your child is 12 months old or so, before making a decision not to have any more children.

Advantages:
- It is a permanent form of contraception.
- If having a laparoscopy, it is effective immediately afterwards.
- It allays concerns about conceiving an unwanted pregnancy.

Disadvantages:
- A laparoscopy requires at least one week's recovery time.
- Not easily reversed. Even if the tubes can be opened again, a pregnancy may not be possible, or an ectopic pregnancy is more likely. You need to be *very* sure that you don't want any more children. Take into consideration if an existing child dies, or if your current relationship ends.
- May entail a period of grief for the loss of your fertility, which is normal, even though you do not want any more children.

Settling in with your new baby

It is common to worry that your baby is not behaving the way they should, although their behaviour usually has more to do with their individual personality than what you are or aren't doing. Most babies don't move into a regular, predictable pattern until 8 to 12 weeks, so going with the flow, and knowing it will eventually change, can help keep your sanity in the early weeks.

Newborns sleep about 16 to 19 hours a day, but not all at once. When awake, they feed and may be unsettled or cry, not wanting to be entertained for long. Their feeding and sleep cycles are constantly changing, making baby-led, or demand, feeding the best way to encourage them into a predictable routine. If you try to feed a baby who is not ready, they won't feed well and will wake sooner for another feed. If feeds are put off because it is too soon after the last one, the baby may be too exhausted from excessive crying to feed well. Very young babies are not trying to manipulate you, they are simply relying on their survival instincts. Therefore, accepting their behaviour rather than trying to change it usually makes everyone feel better about what is going on.

Babies need to know that their needs will be met. Leaving your baby to cry before they are six months old in the hope they will fall asleep does not build trust and only makes them more tired and frustrated, and therefore more likely to cry. When your baby is older than six months you may choose controlled crying techniques (now called 'controlled comforting'), which try to teach them to fall asleep by themselves. This is not proven to be detrimental to a child's psychological health and is entirely a personal choice.

Did you know?
Newborn babies cry for an average of 1.6 hours every 24 hours, ranging from 30 minutes to 3 hours!

SLEEPING AND FEEDING PATTERNS

Newborns normally bunch up feeds at certain times and spread them out at others. The most common pattern over a 24-hour period has 3 phases:
1. **Regular phase** – The baby has two or three feeds, three to four hours apart.
2. **Wakeful phase** – The baby feeds frequently (or constantly) every one to two hours, over two to six hours, and is unsettled and crying.
3. **Sleeping phase** – The baby sleeps for four to six hours, before starting the regular phase again.

Did you know?
The length of time between feeds is measured from the beginning of one feed to the beginning of the next feed. So if you start feeding at 3 pm (for 1 hour) and the next feed starts at 6 pm, they are 3 hours apart.

Young babies can't tell night from day and their wakeful phase may be from midnight till 4 am, until their biorhythms adapt. Over time the wakeful phase slowly moves to the early evenings, sometime between 4 pm and 11 pm. Some subtle things you can do at night to let your baby know it is time for sleep include:
- Feeding by dimmed light. Some women use a torch to change and organise their baby, then turn the light off to feed.
- Turning off music or the TV (or wearing headphones).
- Limiting eye contact and communication to let your baby know it is not a time to play.
- Only changing your baby's nappy if it is very wet or soiled. Otherwise wait till morning.
- Sleeping with your baby and/or feeding them in bed.

Sleep cycles

Everyone has repetitive sleep cycles. Adults and children average 90 to 100 minutes, but newborns average 40 to 50 minutes. Each sleep cycle is made up of phases:

- **Light non-REM sleep** – This comprises two stages. Stage 1 is smooth breathing and relaxation, and stage 2 is drifting into sound sleep. Babies appear drowsy and very relaxed, their eyelids droop and their eyes may roll upwards.
- **Deep non-REM sleep** – This is a deep sleep that contributes to you feeling rested and rejuvenated. Babies lie very still, in a complete state of relaxation.
- **Rapid eye movement sleep** – REM sleep is the time when we dream and have increased brain activity. Researchers believe this is important for the baby's brain development. Babies can twitch their limbs, move their entire body and breathe irregularly and sometimes slightly faster. They may grimace, make faces, smile or mimic chewing or sucking actions, and their eyelids can flutter.
- **Wake phase** – At the end of each REM phase there is a brief waking period. Adults often don't recall this phase because they have learnt to fall back to sleep. Newborns need to learn how to do this. However, in many cases they wake completely and cry for attention.

GETTING YOUR BABY TO SLEEP

One of the biggest challenges for new parents is getting their baby to sleep. The trick is to recognise your baby's tired signs, which can take a little experience, and then act on them to help your baby wind down and fall asleep with a minimum of fuss. Tired signs can include:

- Grunting, grizzling, fussing, whimpering, whinging or intermittently crying.
- Sucking their fists more than usual, for comfort.
- Yawning.
- Jerky or thrashing limb movements, or a slowing down of movements.
- Turning away from distractions or becoming more irritable and upset.
- Frowning.

Trying to keep your baby awake only irritates and overstimulates them; it then takes longer for them to fall asleep. Babies do not appreciate having a toy jangled in their face or being passed from person to person when tired – just as you wouldn't.

NOTE: *A few babies are 'happy wakers' and do not show typical signs of tiredness, or just become less responsive, although not necessarily complaining or upset. It can take a while to recognise this behaviour and it may mean you need to put your baby in their bed to sleep in a regular routine rather than waiting for obvious tired signs. Babies like this still need their sleep – they just don't show it as much.*

Sleep cues
To help your baby go to sleep, you can start using sleep cues to calm and relax them. Hopefully these cues will create a trigger, or body memory, to remind your baby it is time for sleep. If cues are consistently repeated, the baby starts to respond positively, with the most favoured cue being suckling (on the breast, bottle, thumb or dummy), because this relaxes, comforts and tires them. Other cues include:
- Rocking or walking them, or pushing them in a pram.
- Rhythmically patting their bottom or thigh, rubbing their belly or stroking their head.
- Driving them around the block, but be aware of starting a cue you do not plan or wish to continue! A quick-fix solution can quickly turn into an unwanted burden.

If you wish to introduce a new cue, understand that your baby may be confused for a while, and is likely to cry until they adapt, which may take up to seven days.

Cues are usually used until *after* the baby falls asleep, so they may wake suddenly if the cue stops, or wake every one to two hours at the end of each sleep cycle, looking for their preferred cue (often disturbing their parents in the process). Again, this is because they haven't yet learnt to get back to sleep by themselves.

Parents of newborns often resort to just about anything for a bit of extra sleep. If your baby becomes reliant on an inconvenient cue, it may be easier to put up with it for a while until you get to the point that it is a pressing issue for you – that way you will be more committed to changing the cue.

Sleep associations
Sleep associations are physical interactions, routines or sounds that help your baby wind down and relax, letting them know it is time for sleep. Sleep associations need to be started when you think your baby is tired, and generally end with putting them in their bed once relaxed but still awake, so they can drift off to sleep on their own. After a while the interactions become an accepted routine that the baby responds to favourably.

Sleep associations aim to prevent babies from waking frequently at the end of each sleep cycle, so they don't disturb you. You can start incorporating them in the early weeks by taking your baby off the breast (or taking the

bottle away) just before they fall asleep, and then placing them in bed to see if they go to sleep by themselves. Other sleep associations include:
- An evening wind-down routine of a bath (and/or massage), sitting quietly and enjoying a cuddle.
- Wrapping them snugly so they are not woken by jerky movements.
- Playing a piece of rhythmic, calming music, or talking or singing to them.
- Initially using cues (like rocking them), until they become still and quiet, then putting them in bed while awake.

After placing your baby in bed, say goodnight and quietly leave them, avoiding eye contact. Be consistent. Chopping and changing will only confuse your baby. However, you may set up one routine for daytime sleeps and another for the evening bedtime ritual. A good guide is to commit to something for at least seven days; if there is no improvement, consider trying something new. Also, think about what you can do when away from home, and get others who care for your baby to continue these associations.

NOTE: *When a baby is overstimulated and tired they may need to have a good cry for a few minutes when you first put them to bed, to help release, relax and wind down. Of course, if their crying continues, or escalates, you will need to attend to them (until they're old enough to be taught to sleep – if this is your choice).*

It helps if you are flexible with your chosen sleep associations. They are not guaranteed to work every time. If the things you try are not working, this is not a reflection on your parenting, and it doesn't mean they won't work if you try them again at a later stage.

SETTLING YOUR CRYING BABY

New babies communicate by crying and the sound is designed to irritate you so you meet their needs promptly and make the crying stop. Learning how to interpret your baby's hungry cry, tired cry or just a cuddle-me cry can take a little time, but it is normal for a baby to cry:
- Irritably when being changed.
- Upsettingly when being undressed or bathed.
- Intensely if hungry, or their needs are not met fast enough.
- In a bored or hollow way if wanting comfort or entertainment.
- By grunting, grizzling, whinging, or growling if overtired, gradually increasing to a full cry.
- Monotonously when having fussy periods, or more intensely if put to bed at these times.

Most babies have short periods of unexplained crying and 20 to 30% cry for prolonged periods for no apparent reason. Thankfully, this is usually a two to three month phase that your baby grows out of. However, when your baby does cry for no clear reason, and nothing you try soothes or settles them, it can be very upsetting and frustrating; however, it does not mean you are doing anything wrong.

Colic

Unsettled behaviour is commonly misdiagnosed as colic, but it is now recognised as very normal for up to 85% of babies. One theory is that the baby's nervous system is still maturing and can only cope with a certain amount of stimulation, so that by the end of the day, their system overloads, triggering a period of active, irritable, fussy and crying behaviour. This would explain why:
- Crying and unsettled periods tend to happen in predictable cycles.
- It is very hard to comfort babies when they are like this.
- Suggested treatments for 'colic' rarely succeed.
- Babies eventually grow out of it.

Suggesting that colic is due to an undersupply of breast milk is usually incorrect, and weaning a baby to formula, or changing formula brands, generally does not resolve it.

NOTE: If your baby cries intensely and inconsolably, or has a continually high-pitched scream for long periods (an hour or more), you should seek medical attention to make sure they are not ill. **Never** *give your baby sedative medications without the advice of your caregiver.*

Support strategies for crying

If you've changed, fed and burped your baby and they are still crying, perhaps try:
- Cuddling and holding them close in an upright position. Perhaps place them into a baby pouch or sling.
- Breastfeeding them more if they are interested. (If bottle feeding, don't offer unlimited amounts of formula; use a dummy, or allow them to suck their hand.)
- Breathing! When babies cry, parents tend to intermittently hold their breath and tense up. Use your out breath to relax your face, jaw and throat. Drop your shoulders and take your awareness to your body to identify any tense areas.
- Using rhythmic motions of rocking or walking, or use a cradle, pram or rocking chair to do this. Keep your rhythm smooth and slow and your touch gentle and relaxed.
- Laying your baby tummy down across your lap and gently rubbing their back or patting their bottom with a relaxed, rhythmic patting action.

- Quietening the environment or playing soft music.
- Going out for a walk to help you to cope.
- Giving them a relaxing bath or massage, or take a bath together.
- Realising you are in survival mode and letting go of housework.
- Calling in support (your partner, family or friends). You are only human.
- Resting whenever possible; avoid overcommitting yourself.

If you feel you are getting to breaking point, put your baby down somewhere safe (their cot) and go into another room, or outside, for a short time. Breathe deeply, cry if you need to, and gather your thoughts for a few minutes before going back. A baby's prolonged crying can be physically, mentally and emotionally draining, often crushing your confidence and self-esteem in the process. It is important to recognise if you feel you may hurt them in some way, either as an immediate reaction or in mistakenly thinking it is safe, such as shaking them in frustration. Vigorously shaking a baby can cause serious damage to their fragile brain, in some cases killing them.

NOTE: *There is no evidence that playing with a baby by throwing them in the air, bouncing them on your knee or jostling them playfully causes shaken baby syndrome.*

If you are afraid you may hurt your baby, phone your partner, a family member or friend and tell them *exactly* how you are feeling. For immediate support and advice within Australia, call the toll free **Cryline 1800 066 777 (24 hours)**.

CARING FOR TWINS, TRIPLETS OR MORE

Caring for multiples requires a lot more work and organisation. In the beginning you will probably muddle your way through, but as time goes by, you will become more skilled and organised, but you still need plenty of help. If you try to do everything yourself, you will only become emotionally and physically exhausted, which is no good for you or your babies.

Individual or synchronised routines

You may decide to care for your babies as individuals, or try to slowly coax them into similar routines. Whatever you decide, be flexible and willing to adjust, in case your preference is not working. Or just try it again at a later time.

Individual routines – Each baby has their own routines, habits, preferences and idiosyncrasies (even identical twins). Therefore, you might want to allow your babies to wake, sleep and feed to their own personal schedules. However, this can sometimes be difficult (or near impossible) to keep up with, unless you have help.

Synchronised routines – To encourage your babies to get into similar routines, you can try the following:
- When one baby is hungry, wake the other(s) soon after to feed.
- In the beginning, keep a daily written schedule of what each baby is doing. You may see similar patterns emerging and can wake one baby a little earlier, to be more like the other(s).
- When one baby is ready to sleep, try settling all the babies together.
- Be aware that one unsettled baby can prevent the others from going to sleep. Consider separating them when sleeping if this is happening frequently.

Support strategies
- Don't worry about bathing every baby each day. Top and tail them or bath every few days (or alternate days with each baby).
- Don't worry if the housework is left undone. It is enough that your babies are happy and well cared for.
- Have baby equipment in every room to save legwork and minimise the need to leave your babies so you can fetch things.
- Don't get caught up in having separate pieces of equipment (dummies, bottles, etc) for each baby. Siblings are in such close proximity to each other, their germs are permanently shared.
- If your partner is helping, take turns in caring for your babies so that one of you is refreshed.
- If you need a shower and your babies are awake, place them in bouncers in the bathroom with you, or do this while you are hanging out the washing.
- Get out of the house as often as you can. We know this is not easy, but fresh air and human contact is worth the effort.

Emotional considerations
Caring for multiples is rewarding, challenging and a shock – all at the same time. In the early months it can often seem like a relentless chain of work, tiring, isolating and at times depressing. Trips out of the house can seem like planning a military campaign and babysitters are thin on the ground.

You may feel constantly guilty if you think your babies (or partner) aren't getting all the attention they need, or perhaps resentful that your partner can walk out the door and go to work. Fathers can also feel overwhelmed, or unappreciated in their working role. (Read the relationship survival tips earlier in this chapter.) However, caring for your babies can create wonderful feelings of accomplishment and pride. Watching them grow, interact and entertain each other can make you feel very privileged to have them.

Lifestyle and breastfeeding

Expressing and storing breast milk

Expressing breast milk while breastfeeding means coordinating this in between your baby's feeds. Ideally you should express days (or weeks) in advance, so it is less stressful and you can practise it. Aim to restrict your expressing to relaxed days at home, or when your baby is relatively settled. A good guide is to express 20 to 80 ml once or twice a day, and slowly banking up a stored supply.

If expressing all of your baby's feeds, a regular regime is required to keep up your milk supply, generally at least six to eight times in 24 hours. You can express two to four hours during the day and evening, and then have a six-hour sleep overnight.

When away from your baby for more than four hours, express milk to keep up your supply and to replace the milk your baby drank in your absence. If at work, try to express at least twice in an 8 to 10 hour period. If you are only away for a few hours, express when you get home if your baby isn't crying for a feed.

How much milk?

Breastfed babies drink variable amounts at each feed, ranging from 60 to 180 ml. One way to leave your baby's carer with enough milk is to divide it into smaller portions before storing, so more can be heated up if needed. This also avoids discarding large amounts of precious unused milk. If you are unable to supply enough expressed breast milk, you may need to make up the rest with formula.

The amount of breast milk you can express at each session may depend on factors such as:

- **Your individual body** – Some women express 40 to 100 ml (or more), others find it hard to get anything at all, or only 20 to 30 ml at a time. Babies are more efficient at removing milk from your breast, so there is plenty there, it is just not easy to express. Check with your early childhood nurse to make sure you are expressing correctly.
- **Whether you have breastfed, or expressed, within the last hour** – There is generally less milk available than if you waited for two to three hours (or more).
- **How old your baby is** – The amount you produce initially increases as your baby grows, but decreases once they have solid foods and/or formula supplements.
- **How often you express** – The more frequently you express, the more

milk you make over the following 24 to 48 hours. However, if expressing all your baby's feeds, your supply may be low at times. Try swapping from one breast to the other frequently during an expressing session (every 2 to 7 minutes) with shorter expression times (10 to 20 minutes) every 2 to 4 hours.
- **Your let-down reflex** – This may not happen as readily when expressing, perhaps because it is harder to relax. You can try using warm compresses on your breasts, looking at a photo of your baby or smelling a piece of their clothing and/or listening to relaxing music. (See Chapter 13 for more strategies.)
- **The time of day** – Milk production fluctuates, with generally more milk in the mornings and less in the evenings.
- **Your state of mind** – You may have less milk when you are ill, run-down, exercising too rigorously, dieting, anxious, depressed, grieving or trying to do too much.

Hand expressing

Using your hands to express breast milk may take a while to master, and many women find it initially frustrating and tedious. However, if shown the proper technique and with practice, you will eventually get the knack. The advantages are that it:
- Costs nothing and is convenient.
- Can be done anywhere, any time.
- Can be used to express small amounts of milk to relieve overfull breasts or to gently rub milk onto sore nipples.
- Involves skin-to-skin contact, which stimulates a greater milk supply and triggers a let-down reflex.

You'll need a sterile receptacle to express into (a bowl or plastic takeaway container, or express directly into a bottle). Follow these steps:
1. Wash your hands, find a quiet, private place and make yourself comfortable. Have a glass of water handy, as expressing (and breastfeeding) naturally triggers your thirst.
2. Try to stimulate a let-down reflex (see Chapter 13). If it is not noticeable within a few minutes, start expressing anyway.
3. Place the thumb of the hand you are expressing with on the top edge of the areola (above the nipple), where the darker skin meets the normal skin of the breast. Place the next two fingers of that hand underneath the nipple, but back from it, so that these fingers lie on the underside edge of the areola. If your breast is large, you may want to

place your other hand under it for support, but well back and clear of the nipple and areola.
4. Okay, now you are ready to start. Using your thumb and other two fingers, push them back into the breast tissue, and then firmly compress the areola with your thumb and fingers. Release the compression (without moving your fingers off the areola) and repeat the action. Push in and compress. Continue this in a rhythmical cycle. Adjust your fingers slightly if it helps to get a better flow.
5. Pour your expressed milk into a plastic bottle or container for storage.

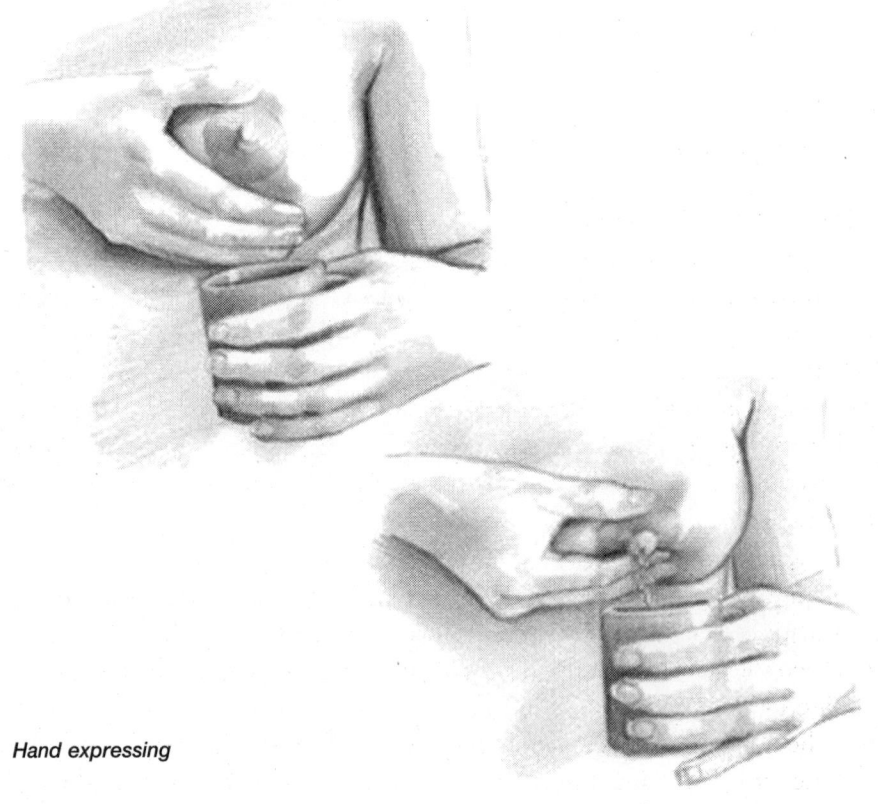

Hand expressing

NOTE: *Avoid pinching or squeezing the actual nipple. You may want to rotate your fingers to other parts of the areola (say, each side of the nipple), or swap hands or start expressing from the other breast if one position becomes tiring or awkward, or the milk flow slows.*

Breast pumps

There are many types of pumps on the market, usually manual or battery operated. Ask your caregiver, or talk with other women about what they used. If you are expressing all the time, you may choose to hire (or buy) an electric pump (through your hospital, a pharmacy or a local branch of the Australian Breastfeeding Association). The pump you choose should come with a set of instructions. If you are unsure, ask your caregiver or early childhood nurse to show you.

- The pump needs to be cleaned and sterilised before and after each use (it remains sterile for 24 hours).
- Make sure your nipple is centred in the middle of the nipple cover to avoid damaging the nipples. Hold it fairly firmly in place to create a seal. If the milk flow slows, reposition it slightly, or swap to the other breast. Avoid having too much suction pressure.
- Use the same techniques for stimulating a let-down as you would for hand expressing.
- Always have frequent rests and suction cycles, to mimic breastfeeding. (Battery-operated and electric pumps do this automatically.)

Storing expressed breast milk

Breast milk can be stored in plastic bottles, containers or disposable milk pouches (available at pharmacies). Do not use glass, as anti-infective agents and proteins stick to it, depriving your baby. When left to stand (or after freezing), breast milk separates into layers, with the thin white milk settling on the bottom, and the creamier, yellow milk forming on the top. It is normal for stored breast milk to have tiny white clumps in it, especially once defrosted. This does not mean the milk is off. If you have expressed and stored your milk correctly, it is safe for your baby to drink.

When banking your milk bit by bit:
- Express the first amount and place it into a sterilised container. Label it with the date and time (you can write on masking tape).
- Place the expressed milk in the fridge to cool before placing it in the freezer.
- When you next express, place the warm milk in the fridge to cool. Once it is cold, add it to the frozen milk. You can continue to add to previously frozen milk for up to one week after expressing.

Fresh breast milk can last for up to:
- Three to five days in the back of the body of the fridge (not the door of the fridge).
- Two weeks in a freezer compartment inside a fridge (a common design in smaller fridges).
- Three months in a separate freezer section of a fridge (with its own door).

- Six months in a deep freezer (at less than 0°C).

NOTE: *This is counted from the time of the first expression, if banking your milk.*
Previously frozen and thawed breast milk can last for up to:
- One hour at room temperature.
- 12 to 24 hours in the body of the fridge.

Any unused breast milk should be discarded after this time. If your baby does not finish the bottle within one hour, the remainder must be discarded. You cannot refreeze unused breast milk once it has been defrosted.

Defrosting and warming stored breast milk

Freshly expressed breast milk can be given at room temperature. Cooled milk in a bottle from the fridge can be stood in a container of warm water for a few minutes. If the milk is frozen, defrost it by placing the bottle into a container of hot (or fairly warm) water from the tap, or placing it in the fridge for a few hours, before placing in a container of warm water. (**Never** microwave breast milk; this affects its nutritional value.) Always test the temperature of the milk by dripping some on your arm before giving it to your baby.

Support strategies
- Educate anyone looking after your baby about how to defrost and manage your expressed breast milk.
- Rotate your stored breast milk so that you use the oldest milk first and the freshest milk last.

BREASTFEEDING WHILE OUT AND ABOUT

Breastfeeding your baby when away from home is something you will need to do at some stage, although it may take a while before you feel confident enough to venture out. Even if your baby latches like a dream, it can still feel awkward breastfeeding in front of others. Some strategies other women have found helpful include:
- Practising how you will feed your baby at home. Learn to unclip (and clip) your bra with one hand under your top (while not looking and holding your baby).
- Taking a light scarf, shawl or muslin cloth to throw over your shoulder and your baby while feeding.
- Wear a top that pulls up, rather than a shirt that unbuttons. Dresses are not really practical, unless you can access your breasts easily.
- Feeding your baby before they become too distressed.

- Finding out about mothers' rooms in shopping centres, movie theatres and other places you visit. Perhaps ring beforehand. Many cafes/businesses now have 'Breastfeeding welcome here' stickers.
- Only socialising with family and friends who support you feeding your baby in front of them.

In most cases you can find a relatively private space to feed your baby (eg. a corner table in a restaurant, a park bench or the car). Be aware that it is not against the law in any State to breastfeed your baby in public.

Breastfeeding with work or study

If returning to work or study, you can still give your baby breast milk and breastfeed. The main advantage is that your baby will tend to be healthier and is less likely to get ill as well as continuing your special feeding relationship. Talk with your employer or lecturer about how you can facilitate this. By law, you should not be discriminated against because of your family responsibilities. Some workplaces are now accredited as breastfeeding-friendly by the Australian Breastfeeding Association.

A few things to consider are:
- Having a private room to express in.
- Having a fridge (or freezer) to store milk in each day. You also need an insulated bag to transport your milk.
- If childcare is on site or close by, consider going to your baby (or having them brought to you) for feeding.
- Delaying your return until your baby is having less breastfeeds and more solids (after six months). Perhaps work shorter hours, part-time or from home.
- Combining the use of formula with expressed breast milk if your milk supply is low.
- Giving expressed breast milk in a bottle occasionally before returning to work, to get your baby used to having a bottle.

Weaning your baby from the breast

If you wean your baby from the breast before they are 12 months old, you need to substitute formula milk until their first birthday. A few babies wean themselves, often for no apparent reason, which can be very distressing if you are not ready, but there is generally little you can do to stop this happening. Try to wean your baby slowly (unless advised otherwise by a health professional). Weaning rapidly can cause blocked ducts, mastitis or a breast abscess. If you do wean quickly, consider expressing small amounts of milk for comfort, and decreasing the frequency and amounts you express over days or weeks.

How quickly you stop breastfeeding depends on your baby's age, how many feeds they are having and how willing they are to give it up. If your baby is mostly breastfeeding (with not many solids), then allow up to four weeks. As a guide:

- Start with dropping the feed your baby relies on **least** and substitute this with a bottle (or cup) of formula. Your breasts may feel overfull for two to five days or so.
- When your breasts adjust, eliminate another feed. Again replace this one with formula and wait for your breasts to adjust. Then drop the third feed, and so on.
- You may prefer to stop one feed every second day for one week, then every day for the next week. Then stop a second feed every second day for the third week, and then every day for week four, and so on.
- If your baby is not accepting the bottle readily, plan to stop feeds that are due when your partner is around (or your baby is in childcare), or feed them while in their bed or bouncer so they are not in their familiar breastfeeding position.
- If you use breastfeeding to settle your baby to sleep, use other cues or sleep associations.
- If your baby is unwell, delay weaning until they are feeling better.

Returning to work or study

Partner returns

Fathers usually try to have some time off work around the birth of their baby. However, the unfortunate reality is that someone has to work to pay the bills, which inevitably creates a myriad of issues for both of you. As the time approaches, try to put aside some time to identify your concerns and prioritise each other's needs, depending on your work commitments. If running a business, aim to structure things to help facilitate the new family. Some strategies can be:

- Working from home for various periods of time.
- Limiting or delaying trips away for a while. Look at telephone and video conferencing options. If you do need to leave, make sure someone else can help your partner.

- Swapping shifts with co-workers.
- Staggering leave over a period of time.
- Taking paternal or family leave and/or working part-time. Look into long service leave or sabbaticals.
- Trying to leave work earlier, or accumulating a day off every week or two.

If you work from home, it can be a challenge to juggle your roles of partner, father and financial provider. Try to arrange your daily commitments around the needs of your family. Endeavour to set boundaries for when work starts and finishes, especially if you find it hard to drag yourself away.

Emotional considerations
As the father, you may feel:
- Sad to leave your new baby. Perhaps disappointed, if you miss their first smile, steps, etc.
- Resentment and pressure to be the provider.
- Relief to be back at work.
- A deep sense of guilt in leaving your partner to fend for herself.
- Frustrated or annoyed, if expected to care for your baby when you come home; perhaps shocked and overwhelmed by how much longer your working day is now.
- Excited and looking forward to seeing your new baby each day; feeling a new sense of purpose in your life.
- Glad you didn't take the option of being a stay-at-home dad.

As the mother, you may feel:
- Sadness and grief; the lovely babymoon is over and now it is time to cope with the real world; missing your partner's help, support and companionship.
- Isolated and very much alone.
- Overwhelmed and teary for the first day or so until you settle into a routine.
- Relief and contentment. You prefer to take the reins by yourself.
- Resentment that he can leave the house and return to his normal life.
- Uncomfortable or upset with the loss of financial control.

MOTHER RETURNS
When mothers return to work, they may be surprised at the emotional difficulties involved when leaving their baby. It can be very hard to do it all and

invariably you feel torn between your many roles. Juggling your career, running the household and caring for your baby (and possibly other children) means there is a never-ending list of things to do. Many working mothers find they learn to be highly organised because that's what it takes to keep the ball rolling every day.

Support strategies

Organising quality childcare is a priority. Knowing your baby is in good hands makes you feel more comfortable and less likely to worry. Here are some support strategies to consider:

- Leave your baby in care for a couple of hours at a time, or half-days, before returning to work to help you both adjust.
- Negotiate for flexibility at work. Job sharing, working part-time or from home may be options.
- If self-employed, consider setting up a nursery at work or perhaps employing a nanny at home or the office (if you can afford this).
- If studying, ask about taking your baby to tutorials, especially when they are young and tend to sleep a lot.
- Prepare everything in advance. Label your baby's bottles, dummies and clothes if using childcare. Get up a little earlier and allow an extra half-hour to prepare and say goodbye to your baby.
- Ring from work to find out how your baby is, especially if there were tears when you walked out the door.

Emotional considerations

It is normal to experience a rollercoaster of emotions when returning to work. Worrying about your baby and feeling guilty is pretty much par for the course. Fortunately, as everyone settles into the new routine, it becomes much easier. Some common emotions are dealt with in 'Stay-at-home dads' on the next page, others include:

- Having second thoughts about returning to work.
- Feeling tired and finding it hard to be a supermum.
- Concern, if your baby doesn't seem happy in childcare.
- Being unable to concentrate on work because of worry or guilt.
- Feeling frustrated and concerned because your baby is frequently ill and you need to take time off.
- Feeling upset if the carer is not doing everything the way you prefer.
- Being happy and content; feeling you are a better mother, with increased self-esteem.

STAY-AT-HOME DADS

Choosing to be a stay-at-home dad is something that may be approached with enthusiasm, uncertainty or perhaps reluctance. However, taking on the primary care role presents a unique chance to bond with your child, even though dealing with their day-to-day care can feel daunting (as it does for many women).

Surviving early parenthood in a female-dominated environment is the main challenge, along with moving against social expectations. Your friends, family and work colleagues may also find the concept confronting, perhaps making you feel the need to justify your choice (sometimes constantly) and possibly questioning your masculinity.

Planning support strategies and communicating openly with your partner can help make the transition easier for you both. Talk about how you both really feel, and regularly discuss and reassess the situation as you adjust to the arrangement. As the time draws near, many emotions can be experienced.

Emotions for the woman may include:
- Guilt. How can I leave my baby? Will they be all right? Am I a bad mother?
- Jealousy that your partner may have a closer relationship with your child.
- Tears, not wanting to leave. Am I doing the right thing?
- Concerned. Will my baby adjust to using a bottle (if breastfeeding)?
- Excitement or relief. You may look forward to, and enjoy, returning to work. There are many men who feel this way, so why shouldn't you?

Emotions for the father may include:
- Will I be able to do this? What if I can't cope?
- What will people think of me? Will I be able to ask for help?
- Will the baby take to the bottle easily (if normally breastfed)?
- Feeling alienated as a man in a woman's domain.
- Wishing it were you walking out the door and not her.
- Excited and privileged at the prospect of caring for your child.

Planning for your new role will help you to feel more in control of the situation and hopefully reduce any hiccups (metaphorically speaking anyway!):
- If breastfeeding, the mother needs to express and store her milk. If this is not working, you may need to accept that your baby has formula at times. Offer the baby a bottle on occasions during the weeks leading up to the mother's return to work so they get used to it.

- Familiarise yourself with the location of neighbouring chemists, doctors, hospitals, toy libraries, parks, supermarkets and your early childhood centre.
- Participate in local parents' groups, gymbaroo or infant swimming classes. Be prepared to be the solo man in the group.
- Find out if other fathers in your area are doing the same. Consider placing a local ad or posting on an online discussion forum.

When caring for your new baby, some common issues you may confront can include:
- Gaining acceptance by other mothers and from family and friends.
- Finding meaningful social support. Isolation can lead to depression. Seek help if you feel you are not coping. It is essential for your sanity to link up with other parents.
- Being prepared for the question 'What do you do?' and trying not to be defensive about it.
- Realising that caring for a baby is a lot of work. If you think otherwise, you're in for a shock.

Enjoy every hug and tickle and each smile your baby gives you, and watch your child blossoming from your love.

Variations

BREAST MILK SUPPLY

One of the main concerns for breastfeeding women is whether they have enough milk. This is often a false perception, but provoked by myths or well-meaning advice, which leads to many women giving up their breastfeeding early as a solution to a nonexistent problem. As a guide, the following **do not** indicate a reduced milk supply:

- The baby constantly sucking their fists. This is a normal physical reflex when hungry, restless, bored and overtired.
- The baby being unsettled and crying. This is normal for babies under four months.
- You don't feel a let-down, or can't express breast milk. This is normal for many women with a plentiful milk supply.
- You have small breasts. This has nothing to do with the ability to breastfeed.
- The baby stops pooing so frequently. This pattern change is very normal.

- It takes a long time to feed your baby. Some babies take longer than others.
- The baby wants to feed frequently. Babies do this for a day or so when going through a growth spurt, usually around five to six weeks and again at three to four months.

If your baby is alert and bright-eyed when awake, and has 6 wet nappies every 24 hours, they are getting enough milk.

True undersupply – reversible

It is possible to experience a true undersupply of breast milk, which is often temporary and generally readily reversible within a few days, but can sometimes take one to three weeks to rectify. Factors that contribute to a true undersupply can be:

- Incorrect positioning on the breast, sore nipples and/or engorgement.
- Infrequent feeding; limiting the length of feeds or using a nipple shield.
- Exhaustion, doing too much.
- Stress, distress, grief, depression or intense homesickness.
- Becoming ill for more than a few days; excessive vomiting and diarrhoea.
- Exercising too vigorously, rapid weight loss or strict dieting.
- Feeling anxious, pressured or embarrassed about feeding, which may inhibit a let-down reflex.
- Expressing all your baby's feeds for many weeks.
- Hormonal changes such as starting periods, the contraceptive pill or conceiving a subsequent pregnancy.
- Smoking.
- Selected medications (some antidepressants) or herbal remedies.

Physical signs of a low milk supply are the baby:
- Having less than 6 wet nappies in 24 hours.
- Experiencing constant, gradual weight loss, and/or being still below their birth weight by four weeks of age (or older); or their weight gain is less than 500 g a month.
- Having loose, wrinkled skin around their upper thighs and bottom, rather than looking 'full'.
- Pooing infrequently, and when the poo does come it is a small, green-coloured splat or staining of the nappy, rather than a large, soft amount.

NOTE: *If your baby is lethargic, floppy, pale, sleeps much of the time, is reluctant to feed, has hardly any wet nappies and/or a fever, seek medical attention as soon as possible.*

Ways to help increase your milk supply include:
- Feed, feed, feed your baby on demand, whenever they are alert or awake, but let them sleep in between. This may be every 1 to 3 hours for 24 to 48 hours or longer.
- Not giving supplements of formula milk or dummies (at this stage anyway).
- Seeing a midwife or lactation consultant to make sure your baby is attaching correctly and you are experiencing a let-down.
- Offering your baby both breasts each feed, remembering to start on different sides at each feeding session but being aware of not changing sides too soon.
- Eating well and resting as much as possible.
- Stopping (or cutting back on) smoking.
- Addressing your feelings and concerns. It may help to talk with someone you trust or to seek professional counselling. Try some techniques for helping a let-down reflex (in Chapter 13).
- Surrounding yourself with others who give you plenty of positive practical and emotional support.
- Using natural therapies, such as herbal teas with fennel, fenugreek seeds, blessed thistle, nettle and/or raspberry leaf, or homeopathic remedies (China or Phosphoric acid). See your practitioner.

Medications have varying degrees of success and should only be used as a last resort for true undersupply. The main types prescribed are metoclopramide (Maxalon), domperidone (Motilium) or sulpiride (Dolmatil), which aim to increase the prolactin hormone. They usually take a week before the milk supply increases, if they are going to be successful. Side effects can include restlessness, drowsiness, fatigue, insomnia, headaches, dizziness, and/or diarrhoea. Effects for the baby are unknown at this stage. Discuss their use with your caregiver. Other approaches using oxytocin, iodine or thyrotropin-releasing hormone have not shown any benefits and are no longer recommended.

True undersupply – ongoing

If the above measures don't show much improvement, it becomes apparent that the undersupply is ongoing, possibly for similar reasons to reversible undersupply or perhaps for no known reason. Less than 1% of women have a physiological problem (usually related to metabolism) that prevents them from producing enough breast milk. Another cause may be previous breast surgery that involved the total removal of the nipple and resituating it.

Support strategies for ongoing undersupply should only be necessary if

your baby is not gaining weight at a satisfactory rate, despite all your efforts to increase your supply. These may include:
- Starting to give small amounts of formula (30 to 60 ml) after 2 or 3 breastfeeds in a 24-hour period, while continuing to breastfeed frequently; or giving one bottle of formula in the evenings and breastfeeding regularly for the rest of the time.
- Starting the baby on solids if they are old enough (at least four months).
- Using a supply line. This is a small pouch containing expressed breast milk or formula, worn around the neck and with two fine tubes coming from the bottom of the pouch and taped to the breasts with their ends sitting in line with the nipples. Essentially the baby breastfeeds and drinks milk from the pouch simultaneously. This needs to be used under the guidance of a lactation consultant.

Oversupply

It is common to have a temporary oversupply of breast milk, usually during the first six weeks but sometimes continuing for longer. Physical signs of oversupply include:
- Constantly full breasts and frequent leaking breast milk.
- The baby putting on weight very quickly, pooing frequently, vomiting dramatically and possibly gasping at the breast if the flow is too fast, especially during a let-down.

While there is no urgent need to do anything, you may wish to:
- Try feeding from one breast at each feed for a while, perhaps putting the baby back to that breast if they are hungry again within an hour. Try not to feed from the second breast for at least two hours.
- Try feeding in different positions if the milk is flowing fast, such as you lying down or the football hold.
- Press the heel of your hand into the nipple of the other breast during a let-down.
- Consider using a dummy between feeds for your baby to suck on for comfort.
- Try natural therapies. Herbalists may recommend parsley and sage, while homeopaths may suggest Belladonna, Bryonia or Calcarea carbonica. Consult with your practitioner and take care not to take too much in case you lower your supply excessively.

NOTE: *Do not cut back on drinking fluids. This does not work and only dehydrates you.*

Conclusion

The process of conceiving, nurturing and birthing your baby, as well as the life-long relationship of parenting can be an overwhelming and unpredictable journey, with many highs and lows, but a fantastic experience where you continue to learn along the way.

The monumental event of having a baby brings the commitment of raising a child. This new person needs to be loved and cared for, presenting parents with many challenges that ultimately change their priorities and responsibilities. Our hopes and dreams are invested in each baby's future, as they grow in our family, community and world to become the next generation.

Congratulations and enjoy your new baby(s),

Sandra and Catherine

Visualisation techniques

Visualisation can be a powerful tool in many life situations. It us_
to create clear images, or positive thoughts, of situations you wisn
reinforce in your subconscious. You may feel comfortable using visua_
wonder what they mean or how to do them correctly. However, they are v_
to use and you don't really need to see anything, just think about a scenario you v_
to experience.

You can create your own visualisation, adapting it for what you want to achieve. Some people write out their visualisation and then get someone else to read it to them (with a gentle, soothing voice). However, for many visualisations, the key is to listen to them repeatedly, over several weeks, so the message becomes a part of your consciousness. Therefore, recording them may be better. A few points to remember for the person who is speaking include:

- Begin in a normal, relaxed tone of voice.
- Allow your voice to become quieter, speaking slower as the visualisation progresses.
- Speak slowly (but not too slowly) and pause every now and then for emphasis. Phrasing for emphasis is important for formulating a hypnotic suggestion. For example, 'Now let yourself drift . . . relax . . . all your muscles are heavy . . . be conscious of breathing in . . . and out.'

You may wish to play relaxing background music or nature sounds (such as running water) while recording, to help with relaxation.

Before you actually visualise:
- Turn the phone down, or off.
- Allow yourself at least 15 to 20 minutes.
- Remember, there is no right or wrong way to visualise.
- If you fall asleep, it doesn't matter. The relaxation objective has obviously worked!
- Make sure you are comfortable.
- Empty your bladder.

STARTING

Visualisations need to start with a relaxation exercise of some sort to calm the body and quieten the mind. This makes suggestions more likely to be accepted by the subconscious. Your relaxation exercise can be a quick head-to-toe check to sense whether all your muscles feel relaxed, or a systematic relaxation, moving up (or down) sections of the body, taking a few minutes (see Chapter 1).

Once the relaxing session is completed, you can move into the purpose of the visualisation and what you wish to achieve. The following is a guide for some visualisations that can be useful, and small snippets of wording to get you started.

Insomnia

The stillness of night can provide an opportunity for practising relaxation techniques which may be used during labour (and hopefully help you get back to sleep!). Start with a systematic muscle relaxation. Then start imagining yourself somewhere calm – on a beach, under the ocean with fish swimming around you, or in space, floating weightlessly. Describe what you see, how you feel there, the warmth of the etc. You can also include things like, 'Feel your body heavy and relaxed . . . dy for sleep . . . drift with your breathing . . . sleeping . . . relaxed and drifting . . .'

Stress
Winding down from stress, releasing tension and providing a quiet inner space can be achieved with visualisation. It can also help you modify, or change, lifestyle habits (such as smoking or drinking alcohol). Some people try to visualise their life as they want it to be, to help create a calmer, more positive approach and to feel more empowered when faced with difficult situations or cravings.

Prelabour and labour
You can create a labour and birth scene in your mind, to help you develop coping strategies to nurture a positive approach, especially if you are fearful or anxious, so labour can be seen as a normal, healthy process, instead of a negative experience. Labour visualisations can also be used to say 'I am ready' if the baby is overdue, or to help contractions intensify during prelabour. A visualisation may not start labour, but many women have appreciated its ability to calm and centre them.
NOTE: *Don't underestimate the power of suggestion (visualisation). This prelabour tool is only recommended after 37 weeks of pregnancy.*

Your visualisation may start with the following: 'Imagine yourself at home . . . maybe in bed, or in the shower, or milling around the house . . . With the next breath out, see yourself having mild, period-like pains . . . a cramping that comes and goes . . . As the day progress, the prelabour continues . . . you now start to move into established labour . . . Imagine your cervix softening . . . thinning . . . opening. See and feel yourself in labour . . . moving and working with the contractions . . . using different positions . . . Relax your body between each contraction . . . Be conscious of your breathing . . . deep and relaxed . . . Do not resist it . . . work with the contractions . . . work with the pain . . . let go of time . . . your concerns . . . your anxieties . . . your expectations (state what your issues are and then give them positives, or state strategies to deal with them).'

The third stage
If your placenta is not coming away readily after the birth, you may wish to visualise this happening, as a simple, noninvasive method before medical interventions are suggested. 'See the inner walls of your uterus shrinking . . . forcing your placenta off the uterine wall. Your placenta is coming away . . . heavy . . . peeling the membranes off the uterus . . . the sac that contained your baby . . . See your placenta sliding down . . . out through your cervix and into the vagina to be delivered. Your uterus continues to contract . . . sealing off the blood vessels where the placenta used to be . . . the blood flow slowing to a trickle . . . the third stage is now complete.'

Breastfeeding
Relaxing your mind and body can facilitate a let-down and the release of milk, especially when you are feeling anxious or stressed, or expressing milk for your baby. 'Imagine your breasts full of milk . . . you feel your nipple being gently pulled within your baby's mouth [insert your baby's name where appropriate] . . . your beautiful baby milks your breasts . . . and with the next breath out you see the milk releasing

down . . . flowing down and out of your breast to your child . . . its richness flows into your baby.'

Closing
It is important to close your visualisation and bring yourself back slowly, to give yourself time to reflect on what you have visualised. This can be: 'Slowly breathing in and out and becoming aware of your body, hearing sounds around you, stretching, opening your eyes, slowly in your own time.'

Acupressure point	Used for	Used when
Hip point	To encourage an efficient labour.	• After 38 weeks of pregnancy. • During labour.
Buttock point (BL32)	• Preparing for labour. • Augmenting contractions after the waters have broken. • Helping with pain relief and backache during labour. • Dilating a thick anterior lip of cervix before pushing.	• After 38 weeks of pregnancy. • During prelabour, labour or after the waters have broken, but no contractions yet.
Wrist point (PC6)	• Morning sickness. • Nausea during late pregnancy. • Vomiting during labour. • Nausea and vomiting side effects after medicated pain relief and/or a caesarean.	• Pregnancy. • Labour. • After the birth.
Ankle point (SP6)	• Augmenting contractions after the waters have broken. • Labour progressing slowly. • Helping the placenta to come.	• Prelabour. • Labour (dilating and pushing phases). • The third stage of labour. *NOTE: Not to be used before labour.*
Hand point (LI4)	• Letting go (physically and emotionally). • Softening, thinning and opening the cervix. • Stimulating, regulating and intensifying contractions. • Dilating a thick anterior lip of cervix before pushing. • Helping the pushing urge or stimulating contractions during second stage. • Helping the placenta to come.	• Prelabour. • Labour (dilating and pushing phases). • The third stage. *NOTE: Should not be used if having medications to induce or augment labour contractions (Syntocinon drip or prostaglandins), as the uterus may become overstimulated.*

How to use the point

Locate the hip point by moving the fingers in a direct, horizontal line from the top of the buttock cleft, out towards the hips. When this line is progressively pressed, a tender point is reached, around two-thirds out from the buttock cleft, and one-third in from the hipbone. The hip point is often used in combination with the buttock point (described below). Pressure can be applied on and off for 30 seconds or so, before moving across to stimulate the buttock point, then finishing with downward massage strokes (this may be repeated several times).

Locate the buttock points with your thumbs, just above the woman's buttocks and about one finger-width either side of her spine. You should be able to feel a small depression here. Many woman can direct the person performing the acupressure, because once the thumbs are in the correct place, they usually 'feel right'. The buttock point is easier to get to if the woman is kneeling on all fours or leaning against the wall, table or bed. If used during labour, pressure is applied during the contractions, possibly in combination with the hip point (as described above). For pain relief as the labour intensifies, you can progressively apply pressure down (one thumb-width at a time), moving closer to the spine until the thumbs arrive at the top of the buttock cleft. For an anterior lip of cervix, strong pressure may be applied with the knuckles during a contraction, perhaps breathing with her, to help her resist the urge to push.

Locate the wrist point on the inside of the arm, about three finger-widths above the wrist crease, between the tendons (use the width of the woman's fingers to provide the correct measurement, not someone else's fingers). Apply pressure firmly, until you feel some relief. This may take up to five minutes. Repeat the pressure when necessary, on one or both wrists. You may prefer to use wristbands for seasickness, which work by applying pressure to this point (purchased from chemists).

To locate the ankle point, measure four of the woman's finger-widths above the high point of her inside anklebone, just behind the border of her tibia bone (at the front of the lower leg). Apply pressure with the index finger (or thumb) for about one minute, on both legs at a time. Pressure time is often interspersed with rests of three to four minutes, before repeating, perhaps several times if the woman's body is slow to respond. Some women find this point feels tender, needing to 'breathe through' the pressure time, as they would for contractions. Once the contractions start, do not stimulate the ankle point further. You may want to move onto using the hand or buttock points (unless the labour slows or stops and the contractions need to be stimulated again).

To locate, bring the woman's index finger and thumb together to form a crease. The point is on the top of her hand (not the palm), at the end of the crease, on the high point of the muscle. Apply pressure with the thumb at different times throughout the day, if labour has not started yet (or during prelabour); or at regular intervals to regulate and strengthen contractions during labour. May be used in combination with the buttock point for an anterior lip, or the leg and neck points to help with the second stage of labour.

NOTE: Once the point is located, start with light pressure, gradually building up to be quite firm (but not pailful). When a point is stimulated correctly, numbness, heaviness, warmth, tingling, aching or buzzing is usually felt around the point. If pain is felt, the pressure needs to be repositioned, or another point used. Consult a qualified acupuncturist before using acupressure on areas of the body with previous injuries.

Acupressure point	Used for	Used when
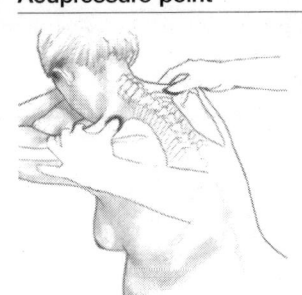 Neck points (GB21)	• Pain relief during labour. • Helping with pushing and progress during second stage.	Dilating and pushing phases of labour. NOTE: Should not be used during pregnancy, only during labour.
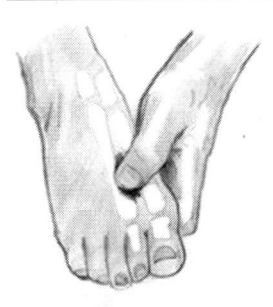 Foot point (LV3)	• Regulating and intensifying contractions. • Helping with pushing and progress during the second stage. • Helping the placenta to come. • Controlling the bleeding after the birth.	• Prelabour. • Labour (dilating and pushing phases). • The third stage. • Soon after the birth. NOTE: Should not be used if having medications to induce or augment labour contractions (eg. Syntocinon drip or prostaglandins), as the uterus may become overstimulated.
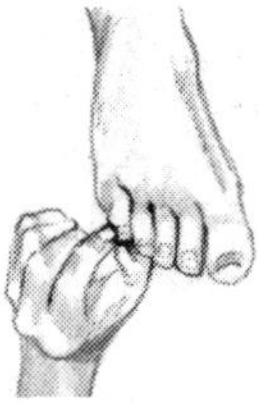 Toe points (BL67)	Turning the baby from a posterior to anterior position, or from a breech to head down position.	• Last weeks of pregnancy. • Prelabour. • Labour (dilating phase).
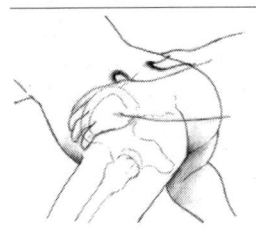 Lower spine points (BL23)	• Turning the baby from a posterior to anterior position. • Helping relieve back pain during the first or second stages of labour.	• Last weeks of pregnancy. • Prelabour. • Labour (dilating and pushing phases).
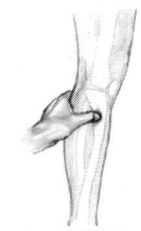 Leg point (ST36)	Helping with pushing and progress during the second stage.	Pushing phase of labour.

How to use the point

To locate, the woman needs to lean her head slightly forward. The person applying the pressure runs their finger down the back of her neck until a prominent bone is felt at the base of the neck. The neck points lie midway along imaginary curved lines that run from this bone to the top of each shoulder joint, at the highest point of the shoulder muscles. Apply firm, downward pressure with your thumbs, knuckles or elbows, to both shoulder points at the same time, starting at the beginning of each contraction and gradually building the pressure up. Release the pressure once the contraction has subsided. A gentle rub or massage of the shoulders and neck can help her relax between contractions, reminding her to release any tension. (If you use your thumbs, the pressure needs to come down through your arms, to avoid sore, tired thumbs.) The woman usually needs to be in an upright or kneeling position to use neck points, but it may be possible to use them if she is lying on her side. Neck points may be combined with leg and hand points during the second stage of labour.

Locate the point in the angle formed from the bones leading from the large and second toes on the top of the foot. This can feel tender, although this makes it easier to locate correctly. Apply pressure at regular intervals.

Locate the points on the outside edge of the little toes, near the outer corner of the toenails. The person applying the pressure uses their index fingers (or thumbs) on both toes at the same time. You may want to use the tip of a pen with the lid on, or another blunt point. During labour, apply pressure as the contractions start, easing off as they subside. The toe points may be used in combination with the lower spine points to help a posterior labour.

Locate the lower spine points by drawing an imaginary line across the woman's back, from the top of her hipbones. Find a space between the two vertebrae just above this imaginary line. Apply firm pressure during the contractions to help relieve back pain and hopefully encourage the baby to rotate. Lower spine points can be combined with toe points to help a posterior labour.

Locate the point on the front of the woman's leg, about four finger-widths below the lower edge of her kneecap, and about one finger-width out from her tibia, or shinbone. Apply pressure during the contractions. The leg point may be combined with neck and hand points during the second stage.

Natural therapies

The therapy	How it is used
Acupuncture – A branch of Chinese medicine based on the belief that the body's energy flows (qi – pronounced *chi*); 12 main channels (or meridians) run through the body, corresponding to the main organs. Acupuncturists strive to encourage proper chi circulation by manipulating chi gateways just below the skin, with fine needles to restore the balance of energy in the body and stimulate healing. Sometimes acupuncture is combined with herbs or homeopathic remedies to be more effective.	The practitioner feels your pulse to gauge your chi. Hair-thin needles are inserted by gently piercing the skin to reach the necessary chi gateways called acupoints. Occasionally, the needles are electrically charged with a TENS machine to increase the stimulation. Your acupuncturist may require you to re-evaluate your lifestyle by improving your diet, exercising, reducing stress and stopping addictive substance use (if applicable).
Acupressure – Works on similar principles as acupuncture.	Certain acupoints are stimulated using deep, focused pressure on the surface of the skin from the thumb, finger or elbow (instead of needles). Can be given in the form of a Shiatsu massage (see Shiatsu) or using moxibustion.
Alexander technique – Focuses on improving physical and psychological wellbeing by correcting the way the body is held and used. Aims to lengthen muscles to relieve tension and improve circulation, lymphatic drainage, digestion, breathing and mental attitude.	The trained instructor works with you to determine your body's distortions and enhance awareness of your posture, balance and movement during normal daily activities.
Aromatherapy – Uses essential oil extracts from flowers, herbs and trees to treat various physical and mental conditions. The therapeutic properties of oils are aimed at restoring harmonious balance of energy within the body to combat ill health. Essential oils are highly concentrated (and usually expensive), with dosages measured in drops.	Can be absorbed into the bloodstream through skin contact, or inhalation via the lungs. Often added to a bath, inhaled by drops in a vaporiser or burner or on a handkerchief or tissue, added to plain carrier oils for massage or water and soaked in cloth compresses applied to the skin.

Preconception, pregnancy, labour & post birth	Precautions
Preconception – Male and female fertility, fatigue, stress, to help give up smoking, and general wellbeing. **Pregnancy** – Back pain, high blood pressure, fluid retention, carpal tunnel, sciatic pain, sinusitis, colds, flu, constipation, haemorrhoids, insomnia, morning sickness, headaches, turning the position of the unborn baby, inducing labour. **Labour** – Pain relief, increasing the strength of the contractions. **Post birth** – Recovery after a caesarean, haemorrhoids, fluid retention, mastitis, balance and general wellbeing.	Certain points need to be avoided during pregnancy. Clean, sterile, single-use needles need to be used to prevent cross infection of viruses such as Hepatitis B, C and HIV/AIDS from other patients.
Preconception – Fatigue, stress, balance and general wellbeing. **Pregnancy** – Breathlessness, heartburn, back pain, fluid retention, carpal tunnel, sciatic pain, sinusitis, haemorrhoids, insomnia, morning sickness, headaches, inducing labour. **Labour** – Stimulating labour contractions, nausea and vomiting, anterior lip, pain relief, posterior labour, help with pushing phase. **Post birth** – Balance and general wellbeing. *NOTE: Refer to acupressure points appendix for images and instructions on how to use specific points.*	Some acupressure points should not be stimulated during pregnancy and should be used with care if you have a previous injury to the area where the specific point is intended for use. Consult your practitioner.
Preconception – Backache, muscular stiffness, aches, pains, stress, anxiety, insomnia, digestive disorders and circulatory problems. **Pregnancy** – Support and prevent muscle pain and discomfort, corrects posture when sitting, standing, walking and lifting items. **Labour** – Teaches upright positions for labour and birth, awareness of breathing and muscle tension during and after contractions. **Post birth** – Body awareness to help with backache and muscle tension. Correct instructions for lifting and carrying your baby.	Generally regarded as safe during pregnancy.
Preconception and first 12 weeks of pregnancy – Should generally be avoided. **After 12 weeks of pregnancy** – Backache, muscular stiffness, aches, pains, stress, anxiety, depression, low spirits, insomnia, nausea, skin conditions, digestive disorders, circulatory problems, swelling, high blood pressure, varicose veins, haemorrhoids, headaches, colds, flu, constipation. **Labour** – Stimulate contractions, calming, optimism, confidence, assisting with stamina, exhaustion, pain relief. **Post birth** – Breast engorgement, hormonal balance, stimulate the immune system, backache and muscle tension, memory, tiredness, fatigue, aphrodisiac.	Essential oils enter the bloodstream and can cross the placenta to the unborn baby and pass through breast milk. There is little research on their side effects and much information is conflicting. Because the risks to the unborn baby are unknown, it is advisable not to use these oils before 12 weeks of pregnancy or when trying to conceive (or on babies under 2 years). **Essential oils to avoid during pregnancy include:** aniseed, basil, birch, bitter almond, camphor, cassia, cedarwood, cinnamon, clary sage (for labour only), clove, comfrey, cypress, eucalyptus, fennel, hyssop, juniper berry, jasmine, marjoram, melissa, mugwort, mustard, myrrh, nutmeg, oregano, parsleyseed, pennyroyal, peppermint, rose (for labour only), rosemary, sage, tarragon, thyme, wintergreen, wormwood. *NOTE: Consult your aromatherapist. Some oils should not be used if you have high blood pressure, asthma or epilepsy.*

The therapy	How it is used
Art therapy – The spontaneous use of art to produce images or sculpture by willing participants (you don't need to have any talent!). Aims to heal emotional stresses and concerns by allowing the creative expression of feelings, thoughts, concerns, fantasies and emotions through art.	There is an increasing trend for art therapy to be incorporated into childbirth education classes to help identify concerns and approaches to labour and birth. The session may start as a relaxation or visualisation, followed by expression using art with drawing, painting or using clay or plasticine to sculpt.
Autogenic training and biofeedback – A form of relaxation therapy based on exercises to help relax nerves and muscles, increase circulation and regulate the heart rate. Uses conscious breathing, creating warmth in the abdomen and coolness in the forehead. Phrases are learnt and with repetition result in physical changes. Biofeedback evolved from autogenic training. Both methods rely on you believing that once your body is relaxed, it is capable of healing itself by releasing stress.	Systematic structured courses are done with a trainer qualified in autogenic methods (ideally with a background in counselling). The trainer teaches the technique to reach a state of near hypnosis and deep relaxation, allowing your body to deal with stress, tension, migraines, concerns and trauma. It may progress onto autogenic meditation for visualisation, to allow deeper access to the subconscious. Biofeedback systematically teaches exercises while your heart rate, brain waves and temperature are monitored by machines. This helps you identify body signals when changes are achieved. Eventually the exercises are done without the trainer and the machines.
Bach flower remedies – Essences of various English wildflowers whose healing energy is used to reconnect the body and soul, treating you as a whole to help correct illness. **Bush flower essences** are the Australian equivalent.	Used to treat the mood and state of mind (or outlook), not the actual physical condition, addressing negative emotions and mental conflicts to restore balance and harmony to facilitate your body to heal itself. A common remedy is Rescue Remedy (or Australian Emergency Essence) for shock, trauma, stress, and labour pains. Remedies are usually a liquid concentrate (called stock), preserved in alcohol or vinegar. They are generally obtained through health food stores, natural pharmacies or some natural health practitioners.
Bowen technique – Addresses the body as a whole, rather than just the presenting symptoms, to embrace your physical, chemical, emotional and mental aspects. Aims to balance and stimulate energy flows, frequently resulting in a deep sense of overall relaxation to allow the body to heal itself.	Uses a system of gentle, precise movements on the skin (or through light clothing) across muscles, nerves and connective tissue on specific areas of the body, with frequent pauses to allow the body time to respond to the moves. Thought to cause the neuromuscular system to reset tension levels and stimulate energy flow to promote natural healing. Combines moves, both in placement and in combination to address the body as a whole, or target a specific problem.
Chiropractic – Recognised as a form of manipulative medicine, with the primary concern being to diagnose the origin of the complaint, rather than trying to treat or control the presenting symptom(s). Uses the relationship between the nervous system and the mechanical framework of the body (skeletal system, joints, muscles and ligaments) to realign bones and relieve muscle spasm, pain, immobile joints, ligaments and tendons.	Your bones are manipulated by your practitioner with precise pressure, usually while you are positioned or lying on an examination table.

Preconception, pregnancy, labour & post birth	Precautions
Used at any time to express feelings. May be helpful for people who find it difficult to recognise and express their emotions. Allows for a release of tension and to acknowledge factors causing inner stress. May identify issues and lead to clarity, focus and management strategies. Some find the therapy confronting or awkward, while others enjoy it, or use it in their daily lives to some degree.	Art therapists (or art psychologists) should ideally have a background in psychology.
Used to deal with addictions, pain management, headaches and insomnia.	Some exercises are unsuitable for pregnant women and need to be modified. Seek the advice of your caregiver before participating in biofeedback sessions during pregnancy.
Preconception – For emotional stress of day-to-day life, emotions when trying to conceive (perhaps disappointment, resentment or guilt). **Pregnancy and labour** – To combat fear (of losing control or failure), panic, shock, the inability to make choices, nervousness, self-doubt, feeling inferior, impatience with self or others. **Post birth** – Transition to parenting and various emotions after the birth.	Safe to use during pregnancy, labour and birth. It is not possible to overdose or experience side effects from an inappropriate remedy. If one remedy doesn't work, just try another. Self-treating is generally acceptable; however, if you feel unfamiliar with the remedies, seek a practitioner trained in the therapy. The small amount of alcohol used to preserve the stock is not believed to be sufficient to cause harm during pregnancy, but alternatives can be used (such as vinegar or glucose water).
Preconception and pregnancy – Sciatica, back pain, carpal tunnel, sprains, joint problems, migraines, stress, tension, neck strains, repetitive strain injury, heartburn. **Post birth** – Often preferred because its gentle and precise technique does not use undue force and pressure. Can be used to help realign or 'reset' the body after birth. **Baby** – May be used to stimulate the respiratory system of newborns who have a degree of respiratory distress or reflux after birth.	Thought to be safe to use during pregnancy. Your practitioner should have experience working with pregnant women as the ligaments and joints are more flexible and easily strained during pregnancy.
Preconception and pregnancy – For circulation, lymphatic drainage, nervous and digestive systems, back, sciatic pain, pelvic discomfort, symphysis pain and muscle spasm. **Post birth** – May be performed between four to six weeks after the birth, before the ligaments and muscles lose their flexibility to realign the body. **Baby** – An increasing trend towards treating unsettled, irritable babies who may have experienced a complicated birth with gentle chiropractic manipulations of the baby's skull and spine.	Pregnant women often need repetitive sessions of chiropractic treatment, because their ligaments and muscles are softened due to the hormone progesterone, making their bones prone to slipping easily out of alignment. Your chiropractor should be experienced in dealing with pregnant women or young babies.

The therapy	How it is used
Colour therapy – Based on the belief that colour has therapeutic properties to alter emotions and psychological conditions. Each colour (red, orange, yellow, green, blue, indigo and violet) is based on seven energy centres, affecting certain parts of the body to restore balance and physical wellbeing.	Uses coloured lamps, wearing certain coloured clothes and even eating certain coloured foods, according to the symptoms.
Counselling and psychotherapy – Involves the sharing of problems, feelings and emotions on a one-to-one basis. The practitioner is an objective listener, facilitating your exploration of issues without making judgments, or expressing their own points of view.	Having an objective professional to bounce things off can help you find solutions and resolutions to issues. Sessions should ideally be in a quiet environment, where you feel safe to discuss anything personal. One or a few sessions may be required, or long-term therapy, depending on the issue(s).
Dance therapy – Involves movement and rhythm to music to explore feelings and emotions. Aims to promote an interaction between your mind and body to encourage creative expression and relieve tension and stress.	Can either be structured and repetitive, or free and spontaneous. The sessions are usually done in groups using peer support to increase the satisfaction of the therapy.
Diet therapy – Used as a tool to treat and prevent illness. Based on 'You are what you eat' with the belief that disease is often due to vitamin and mineral deficiencies.	Your practitioner assesses your diet, taking into account any food allergies or deficiencies. They may prescribe vitamin and mineral supplements. However, care needs to be taken to avoid toxic high doses during pregnancy (see vitamins and minerals Chapter 1).
Healers – People who believe they have a gift to transfer power from themselves to heal another person. It is not really understood how healing works, but it is thought your brain waves are stimulated to speed up the body's ability to heal itself, rectifying imbalances and promoting a feeling of relaxation and wellbeing.	Normally done on a one-to-one basis, with sessions lasting up to an hour or so. May involve the healer laying their hands on or just above the person or may be performed on a psychic level, with no touch involved or perhaps not even being present (distant healer).

NATURAL THERAPIES 535

Preconception, pregnancy, labour & post birth	Precautions
Used for anxiety, depression, stress and health conditions to calm and sooth. For example, blue is recommended to help with high blood pressure; red is advised for fatigue, depression and headaches.	Thought to be safe for pregnant women. Colour therapists believe that improper use can be confusing or disturbing.
Preconception and early pregnancy – May help with lifestyle changes, such as giving up smoking or dealing with a past pregnancy loss or infertility issues. **Pregnancy** – May be needed for personal, relationship, financial or health issues, for lifestyle changes. **Parenting** – This is a time of dramatic change, sometimes one of crisis for new parents. Counselling may be needed to help with stress, depression, grief or feelings of trauma after the birth or after a pregnancy loss.	The therapist should be trained in some form of psychology. Ideally you should feel at ease with your counsellor.
Preconception and pregnancy – To improve fitness, flexibility, balance, coordination, circulation, fluid retention, breathing, digestion and increase self-confidence. Many women use belly dancing to help with pelvic discomforts. In ancient cultures, women belly danced to show the pregnant women how to pelvic rock her baby down and out – a skill that may be handy in labour!	Thought to be safe during pregnancy, presuming the woman is well enough to participate in exercise. Formal dance therapy is generally conducted by a teacher trained in dance therapy and counselling.
Preconception – To achieve optimum health for fertility. **Pregnancy** – For health or metabolic disorders such as diabetes, miscarriage prevention, depression, stress, viral illnesses, unborn babies who are small for dates, high blood pressure. **Post birth** – For postnatal depression, stress, viral illnesses and metabolic disorders.	Usually carried out by a clinical nutritionist (doctors who specialise in nutrition) or a dietician. Some natural therapists (eg. naturopaths) also have extensive training in diet therapy. A trained professional should always supervise any dietary treatments during pregnancy.
Used to treat stress-related conditions as well as depression, phobias, eating disorders and some medical conditions, with varying results.	Healers generally have no formal training, believing their power is a natural gift. Therefore, there are many people who pretend to be healers. Ideally, your healer should be registered with a professional organisation and you should feel comfortable with them. It may be advisable to ask for references, or go with the recommendation of a friend.

The therapy	How it is used
Herbal medicine – Aims to balance the energies in the body using herbs, treating the cause of the illness rather than the symptoms by stimulating the immune system to aid your body to heal itself. There are thousands of different herbs available, encompassing many cultures and societies.	Created from whole plants as it is thought this avoids the side effects of medical drugs, which are only synthesised from plant extracts. May be used in teas or infusions, creams, ointments, compresses or liniments, syrups, powders, poultices, capsules, tablets or tinctures (herbs suspended in alcohol), depending on the condition being treated. Herbs are often more effective if combined with other therapies such as acupuncture and lifestyle changes.
Homeopathy, tissue or cell salt – Based on the principle 'Like cures like', it stimulates (rather than suppresses) symptoms to assist your body's natural healing process. Remedies are based on small doses curing disease, where large doses produce symptoms of the disease. Extreme dilution of the medicine aims to enhance its curative properties and reduce any 'poisonous' or undesirable side effects. **Tissue salts** is another branch of homeopathy (or cell salts or biochemic salts).	A complex therapy in which your practitioner considers a wide range of aspects including appetite, emotions, sleep patterns, moods, posture, complexion, dietary preferences and lifestyle factors, as well as the condition. Therefore, different remedies may be prescribed to different people with the same illness. **Tissue salts** come in tablet form and are usually dissolved under the tongue (rather than swallowed). They are not as potent as homeopathic remedies and are usually self-prescribed.
Hydrotherapy – The therapeutic use of water, based on water having curative and restorative properties, both physically and psychologically. Flotation tanks may be used to reduce environmental stimulants and help relaxation.	The water is normally warmed and can sometimes be propelled with jets (spa), to stimulate your circulation and provide localised massage. Bathing or swimming allows for exercise with buoyancy, minimising strains on joints and muscles and the added benefit of feeling weightless.
Hypnosis – Hypnosis uses repeated instructions to bring you into a state of deep relaxation, so your subconscious is free to explore psychological or emotional problems, making you open to suggestions from the therapist.	A hypnotised state aims to address emotional and behavioural problems, as well as bodily functions and addictions to restore you to a normalised balance. Hypnosis may be used for pain relief for medical treatments, particularly dental surgery; children often respond well to this form of treatment.
Iridology – Diagnosis of diseases by studying the iris (or coloured part) of the eye. This is individually unique, like fingerprints. Iridology dates back to the time of Hippocrates (about 400 BC) and is believed to reflect the health of the body's organs. Natural therapists (such as herbalists and homeopaths) may use iridology to complement their other therapies.	Weaknesses are diagnosed by noting spots, changes in colour, unusual patterns and markings on the iris and charting them on an 'eye map' (or photographing them). The therapy aims to detect health problems before symptoms actually appear.

NATURAL THERAPIES

Preconception, pregnancy, labour & post birth	Precautions
Preconception – To help fertility, menstrual problems and optimise health before conception. **Pregnancy** – Morning sickness, varicose veins, haemorrhoids, constipation, heartburn, urine infections, colds, herpes, fluid retention, high blood pressure. **Post birth** – For healing, hormonal balance, milk supply. NOTE: Small amounts of garden (or dried) herbs used in foods and normal herbal teas are generally safe to use throughout pregnancy and while breastfeeding. Be aware that herbal treatments, aromatherapy essential oils and homeopathic remedies are all very different and have different potencies and uses, even though they can have similar names.	Herbs during pregnancy should be supervised by a qualified herbalist experienced in dealing with pregnant women and recognised by a professional body. **Some herbs to avoid include**: aloe vera, arbor vitae, autumn crocus, angelica, barbery, black cohosh, blue cohosh, broom, bryony chinchona, cotton root, dhea, dong quai, feverfew, ginseng, goldenseal, greater celandine, juniper, kava kava, lethroot, life root, marjoram, mistletoe, motherwort, mugwort, myrrh, nutmeg, parsley leaf (if used vaginally), pennyroyal, poke root, rue, sage, senna, shepherd's purse, squaw vine, tansy, thuja, thyme, wormwood, yarrow. **Some herbs to avoid when breastfeeding:** aloe vera, black cohosh, borage, dhea, feverfew, kava kava, parsley, sage, senna, wormwood.
Preconception, pregnancy, labour & post birth – Remedies can be used for nearly all types of ailments. Many women obtain a homeopathic labour kit from their practitioner before their due date, containing a range of remedies and a written list of the various conditions and/or emotions they can be used for. Cell salt may help with muscular pains, cramps and labour pain. Some women self-prescribe low potency homeopathic remedies and cell salts (obtained from homeopathic pharmacies, herbal dispensaries or health stores) with directions on the bottle.	Homeopathic treatments and cell salts are believed to be safe to use during preconception, pregnancy, labour and after the birth, as well as for babies, with no known side effects. Ideally, remedies need to be prescribed and supervised by a qualified practitioner to obtain the best responses.
Pregnancy – Generally regarded as safe during pregnancy, with some pools offering specialised classes for pregnant women and new babies. If doing aqua aerobics, let your teacher know that you are pregnant and seek the advice of your caregiver about exercising in general before starting.	If using hydrotherapy at home, be aware of having your bath or spa around body temperature or less (about 37°C), as you shouldn't overheat your body during pregnancy.
Preconception and pregnancy – Increasingly used to help give up or modify addictions such as smoking. Is becoming a popular method for pain relief during labour (called 'hypnobirthing'). Can also be used for stress management and insomnia. **Post birth** – May help with the release of let-down reflex when breastfeeding.	Therapists should be reputable and recognised by a professional association, with qualifications in counselling to enable them to resolve any emotional issues. Hypnosis is capable of putting you into a vulnerable state. It is important you have a level of trust and feel comfortable with your therapist.
Preconception, pregnancy and post birth – Can be used for general health reasons.	There are no problems with using iridology during preconception, pregnancy and after the birth but if serious health problems are found, you may need to be referred to another caregiver for further investigations and treatment.

The therapy	How it is used
Kinesiology – Gently tests the muscles to identify weaknesses in your body and detect physical and emotional imbalances before they manifest into serious health problems. Kinesiologists are usually practitioners in other fields such as chiropractic, osteopathy, naturopathy, medicine or shiatsu.	Your therapist gently tests up to 40 muscles at certain points to assess circulatory, digestive, lymphatic, respiratory and nervous systems as well as emotional and psychological states. They apply pressure while you resist by applying counterpressure. The process is generally quick and there should be no pain involved. If a problem is identified, light acupressure is usually applied to restore energy and balance to the body. Sometimes dietary changes are suggested.
Massage – Western massage techniques focus on stimulating and lengthening muscles to relieve spasm and tension, and encourage relaxation and healing due to incorrect movement, posture, stress and strain. Eastern massage involves stimulating points to encourage the flow of energy along the body's meridians, similar to acupuncture or acupressure (see Shiatsu).	Your therapist uses their hands, arms and elbows (and sometimes feet) to stroke and knead your muscles in various areas of your body, usually while you lie on a massage table. It is generally done with you being naked or just wearing underpants, with the therapist using towels over the body to provide privacy as needed.
Naturopathy – A lifestyle and health philosophy based on the belief that your body has the ability to heal itself when free of toxins which may be accumulated through poor lifestyle habits. Aims to stimulate the body's natural defences to promote equilibrium and allow the body to function at its optimum.	Practitioners believe that the body naturally strives for health, with 7 basic principles: 1. Help nature heal. 2. Do no harm. 3. Find the underlying cause. 4. Treat the whole person. 5. Encourage prevention. 6. Recognise wellness. 7. Act as a teacher. In order to free the body of toxins, naturopaths often recommend restricting what you eat and drink, advising exercise, and possibly using massage, chiropractic manipulations or other natural remedies such as acupuncture, herbs or homeopathy to treat health conditions.
Osteopathy – A manipulative therapy based on the belief that skeletal and organ systems are dependant on one another. If the body is out of alignment, the organs will be dysfunctional, leading to impaired circulation and illness. Some chiropractors are also trained in osteopathy and combine both elements in their treatments.	Similar to chiropractic treatments, but uses more massage and stretching for manipulation, rather than rapid moves or pressure on specific points. Aims to restore balance to your body, allow smooth flow of blood to the organs, efficient functioning of the nervous system, elimination of toxins by the lymphatic system, improving digestion and respiration, and relieving pain.
Reflexology – Based on the belief that energy or chi flows though 10 major meridians (or channels) running the length of the body to the 7000 nerve-endings in the feet and across to the fingertips, called reflex zone therapy. Aims to stimulate your body's natural ability to heal itself.	The reflexologist uses a map of the hands and feet to indicate the appropriate areas for treatment, and then probes the areas feeling for tension (or small pieces of 'debris') that can reflect a weakness in your body. Massage and applying pressure to the points corresponds to various organs and systems in your body, stimulating zones to release trapped energy. After a treatment, a variety of physical reactions may occur that can be positive and negative, because toxins are being eliminated (such as a metallic taste in the mouth), referred to as a healing crisis, where you appear to get worse before getting better.

NATURAL THERAPIES 539

Preconception, pregnancy, labour & post birth	Precautions
Preconception, pregnancy and post birth – Commonly used for allergy testing and related disorders such as eczema, arthritis, asthma, fatigue and hyperactivity, as well as anxiety, depression and phobias. Some people use it to test for health problems to avoid painful or invasive techniques.	Regarded as safe to use during pregnancy.
Preconception, pregnancy and post birth – For reducing tension and stress, relieving depression, fatigue and insomnia; to treat back pain, headaches, muscle strain, carpal tunnel, digestive and circulatory disorders. **Babies** – Baby massage is gaining popularity as a way to treat irritable and restless babies as well as colic, constipation and hyperactivity.	If you are more than 28 weeks pregnant, you will need to be massaged lying from side to side, or the masseur may have a special pregnancy table with a hole in it for your belly, so you can lie on your front safely and without discomfort. If you need to lie on your back, a small, flat pillow can be placed under the right side of your body to tilt the uterus off the large vena cava vein, leading to the heart. This avoids decreasing the blood supply to you and your baby, often making you feel faint and breathless.
Preconception, pregnancy and post birth – May be used to treat a variety of conditions including allergies, arthritis, chronic pain, digestion, thrush, haemorrhoids, varicose veins, insomnia, stress, colds, and viral infections.	As a general rule, pregnant women and babies should only be treated by naturopaths experienced in dealing with these specialised groups of people. Some dietary restrictions may need to be modified or perhaps omitted for women during pregnancy.
Preconception – For neck and back pain, injuries and for general balancing of the body. **Pregnancy** – May help with back, sciatic, rib, symphysis or groin pain, heartburn, reflux, carpal tunnel. **Post birth** – Often performed around four to six weeks after the birth, before the ligaments lose their flexibility, to help with back, neck or pelvic pain. **Babies** – Increasingly being used for small babies who may be irritable or unsettled after experiencing a difficult birth (often referred to as cranial osteopathy), through gently manipulating the bones in the baby's head.	Osteopaths should have about four to five years of training through a reputable college and be recognised by a professional association, as well as skilled and experienced in dealing with pregnant women and babies. Pregnant women may need a few sessions of treatment due to ligaments softening under hormonal influences, making the bones prone to slipping easily out of alignment.
Preconception – For relieving stress, pain, discomfort and minor ailments; helping the body to detox in readiness for conception. **Pregnancy** – For nausea, vomiting, constipation, haemorrhoids, backache, heartburn, swollen ankles, insomnia, anxiety. **Labour** – See Chapter 9 for points to use during labour.	Reflexology is regarded as safe to use during pregnancy and for small children. Let your therapist know that you are pregnant, as it is believed that certain points should be avoided during the first 12 weeks of pregnancy.

The therapy	How it is used
Shiatsu – A form of massage originating from Japan, the word *shiatsu* meaning 'finger pressure'. Uses pressure on points along the 12 main meridians (or channels) that correspond with the main organs in the body, working on the same principles as acupuncture, but less invasive. Aims to stimulate and balance energy flow to organs, enabling the body to heal itself and work effectively.	Your practitioner determines the source of the illness through assessing movement, build, posture, listening, smell, facial expression, touch and questions of the client. They then use hand pressure, massage and manipulation to adjust your body's energy flow to restore balance and promote immunity and health. Dietary advice and exercises may also be included.
T'ai chi – Means 'supreme and ultimate power'. A physical and mental discipline aimed at promoting health and wellbeing.	There are 128 postures (called forms) that are worked through in a specific order at a slow pace. The postures run together in a flowing movement, correcting posture, regulating breathing and improving circulation, muscle strength, flexibility, co-ordination and body tone. Aimed at facilitating the release of toxins, healing pain and promoting health. The meditative aspects aim to reduce stress and relax you, boosting energy levels and reducing anxiety. T'ai chi teachers encourage discipline and commitment, as well as spiritual guidance. The moves are complex and generally taught over a period of time in a class situation, taking about 30 minutes to work through. Shortened sessions can be learnt, which take about 10 minutes.
Yoga – Means 'union'; uniting the body, mind and spirit. Designed to calm, strengthen, protect and cure. Some styles are more powerful and active, aiming to improve cardiovascular health, flexibility and co-ordination through a serious of exercises. Hatha yoga is gentle yoga, used primarily for relaxation and breathing control, toning muscles and body systems.	Normally taught by a yogi in a group situation. After a while many people use yoga exercises on their own at home. Sometimes diet, nutrition and relaxation techniques are incorporated into the classes.

Preconception, pregnancy, labour & post birth	Precautions
Preconception – For general wellbeing and a wide range of physical and emotional conditions including stress. **Pregnancy** – Insomnia, nausea, vomiting, headaches, tiredness, breathlessness, haemorrhoids, carpal tunnel, heartburn, oedema (swelling), colds. **Labour** – Inducing labour, strengthening contractions, help with exhaustion, moving the baby from a posterior position, pain relief, helping to release the placenta. **Post birth** – General relaxation, depression, constipation. **Baby** – Colic, constipation, diarrhoea, vomiting (or positing); may help with overall calming and relaxing.	Believed to be safe for use in pregnancy, but certain points should be avoided during the first 12 weeks of pregnancy, to avoid potential miscarriage. Let your practitioner know that you are pregnant.
Preconception and pregnancy – To prevent or treat backache, constipation, depression, haemorrhoids, headaches, heart burn, indigestion, anxiety, insomnia, nausea, vomiting, oedema, sciatica, symphysis pubis pain and varicose veins. **Labour** – Inducing labour and pain relief. **Post birth** – For depression, stress, anxiety, back pain.	Regarded as safe for pregnant women.
Preconception – For general fitness, strengthening the body and well being. **Pregnancy** – Improving muscle strength, general fitness, backache, carpal tunnel, constipation, depression, haemorrhoids, headaches, heartburn, indigestion, stress, anxiety, insomnia, nausea, vomiting, oedema, sciatica pain, symphysis pubis pain, varicose veins. Certain positions may be suggested to turn a breech baby. **Labour** – Prenatal yoga may teach postures or positions for labour to strengthen the mind and body, to help prevent fear or anxiety and for pain relief. Calm, deep breathing is taught to help relax the mind and body for contractions. Some yoga positions help to open the pelvis. **Post birth** – To help with recovery, strengthening of the muscles and to relieve stress and anxiety.	If performed correctly, yoga is believed to be safe for pregnant women; however, some exercises may need to be modified. If you haven't done yoga before, it is generally recommended that you wait until after 12 weeks of pregnancy before starting classes. Let your instructor know that you are pregnant.

Birth plan

This worksheet is designed for the woman, her partner, support person and caregiver to promote discussion and create a clear understanding of your preferences. Create your own birth plan by ticking the information that applies to you or use it to write your own. We have included some options for caesarean birth.

Our/my full names ....
I/we like to be called ....
Our/my support person's name(s) ....
Their relationship to me/us ....
Name(s) of other child(ren) ....

CHOICE OF CAREGIVER, SUPPORT AND BIRTHPLACE

My chosen caregivers are:
- ☐ Private midwife.
- ☐ Hospital-based midwife.
- ☐ Birth centre midwife.
- ☐ Private obstetrician.
- ☐ Hospital doctors.
- ☐ Local doctor/GP.

My planned place of birth is:
- ☐ The hospital delivery suite (name of hospital).
- ☐ Operating theatre of the hospital.
- ☐ Birth centre.
- ☐ At home.

The people who plan to be present at the birth are:
- ☐ My partner.
- ☐ Friend as support person.
- ☐ Employed support person (doula).
- ☐ Relative(s).
- ☐ Sibling(s).

The environment I prefer includes:
- ☐ The lights dimmed.
- ☐ The room warmed.
- ☐ No unnecessary conversation.
- ☐ I'd like to wear my own choice of clothing.
- ☐ We would like to film (photos and/or video) in the place of birth.
- ☐ Play music (take ours if not supplied).

- ☐ Candles (check on hospital policy for fire restrictions).
- ☐ Burning of aromatherapy (hospitals – you may only be allowed electric burners).
- ☐ My own pillow/blankets.
- ☐ Photos of my child/family/pet where I can see them.
- ☐ My partner/support people with me at all times.

Comments: ....
....

Prelabour and early phase of first stage

What I may need during prelabour and early labour while still at home:

- ☐ For the labour to start of its own accord.
- ☐ To be allowed to go 10 to 14 days past the due date before being induced.
- ☐ To avoid augmentation, unless necessary or I request this.
- ☐ To be reminded this is the beginning and to conserve my energy by resting, sleeping if possible, eating and drinking.
- ☐ Using heat (or cold) packs.
- ☐ Candles or low lighting.
- ☐ Music/videos if this feels appropriate.
- ☐ Phone turned down or off. Put a message 'Don't call us, we'll call you' on the voicemail.
- ☐ My partner/support person with me.
- ☐ Not to let everyone know that prelabour has started, in case it goes for days.
- ☐ A massage.
- ☐ Acupuncture or acupressure.
- ☐ Inflate the pool if birthing at home, fill when labour starts to establish.
- ☐ Bag packed for hospital, full tank of petrol in the car, baby capsule fitted. Partner/support person knows best route to hospital and knows where to park.
- ☐ If my waters break and there are no other signs or labour, I would like to wait . . . . . . hours/days before being induced.
- ☐ Food and drinks to take to the hospital for myself, partner/support person.

Comments: ....
....

Active and Transition Phases of First Stage

During the active and transition phases I would prefer:

- [ ] The freedom to choose positions, use the shower or bath and walk around in labour as desired.
- [ ] Not to be separated from partner/support people at any point unless I request it.
- [ ] The option to return home if I am less than 3 cm dilated and all is well.
- [ ] To wear my own clothes.
- [ ] To wear a hospital gown.
- [ ] No students or nonessential personnel to be in the room (a training midwife working with a senior midwife is acceptable).
- [ ] Not to have internal vaginal examinations unless they are medically necessary or I request them.
- [ ] Not to have my membranes ruptured unless medically indicated or discussed with us.
- [ ] Not to be offered managed pain relief; I will ask for it if I need it.
- [ ] To offer suggestions when I or my partner ask for it.
- [ ] Not to routinely monitor the baby's heart rate continuously, unless there has been meconium staining or we require further information.
- [ ] To intermittently monitor the baby's heart rate using a Doppler or Pinard's earpiece (circle one or both).
- [ ] Providing I and the baby are fine, I would prefer to be free of time limits.

Comments: ....
....

What I may need during this phase from my partner/support person:

- [ ] To offer me fluids or ice cubes to suck on to keep me hydrated.
- [ ] To suggest and physically help me into different labour positions.
- [ ] Walk with me if I need to do this.
- [ ] Remind me to empty my bladder every two to three hours.
- [ ] Emotional support and communication.
- [ ] Breathe with me when I look lost.
- [ ] Provide unconditional support even when I appear snappy, unresponsive or am yelling at you!
- [ ] Remind me to relax between contractions.
- [ ] Use key words/affirmations that we have worked out (let go, release, take the breath deeper, drop your jaw, etc).
- [ ] Communicate with the staff for me so I can focus on my labour, unless we need to make decisions about my care.
- [ ] Not to allow visiting family or friends into the birth room unless I consent.

- ☐ Not to accept any phone calls from family and friends – we will ring them.
- ☐ Allow me to have the pain in labour, remember I have my endorphins, if you are uncomfortable try not to show it.
- ☐ Stay calm.
- ☐ If I ask for drugs, listen to me so we can talk about the decisions we need to make.

Comments: ....
....

If possible, I would like to have the following birthing equipment available:
- ☐ Birthing stool.
- ☐ Beanbags/lots of pillows.
- ☐ Massage implements.
- ☐ Mat.
- ☐ Shower.
- ☐ Bath.

PAIN MANAGEMENT FOR ACTIVE AND TRANSITION PHASES OF FIRST STAGE

I would like to deal with my pain using some or all of the following:
- ☐ Massage.
- ☐ Touch to reassure me.
- ☐ Heat/cold packs.
- ☐ Acupressure or acupuncture.
- ☐ Relaxation techniques.
- ☐ Shower and/or bath.
- ☐ TENS machine (may need to hire this).
- ☐ Breathing techniques.
- ☐ Visualisation.
- ☐ Homeopathy.
- ☐ Walking with and through contractions.
- ☐ Communication and feedback, affirmations, eye contact.

I am open to managed pain relief if I request it. Do not offer it to me. If requested I would prefer:
- ☐ Gas.
- ☐ Narcotic injection (Pethidine).
- ☐ Epidural/spinal/CSE (circle preferred option).
- ☐ I do not have any preferences about pain relief; I would prefer to make my decisions as I labour.

☐ An internal vaginal examination prior to any managed pain relief, to help me make my decision.

Comments: ....
....

SECOND STAGE OF LABOUR AND THE BIRTH

I would prefer the following for the birthing phase:

☐ Squatting.
☐ On all fours.
☐ Standing.
☐ Lying on side.
☐ Semi-reclining.
☐ I do not wish to lie on my back.
☐ Whatever position feels right for me at the time.
☐ I do not wish to be encouraged into another position that suits the caregiver.
☐ I want to push instinctively (not coached or told when to push).

I wish to have the options of:

☐ Being in the shower.
☐ Being in the bath – water birth (check your birthplace's policy).
☐ Sitting on a birth stool or toilet.
☐ Being allowed to rest and wait if I do not have the urge to push straight away, providing the baby and I are fine.
☐ Viewing the birth by using a mirror.
☐ Touching my baby's head as it crowns.
☐ The option of my partner 'catching' the baby.
☐ Risking a tear rather than have an episiotomy (unless a medical emergency).
☐ To have an episiotomy.
Reason being ....

Comments: ....
....

If induction or augmentation becomes necessary, I would prefer if possible to have:

☐ A Foley's catheter inserted.
☐ Prostaglandin gel or pessary.
☐ Having my waters broken.
☐ Having a Syntocinon drip.
☐ Having a combination of these if necessary.

If an assisted birth becomes necessary, I would prefer if possible to have:
- [ ] Forceps.
- [ ] The use of a ventouse (vacuum).

CAESAREAN BIRTH
Depending on the medical circumstances, I would prefer to have:
- [ ] An epidural.
- [ ] A spinal.
- [ ] A general anaesthetic.
- [ ] My partner present if an epidural or spinal is used.
- [ ] My partner/support person close by if a general anaesthetic is used.
- [ ] My child(ren) to wait with our support person (name and relationship to you) in the ward before and/or after the caesarean operation.
- [ ] The sterile screen lowered so I can see my baby being born (epidural or spinal only).
- [ ] A running commentary of the operation to let me know what is happening.
- [ ] My partner to engage me in conversation so I am distracted.
- [ ] A personal stereo to listen to, to relax me during the procedure.
- [ ] The placenta delivered by controlled cord traction rather than manually removed, to reduce bleeding and infection risks.
- [ ] Our baby given to me or my partner as soon as possible.
- [ ] Photos taken in the operating theatre.
- [ ] A videotape of the birth of our child.
- [ ] My baby to stay with me until the suturing is finished.
- [ ] My partner and baby to wait for me in recovery.
- [ ] The opportunity to try to breastfeed my baby in recovery.
- [ ] The means to be taken to the intensive care nursery (if applicable) after leaving recovery, to see my baby.
- [ ] My baby's cord blood donated (if available).
- [ ] My placenta kept for me to look at (when convenient).
- [ ] My placenta kept so I can take it home.

Comments: ....
....

Birth and soon after
Presuming my baby is well, I would prefer:
- ☐ To hold my baby immediately after the birth.
- ☐ To wait until the umbilical cord stops pulsating before it's cut and clamped.
- ☐ My partner to cut the cord.
- ☐ To discover the sex of my baby myself and not be told by others.
- ☐ Skin-to-skin contact with my baby.
- ☐ Not to have my baby's nose and mouth suctioned unless it is necessary (eg. meconium in the amniotic fluid).
- ☐ To contribute to the cord blood donor scheme (if available).
- ☐ To avoid the Syntocinon injection unless necessary.
- ☐ To have Syntocinon to help control the bleeding and deliver the placenta.
- ☐ To be shown my placenta after the birth.
- ☐ To keep my placenta.
- ☐ All the newborn procedures (weighing and measuring) to wait until I have had time to be with and/or breastfeed my baby.
- ☐ My baby to have a vitamin K injection/three oral doses (circle preferred option).
- ☐ Not to give my baby vitamin K (unless necessary).
- ☐ All newborn procedures to be carried out in my presence.
- ☐ Not to have my baby washed with antiseptic solutions.
- ☐ My partner to stay with the baby at all times if I can't be with my baby.
- ☐ To have my stitches attended to soon after the birth (if required).
- ☐ To wait until after I have fed my baby and settled before having stitches (if required).
- ☐ A heat pack for any afterpains/analgesic medications as recommended, if required.

Comments: ....
....

Postnatal days
I would prefer to:
- ☐ Breastfeed my baby.
- ☐ Bottle feed my baby.
- ☐ Breastfeed and bottle feed my baby.
- ☐ Room in with my baby.
- ☐ Go home early and have midwives visit me at home.
- ☐ My partner to room in with me on the postnatal ward (if possible).

Comments: ....
....

Labour Support Guide

What's happening to the woman's body	What the woman may feel
LAST WEEKS AND PRELABOUR • Baby's head heavy in the pelvis • Lightening – baby's head engages • Muscles relax under influence of hormones • Cervix begins to thin, soften and starts to open to around 2 to 3 cm	• Backache and/or sore thighs • Period pain or cramping • Waters may break (call caregiver) • Possibly a mucus show • Bursts of energy • Chatty and excited or introspective • Change in bowels – constipation or diarrhoea • Heavy pelvic pressure • Vomiting or nausea • Nesting instinct – exited or scared • Mild to moderate regular or irregular contractions
MOVING INTO EARLY PHASE OF FIRST STAGE • Contractions become closer more regular and intensify • Cervix opens up to about 3 to 4 cm • Contractions last from 45 to 60 seconds long now • Baby's head moves further into the pelvis	• Contractions increase in length and intensity • Show – mucus plug, or vaginal discharge can be clear, pink or bright red • Membranes may rupture – check for any green or brown discolouration (call caregiver) • Exited, impatient, talkative • Need to be upright or move • Needing to use deeper breaths during the contractions now
ACTIVE PHASE/ESTABLISHED FIRST STAGE • Cervix opening up from 4 to 7–8 cm dilation • Contractions stronger, longer and closer together • Baby's head moving lower	• Contractions need all of your attention • May become restless or sleepy • Needing to breathe and work with them now • Not that interested in conversation • Focus turns inward • Membranes may rupture • 'Show' with blood may come • Dependant on your companion • Starting to feel you need to be at your birthplace or have your caregiver with you • Thinking about pain relief

What you can do	What the partner/support people can do
- Swim, walk, rest or sleep - Carry on as normal - Keep eating and drinking - Arrange to have a massage - Try to resist telling everyone. - Relax and enjoy it! - Remember, it is just the beginning. It can still take many hours or days yet! - Pack bag for hospital - Baths, showers, heat packs NOTE: *Do not have a bath if your waters have ruptured and you are not having contractions.*	- Massage - Organise an evening out or a candlelit dinner for two - Hire videos - Check route to hospital, petrol in car, capsule fitted - Cuddles – talk about how you both are feeling - Prepare to take time off work - Organise last minute preparations - Organise siblings - Take a photo - Rest if she doesn't need you
- Contact caregiver, prepare to leave (second or subsequent babies) - Pelvic rocking - Keep eating if you feel like it - Drink after each or every other contraction - Watch for regularity in contractions - Think about this new person coming into your life - Visualise the cervix thinning and opening - Go for a walk - Take a shower or use heat packs	- Call caregiver and take her to birthplace (second/subsequent babies) - Encourage relaxation - Burn aromatherapy oils (ask first) - Massage – use acupressure points - Encourage walking, light snacks and drinks; be sure to eat yourself - 'Bodycheck' between contractions, remind her to relax her body - Remind her to empty bladder - Heat/cold packs - Tie her hair back - Offer love and encouragement - Take a photo
- Contact your caregiver, prepare to leave (first babies) - Empty your bladder before you go and every two hours - Drink, suck ice or lollies after every contraction - Breathe with open relaxed jaw and throat - After every contraction breathe in and release that contraction - Pelvic rocking - Listen to your body – go with it - Think of, and talk to your baby! - Change positions frequently - Get on 'all fours' for backache - Shower or bath needed now - Heat packs	- Call her caregiver and take her to the birthplace (first babies) - Breathe with her, remind her to take the breath deep into her body. - Eye contact if she looks lost - Heat packs to lower back and abdomen - Rub back with warm oil (rub between your hands first to warm) - Foot and shoulder massage - 'Bodycheck' after every contraction, make sure she relaxes her body - Offer her fluids after each or every other contraction - Remind her to urinate every two hours - Suggest and physically help her into other positions - Stay calm and look after yourself

What's happening to the woman's body	What the woman may feel
MOVING INTO THE END OF FIRST STAGE/TRANSITION	
• Cervix opens from 7–8 to 10 cm or fully dilated • Contractions very strong, close together 1 to 2 minutes apart or back to back with little or no rest between • Contractions lasting mostly 60 to 70 seconds long	• 'Panicky' • Leg cramps and shaking • Nausea and/or vomiting • Need to open your bowels • Heavy bloodstained show • Hot and perspiring or cold and shivery • Pressure in the lower back • Feelings of being out of control • Not wanting to do this anymore • Pressure in your bottom as your baby's head moves lower • Needing to make more noise and possibly some grunting noises • Wanting this baby born *now* • Asking for pain relief, perhaps not really wanting it if you are nearly there; difficulty staying in the 'here and now'
THE RESTING AND PUSHING PHASES OF SECOND STAGE	
• Cervix fully dilated • Baby descends and rotates in the pelvis • Contractions five or more minutes apart • Urge to push • No urge to push (resting phase) • Your baby moves out of the uterus, through the pelvis and down the vagina • Pushing for 20 minutes to 2 hours • Baby's head crowns • Birth of the baby	• Baby moving down the birth canal • Urge to push or • No urge to push – rest and wait • Pushing – cannot resist the urge • Possibly need direction to help push • May open bowels • Towards the end of second stage the head is seen with pushing and moves back when the contraction finishes • Feeling frustrated – remember it is better that your baby takes time, so your body can stretch with the head coming out • The top of the baby's head is clearly visible and does not move back now, the perineum is stretched to the maximum • Burning and stretching as baby's head crowns • You pant the head out • You wait for your baby to rotate around so the shoulders can emerge, top shoulder out, and body follows • You may feel awe, numb, relief, love, exhaustion, shock, quietness, disbelief – all that and more!
THIRD STAGE	
• The uterus contracts, the placenta separates and comes down and out of the vagina • Delivery of placenta – usually within 5 to 30 minutes • Probably an injection of Syntocinon, as the baby is being born, to speed up delivery of the placenta and control the bleeding	• Mild contractions or cramping afterpains • Some bleeding • Sore bottom and perineum • Not wanting to be touched or moved for a while • Lengthening of the umbilical cord • Heaviness in pelvis • Relief, joy, shock that your baby is finally here

LABOUR SUPPORT GUIDE

What you can do	What the partner/support people can do
• Try to keep focused and calm; if you need to release sounds then let it go • Know it's all right to feel out of control • Maintain eye contact with partner or keep eyes closed to focus • Get into the bath or the shower • Sip fluids regularly • Relax – know your baby is arriving soon • Cry and complain • Try to remember that you will probably not find a comfortable position • Trust your body, the process is normal	• Eye-to-eye contact if she needs and wants it • Allow her to be noisy and out of control; reassure her this is good • Be quiet if she finds talking annoying • Encourage her to stay in the here and now, let go of the idea of 'how long?' • Maintain tranquillity around her • Breathe with her • Tell her to release sounds if she needs to • Stay close and stay calm • Let her direct you • Thigh or shoulder massage if she wants to be touched • Cold washer or spray to face • Offer fluids or ice chips • Be open and flexible to her needs
• Go with your body – push only when you have a contraction to avoid exhaustion • Relax between pushes • Drink between the contractions • Let gravity assist you and your baby try upright positions, eg. standing, squatting • Get on all fours if the baby is coming too fast • Get into the bath or shower • Let your vagina open – you're doing well! • When you feel the stinging, burning sensations, pant – pant your baby's head out to help avoid tearing • Touch your baby's head as it emerges • Enjoy the feeling of bliss when your baby enters your arms • Feel relieved – you've done it! • Cry	• Physical support – help with positioning • Help her into the bath • Organise a mirror if she wants one • Tell her when you can see the baby's head • Help her to feel the baby's head • Maintain eye contact – pant with her! • Encourage her to relax the pelvic floor and let go • If she says, 'It's stinging/burning', tell her the baby is coming! • Wipe her brow. It's hard work! • Offer drinks between contractions • Tell her how wonderful she is • Be in awe of a labouring and birthing woman • Help 'catch' the baby if it is appropriate and she doesn't need you to hold her • Cry • Take photos if she wants them • Cut the cord if appropriate
• Remain in an upright position to help placenta come away • Give gentle pushes, with a contraction or cramping • Put baby to the breast if you both feel like it • Hot cup of tea or drink • Take some mild pain tablets or use heat packs	• Offer warm drinks and something to eat • Assist her into a position to help birth placenta • Once placenta comes away, help her to be comfortable to feed the baby • Take photos • Make phone calls • Help her into the shower when she is ready • Feel relief and joy

Support resources

Birthnet Pty Ltd – for more information on all areas relating to preconception, pregnancy, birth and early parenting, see our website www.birth.com.au

PRECONCEPTION, SEXUAL HEALTH, CONTRACEPTION

Australian Women's Health Network (AWHN)
www.awhn.org.au

Australian Federation of Men's Health & Wellbeing Associations Inc.
www.menshealthandwellbeing.org.au

Sexual Health and Family Planning Australia
National tel: (02) 6230 5255 (ACT)
www.fpa.net.au

Family Planning Australia ACT
Tel: (02) 6247 3077
www.shfpact.org.au

FPA Health (NSW)
FPA NSW Healthline: 1300 658 886
www.fpahealth.org.au

Family Planning Welfare Association of Northern Territory
Tel: (08) 8948 0144 (Darwin)
Tel: (08) 8953 0288 (Alice Springs)
www.fpwnt.com.au

Family Planning Queensland (FPQ)
Tel: (07) 3250 0240
www.fpq.asn.au

Family Planning Australia (SA)
Tel: (08) 8210 8180

Family Planning Tasmania Inc.
Tel: (03) 6228 5244
Health hotline: 1800 007 119
www.fpt.asn.au

Family Planning Victoria Inc. (FPV)
Tel: (03) 9257 0123 (clinic)
www.sexlife.net.au

Family Planning Association Western Australia (FPWA)
Free call: 1800 198 205
www.fpwa-health.org.au

Family Planning Association New Zealand
National Office tel: (04) 384 4349
www.fpanz.org.nz

Natural Family Planning Australia
Free call: 1800 114 010
Northern Territory: 1800 812 722
www.natfamplan.com.au

Women's Information & Referral Centres
Counselling, advice and information.
ACT   (02) 6205 1075
NSW   (02) 9334 1160 Free call: 1800 817 227
      www.women.nsw.gov.au
NT   (08) 8951 5880
QLD   (07) 4051 9366 Free call: 1800 177 577
      www.womhealth.org.au
SA   (08) 8303 0590 Free call: 1800 188 158
      www.wis.sa.gov.au
TAS   (03) 6233 2208 Free call: 1800 001 377
      www.dpac.tas.gov.au
VIC   (03) 9654 6844 Free call: 1800 136 570
      TTY for deaf (03) 9654 5124
      www.vicnet.net.au/~wire
WA   (08) 9264 1900 free call: 1800 199 174
      www.wa.gov.au/wpdo

INFERTILITY
ACCESS Australia Infertility Network
Tel: (02) 9670 2380
Outside NSW 1800 888 896
www.access.org.au

Fertility New Zealand
Tel: 0800 333 306
www.fertilitynz.org.nz

Natural Fertility Management Pty Ltd
The Jocelyn Centre tel: (02) 9369 2047
www.fertility.com.au

New Zealand Natural Fertility Management Pty Ltd
Tel: (03) 381 4924

ADOPTION
All States have government welfare departments and private adoption agencies. Various government contacts can be found at: http://www.aacasa.org.au

WORK, ENVIRONMENT, DISCRIMINATION
Environment Protection Authority (EPA)
Tel: (02) 9716 0014
www.lead.org.au

Human Rights and Equal Opportunity Commission
Tel: (02) 9284 9600
www.humanrights.gov.au

National Occupational Health & Safety Commission (NOHSC)
Tel: (02) 6279 1000
www.nohsc.gov.au

MEDICATIONS, ALCOHOL AND DRUGS

National Prescribing Service Limited (NPS)
Australians can ask health experienced drug information specialists about their medicines.
Tel: 1300 888 763
www.nps.org.au

Medications in Pregnancy & Lactation Service (NSW)
(Mothersafe) Information about drugs, medications, infections, radiation, occupational health exposures.
Tel: (02) 9382 6539 Mon–Fri 9 am–4 pm (EST)
Free call: 1800 647 848 (rural areas)

Australian Drug & Information Service (ADIS)
ACT (06) 205 4545
NSW (02) 9361 8000 Free call: 1800 422 599
NT   (08) 8922 8399 Free call: 1800 629 683
     (08) 8951 7580 (Alice Springs)
QLD (07) 3236 2414 Free call: 1800 177 833
SA   (08) 8363 8618 Free call: 1300 131 340
TAS (03) 6233 6722 Free call: 1800 811 994
VIC (03) 9416 1818 Free call: 1800 888 236
WA   (08) 9442 5000 Free call: 1800 198 024

Australian Drug Information Network (ADIN)
www.adin.com.au

Alcohol & Other Drug Council of Australian (ADCA)
National resource centre tel: (02) 6281 1002
www.adca.org.au

Family Drug Support (FDS)
Hotline: 1300 368 186
www.fds.org.au

New Zealand Alcohol & Drug Helpline
Tel: 0800 787 797
www.adanz.org.nz

SMOKING

Australian Quit Line
Tel: 131 848 (24 hours)
www.quitnow.info.au

New Zealand Quit Line
Tel: 0800 778 778
www.quit.co.nz

HIV/AIDS, Hepatitis C

Australian Federation of AIDS Organisations (AFAO)
Tel: (02) 9557 9399
www.afao.org.au

AIDS Action Council of ACT
Tel: (02) 6257 2855
www.aidsaction.org.au

AIDS Council of NSW (ACON)
Tel: (02) 9206 2069
Free call: 1800 063 060
www.acon.org.au

Northern Territory AIDS & Hepatitis C Council (NTAC)
Tel: (08) 8941 1711
www.ntac.org.au

Queensland AIDS Council (QuAc)
Tel: (07) 3017 1777
Free call: 1800 177 434 (outside Brisbane)
www.quac.org.au

AIDS Council South Australia
Tel: (08) 8362 1611
Free call 1800 888 559
www.aidscouncil.org.au

Tasmanian Council of AIDS, Hepatitis and Related Diseases Inc. (TasCAHRD)
Support line: 1800 005 900
www.tascahrd.org.au

AIDS Council Victoria
www.vicaids.asn.au

WA AIDS Council (WAAC)
Tel: (08) 9482 0000

New Zealand AIDS
Hotline: 0800 802 437
Auckland tel: (09) 358 0099
www.everybody.co.nz/sexfiles/cont.html

Hepatitis C Council of NSW
Tel: (02) 9332 1853
Free call: 1800 803 990
www.hepatitisc.org.au

Hepatitis C Council of Qld
Tel: (07) 3229 3767 (metro area)
Free call: 1800 648 491
www.hepatitisc.asn.au

Pregnancy support
Pregnancy National Helpline:
Tel: 1300 139 313
ACT   (02) 6247 5050
NT   (08) 8981 8526
QLD   (07) 3233 0328
TAS   (03) 6224 2290

Australian Federation of Pregnancy Support Services
National tel: (02) 6257 5200
Helpline: 1300 1393 13 (24 hrs)
www.pregnancysupport.com.au

Pregnancy Counselling Australia
Free call: 1800 650 840
www.birthline.org.au

Caregivers
Australian College of Midwives
National tel: (3) 9804 5071
www.acmi.org.au

Australian Society of Independent Midwives (ASIM)
Tel: (02) 9546 4350
members.ozemail.com.au/~midwife

Childbirth Choices in New Zealand
Maternity Services Consumer Council
Tel: (09) 520 5314
www.maternity.org.nz

Council of Remote Area Nurses of Australia Inc. (CRANA)
Maternity care in the bush
www.crana.org.au

Homebirth Australia
Tel: 1800 222 180
www.homebirthaustralia.org

Lead Maternity Carers (NZ)
For LMC services in your area
Tel: 0800 686 223

Maternity Coalition Inc. (MC)
Consumer advocacy
www.maternitycoalition.org.au

New Zealand College of Midwives
Tel: (03) 377 2732
www.midwives.org.nz

NSW Midwives Association Inc.
Tel: (02) 9281 9522
www.nswmidwives.com

Royal Australian & NZ College of Obstetricians & Gynaecologists (RANZCOG)
Tel: (03) 9417 1699
www.ranzcog.edu.au

Royal Australasian College of Physicians (and Paediatricians) RACP
Tel: (02) 9256 5444
www.racp.edu.au

RACP NZ
Tel: (04) 4 472 6713
e-mail: racp@racp.org.nz

NATURAL THERAPIES

Australian Acupuncture and Chinese Medicine Association Ltd (AACMA)
National practitioner referral 1300 725 334
www.acupuncture.org.au

Australian Association of Professional Homoeopaths Inc.
Tel: 1300 13 2927
www.homoeopathy.org.au

Australian Homeopathic Association (AHA)
Tel: (03) 5979 4697
www.homeopathyoz.org

Australian Natural Therapists Association Ltd
(07) 5491 9850
www.anta.com.au

Australian Osteopathic Association (AOA)
Tel: (02) 9440 2511
www.osteopathic.com.au

Australian Society of Teachers of the Alexander Technique (AUSTAT) Inc.
Free call: 1800 339 571
alexandertechnique.org.au

Chiropractors Association of Australia (CAA)
www.chiropractors.asn.au

International Federation of Aromatherapists (Australian Branch) Inc.
www.ifa.org.au

National Herbalists Association of Australia
Tel: (02) 9555 8885
www.nhaa.org.au

GENETIC TESTING

Genetic information & testing in Australia
Tel: (02) 9926 7324
www.genetics.com.au

Genetic information & testing in New Zealand
Auckland free call: 0800 476 123
Wellington free call: 0508 364 436
Christchurch free call: 0508 364 436 (South Island callers)

Miscarriage and stillborn baby support
Bonnie Babies Foundation
24-hour counselling in Australia
Tel: (03) 9758 2800
www.bbf.org.au

SANDS Australia
ACT (02) 6287 4255
NSW (02) 9721 0124
QLD (07) 3254 3422 Rural: 1800 228 655
SA (08) 8277 0304
TAS (03) 9517 4470
VIC (03) 9899 0217
WA support line: 1800 686 780 Rural: 1800 199 466
www.sands.org.au

Miscarriage Support New Zealand
Nth Auckland tel: (09) 428 0222
Wellington tel: (04) 384 4272
www.miscarriagesupport.org.nz

SIDS Australia (Sudden Infant Death Association)
Tel: 1800 651 186 (24-hour support line)
www.sidsandkids.org

Bereavement CARE Centre
Counselling Advice Referral Education
Tel: 1300 654 556
www.bereavementcare.com.au

Premature babies
Preterm Infants' Parents Association (PIPA)
Qld & northern NSW
Tel: (07) 3354 4638, (07) 3209 9896
www.pipa.org.au
Other websites:
www.parentcare.org.nz
www.austprem.org.au
www.preemie-l.org

Twins and more
Australian Multiple Birth Association (AMBA)
National tel: (02) 9875 2404
www.amba.org.au

Twin to Twin Transfusion Support
www.twin-twin.org

Breastfeeding
Australian Breastfeeding Association (ABA)
ACT (02) 6258 8928
NSW (02) 9639 8686

QLD (07) 3844 8977
SA   (08) 8411 0050
VIC (03) 9885 0653
TAS (03) 6223 2609
WA   (08) 9340 1200
www.breastfeeding.asn.au

La Leche League (NZ) breastfeeding counsellors
Tel: (4) 471 0690
www.lalecheleague.org/LLLNZ
Plunketline free call: 0800 933 922 (24 hrs/7 days)
www.plunket.org.nz

Parent lines
ACT (02) 6278 3995
NSW 132 055
NT   (08) 8953 0785
QLD 1300 301 300
SA   1300 364 100

TAS Parent Information Telephone Assistance (PITAS)
Free call: 1800 808 178
VIC 132 289 or 136 388 (24 hrs/7 days)
WA   (08) 9272 1466 (24 hrs)

Family crisis care
NSW (02) 9622 0522 Mon–Fri 6 pm–11 pm, Sat, Sun and public hols 10 am–11 pm
NT   (08) 8981 9227 (24 hrs) Free call: 1800 019 116 (24 hrs)
SA   131 611 Mon–Fri 4 pm–9 am, 24 hrs weekends & public holidays
VIC (03) 9329 0300 (24 hrs)
WA   (08) 9223 1100 (24 hrs) Free call: 1800 643 000 (24 hrs)
If you require assistance outside these times (or in other States) contact the National Lifeline: 131 114.

Cryline
When you are not coping with your baby's crying
National tel: 132 111
Free call: 1800 066 777

Other parent services
ACT
Queens Elizabeth II Family Centre
Tel: (02) 6205 2333 (24 hrs)

NSW
Karitane
Tel: (02) 9794 1852 (24 hrs)
Free call: 1800 677 961 (24 hrs)
www.swsahs.nsw.gov.au/karitane

Tresillian
National tel: (02) 9787 0800
Helpline: (02) 9787 5255 (24 hrs)
Free call: 1800 637 357 (24 hrs)
Dial-a-Mum counselling service; trained volunteer mothers
Tel: (02) 9477 6777 (8 am–midnight)

QLD
Child Health Information & Advisory Service
Tel: (07) 3862 2333 (24 hrs)

Community Child Health
Tel: (07) 3860 7111

SA
Torrens House
Tel: (08) 8303 1530
www.cyh.com

Sparks Resource Centre
Tel: (08) 8226 2500

TAS
Lady Gowrie
Tel: (03) 6236 9256
Free call: 1800 675 416

VIC
Caroline Chisholm
Tel: (03) 9370 3933 (24 hrs)
Free call: 1800 143 863

WA
WA Parent helpline (08) 9272 1466 (24 hrs)
Parent helpline free call: 1800 654 432 (24 hrs)
Family helpline (08) 9223 1100 (24 hrs)
Family helpline free call: 1800 643 000 (24 hrs)

Relationship Counselling
Tel: (02) 9418 8800
Free call: 1800 801 578
Australia-wide: 1300 364 277
www.relationships.com.au

SINGLE PARENT SUPPORT
National tel: 1300 300 496
SA   (08) 8226 2500 or (08) 8226 2509
TAS   (03) 6263 5464
VIC   (03) 9654 0622
          (03) 9654 0327
WA   (08) 9389 8373

Parents without partners
ACT   (02) 6248 6333
NSW   (02) 9896 1888

QLD (07) 3275 3290
SA   (08) 8359 1552
TAS (03) 6249 5215
VIC (03) 9836 3211
WA   (08) 9389 8350

POST NATAL DEPRESSION
ACT
Queen Elizabeth II Family Centre
Tel: (02) 6205 2333 (24 hrs)

NSW
Dona Maria
Tel: 1300 555 578

QLD
Brisbane Centre for Post Natal Disorders
Tel: (07) 3398 0238 (24 hrs)

SA
Tel: (08) 8303 1183 (24 hrs)
Free call: 1800 182 232

VIC
Post and Ante Natal Depression Association (PANDA)
Tel: (03) 9882 5756

Overcoming Postnatal Depression (OPND)
Tel: (08) 8367 6772

WA
Postnatal Depression Support Association
Tel: (08) 9340 1622

Post Traumatic Stress Disorder (PTSD)
New Zealand tel: 0064 08324 8227
www.tabs.org.nz

Post Natal Psychosis Support
Auckland NZ tel (9) 449 1011

IMMUNISATION AND VACCINATION
Australian Childhood Immunisation Register
Free call: 1800 653 809

Australian Health Insurance Commission
Medicare/immunisation
Tel: 132 011 (local call rate)
www.hic.gov.au

Australian Vaccination Network (AVN)
Tel: (02) 6687 1699
www.avn.org.au

National Child Immunisation Program
Free call: 1800 671 811

HOME AND PRODUCT SAFETY
CHOICE Guide to Baby Products
www.choice.com.au

Infant Nursery Product Association of Australia (INPPA)
www.inpaa.asn.au

Kidsafe Australia
National office (QLD)
Tel: (07) 3854 1829
www.kidsafe.org.au
ACT   (02) 6290 2243
NSW   (02) 9845 0890
         www.kidsafensw.org
NT   (08) 8985 1085
         www.ozemail.com.au/~kidsafen
SA   (08) 8161 6318
TAS   (03) 6249 1933
VIC   (03) 9345 6471
         www.kidsafe.com.au
WA   (08) 9340 8509
         www.kidsafewa.com.au

The Ministerial Council on Consumer Affairs
www.consumer.gov.au

MISCELLANEOUS
Birthrites – Healing after Caesarean & VBAC support
Tel: (08) 9418 8949
www.birthrites.org

Continence Foundation of Australia Ltd
National Helpline 1800 3300 66
www.contfound.org.au

Department of Family and Community Services (FaCS)
Tel: 1300 653 227
TTY for the deaf: 1800 260 402
www.community.gov.au

Manhood
www.manhood.com.au

National Association for Prevention for Child Abuse and Neglect (NapCan)
www.napcan.org.au

National Childcare Accreditation Council Inc.
Tel: (02) 8260 1900
1300 136 554 outside Sydney
www.ncac.gov.au

Further reading

Australian Consumers Association, *The Choice Guide to Baby Products*, Choice Books, Sydney, 2001.
Australian Cord Blood Bank (ACBB), *Questions Most Frequently Asked?*, Sydney Children's Hospital, Randwick, NSW, 2000.
Australian Cord Blood Bank (ACBB), *You Can Save a Life by Giving your Cord Blood*, Sydney Children's Hospital, Randwick, NSW, 2000.
Balaskas, J, *New Active Birth: A Concise Guide to Natural Childbirth*, Thorsons, London, 1989.
Barker, Robin, *Baby Love: Everything You Need to Know About Your New Baby*, Pan Macmillan, Sydney, 2001.
Beech, LB & Robinson, J, *Ultrasound??? Unsound*, AIMS, Preston, UK, Feb 1994.
Bradford, N, *Your Premature Baby – 0–5 years*, Frances Lincoln, London, 2001.
Bradley, RA, *Husband Coached Childbirth*, 4th edn, Bantam, New York, 1996.
Brazelton, TB, *Touchpoints*, Doubleday, Sydney, 1993.
Castro, M, *Homoeopathy for Mother and Baby*, Papermac, London, 1993.
Cohen, NW, *Open Season: A Survival Guide for Natural Childbirth and VBAC in the 90's*, Bergin & Garvey, New York, 1991.
Collinge, A, Daniel, S, & Jones, HG, *Always a Part of Me: Surviving Childbearing Loss*, ABC Books, Sydney, 2002.
Commonwealth of Australia, *7 Helpful Hints for Solving Breastfeeding Problems*, Ausinfo, Canberra, 1998.
Cox, S, *Breastfeeding – I Can Do That! A do it yourself guide*, TasLaC, Lindisfarne, Tas, Vic 1997.
Crawford, K & Walters, J, *Natural Birth after Caesarean: A Practical Guide*, Blackwell Science, Cambridge, UK, 1996.
Cummings, R, Houghton, K & Williams, LA, *Sleep Right, Sleep Tight*, Transworld, Sydney, 2000.
Dick-Read, G, Wessel, H & Ellis, HF, *Childbirth Without Fear: The Original Approach to Natural Childbirth*, HarperCollins, New York, 1994.
England, P & Horowitz, R, *Birthing from Within*, Patera Press, New Mexico, 1998.
Enkin, M, Keirse, MJNC, Neilson, J, Crowther, C, Duley, L, Hodnett, E & Hofmeyr J, *A Guide to Effective Care in Pregnancy and Childbirth*, 3rd edn, Oxford University Press, Oxford, 2000.
Fowler, C & Gornall, P, *How to Stay Sane in Your Baby's First Year: The Tresillian Guide*, revised edn, Simon & Schuster, Sydney, 2000.
Gaskin, IM, *Spiritual Midwifery*, 3rd edn, The Book Publishing Company, Summertown, TN, 1990.
Gillespie, C, *Your Pregnancy – Month by Month*, HarperCollins, New York, 1998.
Gladstar, R, *Herbal Healing for Women*, Bantam, London, 1994.
Goer, H, *The Thinking Woman's Guide to a Better Birth*, Penguin, New York, 1999.
Hale, T, *Medications and Mother's Milk*, 8th edn, Pharmasoft Medical Publishing, Texas, 2000.
Hamilton-Craig, I, *Men's Health*, Pan, Sydney, 1993.
Harper, B & Arms, S, *Gentle Birth Choices: A Guide to Making Informed Decisions about Birthing Centres, Birth Attendants, Water Birth, Home Birth, Hospital Birth*, Healing Arts Press, Vermont, 1994.
Karst, P, *The Single Mother's Survival Guide*, Crossing Press, Freedom, California, 2000.

Kitzinger, S, *The Experience of Breastfeeding*, Penguin, London, 1984.
Kitzinger, S, *The New Pregnancy and Childbirth*, Doubleday, Sydney, 1991.
Kitzinger, S, *The Year after Childbirth: Surviving the First Year of Motherhood*, Oxford University Press, Oxford, 1994.
Laughlin, K, *Stretching & pregnancy*, Simon & Schuster, Sydney, 2001.
Lichy, R & Herzberg, E, *The Waterbirth Handbook: The Gentle Art of Waterbirthing*, Gateway Books, Bath, UK, 1993.
Lim, R, *After the Baby's Birth . . . A Woman's Way to Wellness*, Celestial Arts, Berkeley, California, 1992.
Lipson, T, *From Conception to Birth*, Millennium Books, Sydney, 1994.
Llewellyn-Jones, D, *Everywoman: A Gynaecological Guide for Life*, 9th edn, Penguin, Sydney, 1998.
Lovin, F, *The Best Friends' Guide to Surviving the First Year of Motherhood*, Bloomsbury, London, 1999.
Luke, B & Eberlein, T, *When You are Expecting Twins, Triplets or Quads*, HarperCollins, New York, 1999.
Machover, I, Drake, A & Drake, J, *The Alexander Technique Birth Book*, Robinson, London, 1993.
Mirosch, N, *Going it Alone: The Single Woman's Guide to Pregnancy and Birth*, New Holland Publishers, Australia, 2002.
Naish, F, *Natural Fertility*, revised edn, Sally Milner Publishing, Sydney, 1993.
National Centre for Immunisation Research & Surveillance of Vaccine Preventable Diseases, *Immunisation Myths & Realities: Responding to Arguments against Immunisation*, Commonwealth Government of Australia, Canberra, 2000.
National Health and Medical Research Council, *Postnatal Depression: Not Just the Baby Blues*, Commonwealth of Australia, Canberra, 2000.
NETS Medical Retrieval, *Information for Parents and Families: NSW Newborn Paediatric Emergency Transport Service*, NSW Pregnancy and Newborn Services Network (PSN), Sydney, 2000.
NHMRC, *Infant Feeding Guidelines for Health Workers*, Commonwealth Government of Australia, Canberra, 1996.
NHMRC, *Recommended Dietary Intakes for Use in Australia*, Commonwealth Government of Australia, Canberra, 2002.
NHMRC, *The Australian Immunisation Handbook*, 8th end, Commonwealth Government of Australia, Canberra, 2003.
NHMRC, *Vitamin K for Newborn Babies*, Commonwealth of Australia, Canberra, 2000.
Nilsson, L, Furunhjelm, M, Ingelmann-Sunberg, A & Wirsen, C, *A Child is Born*, revised edn, Faber & Faber, London, 1977.
NSW Health, *Tests to Protect Your Baby*, revised edn, Sydney, 2001.
NSW Health, *Some Infectious Diseases of Children*, Public Affairs and AIDS Infectious Diseases Branch, Better Health Centre, Sydney, 2001.
NSW Department of Industrial Relations, *Maternity at Work*, Women's Equity Bureau (WEB), Sydney, 2001.
Panuthos, C & Romeo, C, *Ended Beginnings: Healing Childbearing Loss*, Bergin and Garvey, New York, 1984.
Peterson, G, *Birthing Normally*, 2nd edn, Shadow and Light, Berkeley, New York, 1984.
Pitchford, P, *Healing with Whole Foods: Asian Traditions and Modern Nutrition*, revised edn, North Atlantic Books, 2002.

Renfrew, M, Fisher, C, Arms, S & Conroy, M, *Breastfeeding: Getting Breastfeeding Right for You*, Celestial Arts, Berkeley, California, 1990.

SANDS NSW, *Miscarriage: Information for Parents and Families*, 2nd edn, Sydney, 1995.

Savage, B & Simkin, D, *Preparation for Birth. The Complete Guide to the Lamaze Method*, Ballantine, 1987.

Sidenbladh, E, *Waterbabies: Igor Tjarkovsky and His Method of Delivering and Training Children Underwater*, A & C Black, London, 1983.

Simkin, P, *The Birth Partner: Everything You Need to Know to Help a Woman Through Childbirth*, 2nd edn, Harvard Common Press, Boston, 2001.

Stephenson-Meere, M, *Baby's First 100 Days*, Doubleday, Sydney, 2001.

St John of God Health Services, *Post Partum Depression and Anxiety – A Self-Help Guide for Mothers*, Pacific Post Partum Support Society, 1998.

Stoppard, M, *The First Weeks of Life*, Viking O'Neil, South Yarra, Victoria, 1989.

Sullivan, K, *Alternative Remedies*, HarperCollins, Glasgow, 1994.

Tracy, AE & Maroney, DI, *Your Premature Baby and Child: Helpful Answers and Advice for Parents*, Berkeley Publishing Group, New York, 1999.

Tupling, H, *Breastfeeding: A New Mother's Handbook*, Watermark Press, Sydney, 1995.

VanDam Anderson, S & Simkin, P, *Birth Through Children's Eyes*, The Penny Press, Washington, DC, 1981.

Wagner, M, *Pursuing the Birth Machine: The Search for Appropriate Birth Technology*, ACE Graphics, Sydney, 1994.

Whitney, EN & Rolfes, SR, *Understanding Nutrition*, 9th edn, Wadsworth Group, Belmont, Tennessee, 2002.

Worwood, VA, *The Fragrant Pharmacy: A Complete Guide to Aromatherapy Essential Oils*, Bantam, Sydney, 1996.

Glossary

afterpains. Cramping of the uterus after the birth, often aggravated with breastfeeding for a short period. More common with second and subsequent babies.

alveoli. Small milk-producing sacs in the woman's breasts.

amniocentesis. A needle passed through the woman's belly to take amniotic fluid from around the baby for testing.

amniotic fluid. The fluid that surrounds the baby while inside their mother's womb.

anencephaly. The medical term for 'the absence of a brain', with the unborn baby's skull and brain not forming.

anterior lip. A swelling of the top of the cervix just before the cervix is fully dilated (or open).

anterior position. The unborn baby's back is facing the front, towards the woman's belly.

antiemetic. A medication that is prescribed to alleviate or prevent nausea and vomiting.

aortocaval compression. When the large blood vessels behind the uterus become compressed by the woman lying on her back in late pregnancy.

areola. The darkened skin around the nipple of the breast.

ARM. Said as A-R-M, meaning 'artificial rupture of membranes', or breaking the waters intentionally.

augmentation. Using interventions or medication to speed up the progress of labour.

bacteriuria. Bacteria present in the urine which may cause an infection.

bicornuate uterus. A piece of tissue or 'septum' inside the uterus (that was present before the pregnancy) that extends from the top of the uterus or fundus, inside the uterus. Also known as a heart-shaped uterus.

biorhythms. The body's innate sense of when night and day are, to regulate sleep patterns.

Braxton Hicks contraction. Practice contractions of the uterus, or 'tightenings', felt usually after about 20 weeks of the pregnancy.

breech. The baby is lying in the uterus with their bottom (instead of the head) down.

brow presentation. A rare position, where the baby's forehead leads the way down the woman's birth canal.

cannula. A small plastic tube inserted in the vein that also can be used to attach a drip to if needed.

caput. An area of swelling on the top of the baby's head that develops with the normal pressure on the cervix during labour.

cephalhaematoma. A blood collection under the baby's skin on their scalp on one or both sides, which dissolves over weeks or months. Usually due to the baby's head rubbing on the woman's pelvis during the birth or forceps or ventouse deliveries.

cervix. The neck or opening to the uterus or womb inside the vagina.

chignon. A large swelling of the baby's scalp that mimics the shape of the ventouse cup.

cholestasis. A liver disorder usually occurring after 20 weeks of pregnancy that suppresses the flow of bile from the liver into the woman's bowel. This causes a build-up of toxins (liver enzymes, bilirubin and bile acids) causing itching and affecting the unborn baby.

chorion. The fine membrane that lines the uterus, encapsulating the amniotic sacs and babies.

colostrum. The first fluid produced by the breasts until the mature milk comes in.

complete breech. Baby lying bottom down in the uterus with their feet crossed down near their bottom.

cord prolapse. The umbilical cord falls down in front of the unborn baby and through the cervix after the waters break, possibly leading to compressing the cord and reducing the blood supply from the placenta to the baby.

CTG. Or 'cardiotocograph', a large electronic machine used to provide a continuous paper readout of the baby's heart rate and contractions.

D&C. Or a dilation and curettage, an operation to evacuate the contents of the uterus.

deflexed head. This describes the unborn baby's head looking forward or slightly up, rather than looking down towards their chest, with their chin tucked in (called 'flexed'). If the baby's head is deflexed, it makes the diameter wider and more difficult for the baby to negotiate the birth canal.

DIC. A rare disorder that involves the body forming blood clots and experiencing internal haemorrhaging.

diuretic. A substance that increases the urine output of the kidneys, making you pass more urine.

Doppler. An electronic device, using sound waves, to detect the baby's heart rate.

DVT. Deep vein thrombosis, where a blood clot forms in the deep veins of the leg (usually the calf).

ectopic pregnancy. Where the baby starts to grow in the fallopian tube, instead of the uterus, causing pain and requiring an operation to remove the pregnancy.

ECV. Or external cephalic version, where the baby is turned by the caregiver through manipulating the outside of the woman's belly.

endometrium. The lining of the woman's uterus that builds each month and then is shed as a period if a baby is not conceived.

endorphins. Natural morphine-like hormones that the body releases to help deal with pain.

engaged. When the baby's head lowers down into the woman's pelvis, in preparation for labour and birth.

episiotomy. A surgical cut of the perineum (lower vagina) with the birth of the baby.

face presentation. A rare position, where the baby's face leads the way down the woman's birth canal.

face to pubes. The baby's head is born with their face looking towards the mother's belly rather than her bottom (not common).

fallopian tubes. Two tubes that lead from the top of the woman's uterus to her ovaries that transport released eggs after ovulation to be fertilised for implantation in the uterus to conceive a baby. Conception takes place in the fallopian tubes.

fetal blood sampling. A sample of blood taken from the baby's scalp during labour, to check their oxygen and blood chemistry levels.

fetal distress. A medical term to describe when the baby is not coping inside the uterus, usually during labour.

flexed head. If the unborn baby's head is flexed (rather than deflexed), the baby is looking down towards their chest, with their chin tucked in, making the baby's crown 'lead the way'. This makes the baby's head the smallest it can be in diameter, assisting them to easily negotiate the birth canal during labour.

fontanelle. The 'soft spot' on top of the baby's head, created by a space in the skull bones, that closes over by the time the baby is 18 months old.

football hold. When breastfeeding, the baby is positioned with their body tucked under your arm.

footling breech. Baby lying bottom down in the uterus with one foot down, the other foot up.

frank breech. Baby lying bottom down in the uterus with their feet up near their ears.

fundus. The very top of the uterus.

haemoglobin. Red blood cells that carry oxygen in the bloodstream, low levels cause anaemia.

HCG. Or human chorionic gonadotrophin, a pregnancy hormone that roughly doubles every 2 to 3 days during the first 12 weeks of pregnancy.

hepatitis. A virus, or infection that inflames the liver, often causing a degree of liver damage.

HPV. Human papilloma virus or wart virus, which can sometimes cause changes in the cells of the cervix.

hydrocephalus. An abnormal health condition for the baby, resulting in fluid accumulating in the baby's brain.

hypospadias. When the opening of the penis is abnormally situated on the underside of the penis, rather than the end of the penis.

internal podalic version. Or IPV, where the baby (usually a second twin), is turned by the caregiver, by grasping their feet via a vaginal examination to be born breech.

ketotic, ketosis, ketones. A complication of dehydration and lack of carbohydrates (or glucose) for energy in the body causing a breakdown in fat stores for energy, leading to an abnormal accumulation of 'ketone bodies' in the blood, body tissues and urine.

labia. The lips of the woman's vulva, or genitals, on either side of her vagina.

let-down. The release of oxytocin from the brain, causing the woman's breast milk to 'eject', or flow freely.

linea nigra. A darkening of the skin as a line down the middle of the belly during pregnancy.

lithotomy position. The woman lies on her back, with feet elevated, knees and thighs bent and apart. Stirrups are usually used to support the woman's feet.

lower segment. As the uterus grows past 24 weeks of pregnancy, a section forms between the upper uterus (or fundus) and the woman's cervix. This is referred to as the 'lower segment' of the uterus.

macrosomic. A baby that has an unusually fat body in relation to their head, often compared to looking like a Buddha. These babies often weigh more than 4.5 kg.

meconium. The first black, sticky poo passed by the baby after birth.

metabolic disorders. A condition where the baby is born with the lack of an enzyme that affects their metabolism, such as galactosemia and phenylketonuria.

molar pregnancy. Or hydatidiform mole. A very rare condition, where the placenta develops abnormally and starts producing fluid-filled cysts, or vesicles that multiply rapidly, and the baby does not develop.

moxibustion. Or moxa, is the burning of chinese herbs and using the heated embers to stimulate an acupressure point.

neural tube defects. When problems occur with the development of the baby's brain, skull and spinal cord during the first six weeks of pregnancy, causing spina bifida or anencephaly (the absence of a brain).

oximeter. A small infra-red light device that is strapped to the body (an adult's finger or a baby's foot) to detect oxygen levels in the blood.

oxytocin. The natural hormone released from the woman's brain that makes her uterus contract.

pelvic rocking. A circular and/or to-and-fro movement of the pelvis, similar to gentle belly dancing.

pelvis. The two bones (that also form the hips), attached to the lower spine and surrounding the non-pregnant uterus.

perineum. The area of muscle and tissue between the woman's vagina and anus.

Pinard's stethoscope. A small plastic, metal or wooden trumpet earpiece, used to listen to the baby's heartbeat.

placenta. Also known as the afterbirth, the organ that provides oxygen and nourishment for the baby inside the uterus.

placenta accreta. A rare complication, where the placenta implants into the wall of the uterus, rather than the lining, making it difficult to detach, or remove, after the birth.

placenta previa. When the placenta implants low in the uterus, close to or covering the woman's cervix.

placental abruption. When the placenta lifts off the wall of the uterus during pregnancy, causing pain and bleeding.

placental insufficiency. The placenta is not functioning to its optimum capacity.

platelets. Small blood cells that play a vital role in helping the blood to clot and control bleeding.

polyhydramnios. The unborn baby being surrounded by an abnormally large volume of amniotic fluid.

posterior position. The unborn baby's back, and the back of the head, is lying against the woman's spine.

postpartum haemorrhage. Also known as a PPH, where the woman bleeds very heavily after the birth, losing more than 500 to 600 ml of blood.

pre-eclampsia. Blood pressure that becomes high enough during pregnancy to cause health concerns for the woman and her baby(s).

prodromal symptoms. The signs of tingling, pain, feeling unwell or irritable, before a herpes sore appears.

progesterone. A female hormone that increases dramatically during pregnancy.

prolactin. A hormone naturally produced in the woman's brain when she breastfeeds, to increase her milk supply.

prostaglandins. Hormones capable of ripening the woman's cervix and/or stimulating labour.

pudendal block. Local anaesthetic is injected into the two pudendal nerves inside the vagina on both sides, for pain relief to the lower birth canal, for forceps or a ventouse delivery.

registrar. A qualified senior doctor close to completing their training in a speciality, such as obstetrics, anaesthesia or paediatrics.

resident. A qualified junior doctor, in training for a speciality such as obstetrics, anaesthesia or paediatrics.

retained placenta. When the placenta does not readily expel from the woman's uterus after the baby is born, usually requiring medical interventions to deliver it.

Rhesus negative blood. The absence of agglutinogens (antibodies) on the red blood cells, classifying a person's blood group as 'negative'. (Eg. O negative, A negative, B negative, AB negative.)

Rhesus isoimmunisation. When the unborn baby's blood (usually Rhesus positive), reacts with the mother's blood (usually Rhesus negative), sometimes making the baby anaemic.

ruptured uterus. A rare complication where the wall of the woman's uterus splits open, causing internal haemorrhaging. This is life-threatening for both the mother and baby.

sacrum. The lower part of the backbone where the pelvic bones are attached.

sepsis. An infection of the blood, which can be life-threatening.

septic work-up. A series of medical procedures performed on a baby in the intensive care nursery involving swab tests, urine samples, blood taken and sometimes a spinal tap to check for infection. The baby may also have antibiotics through the vein for 48 hours, until all the tests come back clear.

septum in the uterus. An unusually formed uterus called 'bicornuate', or heart-shaped, where a piece of tissue extends down inside the uterus from the fundus, a little like a stalactite descending from the roof of a cave.

shoulder dystocia. Difficult birth of the baby's shoulders, with a vaginal birth.

show. A thick plug of mucus that accumulates in the cervix during the pregnancy.

sitz bath. Sitting in a small bowel of warm water, to cleanse or soak the genital area.

SIDS. Sudden infant death syndrome – when a baby dies in their sleep for no known reason.

speculum. A metal or plastic instrument placed into the woman's vagina to check the cervix or take a Pap test.

spina bifida. The baby's spinal cord is exposed through an opening along their spine, sometimes protruding out to create a lump (or bulge).

stress incontinence. The uncontrolled passing of urine.

suppository. A medication that can be inserted into the anus and rectum, and is absorbed through the bowel.

syntocinon. A synthetic form of the natural oxytocin hormone that the woman releases to make her uterus contract.

TENS machine. Uses electrode pads on the woman's lower back to administer electrical impulses for pain relief. May also be used to stimulate acupressure points.

teratogenic. A substance, or effect, that can cause abnormalities in the baby, usually during the first 12 weeks of the pregnancy.

term. Baby born on time (37 to 42 weeks of the pregnancy).

thrombosis. See *DVT*.

tocolytic. Medications used to suppress contractions of the uterus.

tonic contractions. Strong, prolonged, continuous contractions due to the uterus being overstimulated.

trace. The name given to the continuous paper recording of the baby's heart rate during monitoring.

transverse position. Baby lying across-ways in the uterus, or if the unborn baby's head is facing sideways in the birth canal, rather than anterior or posterior.

ureters. Tubes that carry urine from the kidneys to the bladder.

urethra. The tube that carries urine from the bladder when urinating.

uterine rupture. See *ruptured uterus*.

vas deferens. Small tubes that carry sperm from the man's testes to his prostate gland before ejaculation.

vasa previa. A formation of the placenta where there is a 'satellite' lobe that implants away from the main body of the placenta, connected by a large blood vessel implanted in the amniotic sac membrane, that may sit in front of the unborn baby's head and bleed during labour.

velamentous insertion. When the umbilical cord implants in the membrane of the amniotic sac, allowing large blood vessels to run to the placenta, sometimes over the opening of the cervix. These may rupture when the waters break, causing bleeding during labour.

vena-caval compression. When the large blood vessel behind the uterus becomes compressed if the woman lies on her back during late pregnancy.

ventouse. Specially designed surgical cups (either metal or rubber) placed on the baby's head using negative pressure to assist the birth during the pushing phase.

vernix. Thick, white, greasy cream that covers the unborn baby's body, to protect their skin in their watery environment.

vertex presentation. When the crown of the baby's head leads the way down the woman's birth canal (the most common presentation).

Endnotes

Chapter 1
1. Human Rights and Equal Opportunity Commission. *Pregnancy Guidelines*, Commonwealth of Australia, Canberra, 2001.
2. Whitney, EN & Rolfes, S R. *Understanding nutrition*, 9th edn, Wadsworth Group, Belmont, Tennessee, 2002.
3. Lumley, J, Watson, L, Watson, M & Bower, C. 'Periconceptional supplementation with folate and/or multivitamins for preventing neural tube defects (Cochrane Review)', *The Cochrane Library*, issue 4, 2003, John Wiley & Sons, Chichester, UK.
4. Lumley, J, Watson, L, Watson, M & Bower, C. 'Modelling the potential impact of population-wide periconceptional folate/multivitamin supplementation on multiple births,' *British Journal of Obstetrics & Gynaecology*, 2001 Sept;108(9), pp 937–42.
5. Baerwald, AR, Adams, GP & Pierson RA. 'A new model for ovarian follicular development during the human menstrual cycle', *Fertility & Sterility*, 2003 July;80(1), pp 116–22.
6. Guillebaud, J. *Contraception, Your Questions Answered*, 3rd edn, Churchill Livingstone, London, 2000.
7. Shettles, LB & Rorvick, DM. *How to Choose the Sex of your Baby*, Doubleday, New York, 1997.
8. Hurst, T and Lancaster, P. *Assisted Conception Australia and New Zealand 1999 and 2000*, Assisted Conception Series, No. 6, AIWH National Perinatal Statistics, Unit, Sydney, 2001.

Chapter 2
1. Jewell, D & Young, G. 'Interventions for nausea and vomiting in early pregnancy (Cochrane Review)', *The Cochrane Library*, issue 4, 2003, John Wiley & Sons, Chichester, UK.
2. NHMRC. *Listeria-Advice for Medical Practitioners*, Commonwealth of Australia, Canberra, 1992.
Australia New Zealand Food Authority. *Listeria and Pregnancy: A guide to foods which are safe and those at 'higher risk' of Listeria contamination*, 2002.
3. Kramer, MS. 'Aerobic exercise for women during pregnancy (Cochrane Review)', *The Cochrane Library*, issue 4, 2003, John Wiley & Sons, Chichester, UK.
Howells, D. 'Exercise in pregnancy', *Practical Midwife*, 2002 Apr;5(4), pp 12–13.
4. Priest, J & Attawell, K. *Drugs in Conception, Pregnancy and Childbirth*, Thorsons, London, 1996.
5. Gardella, JR & Hill, JA. 'Environmental toxins associated with recurrent pregnancy loss', *Seminars in Reproductive Medicine*, 2000;18(4), pp 407–24.
6. Marcus, M, McChesney, R, Golden, A & Landrigan, P. 'Video display terminals and miscarriage', *Journal of the American Medical Women's Association*, 2000 Spring;55(2), pp 84–88, 105.
7. Koren, G. 'Exposure to electromagnetic fields during pregnancy', *Canadian Family Physician*, 2003 Feb;49, pp 151, 153.
8. Environment Protection Authority. 'Recommendations for limiting exposure to ionising radiation (1995) and national standard for limiting occupational exposure to ionising radiation (RH39)', *Radiation Control Authority NSW*, Sydney, 1995.
NHMRC. *Recommendations for Limiting Exposure to Ionizing Radiation*

(NOHSC:3022 - 1995) *and National Standard for Limiting Occupational Exposure to Ionizing Radiation (NOHSC:1013 - 1995)*, Commonwealth Government of Australia, Canberra, 1995.
9. NSW Environmental Protection Authority. *Lead Safe – A Guide to Keeping your Family Safe from Lead*, EPA, Sydney, 1998.
10. Fortier, JC, Carson, VB, Will, S & Shubkagel, BL. 'Adjustment to a newborn: Sibling preparation makes a difference', *Journal of Obstetric, Gynecologic and Neonatal Nursing*, 1991 Jan/Feb;20(1), pp 73–79.
11. Katz-Rothman, B. *The Tentative Pregnancy*. HarperCollins, London, 1994.
12. Everett, C. 'Incidence and outcome of bleeding before the 20th week of pregnancy: A prospective study from general practice', *British Medical Journal*, 1997 July 5;315(7099), pp 32–34.
13. McLaren, B & Shelley, JM. 'Reported management of early-pregnancy bleeding and miscarriage by general practitioners in Victoria', *Medical Journal of Australia*, 2002 Jan 21; 176(2), pp 63–66.
14. Vazquez, JC, Hickey, M & Neilson, JP. 'Medical management for miscarriage (Protocol for a Cochrane Review)', *The Cochrane Library*, issue 4, 2003, John Wiley & Sons, Chichester, UK.
15. Bamigboye, AA & Morris, J. 'Oestrogen supplementation, mainly diethylstilbestrol, for preventing miscarriages and other adverse pregnancy outcomes (Cochrane Review)', *The Cochrane Library*, issue 4, 2003, John Wiley & Sons, Chichester, UK.
Oates-Whitehead, RM & Carrier, JAK. 'Progestogen for preventing miscarriage (Protocol for a Cochrane Review)', *The Cochrane Library*, issue 4, 2003, John Wiley & Sons, Chichester, UK.
Scott, JR & Pattison, N. 'Human chorionic gonadotrophin for recurrent miscarriage (Cochrane Review)', *The Cochrane Library*, issue 4, 2003, John Wiley & Sons, Chichester, UK.
Scott, JR. 'Immunotherapy for recurrent miscarriage (Cochrane Review)', *The Cochrane Library*, issue 4, 2003, John Wiley & Sons, Chichester, UK.
16. Drakeley, AJ, Roberts, D & Alfirevic Z. 'Cervical stitch (cerclage) for preventing pregnancy loss in women (Cochrane Review)', *The Cochrane Library*, issue 4, 2003, John Wiley & Sons, Chichester, UK.
17. Aronsen, L, Lochen, ML & Lund E. 'Smoking is associated with increased risk of ectopic pregnancy – A population based study', *Tidsskr Nor Laegeforen*, 2002 Feb 10;122(4), pp 415–18.
18. Hajenius, PJ, Mol, BWJ, Bossuyt, PMM, Ankum, WM & Van der Veen, F. 'Interventions for tubal ectopic pregnancy (Cochrane Review)', *The Cochrane Library*, issue 4, 2003, John Wiley & Sons, Chichester, UK.

Chapter 3
1. Young, GL & Jewell, D. 'Antihistamines versus aspirin for itching in late pregnancy (Cochrane Review)', *The Cochrane Library*, issue 4, 2003, John Wiley & Sons, Chichester, UK.
2. Mallol, J, Belda, MA, Costa, D, Noval, A & Sola, M. 'Prophylaxis of striae gravidarum with a topical formulation: A double blind trial', *International Journal of Cosmetic Science*, 1991;vol.3, pp 51–57.
3. McDonald, H, Brocklehurst, P, Parsons, J & Vigneswaran, R. 'Antibiotics for treating bacterial vaginosis in pregnancy (Cochrane Review)', *The Cochrane Library*, issue 4, 2003, John Wiley & Sons, Chichester, UK.
4. Crawley, RA, Dennison, K, & Carter, C. 'Cognition in pregnancy and the first

year post-partum', *Psychology & Psychotherapy*, 2003. Mar;76(pt 1), pp 69–84.
5. Neilson, JP. 'Symphysis-fundal height measurement in pregnancy (Cochrane Review)', *The Cochrane Library*, issue 4, 2003, John Wiley & Sons, Chichester, UK.
Gardosi, J & Francis, A. 'Controlled trial of fundal height measurement plotted on customised antenatal growth charts', *British Journal of Obstetrics and Gynaecology*, 1999 Apr;106(4), pp 309–17.
6. Enkin, M, Kierse, MJNC, Neilson, J, Crowther, C, Duley, L, Hodnett, E & Hofmeyr, J. *A Guide to Effective Care in Pregnancy and Childbirth*, 3rd edn, Oxford University Press, Oxford, 2000.
7. Kieler, H, Axelsson, O, Haglund, B, Nilsson, S & Salvesen, KA. 'Routine ultrasound screening in pregnancy and the children's subsequent handedness', *Early Human Development*, 1998 Jan 9;50(2), pp 233–45.
8. Walkinshaw, SA. 'Very tight versus tight control for diabetes in pregnancy (Cochrane Review)', *The Cochrane Library*, issue 4, 2003, John Wiley & Sons, Chichester, UK.
9. Boulvain, M, Stan, C & Irion, O. 'Elective delivery in diabetic pregnant women (Cochrane Review)', *The Cochrane Library*, issue 4, 2003, John Wiley & Sons, Chichester, UK.
10. Clough, HE, Marson, AG, Williamson, PR, Lopes-Lima, JM, Hutton, JL & Chadwick, DW. 'Carbamazepine versus phenytoin monotherapy for epilepsy (Protocol for a Cochrane Review)', *The Cochrane Library*, issue 4, 2003, John Wiley & Sons, Chichester, UK.
11. Stables, D. *Physiology in Childbearing*, Harcourt-Bailliere Tindall, London, 2000.
12. Roberts, D, Neilson, JP & Weindling, AM. 'Interventions for the treatment of twin–twin transfusion syndrome (Cochrane Review)', *The Cochrane Library*, issue 4, 2003, John Wiley & Sons, Chichester, UK.
13. Huch, R. 'Air travel in pregnancy', *Z Arztl Fortbild Qualitatssich*, 1999 Oct;93(7), pp 495–501.
14. Giangrande, PL. 'Air travel and thrombosis', *International Journal of Clinical Practice*, 2001 Dec;55(10), pp 690–93.

Chapter 4
1. Eason, E, Labrecque, M, Wells, G & Feldman, P. 'Preventing perineal trauma during childbirth: A systematic review', *Obstetrics and Gynecology*, 2000;95(3), pp 464–71.
2. Hopson, JL. 'Fetal Psychology', *Psychology Today*, Sept/Oct 1998;31(5), p. 44.
3. Villar, J, Carroli, G, Khan-Neelofur, D, Piaggio, G & Gülmezoglu, M. 'Patterns of routine antenatal care for low-risk pregnancy (Cochrane Review)', *The Cochrane Library*, issue 4, 2003, John Wiley & Sons, Chichester, UK.
4. www.who.int/child-adolescent-health/NUTRITION/infant_exclusive.htm
5. Golding, J. 'Sudden infant death syndrome and parental smoking: A literature review', *Paediatric & Perinatal Epidemiology*, 1997;vol.11, pp 67–77.
6. Scragg, RKR, Mitchell, EA, Stewart, AW, Ford, RPK, Taylor, BJ, Hassall, IB, Williams, SM & Thompson, JMD. 'Infant room-sharing and prone sleep position in sudden infant death syndrome', *Lancet*, 1996;vol.347, pp 7–12.
7. NSW Consumer Protection Agency. *In Good Hands: Baby Products and You*, Department of Fair Trading, Sydney, 2000.
8. National Health and Medical Research Council (NHMRC). *Care Around*

Preterm Birth: A Guide for Parents, Australian Government Publishing Service, Canberra, 1997.
9. Drakeley, AJ, Roberts, D & Alfirevic, Z. 'Cervical stitch (cerclage) for preventing pregnancy loss in women (Cochrane Review)', *The Cochrane Library*, issue 4, 2003, John Wiley & Sons, Chichester, UK.
10. NETS. *Outcomes for Premature Babies in New South Wales and the ACT: Information for Parents and Prospective Parents*, NSW Pregnancy and Newborn Services Network, Sydney, 2000.
11. Makrides, M & Crowther, CA. 'Magnesium supplementation in pregnancy (Cochrane Review)', *The Cochrane Library*, issue 4, 2003, John Wiley & Sons, Chichester, UK.
    Hofmeyr, GJ, Atallah, AN & Duley, L. 'Calcium supplementation during pregnancy for preventing hypertensive disorders and related problems (Cochrane Review)', *The Cochrane Library*, issue 4, 2003, John Wiley & Sons, Chichester, UK.
    Mahomed, K. 'Zinc supplementation in pregnancy (Cochrane Review)', *The Cochrane Library*, issue 4, 2003, John Wiley & Sons, Chichester, UK.
12. Crowley, P. 'Prophylactic corticosteroids for preterm birth (Cochrane Review)', *The Cochrane Library*, issue 4, 2003, John Wiley & Sons, Chichester, UK.
    Crowther, CA & Harding, J. 'Repeat doses of prenatal corticosteroids for women at risk of preterm birth for preventing neonatal respiratory disease (Cochrane Review)', *The Cochrane Library*, issue 4, 2003, John Wiley & Sons, Chichester, UK.
13. Hofmeyr, GJ & Kulier, R. 'External cephalic version for breech presentation at term (Cochrane Review)', *The Cochrane Library*, issue 4, 2003, John Wiley & Sons, Chichester, UK.
    Hofmeyr, GJ & Gülmezoglu, AM. 'Maternal hydration for increasing amniotic fluid volume in oligohydramnios and normal amniotic fluid volume (Cochrane Review)', *The Cochrane Library*, issue 4, 2003, John Wiley & Sons, Chichester, UK.
    Lau, TK, Lo, KW, Wan, D & Rogers, MS. 'Predictors of successful external cephalic version at term: A prospective study', *British Journal of Obstetrics and Gynaecology*, 1997 July; 104(7), pp 798–802.
14. Hofmeyr, GJ & Hannah, ME. 'Planned caesarean section for term breech delivery (Cochrane Review)', *The Cochrane Library*, issue 4, 2003, John Wiley & Sons, Chichester, UK.
15. Hofmeyr, GJ, Kulier, R. 'Expedited versus conservative approaches for vaginal delivery in breech presentation (Cochrane Review)', *The Cochrane Library*, issue 4, 2003, John Wiley & Sons, Chichester, UK.
16. Kelnar, CJH, Harvey, D & Simpson, C. *The Sick Newborn Baby*, 3rd edn, Bailliere Tindall, London, 1995.
17. Bricker, L & Neilson, JP. 'Routine ultrasound in late pregnancy (after 24 weeks gestation) (Cochrane Review)', *The Cochrane Library*, issue 4, 2003, John Wiley & Sons, Chichester, UK.
18. Demir, N, Celiloglu, M & Thomassen, PAB. 'Prolactin and amniotic fluid electrolytes', *Acta Obsterica et Gynaecologica Scandinavica*, 1991;vol.71, pp 197–200.
19. Kramer, WB, Van den Veyver, IB, Kirshon, B. 'Treatment of polyhydramnios with indomethacin', *Clinical Perinatology*, 1994 Sept;21(3), pp 615–30.
20. Hofmeyr, GJ. 'Amnioinfusion for preterm rupture of membranes (Cochrane

Review)', *The Cochrane Library*, issue 4, 2003, John Wiley & Sons, Chichester, UK.
21. van Dijk, BA, Dooren, MC & Overbeeke, MA. 'Red cell antibodies in pregnancy: There is no "critical titre"', *Transfusion Medicine*, 1995 Sept;5(3), pp 199–202.
22. Palma, J, Reyes, H, Ribalta, J, Hernandez, I, Sandoval, L, Almuna, R, Liepins, J, Lira, F, Sedano, M, Silva, O, Toha, D & Silva JJ. 'Ursodeoxycholic acid in the treatment of cholestasis of pregnancy: A randomised double blind study controlled with placebo', *Journal of Hepatology*, 1997 Dec;27(6), pp 1022–28.
23. Palma, J, Reyes, H, Ribalta, J, Hernandez, I, Sandoval, L, Almuna, R, Liepins, J, Lira, F, Sedano, M, Riikonen, S, Savonius, H, Gylling, H, Nikkila, K, Tuomi, AM & Miettinen, TA. 'Oral guar gum, a gel-forming dietary fiber relieves pruritus in intrahepatic cholestasis of pregnancy', *Acta Obstetricia et Gynecologica Scandinavica*, 2000 Apr;79(4), pp 260–64.
24. Parsons, M, Simpson, M, Ponton, T. 'Raspberry leaf and its effect on labour: Safety and efficacy', *Australian Midwifery Journal of the Australian College of Midwives*, 1999 Sept;12(3), pp 20–25.
25. Simpson, M, Parsons, M, Greenwood, J & Wade, K. 'Raspberry leaf in pregnancy: Its safety and efficacy in labour', *Journal of Midwifery Women's Health*, 2001 Mar/Apr;46(2), pp 51–59.

Chapter 5
1. Hodnett, ED, Gates, S, Hofmeyr, GJ & Sakala, C. 'Continuous support for women during childbirth (Cochrane Review)', *The Cochrane Library*, issue 4, 2003, John Wiley & Sons, Chichester, UK.
2. Deguidice, GT. 'The relationship between sibling jealousy and presence at a sibling's birth', *Birth*, 1986; vol. 13, p. 4.
3. Lumley, J. 'Preschool siblings at birth, short term effects', *Birth*, 1983 Spring;10(1).
4. Price, CA. 'Water birth and land birth: A retrospective study of maternal and neonatal outcomes in one Australian birth centre', unpublished treatise, University of Sydney (Faculty of Nursing), 1995.
5. Beech, BL. *Water Birth Unplugged, Proceedings of the First International Water Birth Conference*, Books for Midwives Press, Cheshire, UK, 1996.
6. Flenady, V & King, J. 'Antibiotics for prelabour rupture of membranes at or near term, (Cochrane Review), *The Cochrane Library*, issue 4, 2003, John Wiley & Sons, Chichester, UK.

Chapter 6
1. O'Sullivan, G. 'The stomach: Fact and fantasy: eating and drinking during labour', *International Anesthesiology Clinics*, 1994;32, pp 31–44.
2. American Society of Anesthesiologists Task Force. 'Practice guidelines for preoperative fasting and the use of pharmacologic agents to reduce the risk of pulmonary aspiration: Application to healthy patients undergoing elective procedures. A report by the American Society of Anesthesiologists: Task Force on Preopertive Fasting', *Anesthesiology*, 1999 Mar;90(3), pp 896–905.
3. Simkin, P. 'Stress, pain, and catecholamines in labor: Part 1, a review', *Birth* 1986;13, pp 227–33.
4. Singata, M & Tranmer, JE. 'Restricting oral fluid and food intake during labour (Protocol for a Cochrane Review)', *The Cochrane Library*, issue 4, 2003, John Wiley & Sons, Chichester, UK.

5. Thacker, SB, Stroup, D & Chang, M. 'Continuous electronic heart rate monitoring for fetal assessment during labor (Cochrane Review)', *The Cochrane Library*, issue 4, 2003, John Wiley & Sons, Chichester, UK.
6. Nielsen, PV, Stigsby, B, Nickelsen, C & Nim, J. 'Intra- and inter-observer variability in the assessment of intrapartum cardiotocograms', *Acta Obstetricia et Gynecologica Scandinavica*, 1987;66, pp 421–24.
7. Umstad, MP. 'The predictive value of abnormal fetal heart rate patterns in early labour', *Australian New Zealand Journal of Obstetrics & Gynaecology*, 1993 May;33(2), pp 145–49.
8. Neilson, JP. 'Fetal electrocardiogram (ECG) for fetal monitoring during labour (Cochrane Review)', *The Cochrane Library*, issue 4, 2003, John Wiley & Sons, Chichester, UK.
9. Morrill, ES & Nickols-Richardson, HM. 'Bulimia nervosa during pregnancy: A review', *Journal of the American Dietetic Association*, 2002, Apr;101(4), p. 448.
10. Hofmey, GJ & Kulier, R. 'Hands/knees posture in late pregnancy or labour for fetal malposition (lateral or posterior) (Cochrane Review)', *The Cochrane Library*, issue 4, 2003, John Wiley & Sons, Chichester, UK.
11. World Health Organisation. *Care in Normal Birth: A Practical Guide*, Maternal and Newborn Health/Safe Motherhood Unit, Geneva, 1996.

Chapter 7

1. Roodt, A & Nikodem, VC. 'Pushing/bearing down methods used during the second stage of labour (Protocol for a Cochrane Review)', *The Cochrane Library*, issue 4, 2003, John Wiley & Sons, Chichester, UK.
2. Mayerhofer, K, Bodner-Adler, B, Bodner, K, Rabl, M, Kaider, A, Wagenbichler, P, Joura, EA & Husslein, P. 'Traditional care of the perineum during birth. A prospective, randomized, multicenter study of 1,076 women', *The Journal of Reproductive Medicine*, 2002 June;47(6), pp 477–82.
3. Carroli, G & Belizan, J. 'Episiotomy for vaginal birth (Cochrane Review)', *The Cochrane Library*, issue 4, 2003, John Wiley & Sons, Chichester, UK.
4. Johanson, RB & Menon, V. 'Vacuum extraction versus forceps for assisted vaginal delivery' (Cochrane Review)', *The Cochrane Library*, issue 4, 2003, John Wiley & Sons, Chichester, UK.
5. Kettle, C & Johanson, RB. 'Continuous versus interrupted sutures for perineal repair' (Cochrane Review),' *The Cochrane Library*, issue 4, 2003, John Wiley & Sons, Chichester, UK.
6. Irion, O & Boulvain, M. 'Induction of labour for suspected fetal macrosomia (Cochrane Review),' *The Cochrane Library*, issue 4, 2003, John Wiley & Sons, Chichester, UK.
7. Bricker, L & Neilson, JP. 'Routine ultrasound in late pregnancy (after 24 weeks gestation) (Cochrane Review),' *The Cochrane Library*, issue 4, 2003, John Wiley & Sons, Chichester, UK.
   Pattinson, RC. 'Pelvimetry for fetal cephalic presentations at term (Cochrane Review)', *The Cochrane Library*, issue 4, 2003, John Wiley & Sons, Chichester, UK.
8. Dodds, SD & Wolfe, SW. 'Perinatal brachial plexus palsy', *Current Opinion Pediatrics*, 2000 Feb;12(1), pp 40–47.

Chapter 8

1. Prendiville, WJ, Elbourne, D & McDonald, S. 'Active versus expectant management in the third stage of labour (Cochrane Review)', *The Cochrane*

Library, issue 4, 2003, John Wiley & Sons, Chichester, UK.
2. Ryan, M. 'Birth centre-labour ward: Do the outcomes differ?', unpublished master of public health treatise, University of Sydney, 1997.
3. McDonald, SJ & Abbott JM. 'Effect of timing of umbilical cord clamping of term infants on maternal and neonatal outcomes (Protocol for a Cochrane Review)', *The Cochrane Library*, issue 4, 2003, John Wiley & Sons, Chichester, UK.
4. Mercer, JS. 'Current best evidence: A review of the literature on umbilical cord clamping', *Journal of Midwifery and Women's Health*, 2001;46(6), pp. 402–14.
5. McDonald, S, Prendiville, WJ & Elbourne D. 'Prophylactic Syntometrine versus oxytocin for delivery of the placenta (Cochrane Review)', *The Cochrane Library*, issue 4, 2003, John Wiley & Sons, Chichester, UK.
6. Fernando, RJ, Sultan, AS, Johanson, RB & Radley S. 'Obstetric anal sphincter injury – A questionnaire survey 2000 (Protocol for a Cochrane Review)', *The Cochrane Library*, issue 4, 2003, John Wiley & Sons, Chichester, UK.
7. Sangalli, MR, Floris, L, Faltin, D & Weil, A. 'Anal incontinence in women with third or fourth degree perineal tears and subsequent vaginal deliveries', *Australian New Zealand Journal of Obstetrics & Gynaecology*, 2000 Aug;40(3), pp 244–48.
8. Harkin, R, Fitzpatrick, M, O'Connell, PR & O'Herlihy, C. 'Anal sphincter disruption at vaginal delivery: Is recurrence predictable?', *European Journal of Obstetrics & Gynaecology & Reproductive Biology*, 2003 Aug 15;109(2), pp 149–52.
9. Nelson, R. 'Operative procedures for fissure in ano (Cochrane Review)', *The Cochrane Library*, issue 4, 2003, John Wiley & Sons, Chichester, UK.

Chapter 9

1. Wongprasartsuk, P, Richards, E, McCandlish, R, Grange, C, Chevassut, A & Popat, M. 'Inhaled pain relief in labour (Protocol for a Cochrane Review)', *The Cochrane Library*, issue 4, 2003, John Wiley & Sons, Chichester, UK.
2. Smith, DA. 'Hazards of nitrous oxide exposure in healthcare personnel', *American Association of Nurse Anesthetists Journal*, 1998 Aug;66(4), pp 390–93.
3. Elbourne, D & Wiseman, RA. 'Types of intra-muscular opioids for maternal pain relief in labour (Cochrane Review)', *The Cochrane Library*, issue 4, 2003, John Wiley & Sons, Chichester, UK.
4. Loughnan, BA, Carli, F, Romney, M, Dore, C & Gordon H. 'The influence of epidural analgesia on the development of new backache in primiparous women: Report of a randomised controlled trial', *International Journal of Obstetric Anesthesia* 1997; vol. 6, pp 203–4.
5. Sudlow, C & Warlow, C. 'Epidural blood patching for preventing and treating post-dural puncture headache (Cochrane Review)', *The Cochrane Library*, issue 4, 2003, John Wiley & Sons, Chichester, UK.
6. Howell, CJ. 'Epidural versus non-epidural analgesia for pain relief in labour (Cochrane Review)', *The Cochrane Library*, issue 4, 2003, John Wiley & Sons, Chichester, UK.
7. Ternov, K, Nilsson, M, Lofberg, L, Algotsson, L & Akeson, J. 'Acupuncture for pain relief during childbirth', *Acupuncture & Electro-therapeutics Research*, 1998; 23(1), pp 19–26.
8. Johnston, RV, Burrows, E, Merrin, MIJ & Burrows, R. 'Transcutaneous electrical nerve stimulation for pain relief in labour (Protocol for a Cochrane Review)', *The Cochrane Library*, issue 4, 2003, John Wiley & Sons, Chichester, UK.

9. Pradhan, P & Johanson, R. 'Intracutaneous sterile water injection for back pain in labour (Protocol for a Cochrane Review)', *The Cochrane Library*, issue 4, 2003, John Wiley & Sons, Chichester, UK.

Chapter 10

1. Steinborn, A, Gunes, H & Halberstadt, E. 'Signal for term parturition is of trophoblast and therefore of fetal origin', *Prostaglandins*, 1995 Nov/Dec;50(5–6), pp 237–52.
2. Mittendorf, R, Williams, MA, Berkey, CS & Cotter PF. 'The length of uncomplicated human gestation', *Obstetrics and Gynecology*, 1990 June;75(6), pp 929–32.
3. Boulvain, M, Stan, C & Irion, O. 'Membrane sweeping for induction of labour (Cochrane Review)', *The Cochrane Library*, issue 4, 2003, John Wiley & Sons, Chichester, UK.
4. National Perinatal Statistics Unit. 'Australia's mothers and babies 2000', *Australian Institute of Health and Welfare*, Perinatal Statistics Series no. 12, Sydney, 2003.
5. Roberts, CL, Tracy, S & Peat, B. 'Rates for obstetric intervention among private and public patients in Australia: Population based descriptive study', *British Medical Journal*, 2000 July15; 321, pp 137–41.
6. Kavanagh, J, Kelly, AJ & Thomas, J. 'Breast stimulation for cervical ripening and induction of labour (Cochrane Review)', *The Cochrane Library*, issue 4, 2003, John Wiley & Sons, Chichester, UK.
7. Fraser, W, Vendittelli, F, Krauss, I & Breart G. 'Effects of early augmentation of labour with amniotomy and oxytocin in nulliparous women: A meta-analysis', *British Journal of Obstetrics and Gynaecology*, 1998;105, pp 189–94. Fraser, WD, Turcot, L, Krauss, I & Brisson-Carrol G. 'Amniotomy for shortening spontaneous labour (Cochrane Review)', *The Cochrane Library*, issue 4, 2003, John Wiley & Sons, Chichester, UK.

Chapter 11

1. Irion, O & Boulvain, M. 'Induction of labour for suspected fetal macrosomia (Cochrane Review)', *The Cochrane Library*, issue 4, 2003, John Wiley & Sons, Chichester, UK.
2. Wilkinson, C & Enkin, MW. 'Manual removal of placenta at caesarean section (Cochrane Review)', *The Cochrane Library*, issue 4, 2003, John Wiley & Sons, Chichester, UK.
3. Roberts, CL, Tracy, S & Peat, B. 'Rates for obstetric intervention among private and public patients in Australia: Population based descriptive study', *British Medical Journal*, 2000 July15; 321, pp 137–41.
4. Hemminki, E. 'Impact of caesarean section on future pregnancy: A review of cohort studies', *Paediatric and Perinatal Epidemiology*, 1996;10(4), pp 366–79.
5. Dodd, J, Crowther, CA & Huertas, E. 'Planned elective repeat caesarean section versus planned vaginal birth for women with a previous caesarean birth (Protocol for a Cochrane Review)', *The Cochrane Library*, issue 4, 2003, John Wiley & Sons, Chichester, UK.
6. Ravasia, DJ, Wood, SL & Pollard, JK. 'Uterine rupture during induced trial of labor among women with previous cesarean delivery', *American Journal of Obstetrics & Gynecology*, 2000 Nov;183(5), pp 1176–79.
7. Myles, TD & Miranda, R. 'Vaginal birth after cesarean delivery in the twin gestation', *Obstetrics and Gynecology*, 2000 Apr 1;95(4: suppl. 1), p. S65.

8. Roberts, RG, Bell, HS, Wall, EM, Moy, JG, Hess, GH & Bower, HP. 'Trial of labor or repeated caesarean section: The woman's choice', *Archives of Family Medicine* 1997;6, pp 120–25.
9. National Health and Medical Research Council. *Report of the Working Party to Investigate Variations in Caesarean Section Rates in Australia, Appendix XXVI*, Australian Government Publishing Service, Canberra, 1984.
10. Appleton, B, Targett, C, Rasmussen, M, Readman, E, Sale, F & Permezel, M. 'Vaginal birth after caesarean section: An Australian multicentre study', *Australian and New Zealand Journal of Obstetrics & Gynaecology*, 2000 Feb;40(1), pp 87–91.

Chapter 12
1. Leboyer, F. *Birth without Violence*. Healing Arts Press, Rochester, NY, 1974.
2. Enkin, M, Keirse, MJNC, Neilson J, Crowther, C, Duley, L, Hodnett, E & Hofmeyr, J. *A Guide to Effective Care in Pregnancy and Childbirth*, 3rd edn, Oxford University Press, Oxford, 2000.
3. Lund, C, Kuller, J, Lane, A, Lott, JW & Raines DA. 'Neonatal skin care: The scientific basis for practice', *Neonatal Network*, 1999 June;18(4), pp 15–27.
4. Golding, J, Greenwood, R, Birmingham, K & Mott, M. 'Childhood cancer, intramuscular vitamin K and pethidine given during labour', *British Medical Journal*, 1992;305, pp 341–46.
5. Paediatric Division of the RACP. 'RANCOG, RACGP & ACMI joint statement and recommendations on vitamin K administration to newborn Infants to prevent vitamin K deficiency bleeding in infancy', *National Health & Medical Research Council*, October 2000, Canberra.
6. Boxall, E, Jefferson, TO, Buttery, J, King, V, Dockerty, J, Trivella, M, Powell, R & Osman, Y. 'Vaccines for preventing hepatitis B in newborn infants (Protocol for a Cochrane Review)', *The Cochrane Library*, issue 4, 2003, John Wiley & Sons, Chichester, UK.
7. Royal Australian College of Physicians. 'Paediatric policy statement on circumcision', *Royal Australian College of Physicians*, September 2002.
8. American Academy of Pediatrics. 'Task force on circumcision: Circumcision policy statement', *Pediatrics*, 1999 Mar;103, pp 686–93.

Chapter 13
1. Steen, M, Marchant, P & Briggs, M. 'Localised cooling treatment for perineal wounds following childbirth (Protocol for a Cochrane Review)', *The Cochrane Library*, issue 4, 2003, John Wiley & Sons, Chichester, UK.
2. Rayburn, WF. 'Clinical commentary: The bromocriptine (Parlodel) controversy and recommendations for lactation suppression', *American Journal of Perinatology*, 1996 Feb; 13(2), pp 69–71.
3. Snowden, HM, Renfrew MJ & Woolridge, MW. 'Treatments for breast engorgement during lactation (Cochrane Review)', *The Cochrane Library*, issue 4, 2003, John Wiley & Sons, Chichester, UK.
4. Joseph, S & Bailham, D. 'Post-traumatic stress following childbirth: A review of the emerging literature and directions for research and practice', *Psychology, Health & Medicine*, 2003; 8(2).

Acknowledgments

Birth: Conceiving, Nurturing and Giving Birth to Your Baby would never have become a reality without the seemingly endless support from our families and friends. This immense project has truly been born from a labour of love, and the patience of our long-suffering partners and children must be acknowledged first and foremost.

To Stephen Robinson. Thank you for being you and believing in me, particularly in my moments of self-doubt. Heartfelt thanks for the many hours of editing and contributing a man's and father's perspective of labour, birth and parenting. My admiration and respect quadrupled during the many hours, days, weeks and months when you were the 'sole' parent during the years of writing. You certainly embraced the roles of cook, cleaner, cricket coach, homework mentor, negotiator and taxi driver for our children. To my children Alice, Liam and Declan – thank you for allowing me to learn all about mothering. I must also thank Marie Burrows for igniting my passion for this work. And to Catherine, thank you for being you and for all your wonderful qualities as a business partner and most importantly as a friend. All my love, Sandra.

To Peter Fitzpatrick, my husband and best friend. Thank you for your love, support and faith in our project. For taking on the burden of provider and househusband, and for tolerating all those lonely nights while I sat up late on the computer, and to my two boys, Hugh and Callum, who always make me smile, I love you all dearly. Also, thanks to my wonderful mum Thea and dad Bill (who sadly is not here to share this), and all my marvellous brothers and sisters and their partners. Coming from a family of nine children is a gift that I treasure. Of course, thank you Sandra, from the bottom of my heart, for your friendship, having the vision and negotiating this long and difficult road over the years with me. Love, Catherine.

A special thanks from both of us to Kate McMaugh. Your invaluable feedback, objective insight into our evolving writing skills and selfless support has kept us on track. Your input is appreciated more than you know. Thanks also to others, whose thoughts and contributions are threaded throughout the writing, including Hilary Hunter, Charles Brooker, Jan Idle, Steve Robinson, Robert Price, Paddy McBride, Sally Reay-Young and Claire Cleaver. Also, thank you to Ian Heads for introducing us to Pan Macmillan.

And last, but never least, thank you to all the women and their partners who have contributed ideas and words of encouragement over the years, and to the many parents and babies we have worked with throughout our careers. You are truly our teachers. We feel privileged to have been with you during life's most amazing journey.

Index

A
Abdomen, baby's 432
Abdominal
　CVS 106, 107
　exercises 444
　muscles 440–441
　pain 469
Abnormalities 102–103, 147
　See also Birth defects
Abortion, threatened 111
Accutane 11
Aches and pains 132–133, 180–181
Aching muscles 73–74
Active management (third stage) 296, 297, 298
Acupressure 61, 93, 129, 204, 258, 261, 265, 347–348, 367, 374
　points 526–529, 530, 531
Acupuncture 116, 129, 177, 204, 344, 347, 367, 389, **530**, **531**
Addictions
　pain relief and 335
　resources to overcome 556
Adipose body fat (BAT) 162, 405
Adoption agencies 555
Adrenaline 321
Advice
　from family and friends 483–484
　professional 482–483
After birth care See Postnatal care
After pains 440
Afterbirth See Placenta
AIDS See HIV/AIDS
Albendazole 72
Alcohol
　managing stress with 26
　pregnancy and 20, 21, 69
　premature birth and 201
　support agencies 556
　vitamin efficiency and 9, 12
Alexander technique 530, 531
Allergies 194, 450
Alopecia 450
Alpha-fetoprotein blood test (AFP) 104
Alpha-tocopherol (alpha-TE) 14, 15
Amenorrhoea 32–33
Amnicator 242
Amniocentesis **106–108**
　potential risks of 102, 111, 212, 213
Amnion (membrane) 165
Amniotic fluid (sac) 49, 115, 120, 121, 122, **165**, 204
　variations in 163, 208–209
　See also Oligohydramnios; Polyhydramnios
Amniotomy 361–363
Anaemia
　blood disorder and 153
　haemolytic 15
　iron deficiency and 16, 17
　prevention of 11
Anaesthetic, general 381, 382, 393
Anal
　fissures 316
　incontinence 315, 316
　sphincter 314
Analgesics 73
Antenatal
　clinic (hospital) 91–92
　depression 154–156
Anterior lip 264–265
Anterior position
　during labour 260, 261
　during pregnancy 186
Antibiotics 15, **70**, 79, 87, 100–101, 124, 203, 259, 386, 465, 468, 469, 470
Antibodies 100, **212–213**
Anti-depressants 155
　PND and 474–475

Anti-epileptics 9, 15, 20, 151–152
Antihistamines 129
Anti-inflammatory drugs 73
　see also NSAIDS
Anus
　baby's 432
　mother's 271
　tear to the 281, 283, 314–316
Anxiety, late pregnancy and 182–183
　see also Emotions
Apgar score 337, 381–382, **407–408**
Areola 126, 191, 447, 466, 509–510
ARM (artificially rupture membranes) 361–363, 373
　See also Breaking waters
Arms, baby's 424, 431
Aromatherapy 348–349, 367, **530**, **531**
Art therapy 532, 533
Ascorbic acid (vitamin C) 12, 13
Aspiration, risk of 251
Aspirin 73, 126
Asthma
　effects on pregnancy 150
　medication in pregnancy 70–71, **150–151**
Astrology, due dates and 56–57
Attachment (breast) 464
Augmentation (labour) 371–373
　how to avoid 375–376
　medical methods of 373–374
　natural methods of 374–375
　VBAC and 401
Australian Breastfeeding Association 560–561
Australian Continence Foundation 316, 564
Australian Cord Blood Bank 301–303
Australian Emergency Essence 349
Australian Sex Discrimination Act (1984) 4
Australian Standards Mark **196**
Autogenic training 532, 533

B
Babinski reflex 429
Baby Health Clinic See Early Childhood Centre
Baby needs (clothes, pram etc.) 196–199
Baby, newborn
　appearance of 422–427
　bathing 410–411
　body temperature of 405
　bonding with your 416
　born before arrival (BBA) 292–294
　enjoying your 522
　feeding your 416–420, 445–456, 500
　holding for first time 274
　holding your 420–421
　marks on 425–427
　measurements of 410
　normal behaviour of 427, 500–507
　overweight 415
　physical checks on 430–432
　premature (preterm) 91, 93, 95, 97, 200–203, 377, **434–435**
　reactions to labour and birth 406
　reviving the 293
　settling in with 500
　settling your 500, 504–506
　siblings and 421–422
　support agencies for 560–563
　underweight 415
　unwell 299, 302, 407, 434–435
　variations for 434
　wrapping the 194, 504
　See also Bottle feeding; Breastfeeding; Crying, baby's; Sleeping, baby's

Baby, pre-birth
　buying for 196–198
　distressed 255, **263**, 269, 285, 373
　female 52, 163, 166
　large 378, 397–398
　male 52, 163–164, 166
　small 207–208
　viable 122
　See also First trimester; Second trimester; Third trimester; Labour
Baby Products, Guide to (CHOICE) 196
Baby's movements See Movements, baby's
Babysitting swaps 481
Bach flower Rescue Remedy 349
Back
　exercises for 170–171, 444–445
　lying on your 160
Backache 170–171
　epidural/spinal and 343, 345
　labour and 231, 232, 233, 349
Balanitis 438
Basal Body Temperature 33
Bassinette 197
Bath (as pain relief) 91, 252, 272, 353
　See also Water birth
Bathing baby 410–411, 506
BBA (baby born before arrival) 292–294
Bearing down 276
　See also Ferguson's reflex
Beauty products 71
Bed-sharing 194–195
　See also Sleeping, baby's
Belly
　cold 216
　growing 133–134
　pain in 180
　piercing 161
Belly button See Navel
Beta-carotene (vitamin A) 10, 11
BFHI (baby friendly hospital initiative) 189
Bilirubin levels 436–437
Birth
　breech 205–206
　by caesarean See Caesarean
　fast 284
　lotus 303
　options for 89–91
　pains after 440
　pelvis, role of in 167
　personal effects for 225–226
　positions for 277–279, **277**, **278**
　privacy during 276
　recovery after 440–476
　support strategies after 305–307
　twins and 290–292
　vaginal See Vaginal birth
　See also Homebirth; Pain relief
Birth centre 92–93, 284
　admission to 238, 239
　labour induction and 359
　packing for 225–227
　travelling to 238–239
Birth defects, medication and **70**, 83, 87
　See also Abnormalities; Genetic
Birth plan 187
　caesarean and 382, 547
　worksheet 542–548
　writing a 230–231, 375
Birth stories 322–323
Birthing
　phase 273–275
　stool 278
Birthmarks
　port wine 427
　spider 426
　stork 426

strawberry 426
traditional 426–427
Black line *See* Linea nigra
Bladder
    emptying 234, 260
    damage to 309–310
    infection of 154, 258, 470
Blastocyst 49
Bleed
    hormonal 110
    implantation 54–55
Bleeding
    after birth 441, 470
    after caesarean 389, 391
Bleeding, baby's 412
Bleeding gums 123–124
Bleeding, heavy
    after birth 284, 294, 304, **311–313**, 391
    during labour 265–266
    in late pregnancy 381
    See also Postpartum haemorrhage
Bleeding nose 128
Bleeding, vaginal
    after cerclage 115
    during labour 249
    early pregnancy 109–111
    late pregnancy 211
Blighted ovum 114
Blisters
    milk 466
    sucking 425
Blood
    disorders 153–154
    supply 49
    type 50, 100
    volume 312
Blood Clot *See* Thrombosis
Blood group test 100
Blood loss *See* Bleeding, heavy
Blood pressure
    after birth 307, 463
    during labour 255, 263
    high 28, 70–71
    in late pregnancy 209–210
    low 312, 342
    medications for 150
    See also Pre-eclampsia
Blood sugar level (BSL) 145
Blood supply, baby's 49
Blood test
    AFP (triple test) 104
    antenatal 85, 93, **100–101**
    for hepatitis 81
    for pregnancy 53
    for rubella 85
    laboratory guidelines for 434
    routine, for newborn baby 433–434
Blood transfusion
    for baby 437
    for mother 312, 470
'Blues', the third-day 458, 471
Body, baby's 424
Body image 139–140, 184–185
Body mass index (BMI) 25–26
    table 25
Bonding (baby) 416
Bones/cartilage 120, 162
Booking (for birth) 96–97
Bottle feed, first 419–420
Bottle feeding 192–194
    baby's poo and 452
    emotions and 454–455
    equipment for 197, 419, 455–456
    newborn 451–455
    positions for 419–420
    settling baby by 503–504
    twins or triplets 454
Bottles, heating 454
    sterilising 455–456
Bottom
    baby's 432
    mother's 441–442
    See also Anus; Bowel

Bowel, baby's 421, 432, 452
    See also 'Poo'
Bowel, mother's
    after birth 442, 463
    pressure on 250
    stimulation of 367–368
    tear to 315
Bowen technique 532, 533
Bradykinin 318
Brain
    development of baby's 8, 49, 51, **121**, 162
    infection of mother's 84
Bras (brassieres), maternity **135**, 191, 226, 447, 451, 512
Braxton Hicks (contractions) 132, 140
Breaking the waters 360, 361–363, 373
    See also Waters breaking
Breast
    abcess of **468–469**, 513–514
    blocked duct of **467**, 513–514
Breast changes 59
Breast milk
    'coming in' 447
    expressing 434, 448, 464–465, **508–511**, **510**, 519
    in oversupply 521
    production, mother's 192
    storing 511–512, 513, 517
    supply 518
    supply line for 521
    undersupply, ongoing 520–521
    undersupply, reversible 519–520
    ways to increase 520
Breast pads 447, 451
Breast pump 197, 455, **510–511**
Breastfeed
    first 416–419
    how to 416–419, **418**, 445–450
    length of 419, 447
Breastfeeding
    at work or out 512–513
    benefits of 188–189
    classes 217
    contraception when 490–500
    diet and 443
    effects on 11, 13, 15, 17, 19, 21, 22, 313
    emotions and 450–451
    myths about 191–192
    settling baby by 503, 505
    social perceptions of 190
    support agencies for 560–561
    tandem 123
    thirst when 509
    twins or triplets 449–450
    weaning from 513–514
    See also Breast milk; Let-down reflex
Breasts
    engorgement of 451, 466
    leaking 123, 447, 486
    size and other variations 192
    sore 59, **466–469**, 494
    weight gain and 65
Breath, baby's
    first 337, 405
    increased rate of 415
    stimulating 408–409
Breathing, baby's
    at birth 407
    difficult, after caesarean 392
    pethidine and 337
Breathing, mother's
    during birth 253, 272–273
    as pain relief 349–350
    pain relief's effect on 333, 336, 344
Breathlessness 171, 312
Breech
    in caesarean birth 205–206
    in vaginal birth 205–206, 290
    position 122, 142, 186, **203–204**
    See also Position, baby's
Bulk billing 92, 93, 94, 95, 96
Burping the baby 419, 420
Buying for baby 196–198

C
Caesarean (caesar) 90, 91, 95, 160, 187, 204, 205–206, 256, 262, 266, 285, 286–287, 290, 292, 309, 311, 341, 367–396
    after baby's death 157
    anaesthetic for 380–382
    consent for 379
    description of 377
    driving after 389
    emotions and 393–396
    home visits after 461
    incisions, types of 383–384
    infection risk, after 391–392
    medical reasons for 377–378
    non-medical reasons for 378
    operation 382–385
    procedures before 378–380
    rates of 390
    recovery from 386–390
    repeat 378, 398, 402–403
    risks for baby 392–393
    risks for mother 390–392
    scar tissue from 383
    sensations during 383
Caffeine
    breastfeeding and 21
    during pregnancy, effects of **20**, **21**, 69
    pre-conception 21
    restless legs and 124
    withdrawal from 20
Calciferol (vitamin D) 14, 15
Calcium intake 14
    osteoporosis and 15
    during pregnancy 15, 64
Cannabis 23
Canula 401
Car
    baby restraint for 197
    travel by 159
Cardiff (count to ten) 188
Caregiver
    after birth, expectations of 307–309
    choosing 89–91, 375
    contact with 98, 100, 141, 185
    during birth, expectations of 279, 378
    during labour, expectations of 254–255, 325, 375–376
    giving information to 99
    information from 99
    labour pain options and 321–322, 325
    newborn care and 430–434, 461, 483
    postnatal checkup with 462–463
    prelabour, expectations of 237–238
    professional associations 558–559
    unexpected outcomes and 463–464
Carpal tunnel syndrome 13, 171–172
Castor oil 367–368
Catheter
    after birth 304, 310, 386
    during birth 260, 379
Caul 270
Caution, during pregnancy 68
Cells, during conception 48
Cephalhaematoma 425
Cerclage *See* Cervix
Cervical incompetence 111, 201
Cervix 30, **30**, **31**
    anterior lip and the 264–265
    changes in 36, 37, 38, 39, 165
    dilation of 206, 232, 233, **245–246**, **247**, 249, 255, 262, 354, 357, 364, 372
    effacement of 232, 357
    for contraception, position of 497–498
    fully dilated 247, 249, 268, **269**
    opening 232–233, **233**, 268
    ripening 232–233, 363, 364, 368
    second stage labour and 279–280

INDEX 587

stitch in (cerclage) 115
thinning of 232–233, **233**
third stage labour and 297
unripe 357
weakened, miscarriage and 111
Change
   adapting to 137–140
   dealing with 2
Checklist (baby's needs) 196–198
Chemicals, exposure to 76
Chest, baby's 431
Chicken pox 78, 79
Childbirth *See* Birth
Childcare, planning 199–200, 516
Childcare Your Guide to 200
Children, other
   after the birth (hospital) 421–422
   at the birth 220–224
   baby and 481
   postnatal depression and 473
   preparing 220
   when to tell 89
   See also Siblings
Chiropractic therapy 532, 533
Chiropractor, paediatric 289
Chlamydia 78, 79
Chloasma 126, 494
   see also 'Mask of pregnancy'
Cholestasis 125, **213–214**, 354
Chorion (membrane) 165
Choroid plexus cysts 149
Chromosomes 31
Cigarettes *see* Smoking
Cilia 30
Circumcision 437–438
'Clap', the *See* Gonorrhoea
Classes, birth (antenatal) 217–218
Cleft lip (harelip) 8–9
Cleft palate 8–9, 431
Clinics *See* Antenatal; Midwives
Clitoris, baby's 52, 432
Clothing
   baby 197
   during labour 225–226
   maternity 125, 134–136
Cobalamin (vitamin B12) 12, 13
Colds, treatment of 128–129
Colic 505
Colostrum 416, 445, 446
Colour therapy 534, 535
Communicating
   after birth 459–460, 480
   during labour 253
   in relationships 2, 42
   See also Emotions
Complications
   after caesarean 390–393
   at birth 90, 91, 200–214
   during pregnancy 223–224, 257–267, 280–295, 309–317, 327
   pregnancy testing and 109
Compound presentation 274, 315
Conceive
   average time to 4
   inability to 47
   preparing to 1–29
   'right time' to 1
Conceiving
   after caesarean 397
   chances of 29
   difficulty 44
   fertility chart and 33–35
   helpful hints for 41–42
   support agencies for 554–555
Condom
   female 490–491
   male 489–490
Constipation 59, **172–173**, 316
Contraception
   after birth 489–500
   support resources for 554–555
Contraceptive pill 33, **494–495**
   breastfeeding and 519
   effect on vitamin intake 12

Contraceptives
   ectopic pregnancy and 116
   fertility and 33
   See also Diaphragm; Family Planning; IUD; Minipill; Pill; Progesterone injections
Contractions
   after induction 359, 360–361, 362, 366
   final 274
   first stage labour 245, 246, 247
   frequent, fast 284
   intensity of 251–252
   prelabour 232, 237, 240
   pushing and 270
   resting between 268
   slowing labour and 372, 373, 374
   timing your 245
   weak (hypotonic) 371, 373
Controlled comforting (crying) 501
Cool packs 309, 451
Coping strategies 276
   See also Birth; Labour; Support strategies
Cord
   blood donation 301–303, 385
   blood, rhesus negative 301
   prolapse 263, **266–267**, 291, 377
   See also Umbilical cord
Cot 197
Cot death *See* SIDS
Counselling
   after miscarriage 113
   couple 67, 474, 480
   for depression 155
   individual 67, 474, **534**, **535**
   postnatal depression 474
Cow's milk formula 193
Cradle 197
Cramping 231, 232, 363
Cravings, food 63–4
CRL (crown to rump length) 49
Crowning phase 272–273
Crying, baby's
   after birth 500–501, **504–505**
   at birth 274, 293
   support strategies for 505–506
   unexplained 504–505
Crying, mother's unexpected 66
Cryline 506
CSE 339, 380
CT scans 76
CTG monitoring 207, 239, 242, 254, **255–257**, 259, 263, 266, 288, 291, 336, 342, 356, 358, 361, 362, 370, 373, 378, 401
Cultural beliefs (birth) 326–327
CVS (chronic villus sampling)
   complications with 111
   procedure for **106**, **107**, 212
Cystic fibrosis (test) 433
Cystitis *See* Urine infection
Cytomegalovirus (CMV) 78, 79

D

D&C 112–113, 115, 313, 470
Dads, 'stay-at-home' 517–518
   See also Partner
Dance therapy 534, 535
Death, baby's (in utero) 157–158
Deflexed, baby's head 372, 398
Dehydration 234, 250, 372
Delivery suite (hospital)
   admission to 238, 239
   packing for 225–227
   privacy of 250
   travelling to 238–239
Dental care, mother's 124
Depression 154–156, 494, 495
   See also Emotions; Postnatal depression
Dermatitis 191
DES (diethylstilbstrol) 115
DHA (dihydroxyacetone) 74

Diabetes
   during pregnancy 151
   gestational 211
   pre-gestational 28, 151
Diagnostic genetic tests 102, 106–108
   See also Screening genetic tests
Diaphragm (cap) 33, 491–492
Diarrhoea
   breastfeeding and 519
   in prelabour 233
Diet
   after birth 443, 460, 519
   during pregnancy 62–64
   five food groups for 5–7
   morning sickness and 61
   preconception 4–5
   therapy 534, 535
   vegan 10–19, 64
   vegetarian 10–19, 64
   See also Cravings, food
Dilation *See* Cervix
Dizziness
   during pregnancy 59
   pain relief and 336, 338
DMPA *See* Progesterone
Doctor *See* Caregiver; GP
Doppler machine 99, 142, 291
   ultrasound and 148
Doula 218
Down syndrome, testing for 101–109
Dreams 138
Drinks
   after birth 306
   during labour 226, 234, 250–251, 375
Drip, intravenous
   after birth 304, 312
   with an epidural/spinal 342
   See also Oxytocin; Syntocinon
Drowsiness
   in baby 337, 346
   in mother 333, 336, 382
Drugs for birth *See* Pain relief
Drugs, hard, effects on pregnancy 20
Due date
   calculating 54
   chart 56–57
   ultrasound for 55
Dummy 198, 503, 505, 521
DVT (deep vein thrombosis) 387, 392, **471**

E

Early Childhood Centre 462, 482–483
Ears, baby's 51, 423, 431
   See also Hearing
Eclampsia 210
ECG (electrocardiographic) machine 257
Ectopic pregnancy 45, 110, 116–117, 493, 499
ECV (external cephalic version) **204–205**, 292
Eczema 125
EDC (estimated date of confinement) 54
Edward's syndrome 105
Effacement 232
Eggs, mother's 30
Ejaculation 31, 46
Electronic fetal monitoring *See* CTG monitoring
Embolus 471
Embryo 49
Emergency arrangements (hospital) 400
   transfer mother or baby 97
Emergency pills 496
Emotions
   after the birth 299–300
   at birth 275
   bottle feeding and 454–455
   breastfeeding and 450–451, 513
   caesarean and 393–396
   complications and 327
   during transition 247–248

fertility cycle and 37, 38, 39
fertility treatment and 47
  induction and 370–371
  in early pregnancy 66–67
  in first stage labour 245, 246, 247, 248
  in late pregnancy 182–183
  in middle pregnancy 137–139
  in second stage labour 272, 273
  labour pain and 320–322, 328–329
  miscarriage and 112, 113, 114
  multiple babies and 507
  newborn baby and 457–459, 460–461
  parenting and 477–479
  partner's 138–139
  post-birth sex and 488–489
  postnatal depression and 472–473
  prelabour and 235–237
  reaction to tests and 108–109
  severe tearing and 315–316
  trying to conceive and 42
  unintended pregnancy and 66
  VBAC and 403–404
  when feeding baby 417
  when returning to work 515, 516, 517
Endoderm 49
Endometriosis 45
Endometrium 30
Endorphins 249, **319**, 325, 331
Engaged (baby's head) 163, 185, **186–187**, 241
English as second language
  during labour 220
  during visits 98
Engorged breasts 451, 466
Environment
  calm, for birth 406
  safe, for labour 250
Environment Protection Authority (EPA) 77
Environmental hazards 75–76
Epidural 91, 93, 95, 206, 247, 258, 262, 264, 269, 271, 278, 289, 309, 315, 325, 327, 338–347, 372, 374
  avoiding 288
  during labour 338–347
  continuous 340
  effects on baby 346, 393
  effects on mother 342–346
  for caesarean 380–381, 387
  procedure for 338, 339–340, **339**, 341–342
  removal of 304
  walking 340–341
  See also CSE
Epilepsy 28, **151–152**
  See also Anti-epileptics
Episiotomy 90, 206, 280, **282–284**, 287, 314
  avoiding an 284, 286
  mediolateral 282
  midline 282
Epstein's pearls 424
Erb's palsy 289
Ergometrine 300–301
Essential oils
  during first trimester 61
  during labour 348–349
Essure (tubal) 499
Examination, newborn 430–434
Exercise
  after birth **443–445**, 482, 519
  during pregnancy 65–66
  for restless legs 124
  See also Overheating
Exhaustion
  after the birth 459, 519
  at the birth 275
  in labour 249, 327
Exposure (e.g. radiation), concerns about 68
Expressing milk 448, 464–465, 508–512, **510**, 519

Expulsion phase of placenta 297
Eyes (eyesight), development of baby's 50–1, 121, 122, 423, 431

F
Facial features, baby's 50–51, 423
Faint, feeling 310, 312
Fainting 59, 311
Fallopian tubes 30, 41
  blocked 45
Family planning, natural (NFP) 497–498
Fat stores, breastfeeding and 65
Father, expectations of 479
Fatigue 59
Feedback (after birth) 463–464
Feeding (baby) 188–194, 416–420
  See also Bottlefeeding; Breastfeeding
Feelings *See* Emotions
Fees, medical (birth) 92, 93, 94, 95, 96
Feet, baby's 424, 432
Female reproductive system 29, 30, **31**
Ferguson's reflex 270
Ferric acid *See* Iron
Fertile days 37
Fertile phase 38
Fertility
  after birth 489
  chart 34–35
  charting 33–39, 497–498
  cycle 37–39
  tests for 40
  treatments 46–47
  weight and 25
Fertility drugs
  ectopic pregnancy and 116
  effects on tests 40
  taking 40
Fever 77
  after birth 469
  in labour 258–259, 343
  See also Temperature
FHS (fetal heart sounds heard) 187
Fimbria 30
Financial considerations 3
First trimester (0–12 weeks)
  visits to caregiver 98–100
  week 3: 48–49
  weeks 4–6: 49–50
  weeks 7–9: 50–51
  weeks 10–12: 51–52
  See also Pregnancy
Fish, mercury in 63
Flagyl (metronidazole) 87, 132
Fluid retention 65, **176**, 361
  See also Oedema
Flying
  while pregnant 158–159
  with newborn 439
  See also Travel
FMF (fetal movements felt) 187
Fetal alcohol syndrome (FAS) 21–22
Fetal distress 269, 377
  See also Baby, pre-birth
Foley's catheter 364–365
Folic acid 12, 13, 332
  in foods 9
  pre-conception and 13
  supplements 8, 9, 20, 153–154
  See also Neural tube defects
Food
  after birth 306
  during labour 226, 250–251
  overcooked, effect on vitamins 11–13, 15
  vitamins in 11, 13, 15, 17, 19
  See also Diet
Food groups, the five 5–7
Forceps 91, 95, 206, 260, 269, 280, 281, 282, **285–288**, 309, 314, 341, 344, 384, 407
Fore milk 447
Foreskin, baby's, care of 438–439
Forgetfulness 137

Formula 192–194, 419, 420
  complementing breastfeed 192, 513, 521
  how much? 451–452
  preparing 452–454
  types of 193–194
  See also Bottle feeding
Full blood count (FBC) **143–144**, 187
Fully-dilated (cervix) 247, 249, 268, **269**
Fundal height 141–142, **185**

G
Gag reflex 120, 428
Galactosaemia 193, 433
Gardnerella 110, 131–132, 169, 470
Gas (laughing, nitrous oxide) 331–334
  effectiveness 332, 374
  effects on baby 333
  effects on mother 333, 334
  use of 91, 94, 325, 327, 331–334
GBS *See* Strep B
Gender *See* Sex, baby's
Genital
  herpes 80, 81
  warts 82, 83
  See also HPV
Genetic
  counselling 28–29, 91, 102, 107, 109
  disorder, risk of 103
  support agencies 559
  testing 101–109, 149–150
  See also Tests
Genitals
  baby's 425, 432
  mother's, after birth 305, 307–309, 441, 463
  mother's, infection of 469
German measles *See* Rubella
Gestational age 185
Ginger, for morning sickness 61
Glucose tolerance test (GTT) 145, 211
Gonads 52
Gonorrhoea 78, 79–80
GP (general practioner) 91, **94–5**, 96, 97, 462, 468, 482, 495
  professional associations 559
Grave's disease 153
  See also Hyperthyroidism
Grief
  loss of baby and 112, 113, 114, 115, 117, 157, 295, 471
  support agencies for 560
Groaning in labour 250
Groin
  baby's 432
  mother's, pain in 132
Group B Strep (GBS) 146–147
Gums, bleeding 123–124

H
Haematomas 311
Haemoglobin
  production 16
  test for 100, **143**, 144
Haemolytic anaemia 15, 212
Haemophilia, baby's sex and 43
Haemorrhoids **173–174**, 305
Hair, baby's 120, 121
Hair, mother's
  changes in 124–125
  dyes 71
  loss 450
  removal 71–72
Hands, baby's 424, 431
Harelip 8–9
Hashish 23
Hay fever 128–129
HCG (human gonadotrophic hormone)
  blood tests for 53, 110
  D&C and 115
  levels of 52, 53, 54

INDEX

Head, baby's
  after birth 422
  appearing (crowning) 272–274
  circumference of 410, 431
Head lice 72–73
Headaches
  after birth 469
  contraceptives and 492, 493, 494, 495
  epidurals/spinals and 344
  in pregnancy 60, 209
Healers 534, 535
Health Care Complaints Commission 464
Health check
  pre-conception 27–28
  pre-existing conditions and 28
Health disorders, infertility and 45–46
Health insurance 3, 95, 96
Health Insurance Commission (HIC) 414
Hearing, baby's 51, **121**
  See also Ears
Heart, baby's, development of 49, 50, 122, 142
Heart disease 28, **152–153**, 176
Heart rate, baby's
  after birth 410
  at birth 407
  during labour 239, 255–257, 342
Heart rate, mothers, during exercise 66
Heartbeat 142, 187
Heartburn 174–175
Heat packs 91, 93, 227, 229, 262, 440
  making 229
Heel prick See Baby, newborn; Blood test
HELLP syndrome 209
Hepatitis A **80**, **81**
Hepatitis B 28, **80**, **81–82**, 302, 413–414
Hepatitis C 28, **82**, **83**, 302, 378
  support agencies 557
Herbs 351, 368, **536**, **537**
Hernias, baby 432
Hexachlorophore 74
Hiccups, baby's 121, **181–182**, 424
Hind milk 447
Hips
  baby's or 'clicky' 432
  mother's, sore 133
HIV/AIDS
  effects and treatment **82**, **83**, 302, 490
  in labour 363, 378
  support agencies for 557
  tests for 28
Homebirth 93, 96
  caregiver's visits after 461
  cord blood donation 302
  induction and 359, 360
  labour and 243, 246, 254, 302, 331, 335
  preparing for 227–229
Homeopathy 351, 368, 374, **536**, **537**
Hospital See Antenatal clinic; Delivery suite
Hospital ward, postnatal 91, 461
Household chores 2, 480
HPV (Human Papilloma Virus) 82, 83
Humidicrib 97
Hydrotherapy 536, 537
Hyperstimulation 345, 359–360, 361, 366
Hypertension 209
  See also Blood pressure
Hyperthyroidism 17, **153**
  congenital 433
  See also Iodine
Hypnosis 351, **536**, **537**
Hysterectomy 314

I

Identification 'bracelets' 409
IgG (and IgM) antibodies 85, 86, 87
Immune system, baby's 122, 163
Immunisation Register 563–564
Implanon 495
Indigestion 174
Induction 187, 243
  See also Labour induction
Infection
  caesarean and 391
  epidural/spinal and 345
  of uterus 102, 469
  signs of 242–243
  water birth and risks of 225
  waters breaking and 242
Infections
  after birth 469–470
  common 77–87
Infertility
  causes of 44–46
  primary 44
  secondary 44
  support resources for 555
  treatments 46–47
Injection
  anti-D immuniglobulin 115
  Hep B (for newborn) 413–414
  iron 144–145
  maxalon 336
  naloxone 336, 337, 415
  narcotics for pain 91, 93, 94, 317, **334**, 372, 374
  vitamin K 15, 16, 411–412
  ZIG 79
  See also Oxytocin; Pethidine; Syntocinon
Insulin 151
Intensive care
  for baby 434
  nurseries 97–98
Intercourse, sexual See Sex
Interferon 83
Intervention
  routine, at birth 408–409
  See also Birth; Labour
In-vitro fertilsation (IVF)
  conception and 46
  gender selection and 43–44
  premature birth and 201
Iodine (iodide) 16, 17
Iridology 536, 537
Iron (ferric acid)
  absorption 17
  deficiency 16
  stores, test for 100
  supplements 144, 154
Isoimmunisation 212–213
IUD (intrauterine device)
  copper 496–497
  progesterone 496–497
IVF See In-vitro fertilisation

J

Jaundice 214, **435–436**
  bilirubin levels and 436–437
  breast milk and 436
  non-physiological 436
  physiological 436

K

ketones 243
ketosis 243, 372
kick chart 181, 188
kicking, baby's See Movements, baby's
kidney stones 13
kidneys
  baby's 209
  mother's 470
kinesiology 538, 539
kneeling (for birth) 278, **278**

L

Labour
  children present at 220–224
  coping with long 236
  food and drinks for 226, 228
  'going into' 244–245
  newborn's reaction to 406
  packing bag for 225–227
  pain during 318–353
  readiness for 357
  recovery from 304
  slowing the 335, 343–344
  support person for 218–220
  vaginal breech 206
  vocalising during 223, 250
  See also Labour first stage; Labour second stage; Labour third stage; Labour fourth stage; Prelabour
Labour, augmented 371–376
  See also Augmentation
Labour first stage 244–267
  accepting 252
  active 245–247
  early 244–245
  emotions during 245, 246, 247, 248
  end of (transition) 247–249
  first baby and 244, 246
  positions in 251
  second or subsequent baby and 244, 246
  slow progress in 262
  support strategies for 250–254
  variations in 257–267
Labour fourth stage 304–317
  emotions during 305
  support strategies for 305–307
  variations in 309–317
Labour induction 211, 243, 354–376
  choosing when to 355–356
  coping with 369–371
  mechanical methods of 361–365
  natural methods of 367–369
  pharmacological methods of 358–361
  rates of 365
  reasons for 354–355
  risks with 365–366
  tests and 356–357
  VBAC and 401
Labour options 91, 92, 93, 94, 95, 96, 157–158
  after baby dying in pregnancy 157–158
Labour second stage 268–295
  crowning phase 272–273
  emotions during 272–275
  pushing (active) 270–272
  resting in 268–270
  support strategies for 271, 272–273, 275–277
  time limit on 280
  twins during 290–291
  variations in 280–295
Labour third stage 296–303
  emotions during 299–300
  expulsion phase 297
  natural vs. active management 297–298
  resting phase 296
  separation phase 296–297
  variations in 309–317
Labourade recipe 226
Lactation consultant 192, 520, 521
Lamicel 365
Laminaria tent 365
Lanugo 121
Laparoscopy 499, 500
Latching (baby to breast) **417–418**, **418**, 446
Lead levels 76
Lead poisoning, symptoms of 76–77
Le Boyer method 406
Leg cramps 175–176
Legs
  baby's 424, 432
  restless 124
Length, baby's 410
Let-down reflex **447–448**, 509
Leukaemia, cord blood and 301–303
LGTT (long glucose tolerance test) 145, 211

Libido 139–140, 488
Lifestyle changes during pregnancy 20, 42, 69
Ligaments (pelvic) 165, 177
Lindane, avoiding 72
Linea nigra (black line) 126, 441
Lips, baby's 424, 431
Listeria (listeriosis) 62–63
Lithotomy position 272, 286
Local doctor See GP
Lochia 441
Lungs, baby's
 checking 431
 formation of 51, 121, 163
Luteal phase 39

M
McRobert's manoeuvre 289
Magnesium (Mg) 16,17
Male reproductive system 31–32, **32**
Marijuana 23
Marks (birth) See Birthmarks
'Mask' of pregnancy 126
Massage
 breasts and 466
 during labour 226–227, 374
 for induction 368
 for pain relief 93, 133, 351
 perineal 168–169, 281, 487
 shiatsu 347–348, 540, 541
 therapy **538, 539**
Mastitis 464, **467–468**, 513
Maternity clothing 134–136
Maternity leave 4
Maxalon 62
Measles 84, 85
 See also Rubella
Mebendazole 72
Meconium 120, 225, 233, 243, 257, 285, 362, 415, **421**
Medicare 3, 92, 93, 94, 95, 96, 365
 card 227
Medication
 category rating system 70
 other types to avoid 173, 175
 prescribed 69–71
Melanocyte stimulating hormone (MSH) 74, 126
Membranes
 artificial rupture of See ARM
 'sweeping the' 363–364
Menadione (vitamin K)
 bloodclotting and 14
 injection to newborn 15
Menopause 32, 45
Menstruation
 after birth 489
 average cycle 32
 conception and 41
 effects on 32–33
 See also Amenorrhoea; Periods
Mesoderm 49
Microwaves 75
Microwaving
 formula 454
 heat packs 229
Midwife, private 96
Midwives (midwifery)
 after birth care 307, 461, 520
 clinic 92
 professional associations 558
 teams 93–94
 See also Caregiver
Migraines 60, 73
Milk, breast See Breast milk
Milk, cow's formula 193
Milk, witches 424
Minipill, the 33, **492–493**
Miscarriage
 0–6 weeks 112–113
 6–13 weeks 112–113
 14–20 weeks 113
 announcing pregnancy and 88
 blighted ovum 114
 concerns about sex and 67

D&C and 115
emotions and 112, 113, 114
fertility and 43
future pregnancies 116
inevitable (spontaneous) 112
late 113
missed (silent) 114
reasons for 111–112
recovery from 116
recurrent 115
support agencies for 560
testing and 102, 107
threatened 109
MMR vaccine 85
Mobile phones 75
Molar pregnancy 110, **571**
Moles 126
MOM (multiple of median) risk factor 105
Mongolian spot 426
Monitor, baby 195, 198
Monitoring
 continuous, during labour 255–257
 late pregnancy **185–188**, 207
 prelabour 239
 VBAC and 401, 402
Morula 48
Morning sickness 60
 acupressure and 61
 medical treatment for 61–62
 natural therapies for 61
 remedies 60–61
 saliva and 59
 vitamin B6 and 13
Mother, expectations of 478
Mothers' groups 462, 482,
Mouth, baby's 424, 431
Movements, baby's 120, 136–137, 162–163, **181–182**, 187
 frequency of 181
Movement during labour 352
Moving after caesarean 387
MRI (magnetic resonance imaging) 76
Multiple birth
 caesarean and 383, 384
 feeding babies after 449–450, 454
 premature 201
 routines after 506–507
 support agencies for 560
 See also Triplets; Twins
Multiple pregnancy
 choosing caregiver for 91, 95
 incidence of 55
Multivitamins 9
Mumps 84, 85
Music during labour 352
Mycoplasma 131
Mylanta 126
Myths of parenting 477–479

N
Nails, changes in 125
Naloxone 336–337, 415
Nappies
 changing newborn's 421
 cloth 197, 198–199
 disposable 197, 199
 wet per day 449, 519
National Australian Immunisation Schedule 413
Natural management (third stage labour) 296, 297–298
Natural therapies 74, 530–541
 aches and pains and 132–133
 after birth 304, 305, 310, 442
 anal fissure and 316
 backache and 171
 bleeding gums and 124
 breast milk supply and 520, 521
 breast pain and 451
 bruising and 311
 colds, sinus and 128–129
 constipation and 172–173
 dehydration and 243

engorged breasts and 466
gardnerella and 131
guide to 530–541
haemorrhoids and 173–174
heartburn and 174–175
induction and 367–369
labour and 227, 258
leg cramps and 175–176
mastitis and 468
metallic taste and 123
miscarriage and 116
posterior position and 260–262, 264
postnatal depression and 475
postpartum haemorrhage and 313
pre-eclampsia and 210
professional associations for 559
raspberry leaf tea 176, 215–216
restless legs and 124
retained placenta and 313–314
skin and 125–128
slow labour and 374–375
stress and 27
stretch marks and 127–128
swelling and 177
symphysis pain and 178
thrush and 130, 466
urinary infection and 154
varicose veins and 179
vulval varicosities and 179
Naturopathy 538, 539
Nausea
 after caesarean 382
 during pregnancy 59, 60
 in labour 233, 250, 257–258
 pain relief and 333, 335–336, 343
 See also Morning sickness
Navel,
 'inny' or 'outy' 425
 sore 180
Neck, baby's 431
Needle See Injection
Nervous system, baby's 121
Neural tube 49
 defects of (NTD) 8, 9
Newborn See Baby, newborn
Niacin (vitamin B3) 10, 11
Nipple
 avoiding damage to the 191, 446, 465
 breastfeeding and the 417–418
 changes during early pregnancy 59
 expressing milk with the 509–510, **510, 511**
 latching on to 417–418, **418**
Nipple shield 465
Nipples, baby's 424, 431
Nipples, mother's
 inverted and flat 191
 sore, cracked 191, **464–466**
 stimulation of 368–369
 thrush in the 465–466
Nitrous oxide See Gas
Nits See Head lice
Noises, clicking (in utero) 216
Nose, baby's 408, 423, 431
Nose bleeds 128
NSAIDS 73, 129
Nuchal translucency (NT) 104, 105
Numbness (limbs) 344

O
Obstetrician
 for caesarean 382
 labour and 254
 private 95, 96, 97, 307
 professional association 559
 See also Caregiver
Occipito 186
Oedema 176
 See also Swelling
Oestrogen 39
 increased levels of 52
 skin changes and 74
Older parents, pre-conception and 29
Oligohydramnios 208–209

INDEX **591**

Oral anti-fungal tablets 131
Organs, baby's, development of 51, 119, 162, 163
Organs, mother's
  after caesarean 391–392
Orgasm
  for induction 369
  during labour 375
Osteopathy 538, 539
Ovaries 30, 31, **31**
Overdosing on supplements, risk of 11, 13, 15, 17, 19
Overdue
  going 355
  waiting when 356
Overdue ('overcooked') baby 164
Overheating 77
Overweight
  baby 397–398, 415
  mother 64
Ovulation
  estimating 41
  prediction kits 40, 497
  signs of 33, 36
Oxygen, baby's
  at birth 273, 274, 279
  inadequate 263, 409
Oxytocin
  different types of 300–301, 447
  injection 296, 298, 312, 314, 317

P

Packing your bag 225–227
Pain
  after birth 305
  'dragging' 132–133
  during caesarean 383
  in breast 451, 466–469
  intense 284
  in uterus 118
  in waist 133
  miscarriage and 113
  See also Aches and pains
Pain, labour
  beliefs and perceptions about 328–329
  endorphins in 319
  expectations of 323–324
  fears and concerns about 321–322, 328–330
  final stage of birth 270–271
  'gate control' theory 319, 353
  helpful tools to overcome 330
  mother's perception of 320
  past experience and 322
  physiology of 318–320
  positive attitude and 329
  threshold 323
  See also Pain relief
Pain relief
  after birth 305, 311
  after caesarean 387, 388
  for VBAC 402
  having twins and 291
  induction and 366, 370
  labour and 331–353
  medical forms of 331–347
  natural therapies for 347–353
  options 91, 92, 93, 94, 95, 96, 248, 262
  slow labour and 374
  social, cultural, spiritual beliefs and 326–327
  stitches and 308, 309
  See also Epidural; Pethidine; Spinal
Painkillers 60, **73**, 305
Palpitations 176
Pap test (smear) 82, 99, 463
Paracetamol **73**, 129, 451, 468
Parenting
  realistic expectations 477–479
  skills 420–421
  support agencies for 560–563
  support strategies for 480–481
  transition to 477–521

Parents' group 482, 518
Partner
  active labour and 246–247, 338
  after the birth 300, 306–307, 458, 460–461, 479
  as primary carer 517–518
  attitudes to pain 324
  BBA and 293
  caesarean and 379, 380, 381, 385, 395–396
  'catching' the baby 275
  during birth phase 273, 275, 276–277
  early stage labour and 245
  labour support role of 219, 235, 252–254
  long labour and 236
  pain relief and 334, 338, 346–347
  postnatal depression and 473–474
  sex after the birth with 488–489
  transition and 248–249
Parvovirus B19 (5th Disease) 84, 85
Patau syndrome 105
Patient Controlled Epidural Anaesthesia (PCEA) 340
Pelvic
  girdle 178
  tilt exercises 171, 444, 445
Pelvic floor
  exercises **167–168**, 179, 180, 441, 442
  muscles **167**, 270, 281, 282, 283
  sex and the 486
Pelvis 167–168, **167**
  pain in 177–178
Penis 31, **32**
Penis, baby's 52, 432
Perineum **168**, 270, 271, 272, 278, 280, 281, 282, 283, 284, 311
  massage of the 168–169
  pain in 305, 315
  See also Tear
Period pain 233
Periods
  delayed 450
  fertility cycle and 37–38
  irregular 489, 492, 493, 495
  missed 32–33
  See also Menstruation
Pethidine 324, 325, 327, 333, **334–335**, 338, 340
  effects on baby 336–337
  effects on mother 335–336, 338
Phenylketonuria (PKU) 433
Pheromones 416
Phimosis 438
Phosphorous (Ph) 16, 17
Photocopiers 75
Photos
  after birth 386
  from ultrasound 147–148
Phototherapy 436–437
Physical activity 24
  effect on menstruation 24
  when to avoid 24–25
Physical changes (woman) 170–179
Physical hazards 77
Physiotherapy 171, 178, 310, 443
  treating painful sex 487
PIH 209
Piles 173–174, 305
Pill, the 33, 494–495
Pinard's stethoscope 122, 142
Placenta
  BBA delivery of 294
  caesarean and the 385
  changes in 165–166
  checking the 299
  disposing of 299
  effect on baby's movement 137
  formation of 49, 121
  in miscarriage 113
  labour and 263
  retained 313–314

  rituals involving 303, 385
  separation of the 296–297, 312
  twins and 55, 58
  weight of 65
Placenta abruption 208, 209, **212**, 263, 311, 377
Placenta accreta 314
Placenta previa 203, **211–212**, 311, 377, 392
Platelets (thrombocytes) 100
Polycystic ovarian syndrome (PCOS) 45
Polyhydramnios 208
'Poo', baby's
  breastfed 447, 448, 519
  first 421
  See also Bowel, baby's; Meconium
Position, baby's
  for comforting 505
  in womb 134, 141–142, 163, **186**, 203–205, 383
  See also Breech; Posterior
Position, mother's
  distressed baby and 263–264
  during pregnancy 160
  epidural and 346–347
  final stages labour 271–272, 327
  in labour 251
  pain relief and 352
  to augment labour 375
Positions, birth (mother's) 277–279
  kneeling 278, **278**
  lying on back 279
  lying on side 278
  on stool 278, **278**
  semi-reclining 279
  squatting, straddling 278, 278
  standing **277**, 278
Posterior, baby
  during pregnancy 186
  in labour 186, **260–262**, 281, 315, 379
Post-fertile phase 39
Postnatal care 91, 92, 93, 94, 95, 96
Postnatal check-up 462–463
Postnatal depression **471–475**
  anti-depressants for 474–475
  natural therapies for 475
  professional help for 474
  psychosis 476
  signs of 472–473
  support agencies for 563
  support strategies for 473–475
Postnatal exercises 443–445, 462
Postnatal psychosis 476
Postnatal ward 91
Postpartum haemorrhage 290, 297–298
  primary 311–313
  secondary 470
Post-traumatic stress disorder (PTSD) 472, **475–476**
Posture, during pregnancy 77, 170–171, 174
Potassium (K) 18, 19
Precipitate birth *See* Birth, fast
Pre-eclampsia 150, 151, **209–210**, 212
Pre-eclampsia toxaemia (PET) 209
Pregnancy
  anembryonic 114
  announcing your 88–89
  birth options after 89–97
  card 227
  confirming 52
  constipation in 172–173
  cravings during 63–64
  depression in 154–156
  diet in 62–64, 448
  dreams in 138
  early pregnancy 67
  ectopic 116–117
  full term 164, **166**
  heterotopic 117
  hormones in 167
  late pregnancy 184–185
  listeria and 62–63

medication in 69–71
middle pregnancy 139–140
miscarriage in 111–116
molar 110, 571
monitoring 185–188
overdue 355
preparing for 4
sex during 67
support resources for 558
taking care during 68
tests during 100–109
tests for 53
travel during 158–160
unplanned 1
viable 46
visit, first 98–100
vitamin intake and 10–19
vomiting during 60, 117–18
work and 2, 3, 4
See also First trimester; Second trimester; Third trimester
Pregnancy Guidelines (booklet) 4
Prelabour
caregiver's questions during 237–238
emotions during 235–237
going home during 240–241
support strategies for 234–235
symptoms of 232–233
variations for 241–243
Premature baby 200–203, 377
care of 434–435
delivery of 91, 93, 95, 97
Premature birth
apgar score and 407
by caesarean 393
causes of 201–202, 213
Premature labour, threatened (TPL) 202–203
Presentation 185–186
brow or face 285
shoulder 265
Product safety resources 564
Progesterone 39
effect on exercise 65–66
increased levels of 52
injections 493–494
Progress, slow, in labour 262, 371–373, 402
Prostaglandins 32, 354
for induction **358–360**, 364, 366, 370
gel 358
injection 312
pessary 358
Prostate gland 32
Puerperal psychosis 471, 476
Puerperium 440
Pulmonary oedema 152
PUPPS 125
Pushing phases (active) 270–273
Pyridoxine 12 (vitamin) 12–13

Q
Quadruple test 104, 105
Quickening 136

R
Rash, heat 125
Raspberry leaf 215–216
Raspberry leaf tea 215, 216, 368
Recovery after birth, mother's 440–476
Rectum, tear to 314–315
Reflexes
Babinski 429
crawling 428–429
gag 428
galant 429
grasp 429
rooting 427–428
startle 420, 428
sucking, swallowing 428
tonic neck 429
traction 429
walking 429, 432

Reflexology 347, 348, 351, 374, **538**, **539**
Rehydration 374
Relationship
counselling 67
effect of pregnancy on 67
realistic expectations in 2
support agencies for 562
survival tips, after birth 479–481
with own father 139
with own mother 138
Relaxation
after birth 482
for augmenting 375
for induction 369
Relaxin (hormone) 127
Religious beliefs (labour) 326
REM (rapid eye movement), baby's 122, **502**
Renal pelvis dilation 149
Reproductive organs, formation of baby's 50, 51, 52
Reproductive system
female 29, 30, **31**
male 31–32, **32**
Resting (after birth) 459–460
Restless legs 124
Resuscitation 293, 385
Retin-A 11
Retroverted uterus 118
Rhesus factor (Rh) 100, 115, 212
after birth 301
after miscarriage 115
Riboflavin 10, 11
Royal Flying Doctor Service (RFDS) 239
Rubella (German measles) 84, 85
miscarriage risk with 111
MMR vaccine for 85
small baby and 207
test for 28
titre test 100, 463

S
Sacrum 118
Safebaby logo **196**
Safety standards, product 196
Saliva
increased during pregnancy 59
test for ovulation 40
Salt (sodium) 18, 19
Scabies 72–73, 125
Scar, caesarean 397, 463
healing of 389
tenderness of 399
tissue 383
Sciatica 170–171
Screening genetic tests (mother) 101, 103
for newborn 433–434
See also Tests
Scrotum (sac) 31, **32**
baby's 425, 432
Second trimester (13–28 weeks)
tests during 143–148
visits to caregiver 141–143
weeks 13–16: 120
week 18: 120–121
weeks 20–24: 121
week 26: 122
week 28: 122
Secretory phase 39
Semen 46
Separation phase of placenta 296–297
'Septic work-up' 259
Serum ferritin 100
Settling (baby) 500–501, 504–506
Sex
after caesarean 389
after miscarriage 116
bleeding after 110
concerns about 140
during early pregnancy 67
during late pregnancy 184–185
for induction 369

no interest in 473
painful, after birth 315, 487
resuming after birth 486–489
See also Contraception
Sex, the baby's
announcing the 279
choosing 43–44
determining through ultrasound 147
disclosing 102
formation of 31, 52
methods of choosing 44
reaction at birth to 275
Sexual desire, fertility cycle and 37, 38, 39
Sexual health support agencies 554–555
Sexual intercourse *see* Sex
Sexuality 139–40, 488–489
and breastfeeding 190
SGA (small for gestational age) 207–208
SGTT (short glucose tolerance test) 145
Shettles method 44
Shiatsu 540, 541
Shingles 78, 79
Shivering (and shaking) 248, 250, 304, 306, 342, 469
Shoes (during pregnancy) 136
Shoulder dystocia 283, **288–290**, 314, 315
'Show', a **165**, 233, 249
Shower
after birth 306, 307
for pain relief 91, 353
Sibling rivalry 484–486
Siblings, baby's
at birth 220–224
newborn and 421–422
preparing 220
reactions 196
See also Children, other; Sibling rivalry
Sickle cell disease 154
SIDS
sleeping and 194, 195, 429
smoking and 22–23
Single parenthood
after birth 481
pregnancy and 1, 66
support agencies for 562–563
Sinus 128
Size, baby's 141–142
Skin, baby's 120, 273, 424, 431
Skin, mother's
changes 125–128
darkening of 126
disorders, treatment of 73–74
itchy 125
tags 127
type, breastfeeding and 191
Slapped cheek syndrome 84, 85
Sleep, baby's
arrangements 194–195
bathing for 506
cues for 503
cycles, newborn 500, 501, 502
in uterus 181
massage for 504, 506
noisy 195
rocking for 503, 504, 505
signs of readiness for 502–503
singing or music for 504, 506
tips to help 501, 502
wrapping for 504
Sleep, mother's
after newborn arrives 459, 473, 481
disorders 13
Small (for dates) baby 207–208
Smell, baby's sense of 120
Smoking
breastfeeding and 23, 192, 519
ectopic pregnancy and 116
effects of, preconception 22
managing stress with 26
premature birth and 201

INDEX 593

small baby and 207
support agencies for 556
the pill and 495
vitamin deficiency and 12
withdrawal from 22
Sneezing, baby 423
Social worker 99
Sodium (Na, salt) 18
water balance and 19
Solids 521
Soy products 64
Soybean formula 193–194
Sperm (spermatoza) 31, 32
test 46
vitamin A and 10
zinc and 19
Spermicide 490, 491
Spider veins (naevi) 127
Spinal anaesthesia (spinal) 338–347
caesarean and 380–381
effects on baby 346
effects on mother 342–345
procedure for 339–340, **339**, 341–342
total 345
Spinal cord, baby's 121
Spotting (periods) 492, 493
Squatting for birth 278
Standing for birth **277**, 278
Star signs *See* Astrology
Startle (Moro) reflex 420, 428
Station, baby's 186
Sterilisation *See* Tubal occlusion; Vasectomy
Sterilising baby's equipment 455–456
Stillbirth 43, 157, 214, **294–295**, 299
support agencies for 560
Stirrups 272, 286, 344
Stitches
after caesarean 385, 386, 387, **388**
anaesthetic for 308
how many? 308
infected 469
post birth 281, 307–309, 442
sex and 487
See also Tear
Straddling position (birth) 278, **278**
Strep B 146–147
effect on baby 146–147, 415
Stress
morning sickness and 61
strategies for managing 26–27
vitamin C and 12
See also Emotions
Stretch marks 127–128, 441
'Strip and stretch' *See* Membranes, 'sweeping the'
Succenturiate lobe 211–212
Sucking
and swallowing action 163, 428
reflex 337, 428
Suctioning
baby's nose and mouth 408–409
baby's stomach 409
Sudden Infant Death Syndrome *See* SIDS
Support person(s)
after birth 300, 306–307, 460–461
attitude to pain 324
caesarean and 379, 380, 381, 385, 395–396
choosing a 219–220
choosing your child's 222, 223
during birth phase 275
during labour 245, 246–247, 248, 338
during transition 248–249
emotions during labour 236–237, 245, 246–247, 248
in long labour 236
pain relief and 334, 338, 346–347
restriction on number of 224
support strategies in birth 276–277

support strategies in labour 235, 252–254
VBAC and 404
Support resources (agencies) 462, 474, **554–564**
Support strategies, after the birth (for mother) 457–458, 462, 480–482
by family and partner 460–461
for sibling rivalry 485–486
self-support 459–460
Surfactant 121, 163
Suture *See* Stitches
Sweating 59, 442
Swelling 176–177
pre-eclampsia and 209
Swimming, after birth 441, 443
Symphysis pubis pain 177–178
Syntocinon
use of 296, 297–298, 300, 301, 312, 314, 317, 359, 362, 370
drip 262, 263, 288, 291, 327, 359, **360–361**, 364, 366, 373–374, 385
See also oxytocin
Syntometrine 301
Syphilis test 100–101

T

T'ai chi 540, 541
Tanning treatments 74
Taste, baby's sense of 163
Tear, tearing
after birth care of 307–309
caesarean and previous 378
episiotomy and 282, 283–284
fear of 272
first degree 280
of cervix 281
of labia 281
second degree 281
severe 311, 314–316
third and fourth degree 281, **314–316**
vaginal 168, 271, 272, 278, 280, **280–282**, 284
Teats *See* Bottle feeding
Teeth, unborn baby's 52, 121
Television 75
Telling people (about your pregnancy) 88–89
Temperature, baby's 405, 409–410, 415
Temperature (mother's)
after birth 306, **469**
change in, during labour 250
contraception and 497
during fertility cycle 37, 38, 39
high or low 36
increased in pregnancy 59
ovulation and 33–36
See also fever
TENS (transutaneous electrical nerve stimulation) 93, **352–353**, 387
Term Breech Trial 205
Term (40 weeks) 164
Terminals 75
Testes 31, **32**
Testes, baby's 163–164
Tests
considerations for 108
future option for 109
in early pregnancy 100–109
in late pregnancy 187–188
in middle pregnancy 143–150
See also Blood test; Genetic testing; Screening
Tetrahydrocannabinol (THC) *See* Marijuana
Thalassaemia 153–154
Thiamine (vitamin B1) 10, 11
Third trimester (29 weeks–birth) 162–216
tests offered during 187–188
visits to caregiver 185–188
week 30: 162
week 32: 162–163

week 34: 163
week 36: 163
week 38: 163–164
week 40: 164
week 41–42: 164, **166**
Thrombocytopenia 84
Thrombosis 471
Thrush **129–131**, 169, 470
in nipples 465
Thyroid
conditions 153
hormones 16, 153
Tiredness (in pregnancy) 59
Toilet
giving birth on the 278
going to after birth 306, 309, 463
going to during labour 260
See also Bowel; Urine
Toxoplasmosis 86, 87
TPL (threatened premature labour) 202–203
Transfer, during birth 97–98, 228–229
Transition phase 247–249
Transverse caesarean incision 383
Travel
by air, for newborn 439
during pregnancy 158–160
overseas, tips for 160
Treatments, 'over the counter' 71
Trichomonas 86, 87
Trimesters *See* First trimester; Second trimester; Third trimester
Triple test 104, 105
Triplets 55, 58
breastfeeding 449–450
caesarean birth and 377, 383
caregiver visits with 98, 143
delivery options for 98
increased calcium for 15
loss of one of 110
non-identical 58
routines for 506–507
support agencies for 560
triamniotic 58
trichorionic 58
weight gain, carrying 65
Trofolastin cream 127
TTN (transient tachypnoea of newborn) 392
Tubal occlusion (tubes tied) 499–500
Tuberculosis 15
Twins
acardiac 58
binovular 55
breastfeeding 449–450
caesarean birth and 377, 383
calcium intake for 15
caregiver visits with 98, 143
conceiving 31, 42
conjoined (siamese) 58
delivery options for 98
diamnitoic 58
dichorionic 58
dizygotic 55
extra helpers at birth for 292
fraternal 55, 58
giving birth to 290–292, 311
health variations for 156
identical 58
identification of 409
loss of one of 110
manipulating second of the 291–292
monochorionic 58
non-identical 58
routines for 506–507
support agencies for 560
transverse 290
uniovular 58
weight gain when carrying 65
Twin-to-twin transfusion 156–157, 263

U

Ultrasound 93, 100–101, 147–150
after bleed 110
anxiety about 149

baby dying and 157
dating 55
detecting twins or more 55
18–20 week 147–148
in labour 266
late pregnancy 187–188, 207, 212, 356
miscarriage and 110, 114
safety of 148–149
3D and 4D 148
Umbilical cord
after birth 297, 425
after caesarean 385
Apgar score and 407
at birth 273, 274, 294, 407
BBA and 293
changes in 166
clamping the 298–299, 425
controlled traction of 297
cutting the 298–299
development of 49, 50
entanglement 156
mechanical induction and 362
prolapse of 266
twins' 291
two vessels in 149–150
vein, injection in 314
See also Cord blood donation
Underwear See Bras; Maternity clothing
Underweight
baby 415
mother 26, 64
Ureaplasma 131
Urinating, baby, frequency of 432, 449, 519
Urine, mother's
infection 154, 258
retention 343
Urine, passing of
difficult, after birth **309–310**, 442, 463
difficult, during labour 260
frequent 59
pelvic floor and 167
Urine tests
during pregnancy 101
for ovulation 40
for pre-eclampsia 209
for pregnancy 52, 53
Uterus 30, **30**, 164
after birth 440
bicornuate 203
caesarean and 383, 384, 385
contracting, after birth 296, 297
during labour 164
fibroids in 311
hyperstimulation of the 345, 359–360
implantation in 49
incarcerated 118
infection after birth 469
inversion of 317
manual exploration of 402
retroverted (tipped) 118
rupture of 399–400
weight gain and 65

V
Vaccination
agencies and support groups 563–564
See also Injections
Vaccine, MMR 85
Vacuum extraction See Ventouse
Vagina, mother's 30, **30**, 167
pain in 180–181
sore 441–442
swollen 305, 311
Vagina, newborn's

appearance 432
discharge from 425
Vaginal
CVS 106, 107
deodorants 74
dryness 450, 486
examinations 239–240, 279–280
lubrication 450
mucus 36, 37, 38, 39
mucus test 46
swab **146–147**, 259
Vaginal birth 268–274
midwife's visits after 461
twins and 290–292
See also Birth; Labour
Vaginal birth after caesarean (VBAC) 396
arguments, for or against 398–400
birth place for 400
caregiver for 400–403
emotions and 403–404
health factors for 397–398
support strategies for 401–402
Vaginal bleeding 109, 188, 211, 249, 265–266
after tests 102
smelly 469
Valsalva manoeuvre 271
Varicose veins 178–179
Vas deferens tube 31–**32**
Vasectomy 498–499
Vasovagal 311
Vegan
diet in pregnancy 64
vitamin intake 11, 13
Vegetarian diet 64
Veins
local anaesthetic in 345
spider 127
varicose 178–179
Venal-carval compression 160, 263
Ventilation (newborn) 409
Ventilator 97
Ventouse (suction) 260, 269, 280, 281, 283, 285–286, **287–288**, 314, 344, 407
Vernix cream 121, 164, 424
Videos
during caesarean 386
pregnancy (ultrasound) 147–148
Viruses 77–87
Vision, blurred 209
Visitors, restricting 447, 458–459, 460
Visits (to caregivers)
information from 99–100
medical history for 99
physical examination during 99
procedures 91, 92, 93, 94, 95, 96
what to expect during 98
See also Caregiver; First trimester; Second trimester; Third trimester
Visual display units 75
Visual focus 353
Visualisation
for breech 205
for induction 369
for pain relief 353
for retained placenta 314
for stress 27, 482
techniques **523–525**
Vitamin
A (retinal or beta-carotene) 10, 11
B1 (thiamine) 10, 11
B2 (riboflavin) 10, 11
B3 (niacin) 10, 11
B5 (pantothenic acid) 10, 11
B6 (pyridoxine) 12, 13
B12 (cobalamin) 12, 13, 64
C (ascorbic acid) 12, 13
D (calciferol) 14, 15, 64
E (alpha-TE) 14, 15

K (menadione) 14, 15
recommended daily intake of 10–19
supplements 8
Vitamin K
after birth 385, **411–413**
deficiency bleeding (VKDB) 411–412
injection 412
oral dose of 412
supplements 152, 412–413
Vocal cords, baby's 120
Vocalising 223
Vomiting
after anaesthetic 382
excessive **117–118**, 519
in labour 233, 250, 257–258
pain relief and 333, 335–336, 343
Vulval varicosities 179

W
Ward, postnatal 90, 91, 93, 95, 385, 414, 461
Warfrin (and Vit K) 15
Water
for pain relief 353
injections 353
Water birth 91, 94, 96, **224–225**, 406
Waters breaking
in labour 249, 267, 269–270, 354
in prelabour 233–234, 238, 241–243
sex and 184
Strep B and 146
twins and 291
See also ARM; Breaking the waters
Weakness (limbs) 344
Weaning 513–514
Weighing (the baby) 410
Weight, baby's 162, 163, 164
after birth 449, 519, 521
at birth 410
average, at birth 164
Weight, mother's, healthy range 25
See also Body Mass Index
Weight gain, mother's
contraceptives and 492, 493, 494, 495
during pregnancy 64–65
fluid retention and 64
Wet lung 392
Wharton's jelly 166
Wind (flatulence) 59
Womb See Uterus
Work
mother's return to 515–516
options 4
partner's return to 514–515
support agencies for 555–556
when to stop 214–215
World Health Organisation (WHO)
on alcohol 21
on breastfeeding 189
on caesarean 390
on induction 365
on labour intervention 262
Worms, intestinal 72
Wrapping, baby 194, 504

X
X-rays 76
See also Ultrasound

Y
Yoga 24, 133, 182, 540, 541
postnatal **443**, 482

Z
Zidovine (AZT) 83
ZIG (zoster immunoglobulin) 79
zinc (Zn) **18, 19**, 64